Practical Care of the Ambulatory Patient

Barry M. Stults, M.D.
Associate Professor of Clinical Medicine
Department of Internal Medicine
University of Utah Medical Center
Salt Lake City, Utah

Willard H. Dere, M.D.
Assistant Professor of Medicine
Department of Internal Medicine
University of Utah Medical Center
Salt Lake City, Utah

1989
W.B. SAUNDERS COMPANY
Harcourt Brace Jovanovich, Inc.
Philadelphia London Toronto Montreal Sydney Tokyo

W. B. SAUNDERS COMPANY
Harcourt Brace Jovanovich, Inc.

The Curtis Center
Independence Square West
Philadel...

Library of Congress Cataloging-in-Publication Data

Practical care of the ambulatory patient.

1. Ambulatory medical care.   I. Stults, Barry M.   II. Dere,
Willard. [DNLM: 1. Ambulatory Care.   2. Medicine.
WB 100 P8937]

RC46.P869   1989   617′.024   88–31919

ISBN 0–7216 2474–X

Editor: William Lamsback
Designer: Terri Siegel
Production Manager: Bill Preston
Manuscript Editor: Judith Gandy
Illustration Coordinator: Peg Shaw
Indexer: Kate Mason
Cover Designer: Ellen Bodner

Practical Care of the Ambulatory Patient   ISBN 0–7216–2474–X

Last digit is the print number: 9   8   7   6   5   4   3   2   1

For Connie, Cheryl, Cynthia, and Sarah,
who made this book possible
and worthwhile.

Barry M. Stults

To Julie and Melissa,
for their love and support.

Willard H. Dere

CONTRIBUTORS

Howard B. Abrams, M.D., F.R.C.P.C.
Assistant Professor of Medicine, University of Toronto;
Attending Physician, Department of Internal Medicine,
Division of General Internal Medicine and Clinical
Epidemiology, Toronto General Hospital, Toronto,
Ontario, Canada
*Preoperative Assessment of Cardiac Patients
Undergoing Noncardiac Surgery*

J. Gary Abuelo, M.D.
Associate Professor of Medicine, Brown University; Co-
Director, Division of Renal Diseases, Rhode Island
Hospital, Providence, Rhode Island
Evaluation of Proteinuria and Hematuria

Arthur S. Banner, M.D.
Associate Professor of Medicine, University of
Pittsburgh; Head, Pulmonary Unit, Montefiore Hospital,
Pittsburgh, Pennsylvania
Evaluation and Management of Chronic Cough

Marshall H. Becker, Ph.D., M.P.H.
Professor of Health Behavior and Associate Dean,
School of Public Health, University of Michigan, Ann
Arbor, Michigan
*Smoking Cessation: A Five-Stage Plan; Understanding
and Improving Patient Compliance*

John L. Bezzant, M.D.
Assistant Clinical Professor of Dermatology, University
of Utah School of Medicine, Salt Lake City, Utah
Topical Corticosteroids

H. William Bonekat, D.O.
Assistant Professor of Medicine, University of California,
Davis; Pulmonary Consultant, University of California
Medical Center, Sacramento, California
Preventing Pulmonary Problems after Surgery

Randall W. Burt, M.D.
Associate Professor of Medicine, Department of Internal
Medicine, University of Utah School of Medicine;
Attending Physician, University of Utah Health Sciences
Center, Salt Lake City, Utah
Cancer Prevention in Primary Care

David E. Bush, M.D.
Assistant Professor of Medicine, Johns Hopkins
University School of Medicine; Active Staff, Division of
Cardiology, Francis Scott Key Medical Center; Active
Staff, Johns Hopkins Hospital, Baltimore, Maryland
Management of the Patient after Myocardial Infarction

Richard L. Byyny, M.D.
Professor of Medicine and Head, Division of Internal
Medicine, University of Colorado, Denver, Colorado
Withdrawal of Corticosteroid Therapy

Thomas H. Caine, M.D.
Professor of Clinical Medicine, Department of Internal
Medicine, University of Utah School of Medicine;
Attending Physician, University of Utah Health Sciences
Center, Salt Lake City, Utah
*Long-term Anticoagulation: Indications and
Management*

David C. Classen, M.D.
Assistant Professor, Department of Medicine, University
of Utah School of Medicine; Attending Physician,
Division of Infectious Diseases, LDS Hospital, Salt Lake
City, Utah
Herpes Simplex and Varicella-Zoster Virus Infections

David M. Clive, M.D.
Associate Professor of Medicine, University of
Massachusetts Medical School; Medical Director,
Dialysis Unit and Program Director, Medical Residency,
University of Massachusetts Hospital, Worcester,
Massachusetts
Renal Complications of Anti-Inflammatory Therapy

Molly Cooke, M.D.
Assistant Professor of Clinical Medicine, University of
California, San Francisco; Attending Physician, Division
of General Internal Medicine, San Francisco General
Hospital, San Francisco, California
Diagnostic Evaluation and Management of Impotence

Willard H. Dere, M.D.
Assistant Professor of Medicine, Department of Internal
Medicine, University of Utah Medical Center; Staff
Physician, Veterans Administration Medical Center;
Attending Physician, University of Utah Health Sciences
Center, Salt Lake City, Utah
*Long-term Anticoagulation: Indications and
Management; Cancer Prevention in Primary Care*

Allan S. Detsky, M.D., Ph.D., F.R.C.P.C.
Associate Professor of Medicine and Health
Administration, University of Toronto; Chief, Division of
General Internal Medicine and Clinical Epidemiology,
Toronto General Hospital, Toronto, Ontario, Canada
*Preoperative Assessment of Cardiac Patients
Undergoing Noncardiac Surgery*

Diane L. Elliot, M.D.
Associate Professor of Medicine, Department of Medicine, Oregon Health Sciences University; Attending Physician, University of Oregon Health Sciences Center, Portland, Oregon
Evaluation and Management of Acute Diarrhea

Kenneth D. Engberg, M.D.
Assistant Professor, University of Minnesota Medical School; Staff Geriatrician, St. Paul–Ramsey Medical Center, St. Paul, Minnesota
Care of the Nursing Home Patient

Stephen A. Eraker, M.D., M.P.H.
Assistant Clinical Professor of Medicine, Department of Medicine, Oregon Health Sciences University, Portland; Staff Physician, Kaiser Permanente, Clackamas, Oregon
Smoking Cessation: A Five-Stage Plan; Understanding and Improving Patient Compliance

Robert H. Fletcher, M.D., M.Sc.
Professor of Medicine and Epidemiology, Co-Director, Robert Wood Johnson Clinical Scholars Program, University of North Carolina at Chapel Hill; Attending Physician, North Carolina Memorial Hospital, Chapel Hill, North Carolina
Mitral Valve Prolapse

Richard Garibaldi, M.D.
Professor of Medicine, Vice-Chairman, Department of Medicine, and Hospital Epidemiologist, University of Connecticut School of Medicine, Farmington, Connecticut
Management of Patients with Chronic Urinary Catheters

Jeremy M. Gleeson, M.B., Ch.B.
Instructor of Medicine, University of Utah Medical Center; Staff Physician, Division of Endocrinology, Veterans Administration Medical Center, Salt Lake City, Utah
Self-Monitoring in Diabetes Mellitus

Richard J. Haber, M.D.
Associate Professor of Medicine, University of California, San Francisco; Chief, Division of General Internal Medicine, and Assistant Chief, Medical Services, San Francisco General Hospital, San Francisco, California
Osteoporosis

David H. Hickam, M.D., M.P.H.
Associate Professor, Division of General Medicine, Department of Medicine, Oregon Health Sciences University; Coordinator of Health Services Research and Development, Veterans Administration Medical Center, Portland, Oregon
Evaluation and Management of Acute Chest Pain; Evaluation and Management of Recurrent Chest Pain

Jeffrey M. Hoeg, M.D., F.A.C.P.
Senior Investigator, National Heart, Lung, and Blood Institute, National Institutes of Health; Director, Lipid Metabolism Clinic, Senior Investigator, Clinical Center, National Institutes of Health, Bethesda, Maryland
Hyperlipidemia: Practical Diagnosis and Management

John H. Holbrook, M.D.
Professor of Internal Medicine and Chief, Division of General Internal Medicine, University of Utah School of Medicine; Attending Physician, University of Utah Health Sciences Center, Salt Lake City, Utah
Periodic Health Examination for Adults

James R. Horning, M.D.
Assistant Professor of Medicine, University of South Dakota School of Medicine; Veterans Administration Hospital, Sioux Falls, South Dakota
Diagnosis and Management of Patients with Urolithiasis

Patrick W. Irvine, M.D.
Assistant Professor of Medicine, University of Minnesota Medical School; Director of Geriatric Medicine and Extended Care, Hennepin County Medical Center, Minneapolis, Minnesota
Care of the Nursing Home Patient

Jay A. Jacobson, M.D., F.A.C.P.
Associate Professor of Internal Medicine, Division of Infectious Diseases, University of Utah School of Medicine; Attending Physician, LDS Hospital, Salt Lake City, Utah
Infectious Diseases and Travel: Risk, Recognition, Remedies, and Prevention

Clifford Johnson, M.D.
Attending Physician, Aultman Hospital, Canton, Ohio
Routine Laboratory Testing in General Medical Practice

Wishwa N. Kapoor, M.D., M.P.H.
Associate Professor of Medicine, Department of Medicine, University of Pittsburgh; Attending Physician, Presbyterian-University Hospital, Pittsburgh, Pennsylvania
Diagnostic Evaluation of Syncope

John P. Kirscht, Ph.D.
Professor, School of Public Health, University of Michigan, Ann Arbor, Michigan
Smoking Cessation: A Five-Stage Plan; Understanding and Improving Patient Compliance

Anthony L. Komaroff, M.D.
Associate Professor of Medicine, Harvard Medical School; Director, Division of General Medicine and Primary Care, Brigham and Women's Hospital, Boston, Massachusetts
Adult Women with Acute Dysuria; Sore Throat in Adult Patients

Gretchen Kunitz, M.D.
Assistant Clinical Professor, Department of Medicine, University of California, San Francisco; Medical Staff, Alta Bates Hospital, Berkeley, California
Diagnostic Evaluation of Lymphadenopathy

Steven P. Kutalek, M.D.
Assistant Professor of Medicine and Clinical Pharmacology, Hahnemann University School of Medicine; Director, Clinical Cardiac Electrophysiology Hahnemann University Hospital; Attending Cardiologist, St. Agnes Medical Center, Philadelphia, Pennsylvania
Management of Ventricular Premature Complexes

Eric B. Larson, M.D., M.P.H.
Professor of Medicine, Division of General Internal Medicine, University of Washington School of Medicine; Chief, Section of General Internal Medicine, University Hospital, Seattle, Washington
Evaluation and Care of the Demented Patient

Steven S. Levine, M.D.
Attending Physician, Nashua Memorial Hospital, Nashua, New Hampshire
Withdrawal of Corticosteroid Therapy

David A. Lieberman, M.D.
Associate Professor of Medicine, Division of Gastroenterology, Oregon Health Sciences University; Staff Physician, Veterans Administration Medical Center, Portland, Oregon
Management of Common Anorectal Disorders by the Internist

Benjamin A. Lipsky, M.D.
Associate Professor, Department of Medicine, University of Washington School of Medicine; Hospital Epidemiologist and Staff Physician, Medical Comprehensive Care Unit, Veterans Administration Medical Center, Seattle, Washington
Diagnostic Evaluation and Treatment of Urinary Tract Infection in Men

Bernard Lo, M.D.
Associate Professor of Medicine and Acting Chief, Division of Medical Ethics, University of California, San Francisco; Attending Physician, Moffitt-Long Hospital, San Francisco, California
Deciding about Life-Sustaining Treatment

Gregory J. Magarian, M.D.
Associate Professor of Medicine, Division of General Medicine, and Director, Medicine Clerkship, Oregon Health Sciences University and Veterans Administration Medical Center, Portland, Oregon
Evaluation and Management of Acute Chest Pain

Juan-Ramon Malagelada, M.D.
Chief of Gastroenterology, Hospital General Vall d'Hebron, Autonomous University of Barcelona, Barcelona, Spain
Diagnosis and Management of Dyspepsia

Keith I. Marton, M.D.
Clinical Associate Professor of Medicine, University of California, San Francisco, School of Medicine; Chairman, Department of Medicine, Pacific Presbyterian Medical Center, San Francisco, California
Unintentional Weight Loss

Kenneth P. Mathews, M.D.
Professor Emeritus of Internal Medicine, University of Michigan Medical School, Ann Arbor, Michigan; Adjunct Member, Scripps Clinic and Research Foundation, La Jolla, California
Urticaria and Angioedema

Jack D. McCue, M.D.
Professor of Medicine, Tufts University School of Medicine, Boston; Vice-Chairman, Department of Medicine, and Chief, Division of General Medicine/Geriatrics, Bay State Medical Center, Springfield, Massachusetts
Evaluation and Management of Vaginal Discharge

Fermin Mearin, M.D.
Hospital General Vall d'Hebron, Autonomous University of Barcelona, Barcelona, Spain
Diagnosis and Management of Dyspepsia

Steven H. Miles, M.D.
Associate Director, Center for Clinical Medical Ethics, and Assistant Professor of Medicine, Pritzker School of Medicine, University of Chicago, Chicago, Illinois
Informed Consent: An Ideal and a Standard of Practice

Joel Morganroth, M.D.
Professor of Medicine and Pharmacology, Hahnemann University; Director, Cardiac Research and Development, The Graduate Hospital, Philadelphia, Pennsylvania
Management of Ventricular Premature Complexes

Richard A. Morin, M.D.
Clinical Assistant Professor of Medicine, University of Nebraska College of Medicine; Hospital Epidemiologist, St. Elizabeth Community Health Center and Lincoln General Hospital, Lincoln, Nebraska
Management of Patients with Chronic Urinary Catheters

Alvin Mushlin, M.D., Sc.M., F.A.C.P.
Associate Professor of Medicine, University of Rochester School of Medicine and Dentistry; Attending Physician, Strong Memorial Hospital, Rochester, New York
Routine Laboratory Testing in General Medical Practice

Harold S. Nelson, M.D.
Professor of Medicine, University of Colorado Health Sciences Center School of Medicine; Acting Head, Allergy-Immunology Division, Department of Medicine, National Jewish Center for Immunology and Respiratory Medicine, Denver, Colorado
Chronic Rhinitis: Diagnosis and Management

Margaret F. Odell, M.S.N.
Diabetes Nurse Practitioner, Division of Endocrinology, University of Utah Medical Center; Clinical Coordinator, Diabetes Research, Veterans Administration Medical Center, Salt Lake City, Utah
Self-Monitoring in Diabetes Mellitus

William F. Owen, Jr., M.D.
Founder, Bay Area Physicians for Human Rights; Consultant, California Medical Association Task Force on AIDS and Sexually Transmitted Diseases; Member, San Francisco Department of Public Health AIDS Medical Advisory Committee; Active Staff, St. Luke's Hospital, San Francisco, California
Medical Evaluation of the Gay Male Patient

Fitzhugh C. Pannill, M.D.
Assistant Professor of Medicine, Yale University School of Medicine, New Haven; Chief, Geriatrics, West Haven Veterans Administration Medical Center, West Haven, Connecticut
Diagnosis and Treatment of Urinary Incontinence

Gary D. Plotnick, M.D.
Associate Professor of Medicine, University of Maryland School of Medicine; Associate Professor of Medicine, Johns Hopkins University School of Medicine; Director of Echocardiography, University of Maryland Hospital, Baltimore, Maryland
Diagnosis and Management of Stable Angina Pectoris

Peter E. Pochi, M.D.
Professor of Dermatology, Boston University School of Medicine; Visiting Dermatologist, University Hospital, Boston; Visiting Physician, Dermatology, Boston City Hospital, Boston, Massachusetts
Management of Acne

Robert J. Quinet, M.D.
Clinical Assistant Professor of Medicine, Louisiana State University School of Medicine in New Orleans; Attending Physician, Section on Rheumatology, Department of Medicine, Ochsner Clinic, Ochsner Foundation Hospital, New Orleans, Louisiana
Management of Regional Low Back Pain

Sheldon M. Retchin, M.D., M.S.P.H.
Associate Professor of Medicine and Chairman, Division of Geriatric Medicine, Department of Internal Medicine, Medical College of Virginia/Virginia Commonwealth University, Richmond; Attending Physician, Medical College of Virginia Hospital; Attending Physician, Hunter Holmes McGuire Veterans Administration Medical Center, Richmond, Virginia
Mitral Valve Prolapse

Alan S. Robbins, M.D.
Associate Professor of Medicine, University of California School of Medicine, Los Angeles; Chief of Staff, Veterans Administration Medical Center, Sepulveda, California
Evaluation of Falls in Elderly Persons

John A. Robbins, M.D.
Associate Professor of Clinical Medicine and Chief, Division of General Medicine, Department of Internal Medicine, University of California, Davis; Attending Physician, University of California, Davis, Medical Center, Davis, California
Preoperative Evaluation of the Healthy Patient

Laurence Z. Rubenstein, M.D., M.P.H.
Associate Professor of Medicine/Geriatrics, University of California School of Medicine, Los Angeles; Clinical Director, Geriatric Research Education and Clinical Center, Sepulveda, California
Evaluation of Falls in Elderly Persons

Anthony G. Salem, M.D.
Associate Professor of Medicine, University of South Dakota School of Medicine; Chief, Medical Service, Veterans Administration Hospital, Sioux Falls, South Dakota
Diagnosis and Management of Patients with Urolithiasis

Leonard H. Serebro, M.D.
Clinical Instructor of Medicine, Louisiana State University School of Medicine in New Orleans; Attending Physician, Section on Rheumatology, Department of Medicine, Ochsner Clinic, Ochsner Foundation Hospital, New Orleans, Louisiana
Management of Regional Low Back Pain

John Wade Shigeoka, M.D.
Associate Professor, Department of Medicine, University of Utah School of Medicine; Chief, Pulmonary Section (Medical Service), Veterans Administration Medical Center, Salt Lake City, Utah
Practical Prescription of Home Oxygen Therapy; Preventing Pulmonary Problems after Surgery

Charles B. Smith, M.D.
Professor and Associate Chairman, Department of Medicine, University of Utah School of Medicine; Chief, Medical Service, Veterans Administration Medical Center, Salt Lake City, Utah
Herpes Simplex and Varicella-Zoster Virus Infections

Kevin Somerville, M.B., F.R.A.C.P.
Senior Registrar, Nuffield Department of Clinical Medicine, Geriatric Medicine Division, Radcliffe Infirmary, Oxford, United Kingdom
Gastrointestinal Complications of Nonsteroidal Anti-Inflammatory Agents

Robert V. Steinmetzer, M.D.
Cleveland Clinic Florida, Fort Lauderdale, Florida
Diagnosis and Treatment of Headaches

Barry M. Stults, M.D.
Associate Professor of Clinical Medicine, Department of Internal Medicine, University of Utah Medical Center; Staff Physician, Veterans Administration Medical Center; Attending Physician, University of Utah Health Sciences Center, Salt Lake City, Utah
Long-term Anticoagulation: Indications and Management; Cancer Prevention in Primary Care

Stephen V. Tang, M.D.
Clinical Instructor in Dermatology, Harvard Medical School; Associate, Brigham and Women's Hospital; Affiliate, Carney Hospital, Boston, Massachusetts
Management of Acne

W. Grant Thompson, M.D., F.A.C.P., F.R.C.P.C.
Professor of Medicine, Chief, Division of Gastroenterology, and Digestive Diseases Research Group, Assistant Dean, Clinical and Community Affairs, University of Ottawa School of Medicine; Chief, Division of Gastroenterology, Ottawa Civic Hospital, Ottawa, Ontario, Canada
Management of the Irritable Bowel

Susan W. Tolle, M.D.
Visiting Scholar, Center for Clinical Medical Ethics,
University of Chicago, Chicago, Illinois
Evaluation and Management of Acute Diarrhea

Richard F. Uhlmann, M.D., M.P.H.
Assistant Professor of Medicine, Division of Gerontology
and Geriatric Medicine, University of Washington School
of Medicine; Medical Director, Senior Care Unit,
Harborview Medical Center, Seattle, Washington
Evaluation and Care of the Demented Patient

Nichols Vorys, M.D., M.M.Sc.
Clinical Associate Professor, Ohio State University
College of Medicine; Director, Midwest Reproductive
Institute, Columbus, Ohio
*Oral Contraceptives: Prescription and Monitoring by
Internists*

Nanette K. Wenger, M.D., F.A.C.P., F.A.C.C.
Professor of Medicine (Cardiology), Emory University
School of Medicine; Director, Cardiac Clinics, Grady
Memorial Hospital, Atlanta, Georgia
*Management of Patients after Coronary Artery Bypass
Surgery*

Richard H. White, M.D.
Associate Professor of Clinical Medicine, University of
California, Davis; Chief, Soft Tissue Rheumatic Disease
Clinic, University of California, Davis Medical Center,
Davis, California
Diagnosis and Management of Shoulder Pain

Dana E. Wilson, M.D.
Professor of Medicine, University of Utah Medical
Center; Division of Endocrinology, Veterans
Administration Medical Center, Salt Lake City, Utah
Self-Monitoring in Diabetes Mellitus

Edward T. Zawada, Jr., M.D.
Freeman Professor and Chairman of Medicine,
University of South Dakota School of Medicine; Chief,
Section of Nephrology, Veterans Administration
Hospital, Sioux Falls, South Dakota
Diagnosis and Management of Patients with Urolithiasis

Bruce L. Zuraw, M.D.
Assistant Member, Department of Basic and Clinical
Research, Research Institute of Scripps Clinic; Staff
Physician, Green Hospital of Scripps Clinic, Division of
Allergy and Immunology, La Jolla, California
Urticaria and Angioedema

PREFACE

Practical Care of the Ambulatory Patient is directed to clinicians who provide primary health care for adult patients. This book does not attempt to provide encyclopedic coverage of the many clinical problems in ambulatory care internal medicine. Instead, the editors have selected a small number of important, and sometimes controversial, clinical topics frequently confronting primary care clinicians. Most of these subjects have been either excluded or presented in limited detail in traditional textbooks of internal medicine and can be adequately reviewed only in speciality or subspecialty texts and journals. As examples of these topics, chapters are included on the management of patients after coronary artery bypass graft surgery, the techniques of monitoring glycemic control in ambulatory diabetics, the management of common anorectal disorders, the management of patients with chronic urinary catheters, care of the nursing home patient, the general medical evaluation of the gay patient, recommendations for travelers, preoperative medical evaluation of surgical patients, problems in clinical ethics, and the role of routine laboratory testing in the care of asymptomatic patients.

Each chapter emphasizes a practical, step-by-step approach to diagnosis and treatment by use of algorithms and other teaching aids. In this era of cost control, appropriate attention is given to the relative efficacy (sensitivity, specificity, and predictive value) and financial costs of diagnostic tests and therapeutic modalities. Each chapter includes an annotated bibliography to provide the reader with ready access to key articles in the medical literature through the middle part of 1988.

We are especially indebted to the authors of the individual chapters—clinically active experts from the United States, Canada, and Europe who have consented to share their expertise on subjects of particular interest to them. We have learned a great deal from our associations with these clinicians, and we believe the readers of this book will benefit as much.

BARRY STULTS
WILLARD DERE

CONTENTS

PART ONE

Cardiology

1

Mitral Valve Prolapse

SHELDON M. RETCHIN, M.D., M.S.P.H.
ROBERT H. FLETCHER, M.D., M.Sc.

Introduction

Mitral valve prolapse (MVP) is a pathophysiologic phenomenon that results from an abnormal coaptation of the two mitral valve leaflets during systole. Known by several synonyms (e.g., Barlow's syndrome, click-murmur syndrome), the typical heart sounds of MVP have been attributed to both cardiac (e.g., pleuropericardial adhesions) and noncardiac (e.g., costochondral motion) anomalies over the past century. It was not until the mid-1960's that the anatomic reason for the findings was first described by using cardiac angiography.

In MVP the posterior leaflet, usually the leaflet responsible for the malalignment, "pops" or "balloons" across an imaginary horizontal line dividing the left ventricle and left atrium. As the posterior leaflet reaches the limit of its prolapse into the atrium it snaps tight, causing the characteristic late systolic click. If the prolapse is complicated by mitral regurgitation, there may be an accompanying late systolic murmur as well. Postmortem studies of patients with MVP show that, in most cases, there is a myxomatous degeneration of the leaflet tissue that results in a weakening of supporting structures and an overall increase in the leaflet area. A much smaller proportion of cases are secondary to systemic diseases of connective tissue: Marfan's syndrome, Ehlers-Danlos syndrome, and others. These conditions, called secondary forms of MVP by some, have a different prognosis that is related to their underlying disease. They will not be discussed here.

Because MVP is prevalent and likely to be detected initially in the ambulatory setting, the appropriate management of outpatients with MVP is a frequent concern. Management strategies address the possibility of serious complications (such as ruptured chordae tendineae, endocarditis, and stroke) and troublesome symptoms (such as chest pain and fatigue). In this chapter, we will first review methods of detecting MVP; we will then consider the complications of MVP. Finally, we will discuss appropriate management strategies for symptomatic patients suspected of having MVP.

Prevalence

With the introduction of M-mode echocardiography in the mid-1970's, MVP was frequently discovered in ambulatory patients. The prevalence of MVP varies with age, sex, and habitus; it is higher in women than in men, highest in the young adult years, and higher in thin than in heavy people. The prevalence in the general population is about 17% in women 20 to 29 years old, 2 to 4% in men regardless of age, and about 1.4% in women above the age of 80. The high prevalence of MVP in young women is partly explained by a slender body habitus; echocardiographic evidence of MVP has been known to disappear with weight gain.

Diagnosis

MVP is often suspected in patients with nonspecific symptoms or is discovered on routine cardiac auscultation in asymptomatic patients. In this section we will describe the typical symptoms attributed to MVP as well as the range of findings on cardiac auscultation. We will then describe how the diagnosis can be confirmed, if necessary, by echocardiography.

Symptoms

As shown in the algorithm in Figure 1–1, approaches to management differ for those who are symptomatic and those who are asymptomatic at presentation. About half of the patients with MVP are both unaware of and previously unaffected by the condition. The remaining patients are found during investigation of complaints that include dyspnea, dizziness, fatigue, lethargy, anxiety, and chest pain. Taken together, these symptoms have been described as a syndrome and often lead physicians to order further diagnostic tests (e.g., echocardiography) or therapeutic interventions (e.g., antibiotic prophylaxis).

There have been numerous attempts to explain the association of MVP with symptoms. For example, chest pain has been attributed to various pathophysiologic mechanisms, such as "tugging" of the inferior left ventricular wall by the prolapsing valve and supporting structures, producing focal ischemia; dysautonomia (i.e., abnormal autonomic neural function) has also been postulated as an explanation for the dizziness and palpitations often encountered. None of these explanations has been very plausible.

The best available evidence, from population-based, well-controlled studies, has shown that symptoms are no more prevalent in patients with MVP than in patients without MVP. Both MVP and nonspecific symptoms of chest pain and fatigue are common, and the likelihood that they would occur together is high. Therefore, we believe that the so-called MVP syndrome is an artifact.

Cardiac Auscultation

The typical sound of MVP is a high-pitched nonejection click, heard best in late systole over the apex. A murmur of mitral insufficiency may accompany the click, or the murmur may be present alone. The murmur may also occur in late systole, or may be pansystolic.

There are two frequent errors in auscultation of the click and murmur of MVP: attributing MVP to a split S_1 and mistaking a midsystolic murmur for a late systolic one. Because the pathophysiologic phenomena of MVP are associated with a redundancy or excess of leaflet material, maneuvers that reduce left ventricular filling pressure will move the click and murmur closer to the first heart sound. The easiest method for reducing left ventricular filling pressure is to have the patient stand from a lying position; occasionally a previously unheard click or murmur of mitral regurgitation will be elicited. Mobility of the click and/

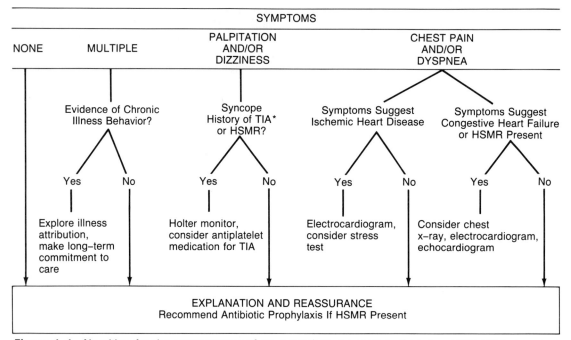

Figure 1–1. Algorithm for the management of an outpatient suspected of having MVP. *TIA, transient ischemic attack; HSMR, hemodynamically significant mitral regurgitation.

or murmur can help differentiate it from a split S_1. The split S_1 also occurs earlier in systole and is louder at the lower left sternal border. The late systolic murmur of MVP can be distinguished from a midsystolic murmur by timing; the late systolic murmur continues into A_2, whereas the midsystolic murmur stops before A_2. The age of the patient is also helpful. A late systolic murmur at the apex is likely to represent MVP in a younger patient, but in the older patient it is frequently due to papillary muscle dysfunction or mitral annulus calcification. Therefore, it has been suggested that an echocardiogram may be helpful in the older patient with an apical systolic murmur.

In the presence of a click or murmur, only a minority of patients have echocardiographic MVP; also, in many patients MVP cannot be detected by auscultation. Therefore, clinical examination is an inaccurate way of making the diagnosis. However, auscultatory findings can provide useful information for management purposes. The respective roles of both cardiac auscultation and echocardiography in the diagnosis and evaluation of MVP are outlined in Table 1-1.

As emphasized in Table 1-1 and Figure 1-1, hemodynamically significant mitral regurgitation has been consistently shown to be the most important risk factor for complications of MVP. What constitutes hemodynamically significant mitral regurgitation? How often is it present in patients with MVP? Many studies indicate that systolic murmurs can be elicited in the majority of MVP patients, yet most of these do not seem to be at risk. There are no clinical data to define at just what point a mitral regurgitation murmur is hemodynamically significant for the purposes of developing endocarditis. Nevertheless, a hemodynamically significant murmur of mitral regurgitation is almost invariably holosystolic, usually with a grade $\geq 3/6$. Moreover, there is reasonable evidence that these murmurs are usually not evanescent and they are rare. According to the Framingham data, a systolic murmur with a grade of 3/6 or greater was present in only about 2% of those with MVP.

Echocardiography

Considerably more than 200,000 echocardiograms are done annually in the United States, many for the detection of MVP. One estimate of the outpatient utilization rate of echocardiography is that MVP may account for one third to one half of outpatient referrals for the procedure. Although echocardiography is without substantial risk to the patient, it is expensive.

Echocardiography has become a gold standard for the diagnosis of MVP because of its anatomic accuracy and precision. Both M-mode and two-dimensional echocardiography have been used to establish the diagnosis, although two-dimensional echocardiography is said to be a more sensitive indicator of MVP. Technical aspects of performing echocardiography for detecting MVP often determine whether MVP is diagnosed. For example, angulating the transducer inferiorly can produce false-positive results. Some echocardiographers now require the prolapse to be holosystolic and to have at least 3 mm of posterior motion, and others use the degree of leaflet

Table 1–1. Comparison of Usefulness of Cardiac Auscultation and Echocardiography for the Diagnosis and Evaluation of MVP

Criterion	Estimated Prevalence	Usefulness
Midsystolic click by cardiac auscultation	17% young women, 2–4% men, 1.4% elderly women	Presence of click is unlikely to be useful
Late systolic murmur	30–50% of those with MVP	Unlikely to be useful, unless severity and duration progress
Holosystolic murmur	Estimated at about 2% of those with MVP	Extremely useful for determining need for antibiotic prophylaxis, risk of serious arrhythmias, progression to significant left-sided heart failure
M-mode echocardiography	0.5–7% of men and 1–21% of women, depending on criteria (e.g., mm of prolapse) and population	Useful for confirming clinical suspicion and for identifying risk factors (e.g., left ventricular enlargement, redundant leaflets) in selected patients, but not as routine part of diagnostic evaluation
Two-dimensional echocardiography	More sensitive than M-mode	Usefulness similar to that of M-mode echocardiography; adds little to diagnostic evaluation

redundancy or thickening to determine the clinical importance of the prolapse. Agreement between M-mode and two-dimensional echocardiography is high, ranging from 80% to almost 100%. Therefore, there is only marginal value for using the two together.

For most illnesses, detection is considered worthwhile if diagnostic confirmation leads to improved prognosis. For MVP, the evidence is not strong that this is the case. Although echocardiography is often ordered when MVP is suspected, its usefulness has not been well documented: a change in management because of the results of the procedure occurs in less than 10% of patients who have echocardiography performed for any reason. Although reported complications are severe and life-threatening, the frequency of these events is so low that active efforts to discover MVP are not warranted. As shown in Table 1–1, echocardiography should not be performed on all patients suspected of having MVP. It should be reserved for ruling out other forms of valvular heart disease (e.g., idiopathic hypertrophic subaortic stenosis) or for evaluating patients with severe symptoms (such as syncope or signs suggesting hemodynamically significant mitral regurgitation). In patients with systolic murmurs thought to be hemodynamically significant, an echocardiogram may be particularly helpful to quantify left atrial and ventricular sizes.

Complications

After numerous reports of high prevalence rates of MVP, several case series were published suggesting that patients with the condition may have an increased risk for serious complications. Many conditions have been associated with MVP, most involving the cardiovascular system: arrhythmias, endocarditis, ruptured chordae tendineae, congestive heart failure, and stroke.

Arrhythmias

Numerous arrhythmias, both supraventricular and ventricular, have been reported in patients with MVP. Among the supraventricular arrhythmias most prominently associated with MVP have been anomalous conduction pathways, such as Wolff-Parkinson-White syndrome. However, patients with uncomplicated MVP (i.e., without hemodynamically signifi-

cant mitral regurgitation) do not appear to be at increased risk for either supraventricular or complex ventricular arrhythmias. Among patients with MVP and significant mitral regurgitation, the evidence suggests that the risk for both types of arrhythmias is considerably increased.

Sudden death has been reported in patients with MVP. The association is inferred from case reports and autopsy studies. However, when the latter evidence is closely examined, the vast majority of sudden deaths associated with MVP occurred because of ruptured chordae resulting from hemodynamically significant mitral regurgitation. The risk of sudden death among MVP patients without significant mitral regurgitation does not appear to be greater than the risk among adults without MVP (about 7 cases per 10,000 persons 45 to 54 years old). On the other hand, MVP patients with hemodynamically significant mitral regurgitation appear to have annual mortality rates of approximately 100/10,000.

Prolongation of the QT interval has also been reported as a risk factor for sudden death among patients with MVP, but rate-corrected prolonged QT intervals do not appear to be more prevalent in MVP patients than in the general population. Although an electrocardiogram would be a method for screening patients with MVP, for either anomalous conduction pathways or prolonged QT intervals, we do not recommend it as a part of the routine evaluation. Because many of the patients with MVP are young women, an electrocardiogram would not provide useful information about other unsuspected conditions (e.g., occult ischemic disease), would likely generate a high rate of false-positive diagnoses, and would heighten patients' concerns about the diagnosis of MVP.

Therefore, unless symptoms (e.g., syncope) or risk factors (e.g., coronary heart disease, mitral insufficiency) warrant further investigation, patients with MVP who have palpitations or dizziness do not require extensive diagnostic work-ups.

Endocarditis

There has been concern that, like other forms of valvular heart disease, MVP might be a risk factor for subacute bacterial endocarditis. Although the risk of endocarditis seems to be increased five- to seven-fold in people with MVP, the absolute risk is low; one estimate is about 2/10,000 per year (compared with approximately 3/100,000 per year in the general population). Those with hemodynamically significant mitral regurgitation and perhaps elderly men seem to be at greater risk.

The American Heart Association recommends antibiotic prophylaxis before procedures associated with a risk of bacteremia for MVP patients with the systolic murmur of mitral regurgitation. We recommend that antibiotic prophylaxis be used for patients with systolic murmurs of grade 3 or above. These murmurs are rare, however. When hemodynamically significant mitral regurgitation is present, these patients should receive standard doses of antibiotics for at-risk procedures, as recommended by the American Heart Association.

Congestive Heart Failure

In follow-up studies, a few patients have been found to have progressively severe congestive heart failure. This is usually caused either by severe dilation of the mitral annulus or by rupture of chordae tendineae, leading to marked mitral regurgitation and "backward" failure. Dilation of the mitral annulus is likely to be insidious in onset. On the other hand, patients with a ruptured chorda tendinea most often have a sudden onset of symptoms (e.g., severe dyspnea) with subsequent rapid deterioration. Both causes of heart failure are rare events and are likely to occur in older patients. Although many patients with MVP complain of dyspnea, and MVP probably represents the most frequent cause of pure mitral insufficiency, most of these patients do not have specific signs of left-sided failure (e.g., rales) or right-sided failure (e.g., jugular venous distention, edema), even in the presence of hemodynamically significant mitral regurgitation; in fact, only 1 to 4% of patients with MVP have been found to have severe enough congestive heart failure by age 80 to require mitral valve replacement. Therefore, it is not useful to pursue the diagnosis of heart failure in the usual MVP patient, unless signs or symptoms warrant it.

Stroke

MVP can apparently cause strokes. The mechanism for stroke in patients with MVP seems to be a hypercoagulable state with formation of noninfective thrombi on the abnormal valves and embolization to the central nervous system. This complication may occur at any age but is more often suspected in relatively young people without evidence of atherosclerosis. Although there are no satisfactory studies of just what the risk is, one estimate is that young patients (i.e., ≤ age 45) with MVP have 4.5 times the risk of stroke compared with similar patients without MVP. Because the incidence of stroke in this age group is extremely rare, approximately 3/100,000 per year, the absolute risk for patients with MVP would be about 1.5/10,000 per year. Therefore, the incidence of stroke is too low to consider preventive therapy in unselected people with MVP.

Management of Symptoms

Chest pain is the most frequent and often the most debilitating symptom attributed to MVP and therefore deserves special mention. The pain is usually nonexertional and is rarely accompanied by dyspnea, diaphoresis, or typical radiation to the jaw or arm. Because patients with MVP are no more likely than the general population to have coronary artery disease unless other risk factors (e.g., strong family history, smoking, unfavorable lipid profile) are present, we do not recommend a formal work-up for ischemic heart disease.

The chest pain seen in patients with MVP can be extremely incapacitating. Some physicians have used beta-blocking agents to manage symptomatic patients. Although selected patients may benefit from this approach, much of the improvement may be a placebo effect. A short-acting beta blocker (e.g., propranolol, 40 mg, twice a day) is recommended as an initial step, for approximately 2 weeks. If the pain is ameliorated, the drug may be continued for another 2 months before slow withdrawal.

Some patients with the typical symptoms of MVP may attribute their complaints to heart disease, despite repeated assurance from physicians and often even in the face of strong diagnostic evidence to the contrary (e.g., normal coronary angiograms). In these cases, a hypochondriacal personality is likely. In patients with numerous symptoms (e.g., chest pain, dyspnea, palpitation) or in those who amplify complaints beyond detectable disease, a somatization disorder should be considered. Attempts to manage these patients with conventional methods of pain control (e.g., analgesics) will likely be met with little success. A long-term commitment from the physician, with routine visits on a periodic basis, should include an exploration of illness attribution (e.g., expectations of cardiac involvement), a review of childhood experiences (family members often have similar complaints), and a history of recent precipitating life events (e.g., anniversary reaction).

Patients who are suspected of having MVP often have a high potential for functional disability. More than half of symptomatic patients who are suspected of having the condition have one or more of the following manifestations of disability: frequent applications for disability insurance, lost income from work, increased absenteeism, sexual dysfunction, and altered family roles. Asymptomatic patients who are found to have late systolic clicks or murmurs on routine auscultation that are not hemodynamically significant are also at risk for functional disability. These patients should be told that they have a heart sound that represents a normal variant. It is extremely important that any diagnostic or therapeutic intervention for these patients be accompanied by sincere reassurance and detailed explanation.

Summary

MVP represents an extremely frequent condition that is often diagnosed in the ambulatory setting. Because MVP is highly prevalent, and because typical symptoms are not specific for the condition, the association of MVP with symptoms is likely to occur by chance alone. Therefore, it is unlikely that most patients with MVP have their symptoms because of MVP. There are numerous reports about potentially serious complications, so it is not surprising that there is concern about long-term risks. However, the overwhelming majority of patients with MVP do not experience serious complications. The small minority who may benefit from increased evaluation and prophylactic interventions can be recognized by the presence of other findings, such as hemodynamically significant mitral regurgitation. Because of the expense of an involved diagnostic work-up as well as the potential for labeling effects, physicians may do well to heed their own cardinal axiom, "Above all do no harm."

Bibliography

American Heart Association, Committee on Prevention of Bacterial Endocarditis. Prevention of bacterial endocarditis. Circulation 70:1123A, 1984.

Clemens JD, Horwitz RI, Jaffe CC, et al. A controlled evaluation of the risk of bacterial endocarditis in persons with mitral-valve prolapse. N Engl J Med 307:776–781, 1982.
> *Because endocarditis is such a rare complication, this case-control study is the best effort evaluating the overall risk of endocarditis for patients with MVP. It also contains a worthwhile appendix explaining the authors' methods. The association of systolic murmurs with risk is emphasized.*

Goldman L, Cohn PF, Mudge GH, et al. Clinical utility and management impact of M-mode echocardiography. Am J Med 75:49–56, 1983.
> *This carefully done study examines the usefulness of the results of M-mode echocardiography and includes clinical assessments about its utility from the clinicians themselves. Only 8% of echocardiograms ordered actually effected a change in medical decision-making! Because MVP is such a frequent reason for ordering echocardiography on outpatients, this study is worthwhile reading.*

Jeresaty RM. Mitral valve prolapse: an update. JAMA 254:793–795, 1985.
> *This is an excellent and concise review of the complications associated with the condition, and emphasizes the overall benign prognosis.*

Kramer HM, Kligfield P, Devereux RB, et al. Arrhythmias in mitral valve prolapse. Effect of selection bias. Arch Intern Med 144:2360–2364, 1984.
> *Both supraventricular and ventricular arrhythmias occur with similar frequency in patients with and without MVP if care is taken to avoid selection bias.*

MacMahon SW, Devereux RB, Schron E (eds). Clinical and epidemiological issues in mitral valve prolapse. Proceedings of a National Heart, Lung, and Blood Institute Symposium. Am Heart J 113:1265–1332, 1987.
> *A portion of the entire issue was devoted to MVP, including sections on disease classification, prevalence, endocarditis, arrhythmias, cerebral ischemia, and mitral regurgitation. Most of the information is taken from the Framingham experience; thus the conclusions are highly generalizable and accurate. For those interested in a detailed and up-to-date review of the literature on the subject, this is the place.*

Perloff JK. Evolving concepts of mitral-valve prolapse. N Engl J Med 307:369–370, 1982.
> *This editorial suggests that MVP be classified into normal and pathologic categories. The author reasons that "normal" MVP represents an echocardiographic finding that is at "one end of the gaussian curve of normal distribution. . . ."*

Procacci PM, Savran SV, Schreiter SL, et al. Prevalence of clinical mitral-valve prolapse in 1169 young women. N Engl J Med 294:1086–1088, 1976.
> *This is one of the early studies that used M-mode echocardiography to detect MVP in asymptomatic female volunteers.*

Quill TE, Lipkin M, Greenland P. The medicalization of normal variants: the case of mitral valve prolapse. J Gen Intern Med 3:267–276, 1988.
> *This excellent review provides a perspective on MVP by comparing it with previous "overlap syndromes" such as hypoglycemia and irritable colon. The authors point out that the prognosis for persons with MVP has been spuriously pessimistic. They emphasize that the majority of patients diagnosed with MVP have a normal variant and should be reassured.*

Retchin SM, Fletcher RH, Earp JA, et al. Mitral valve prolapse: disease or illness? Arch Intern Med 146:1081–1084, 1986.

This historical cohort study followed up more than 150 outpatients. Despite a relatively young study population, both patients with and without MVP by echocardiography had high rates of functional disability "due to heart disease": loss of income, sexual dysfunction, application for public assistance, and even retirement. Most specifically referred to MVP as the reason for the disability.

Retchin SM, Fletcher RH, Waugh RA. Endocarditis and mitral valve prolapse: what is the "risk"? Int J Cardiol 5:653–659, 1984.

Using vital statistics on the number of cases of endocarditis in the United States and data on the prevalence of MVP in the general population, this article reveals that the risk for MVP patients is greatly overestimated. The discussion includes suggestions about possible sources for the overestimate: exaggerated prevalence and an overstated incidence of endocarditis with MVP.

Savage DD, Devereux RB, Garrison RJ, et al. Mitral valve prolapse in the general population: II. Clinical features: the Framingham study. Am Heart J 106:577–581, 1983.

The authors used data from the Framingham cohort to show that MVP patients in the general population (i.e., unselected) have similar prevalence rates of symptoms (e.g., chest pain) as those without MVP.

2

Diagnostic Evaluation of Syncope

WISHWA N. KAPOOR, M.D., M.P.H.

Introduction

Syncope is defined as a sudden, temporary loss of consciousness, associated with a loss of postural tone, and followed by spontaneous recovery. Syncope is a common medical problem. In reported series, 12 to 37% of healthy young adults had had at least one episode of fainting. In our own community survey in Pittsburgh, 25% of all adults contacted noted at least one syncopal episode during their lifetime.

The differential diagnosis for syncope has a broad scope (Table 2–1). Some of the disorders such as vasodepressor syncope are benign problems that may have few consequences; others such as ventricular tachycardia are life-threatening if not evaluated and treated properly. Table 2–2 gives the number of patients with various causes of syncope among a total of 204 patients seen in our medical center. Of the noncardiovascular causes, vasodepressor syncope, situational syncope, and orthostatic hypotension were the most common. Ventricular tachycardia and sick sinus syndrome were the most frequent cardiovascular causes of syncope. These frequencies may vary according to age and may be different in community hospitals and in outpatient settings.

Because of the serious nature of many of the entities causing syncope and the broad scope of the differential diagnosis, a large number of tests—in addition to the history, physical examination, and basic laboratory analyses—are used for the evaluation of patients with syncope. These tests include a 12-lead electrocardiogram (ECG), carotid sinus massage, prolonged electrocardiographic monitoring, echocardiogram, cardiac catheterization, electrophysiologic studies, and a neurologic evaluation including electroencephalogram (EEG), head computed tomography (CT) scan, radionuclide brain scan, and cerebral angiography. Utilization of a large number of these studies in any one patient can result in considerable cost to the patient. Therefore,

Table 2–1. Causes of Syncope

Noncardiovascular Causes	Cardiovascular Causes
Vasodepressor reactions	Reduced cardiac output
Situational syncope	Obstruction to left ventricular outflow: aortic stenosis and hypertrophic cardiomyopathy
Micturition	Obstruction to pulmonary flow: pulmonic stenosis, pulmonary hypertension, pulmonary embolism, tetralogy of Fallot
Defecation	Pump failure: massive myocardial infarct
Cough	Cardiac tamponade
Orthostatic hypotension	Atrial myxoma
Drugs	Aortic dissection
Cerebrovascular disease	Arrhythmias
Carotid sinus syncope	Bradyarrhythmias
	Second- and third-degree atrioventricular block
	Ventricular asystole
	Sick sinus syndrome
	Glossopharyngeal neuralgia with asystole
	Tachyarrhythmias
	Ventricular tachycardia
	Supraventricular tachycardia

Table 2–2. Causes of Syncope
in 204 Patients

Cause	No. of Patients
Cardiovascular	53
Ventricular tachycardia	20
Sick sinus syndrome	10
Bradycardia	2
Supraventricular tachycardia	3
Complete heart block	3
Mobitz II atrioventricular block	2
Pacemaker malfunction	1
Carotid sinus syncope	1
Aortic stenosis	5
Myocardial infarction	2
Dissecting aortic aneurysm	1
Pulmonary embolus	1
Pulmonary hypertension	2
Noncardiovascular	54
Vasodepressor syncope	9
Situational syncope	15
Drug-induced syncope	6
Orthostatic hypotension	14
Transient ischemic attacks	3
Subclavian steal syndrome	2
Seizure disorder	3
Vagal reaction with trigeminal neuralgia	1
Conversion reaction	1
Unknown	97

Adapted from Kapoor et al. Reprinted, by permission of The New England Journal of Medicine (309; 197–204, 1983).

it is prudent to develop an approach that would decrease the cost of care yet lead to an accurate diagnosis.

This chapter will review an approach to the evaluation of patients with syncope that emphasizes selective use of diagnostic tests, with the initial history, physical examination, and ECG being the cornerstones of the evaluation.

Diagnostic Approach

A careful, detailed initial history and physical examination and ECG are critical and will establish or suggest the majority of causes of syncope. Figure 2–1 shows an algorithm in which the initial history and physical examination are used to guide the further work-up of patients.

Causes Established by History and Physical Examination

The initial history and physical examination by themselves can lead to a diagnosis of specific causes of syncope, such as vasodepressor, situational, and drug-induced syncope, and orthostatic hypotension.

VASODEPRESSOR SYNCOPE

Vasodepressor syncope occurs in all age groups, although it is more common in younger patients and rare in the elderly. Vasodepressor syncope occurs in response to sudden emotional stress or in a setting of real, threatened, or fantasized injury. Some of the situations commonly leading to vasodepressor syncope include pain, the sight of blood, instrumentation, and venipuncture. Vasodepressor syncope occurs primarily with the patient in the standing position and less frequently, in the sitting position. Patients usually experience several minutes of prodromal symptoms including weakness, pallor, sweating, nausea, increased peristalsis, yawning, belching, and dimming of vision, followed by a loss of consciousness associated with hypotension and bradycardia. The patient's blood pressure, pulse, and mental status return to normal within minutes. Syncope may recur when the patient stands up.

The criteria for diagnosis of vasodepressor syncope include typical clinical presentation and a precipitating factor for the syncope. Generally, a careful history and physical examination are sufficient for evaluation of these patients.

SITUATIONAL SYNCOPE

Micturition Syncope. Classically, micturition syncope occurs in healthy, young to middle-aged men. Syncope usually occurs in the middle of the night during or immediately after voiding, often without premonitory symptoms. The reported predisposing factors include excessive alcohol consumption, recent viral infection, fatigue, or recent reduced food intake. Micturition syncope is usually not recurrent; however, recurrent syncope has been reported with bladder neck obstruction, severe chronic orthostatic hypotension, and atrioventricular block. In our own study, a group of older patients with micturition syncope was described; the majority were women and most had orthostatic hypotension.

Further work-up of these patients is generally not needed.

Defecation Syncope. Syncope occurring during defecation has been reported in elderly patients and usually is not recurrent. The

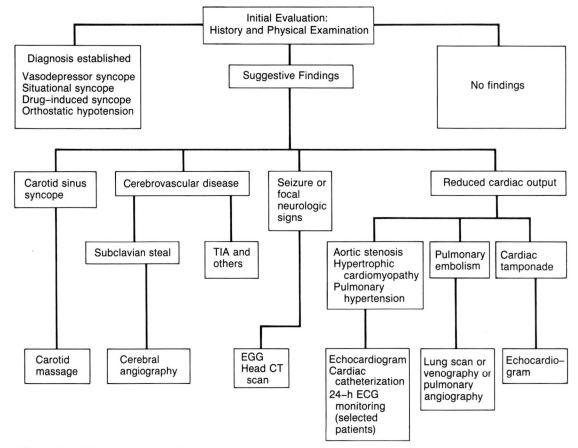

Figure 2–1. *Flow sheet for evaluation of syncope. An approach to the evaluation of patients with syncope based on data available from the initial history, physical examination, and ECG.*

mechanism of defecation syncope is unknown, but physiologic responses similar to those causing micturition syncope may be responsible. In our own study, defecation syncope had a multifactorial etiology, and possible predisposing factors included gastrointestinal illnesses, arrhythmias, and orthostatic hypotension.

Cough Syncope. Syncope occurring in association with a paroxysm of severe cough is defined as cough syncope. Patients with cough syncope are usually middle-aged men who are mildly obese, or heavy alcohol users who often have associated pulmonary conditions such as chronic obstructive pulmonary disease, asthma, bronchiectasis, pneumoconiosis, sarcoidosis, or tuberculosis. Cough syncope has very rarely been associated with hypertrophic cardiomyopathy and herniation of cerebellar tonsils. Diagnosis and therapy of underlying pulmonary disease are needed in these patients.

DRUG-INDUCED SYNCOPE

Drugs can lead to syncope by at least four different mechanisms:

1. Postural hypotension. In this category are antihypertensive drugs, diuretics, nitrates and other arterial vasodilators, L-dopa, and phenothiazines and other tranquilizers. Severe or symptomatic orthostatic hypotension (discussed later) related to the use of a specific drug is needed to classify a syncopal event as drug-induced.

2. Anaphylactic reaction. Drugs may lead to a reaction with associated symptoms of anaphylaxis and hypotension resulting in syncope.

3. Drug overdose. Drug overdoses most often lead to coma and prolonged loss of consciousness, although occasionally they may lead to syncopal episodes. Specific examples include lithium toxicity with arrhythmias, and tricyclic antidepressant or digitalis toxicity, which may lead to arrhythmias and syncope. In these instances, measurement of specific drug levels may be helpful in making a diagnosis.

4. Ventricular tachycardia. This group of drugs includes those leading to prolongation of the QT interval and to torsades de pointes,

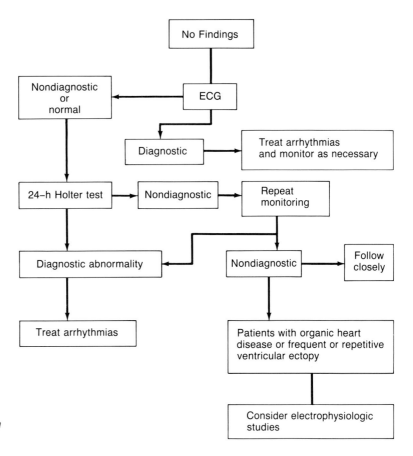

Figure 2-1 *See legend on opposite page*

a special form of ventricular tachycardia. The drugs most often implicated in leading to torsades de pointes include quinidine, disopyramide, procainamide, phenothiazines, and tricyclic antidepressants. In addition, drug-induced hypokalemia and hypomagnesemia may lead to a prolonged QT interval and development of torsades de pointes. Diagnosis of this arrhythmia in patients with a prolonged QT interval requires an ECG and electrocardiographic monitoring.

ORTHOSTATIC HYPOTENSION

Orthostatic hypotension is a common cause of syncope and is seen frequently in the elderly population. One study found a blood pressure drop of 20 mmHg or more in 24% of community dwellers more than 65 years of age. Similarly, orthostatic hypotension is a common problem in elderly nursing home residents. Orthostatic hypotension may be aggravated by the use of antihypertensive, diuretic, or vasodilator drugs, or other medications causing syncope. Postural hypotension occurs in a variety of clinical situations including volume depletion, decreased venous return, and use of pharmacologic agents, and it may be a symptom of central and peripheral nervous system disorders (Table 2-3).

To implicate orthostatic hypotension as causing syncope, the orthostatic blood pressure

Table 2-3. *Causes of Orthostatic Hypotension*

Volume depletion or venous pooling
Prolonged bed rest
Prolonged standing
Dehydration
Acute blood loss
Severe varicose veins
Adrenal insufficiency
Medications
Antihypertensives
Diuretics
Nitrates
Arterial vasodilators
Calcium channel–blocking agents
Phenothiazines
Others
Neurologic diseases
Neuropathy
Spinal cord disease
Surgical sympathectomy
Idiopathic postural hypotension
Shy-Drager syndrome

drop should be severe (systolic blood pressure fall to less than 90 mmHg) or should be associated with symptoms of dizziness or syncope, or both.

Blood pressure in the supine position should be measured after the patient has been lying down for an adequate period (some authors recommend 15 to 20 minutes). Standing blood pressure should be measured at 2 and 5 minutes. Because orthostatic hypotension can vary with time, multiple orthostatic blood pressure measurements may give diagnostically important information.

Once the diagnoses are established by history and physical examination, appropriate treatment includes management of associated diseases, discontinuation or alteration of drugs causing syncope, and the evaluation and treatment of orthostatic hypotension.

Causes Suggested by History and Physical Examination

The initial history and physical examination may suggest specific causes of syncope that will require confirmatory tests for diagnosis (Fig. 2–1). The entities in this category include the following.

CAROTID SINUS SYNCOPE

When syncope is associated with hyperextension of the neck, head turning, tight collars, carrying shoulder loads, shaving, or other maneuvers spontaneously stretching the carotid sinus, a diagnosis of carotid sinus syncope should be considered. Although 10% or more of normal healthy older individuals may have hyperactive carotid sinus reflexes, actual carotid sinus syncope is rare, occurring in only 5 to 20% of persons with a hyperactive reflex. Carotid sinus syncope occurs more often in men in the seventh and eighth decades of life. Occasionally thyroid tumors, carotid body tumors, and inflammatory and malignant lymph nodes may precipitate carotid sinus syncope. Drugs such as digoxin, propranolol, and methyldopa may also precipitate this syncope.

There are two types of responses to carotid sinus stimulation. (1) The cardioinhibitory type is manifested by bradycardia or asystole with or without hypotension; this type is most prevalent, accounting for 50 to 70% of all cases of carotid sinus hypersensitivity. (2) The vasodepressor reflex produces hypotension without significant bradycardia. Often, the response is a combination of the cardioinhibitory and vasodepressor types.

In patients suspected of having carotid sinus syncope, carotid massage is needed for diagnosis. Carotid massage should be performed in elderly patients *only* if other diagnostic studies have not been helpful, because rare transient and permanent neurologic deficits have been precipitated by this maneuver. Electrocardiographic monitoring and frequent blood pressure determinations should be done during the procedure. The test is performed with the patient in the supine position and is repeated in sitting and standing positions if carotid sinus hypersensitivity is strongly suspected. A sinus pause of 3 seconds or more or a decrease in systolic pressure of 50 mmHg or more with no significant decrease in pulse rate represents a positive test diagnostic of a hypersensitive carotid sinus. The diagnosis of carotid sinus syncope is justified when an individual has a hyperactive carotid sinus reflex and when syncope is clearly related to activities that press on or stretch the sinus. In our study, 1% of patients were found to have carotid sinus syncope.

CEREBROVASCULAR DISEASE

Cerebrovascular disease is an uncommon cause of syncope. In patients with vertebrobasilar transient ischemic attacks or subclavian steal syndrome, syncope and drop attacks are almost always associated with other neurologic signs and symptoms of vertebrobasilar ischemia such as vertigo, visual disturbance, and sensory and motor findings. In patients with symptoms of vertebrobasilar ischemia, underlying etiologies such as atherosclerotic disease, migraines, vasculitis, and embolic diseases need to be considered and investigated.

In patients with a difference in blood pressure of 20 mmHg or more between the two arms or a decrease in pulse intensity in one arm, a diagnosis of subclavian steal syndrome should be considered (aortic dissection may also lead to differences in blood pressure or pulse between the two arms and should be considered).

The diagnosis of subclavian steal syndrome requires cerebral angiography. Vertebrobasilar transient ischemic attack is a clinical diagnosis, and neurologic symptoms of vertebrobasilar ischemia are usually present at the time of syncope. If associated carotid artery disease is suspected, noninvasive flow studies, digital subtraction angiography, or carotid angiography may be useful for diagnosis and potential therapy. These studies are not generally needed for the evaluation of syncope.

SEIZURE DISORDER

In patients with symptoms compatible with a seizure as a cause of loss of consciousness such as an aura, postictal state, or tonic-clonic movements, a sleep EEG is needed. A head CT scan may also be needed as part of the work-up. In addition, in patients with syncope and focal neurologic signs or symptoms, an EEG and CT scan are needed to determine the underlying cause of the symptoms.

REDUCED CARDIAC OUTPUT SECONDARY TO STRUCTURAL ABNORMALITIES

Structural abnormalities leading to decreased cardiac output include aortic stenosis, hypertrophic cardiomyopathy, acute myocardial infarction, aortic dissection, cardiac tamponade, and atrial myxoma. Pulmonary embolism, pulmonic stenosis, pulmonary hypertension, and tetralogy of Fallot, which obstruct the pulmonary outflow, may also cause syncope. Patients with aortic stenosis, pulmonary hypertension, or idiopathic hypertrophic subaortic stenosis may present with exertional syncope.

Diseases resulting in syncope from structural abnormalities of the heart are suspected on the basis of a history and findings on physical examination, which may disclose cardiac murmurs and other cardiovascular signs of these entities. In patients with these specific findings, further evaluation for definitive diagnosis and for determination of the severity of these diseases requires an echocardiogram or cardiac catheterization, or both. If aortic dissection is suspected, an emergency aortogram is needed. For diagnosis of acute myocardial infarction, monitoring in a cardiac care unit, serial ECGs, and cardiac enzyme determinations are needed. Of elderly patients with myocardial infarction, 5 to 12% may present with syncope rather than chest pain.

Approximately 10 to 15% of patients with pulmonary embolism present with syncope associated with other symptoms of thromboembolism. Syncope is more often associated with massive embolus. In patients with syncope who have a sudden onset of dyspnea, pleuritic chest pain, or other findings of pulmonary embolism, a lung scan (ventilation and perfusion) is needed. If the lung scan findings are indeterminate, pulmonary angiography may be needed for diagnosis of possible pulmonary embolism.

No Cause Established or Suggested by History or Physical Examination

In a substantial number of patients (approximately 65% in our study), the initial history and physical examination do not establish or suggest a specific cause of syncope. In the majority of these patients, a search for possible arrhythmias as a cause of syncope is needed (Fig. 2–1). For this purpose, the ECG, electrocardiographic monitoring, and electrophysiologic studies have been utilized. In this group of patients, the EEG and brain scans have also been used and will be discussed later.

ELECTROCARDIOGRAM

The 12-lead ECG and rhythm strip are often needed in the diagnostic evaluation of syncope, especially if the initial history and physical examination do not disclose or suggest a possible etiology. The incidence of diagnostic abnormalities on an initial ECG is low, but when found, these abnormalities may eliminate the need for extensive evaluation. Important diagnostic findings derived from both the initial ECG and prolonged electrocardiographic monitoring are similar (discussed later). In our own study, 5% of patients had a diagnosis established by findings on the initial ECG or a rhythm strip.

For patients with diagnostic findings from the ECG, admission to the hospital is needed for further monitoring and therapy of arrhythmias. Further evaluation is often needed for patients in whom the initial ECG does not show an arrhythmia or myocardial infarction as a potential cause of syncope. Although data are not available for young, healthy individuals with one unexplained syncopal episode, the yield of further work-up in this population is low if careful initial history, physical examination, and ECG are normal.

For most patients, a decision regarding admission to the hospital needs to be made. There are no reported studies addressing the need for hospitalization in patients with syncope. Patients with evidence of prior myocardial infarction, congestive heart failure, history of ventricular tachycardia, or bifascicular block generally require admission, electrocardiographic monitoring, and a rapid evaluation for detection and treatment of possible arrhythmias. If results of bedside monitoring are negative, another 24 to 48 hours of ambulatory monitoring is needed, although the incremental yield of this additional monitoring has not been studied.

PROLONGED ELECTROCARDIOGRAPHIC MONITORING

Prolonged electrocardiographic monitoring is indicated when the initial evaluation, including an ECG, is suggestive but not diagnostic of an arrthymia or if no etiology of syncope can be determined from the initial evaluation. However, the following limitations should be recognized.

First, there is a poor correlation between symptoms reported during monitoring and concurrent electrocardiographic findings. Arrhythmias may be excluded as a cause if the patient has syncope during monitoring but no concurrent rhythm disturbance. However, most patients do not have syncope during monitoring; in our study, this occurred in only 3% of patients. Symptomatically important arrhythmias were found in only 2.5% of patients when dizziness occurred during monitoring. Therefore, presumptions regarding the cause of syncope based on asymptomatic findings are frequently necessary because of the prognostic importance and sporadic nature of the arrhythmias.

Second, the optimal duration of electrocardiographic monitoring has not been determined. One study suggested that patients should be continuously monitored until the symptoms recur. This approach is impractical.

Third, the yield of prolonged electrocardiographic monitoring is variable, showing transient arrhythmias as a potential cause of syncope in only 10 to 64% of patients.

Despite these shortcomings, prolonged electrocardiographic monitoring is a useful diagnostic test in the evaluation of patients with syncope if its cause cannot be determined by the history, physical examination, and ECG. In our study, prolonged electrocardiographic monitoring yielded a potential diagnosis in 12% of patients.

Prolonged transtelephonic monitoring is occasionally used in the evaluation of syncope, although the usefulness of this test has not been well studied. Because this test requires the patient to be alert to use the electrodes to record a symptomatic episode, it is not expected to be useful in patients with loss of consciousness. Our own limited experience suggests that this modality is very rarely if ever useful for this evaluation.

The information derived from prolonged electrocardiographic monitoring can be classified in the following manner:
1. Symptomatic arrhythmias. As noted above, symptoms during monitoring are rare, but if arrhythmias are found simultaneously with symptoms, they are the most definitive evidence for the cause of syncope.
2. Transient asymptomatic serious arrhythmias. A decision regarding management of the patient frequently has to be made on the basis of asymptomatic arrhythmias. There are no agreed upon criteria for assigning a cause of syncope based on asymptomatic findings. The following criteria were used in our prospective study:
   a. Bradyarrhythmias
      i. Symptomatic sinus bradycardia or pauses
      ii. Sinus pauses greater than 2 seconds
   b. Atrioventricular block
      i. Mobitz II atrioventricular block
      ii. Complete heart block
   c. Tachyarrhythmias
      i. Symptomatic or sustained ventricular tachycardia ($\geq$ 30-second duration)
      ii. Asymptomatic ventricular tachycardia of more than five beats
      iii. Symptomatic supraventricular tachycardia

Because of a poor correlation between symptoms during ambulatory monitoring and concurrent electrocardiographic findings, it is frequently difficult to state definitively that an abnormality on subsequent monitoring can explain a prior symptom. Therefore, it may be necessary to infer probable diagnoses from findings during asymptomatic periods. Our criteria, based on asymptomatic findings, were arrived at after extensive review of the literature on findings in normal healthy subjects. For example, sinus pauses of more than 2 seconds occur in 1 to 4% of normal persons, and thus pauses longer than 2 seconds in patients with a history of syncope suggest a diagnosis of sick sinus syndrome. Similarly, ventricular tachycardia has been reported in up to 2% of normal persons, and when present it is usually isolated and consists of less than five beats. Therefore, in patients with a history of syncope, asymptomatic ventricular tachycardia of more than five beats was considered a potential indicator of longer periods of ventricular tachycardia.

3. Exclusion of arrhythmias as a cause of syncope. Rarely, electrocardiographic monitoring may provide objective evidence to exclude arrhythmias. This occurs when the patient has a syncopal episode and has no significant concurrent electrocardiographic findings.

Although a normal result from 24-hour ambulatory monitoring decreases the likelihood of arrhythmias as a cause of syncope, it clearly does not exclude arrhythmogenic syncope.

ELECTROPHYSIOLOGIC STUDIES

The indications for and the utility of results obtained from electrophysiologic studies are controversial and not completely established. Previous studies used this test in the following types of patients:

1. Those with recurrent syncope with severe bradycardia (< 40 beats per minute) to document prolonged sinus node recovery time as evidence for sick sinus syndrome
2. Those with syncope of unknown origin after thorough evaluation, when bifascicular block is documented on an ECG
3. Those with syncope of unknown etiology, when there is underlying coronary or valvular heart disease, or in patients with brief episodes of unsustained ventricular tachycardia
4. Those with recurrent syncope of unknown origin

Based on the criteria used in reports on electrophysiologic studies, the following findings can be considered as presumptive evidence of a cause of syncope:

1. Ventricular tachycardia. Inducible ventricular tachycardia is the abnormality found most frequently in patients with unexplained syncope who undergo electrophysiologic studies. Sustained, monomorphic ventricular tachycardia seems to be specific to patients who probably have had spontaneous ventricular tachycardia. Therefore, a finding of sustained monomorphic ventricular tachycardia constitutes a presumptive diagnosis of the patient's prior syncope. Induced polymorphic, nonsustained ventricular tachycardia, on the other hand, is probably a nonspecific response and may be due to an aggressive ventricular stimulation protocol. The exact significance of this type of ventricular tachycardia is unclear, and this finding may not justify a presumptive diagnosis of prior syncope.
2. Sinus node disease. A corrected sinus node recovery time greater than 525 ms suggests

sinus node dysfunction. The diagnosis of sinus node disease, however, most often rests on the finding of bradyarrhythmias on prolonged ECG monitoring and correlation with symptoms during monitoring. The sensitivity of sinus node recovery time for diagnosis of sinus node disease is low (estimated to be approximately 50%).

3. Atrioventricular block. A prolonged H-V interval (> 55 ms) may be associated with an increased risk of subsequent complete heart block, but moderate H-V prolongation is common in patients without a history of symptomatic heart block. Various studies of syncope have used different criteria for the H-V interval as being diagnostic, including an H-V interval greater than 55, 75, or 100 ms. Marked prolongation of the H-V interval (> 100 ms) is uncommon, and in patients with syncope of unknown cause may justify a trial of ventricular pacing.
4. Supraventricular tachycardia. The finding of induced supraventricular tachycardia may occasionally be useful in the management of patients with syncope of undetermined etiology; false-positive results are common, however, and the findings should be interpreted in view of the patient's clinical symptoms. Supraventricular tachycardia that may be significant generally leads to sudden hypotension and syncope.
5. Other findings. Abnormalities of atrioventricular node refractory periods and abnormalities induced by various pharmacologic agents are generally difficult to interpret in terms of the cause of a patient's syncope.

Studies of the use of electrophysiologic testing for syncope generally have found that more than 50% of the patients with syncope of unknown origin had abnormalities that were considered to be diagnostic and that led to specific therapy. In all but two of the follow-up studies, the patients with positive tests leading to specific therapy had a lower rate of recurrent syncope than those with negative tests. These results imply that therapy directed at electrophysiologic abnormalities may be effective in minimizing the risk of recurrent syncope, although controlled randomized trials are needed to determine the ultimate role of electrophysiologic studies in syncope.

ELECTROENCEPHALOGRAPHY

The differential diagnosis between syncope and a seizure disorder can occasionally be very difficult, especially if the episode has not been witnessed. An EEG is indicated when a seizure disorder is suspected clinically or if there is a focal neurologic deficit on physical examination. In addition, in patients with recurrent unwitnessed episodes of syncope of unknown origin, an EEG may occasionally be useful. The EEG can provide information regarding only a convulsive tendency or the possibility of a focal abnormality. If such findings are detected, neurologic evaluation and further testing with a CT scan of the head or angiography, or both, may be needed. Nonselective use of the EEG, however, is not warranted in the evaluation of patients with syncope.

Brain Scans, CT Scans of the Head, Cerebral Angiography

Radionuclide brain scans and CT scans of the head rarely help in the diagnosis of a cause of syncope. If a seizure disorder or focal neurologic findings are present, these tests are warranted. In our retrospective study of 121 patients, an EEG (done in 67 patients) and CT scan (done in 39 patients) were not useful in assigning a cause of syncope in any patient. In our prospective study of 204 patients, an EEG and CT scan were useful in the evaluation of one patient who had focal neurologic findings. The findings of cerebrovascular atherosclerotic disease on cerebral angiography do not help to establish the cause of syncope because such findings may be common in elderly asymptomatic patients.

Glucose Tolerance Test

Hypoglycemia can lead to alteration of consciousness that is gradual and associated with symptoms of excessive autonomic tone. In patients with syncope as defined here, a glucose tolerance test is not generally useful. In our studies, a 5-hour glucose tolerance test has not uncovered hypoglycemia as a cause of syncope in any patient.

An Overall Strategy for Evaluation of Syncope

The flow sheet in Figure 2–1 summarizes the approach to the evaluation of patients with syncope. All patients in whom a diagnosis cannot be established should be periodically re-evaluated for new clues to the etiology of their syncope. Patients having recurrent episodes of syncope of unknown cause may require repeated evaluation following the same scheme as outlined, although the yield of repeat evaluation is low. In our study of 433 patients, eight new diagnoses were established through evaluation of recurrences in patients in whom a cause was not assigned at initial evaluation.

With these guidelines, a cause of syncope can be established in 50 to 60% of the patients with syncope. Table 2–4 shows the results of diagnostic tests in 400 patients evaluated in our medical center. This table emphasizes the central role of history and physical examination. Approximately half of the patients had a cardiovascular cause, the other half, a noncardiovascular cause. The experience at our medical center indicates that using these various diagnostic modalities in a less goal-directed fashion does not increase the diagnostic yield but does increase potential cost to and discomfort of the patient.

Prognosis

Our initial report noted a mortality of 14% and an incidence of sudden death of 8% in patients with syncope. As shown in Figure 2–2, the 1-year mortality of 30% of patients with a cardiovascular cause of syncope was significantly higher than the 12% for patients with a noncardiovascular cause or 6.4% for patients with syncope of unknown origin. The incidence of sudden death of 24% for patients with a cardiovascular cause was also higher than the 4% for patients with a noncardiovascular cause or 3% for patients with syncope of unknown origin. These data have been confirmed by other studies, which show a mortality of 18 to 33% for patients with a cardiovascular cause of syncope compared with 6 to 12% for the other two groups. The incidence of sudden death has not been examined in any other study.

Table 2–4. *Success of Diagnostic Test in Establishing a Cause of Syncope in 400 Patients*

Technique	%
History and physical examination	30
Electrocardiogram	5
Electrocardiographic monitoring	12
Electroencephalography	< 1
Carotid massage	1
Electrophysiologic studies	2
Cardiac catheterization	3
Cerebral angiography	< 1
Stress test	< 1

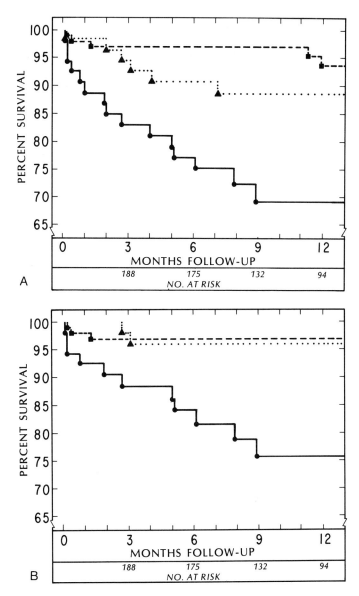

Figure 2–2. A: *Comparison of cumulative survival of patients with syncope with a cardiovascular cause (circles), syncope with a noncardiovascular cause (triangles), and syncope of unknown cause (squares) (Kaplan-Meier estimates).* B: *Comparison of cumulative incidence of sudden death of patients with syncope with a cardiovascular cause (circles), syncope with a noncardiovascular cause (triangles), and syncope of unknown cause (squares) (Kaplan-Meier estimates). From Kapoor et al. Reprinted, by permission of The New England Journal of Medicine (309; 197–204, 1983).*

In our study of 433 patients, 146 had one or more episodes of recurrent syncope during the mean follow-up period of 30 months. The rate of recurrence in patients with an initial diagnosis of cardiac cause was similar to that for patients with a diagnosis of noncardiac cause or syncope of unknown origin (31 to 43%). In only eight patients with an initial diagnosis of syncope of unknown origin was a new diagnosis assigned based on an evaluation of recurrence. Our study also showed that recurrence is not a predictor of increased mortality or sudden death.

Bibliography

Branch WT, Jr. Approach to syncope. J Gen Intern Med 1:49–58, 1986.
This is a review of the pathophysiology of and diagnostic testing in syncope.
Day SC, Cook EF, Funkenstein H, et al. Evaluation and outcome of emergency room patients with transient loss of consciousness. Am J Med 73:15–23, 1982.
An evaluation of 198 emergency room patients showed that causes of syncope and seizure were defined in more than 80% of the cases. Prognostic implications of various clinical findings are discussed.
DiMarco JP. Electrophysiologic studies in patients with unexplained syncope. Circulation 75(Suppl III):140–143, 1987.
This article highlights some of the problems with the use of electrophysiologic studies.
Eagle KA, Black HR, Cook EF, et al. Evaluation of prognostic classifications for patients with syncope. Am J Med 79:455–460, 1985.
This article compares the results of a study done in Pittsburgh to those done at Yale New Haven Hospital and Brigham and Women's Hospital. The article points to small differences in the prognosis of patients at

different hospitals and indicates that patients with a cardiovascular cause of syncope have a worse prognosis in all three different settings.

Gibson TC, Heitzman MR. Diagnostic efficacy of 24-hour electrocardiographic monitoring for syncope. Am J Cardiol 53:1013–1017, 1984.

This paper discusses the results of electrocardiographic monitoring in a large group of patients referred because of syncope. It notes that symptomatic correlation during monitoring is rare.

Kapoor WN. Use of electrophysiologic studies in unexplained syncope. Pract Cardiol 13:53–63, 1987.

This article reviews the indications, diagnostic criteria, cost, and complications of electrophysiologic studies in unexplained syncope.

Kapoor WN, Cha R, Peterson JR, et al. Prolonged electrocardiographic monitoring in patients with syncope. Importance of frequent or repetitive ventricular ectopy. Am J Med 82:20–28, 1987.

Problems of lack of symptomatic correlation and prognostic implications of arrhythmias are discussed.

Kapoor WN, Karpf M, Levey GS. Issues in evaluating patients with syncope. Ann Intern Med 100:755–757, 1984.

Important issues in diagnosis and management are discussed.

Kapoor WN, Karpf M, Maher Y, et al. Syncope of unknown origin: the need for a more cost-effective approach to its diagnostic evaluation. JAMA 247:2687–2691, 1982.

An extensive evaluation of patients with syncope of unknown origin led to 13 new diagnoses in 121 patients. Electrocardiographic monitoring and electrophysiologic studies were the most useful tests.

Kapoor WN, Karpf M, Wieand S, et al. A prospective evaluation and follow-up of patients with syncope. N Engl J Med 309:197–204, 1983.

History, physical examination, and ECG are the cornerstones of evaluation. Patients with a cardiovascular cause have a poor prognosis.

Kapoor WN, Peterson J, Wieand HS, et al. Diagnostic and prognostic implications of recurrences in patients with syncope. Am J Med 83:700–708, 1987.

Of 433 patients, 34% had recurrences over a mean follow-up of 30 months. There was no significant difference in recurrence rate in the three diagnostic groups. Recurrence was not a predictor of mortality or sudden death.

Kapoor W, Snustad D, Peterson J, et al. Syncope in the elderly. Am J Med 80:419–428, 1986.

The elderly more often have arrhythmias. Prognosis of patients with a cardiovascular cause is similar whether they are elderly or young.

Lipsitz LA. Syncope in the elderly. Ann Intern Med 99:92–105, 1983.

This article reviews the pathophysiology, causes, and diagnostic evaluation of syncope in the elderly.

McAnulty JH. Syncope of unknown origin: the role of electrophysiologic studies. Circulation 75(Suppl III):144–145, 1987.

This article reviews the usefulness and problems of electrophysiologic studies in the evaluation of patients with syncope.

Silverstein MD, Singer DE, Mulley AG, et al. Patients with syncope admitted to medical intensive care units. JAMA 248:1185–1189, 1982.

Patients admitted to medical intensive care units are generally sicker than those going to an emergency room. The cause of syncope was not assigned in 47% of the patients. Patients with a cardiovascular cause of syncope had a worse prognosis than other groups.

3

Management of the Patient after Myocardial Infarction

DAVID E. BUSH, M.D.

Introduction

Despite advances in our understanding of the pathophysiology of coronary artery disease, approximately 1.5 million people suffer a myocardial infarction in the United States annually, of whom 0.5 million die. Patients recovering from a myocardial infarction are a heterogeneous group in terms of their risk for major complications such as recurrent myocardial infarction and life-threatening arrhythmias. The overall 1-year mortality for patients discharged from the hospital after an acute myocardial infarction is approximately 10%; most deaths occur within the first 3 months. It is possible with currently available techniques to identify patients who have both higher and lower risks than average for reinfarction and death. Stratification of patients according to their predicted risk for subsequent complications allows the most effective use of the available diagnostic and therapeutic options. Stratification begins during hospitalization but is continually refined in the convalescent phase as additional information becomes available. The need for diagnostic and therapeutic interventions is best decided in light of the patient's predicted risk for subsequent events. However, even patients assigned to low risk categories will benefit from a strategy designed to reduce certain risk factors such as smoking, elevated cholesterol levels, and hypertension.

Clinical and Pathologic Predictors of Outcome after Myocardial Infarction

The pathologic features that influence the clinical course after an infarction include in-farct size, infarct type, and the extent and distribution of coronary artery disease. Commonly available noninvasive techniques can provide an assessment of ventricular function, electrical stability, and residual myocardial ischemia. Patient management can be optimized by coupling these noninvasive tests with an understanding of the pathophysiology of myocardial infarction.

Infarct Size

One of the major features that predict outcome after myocardial infarction is lesion size. The true infarct size is the sum of all injury to the left ventricle, both new and old. Pathologic studies demonstrate that cardiogenic shock is seen when more than 40% of the left ventricle is infarcted.[1] Thus, a system to classify infarcts according to their size would be expected to yield clinically useful information about prognosis. Killip devised a classification scheme that categorizes patients according to the degree of left ventricular dysfunction at the time of presentation.[2] This system has proved to be useful in determining outcome because it is a means of clinically assessing infarct size. Class I infarcts produce no congestive heart failure and have less than a 5% in-hospital mortality. Infarcts that produce mild to moderate heart failure are class II and are associated with a 10 to 15% mortality. Class III infarcts produce acute pulmonary edema and have mortalities of 35 to 40%. In patients with cardiogenic shock (class IV), the mortality frequently exceeds 80%.

The ejection fraction can be viewed as another means to infer infarct size. Like the true infarct size the ejection fraction also reflects any previous injury to the left ventricle. Studies correlating ejection fraction with prognosis have generally found that ejection fractions of greater than 40% are associated with good prognoses (< 10% 1-year mortality), ejection fractions in the 30 to 40% range have intermediate prognoses, and ejection fractions of less than 30% have much poorer prognoses. The relationship of the ejection fraction to infarct size is not a linear one (Fig. 3–1). Infarcts involving up to 15% of the left ventricle may cause little or no change in the ejection fraction. However, because left ventricular dysfunction and infarct size reflect the sum of all infarct damage, small infarcts when added to pre-existing damage can result in marked deterioration in left ventricular function (Fig. 3–1). The use of the Killip clinical classification in combination with an imaging study to calculate the ejection fraction (two-dimensional echocardiogram or radionuclide ventriculogram) may be a better predictor than the use of either method alone.

Infarct Location

The location of an infarct is another easily assessable clinical feature that has bearing on prognosis. Infarctions involving the anterior and anteroseptal walls, which typically result from occlusions of the left anterior descending coronary artery, have poorer outcomes than other types of infarction.[3] Differences in infarct size between anterior and inferior infarctions may account for some of this difference in prognosis. However, it has been suggested that anterior wall infarction has a poorer prognosis even when matched for infarct size.[4] One possible explanation for the observed difference in mortality between inferior and anterior myocardial infarctions is the predilection for infarct expansion in the latter. Infarct expansion, acute thinning, and dilatation of the infarct region are seen predominantly in anterior infarctions. Infarct expansion is the precursor to several major sequelae of myocardial infarction including left cardiac dilatation, ventricular aneurysm, and cardiac rupture.[5]

Inferior myocardial infarctions more commonly have bradyarrhythmias and heart block than do infarcts at other locations. In the setting of inferior infarction these rhythm disturbances typically result from ischemia to the atrioventricular node, which tends to be transient, usually resolving in less than a week. When ischemic injury occurs in the peripheral bundles, such as that seen typically during anterior myocardial infarction, the conduction disturbances are more often permanent.

Q Wave versus Non–Q Wave Infarction

Whether or not patients who suffer myocardial infarction develop pathologic Q waves can

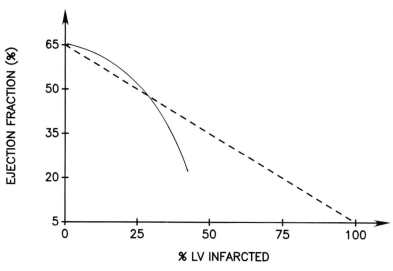

Figure 3–1. Estimated relationship of infarct size to left ventricular ejection fraction. Infarct damage is cumulative in its effect on left ventricular function. A small infarct may have little effect on a previously normal ventricle but a large effect on a previously damaged ventricle. The relationship between the pathologically determined infarct size and ejection fraction is not linear as would be predicted by the dashed line.

give important clues about prognosis. Non–Q wave infarctions occur in approximately 25% of patients admitted to a coronary care unit with an acute myocardial infarction. Patients with non–Q wave infarctions tend to have smaller infarctions, better left ventricular function, and a more favorable in-hospital prognosis when compared with patients having Q wave infarctions. However, in the posthospital phase, non–Q wave infarction is more often associated with recurrent angina, myocardial infarction, and sudden death.[6]

Pathologically, non–Q wave infarctions are more frequently nontransmural, whereas Q wave infarctions more often tend to be transmural. However, there are other pathologic differences between Q wave and non–Q wave infarctions. The infarct-related artery in a non–Q wave infarction is more likely to be patent with a critical stenosis, whereas Q wave infarctions more often tend to have total occlusions. In this regard patients with non–Q wave infarctions can be likened to patients who have received successful thrombolytic therapy for an acute myocardial infarction; in one case the thrombolysis is spontaneous, whereas in the other it is induced. In the setting of non–Q wave infarction by whatever means, there typically remains a substantial region of ischemic myocardium. This residual ischemic myocardium is the substrate for recurrent infarction and arrhythmias and confers an unfavorable prognosis on non–Q wave myocardial infarction despite the smaller initial infarct size. Recognition of this fact should lead to a particularly careful evaluation of these patients for residual ischemic myocardium and the potential need for a revascularization procedure. There has been some recent evidence that diltiazem may be of prophylactic benefit in preventing recurrent infarction during the hospital phase of non–Q wave infarction.[7]

Extent and Distribution of Coronary Artery Disease

The prognosis for a patient surviving the initial phase of a myocardial infarction is closely linked to the extent of remaining coronary artery disease. More than two thirds of patients with infarctions have significant coronary artery disease in at least two vessels. It is precisely these noninfarcted regions that must take on the burden of compensating for the myocardial mass that was lost because of infarction. It is therefore not difficult to under-

stand why stenoses in regions remote from the infarction site can be associated with particularly poor outcomes. This concept has been validated by studies examining the outcome in patients with postinfarction ischemia. It was found that mortality is significantly higher in patients with ischemia distant from the vascular distribution of the infarct.[8] These same studies demonstrated that the standard electrocardiogram (ECG) proved to be a reliable predictor of whether the same or a different vascular distribution was involved. Thus, in the setting of postinfarction angina, additional information regarding prognosis can be obtained by noting whether the electrocardiographic changes with pain occur in the same or different leads compared with those of the original infarction.

Ventricular Arrhythmias

Many unanswered questions remain about the management of ventricular arrhythmias in patients after myocardial infarction.[9] An estimated 5% of patients who survive the initial phase of a myocardial infarction will experience sudden cardiac death within the first year. Those who survive the first year after a myocardial infarction remain at risk for sudden death in subsequent years, at the approximate rate of 3% per year. Some clinical features do help identify patients at higher risk for late ventricular tachycardia:

- Congestive heart failure
- Large anterior infarction
- Right bundle branch block
- Left ventricular aneurysm
- Ejection fraction < 40%

Despite the considerable efforts that have been made to address the major diagnostic and therapeutic issues in this group of patients, our understanding of how best to manage them remains incomplete.

Sustained ventricular tachycardia or ventricular fibrillation occurring in the late phase after a myocardial infarction is associated with an increased risk of sudden cardiac death. One unresolved issue is when does *late* begin. There is general agreement that ventricular tachycardia/ventricular fibrillation,which occurs within the first 72 hours after a myocardial infarction, is early and thus not necessarily associated with an increased risk of subsequent sudden death. Generally, a somewhat arbitrary time of around 5 to 7 days is taken to divide early from late arrhythmias.

Another issue of controversy is whether there are benefits to treating complex ventricular ectopy (Table 3–1) besides sustained ventricular tachycardia or ventricular fibrillation. Several studies examining the incidence of death in postinfarction patients with and without complex ventricular ectopy have shown that complex ventricular ectopy does identify a group of patients at higher risk for death. However, these same studies have failed to demonstrate that patients with complex ventricular ectopy are at higher risk for sudden cardiac death than those without such arrhythmias. Indeed, most studies have found about the same rates of sudden death among those with and without complex ventricular ectopy. Complex ventricular ectopy is associated with a higher incidence of death, but not necessarily sudden death. Thus, complex ventricular ectopy seems to be more of a nonspecific marker for poor outcome than a specific predictor of subsequent life-threatening ventricular arrhythmias.

Patients who have ventricular fibrillation or sustained ventricular tachycardia benefit from antiarrhythmic treatment. The benefits of such therapy in patients with asymptomatic complex ectopy (excluding sustained ventricular tachycardia) are less clear. There may be some benefit to treating these patients with antiarrhythmic agents, although the benefit appears to be small and probably of limited duration. In all patients with significant ventricular arrhythmia it is important to evaluate ischemia as the possible cause. Arrhythmias that occur because of ischemia are more likely to respond to anti-ischemic therapy than to antiarrhythmic therapy. An approach to management of these patients is outlined in Figure 3–2.

When a decision is made to treat a patient for an arrhythmia, a means of assessing the adequacy of the therapeutic response should exist. Thus for patients who have symptomatic but not life-threatening arrhythmias, the response to therapy can be assessed on the basis of symptoms. This group of patients often responds well to treatment with beta blockers, which are both antiarrhythmic and anti-ischemic. There is a considerable amount of spontaneous variability in the occurrence of most arrhythmias. Holter monitoring can be used as a method of monitoring the effectiveness of antiarrhythmic therapy only when the frequency of the arrhythmia is sufficient to allow the detection of a treatment response. When the frequency of the arrhythmia to be treated is low, the response to programmed electrical stimulation is the best means of assessing the adequacy of a given therapeutic intervention.

Diagnostic Testing

As outlined in the preceding sections, the clinical presentation and hospital course can provide much useful information about the patient's prognosis. These clinical observations should be supplemented, in most instances, by Holter monitoring, a ventricular function study, and an exercise study (Table 3–2).

Holter Evaluation

The predischarge assessment of every patient recovering from a myocardial infarction should include a 24-hour Holter study, which should be performed no earlier than 5 to 7 days after the myocardial infarction. In addition to providing information about arrhythmias, the Holter study may also be able to identify patients experiencing silent myocardial ischemia. There is evidence that such patients are at even higher risk of poor outcome than patients with exclusively symptomatic ischemia.[10]

Ventricular Function Studies

Ventricular function is one of the key determinants of outcome. Thus patients with impaired ventricular function may warrant more aggressive treatment than those with normal ventricular function.

Exercise Testing

Exercise testing before discharge from the hospital has been quite valuable in the man-

Table 3–1. Lown Classification
of Ventricular Ectopy

Simple	Complex
Class 1: < 30/h	Class 3: multiform complexes
Class 2: > 30/h	Class 4A: couplets
	Class 4B: runs of 3 or more (ventricular tachycardia)
	Class 5: R on T

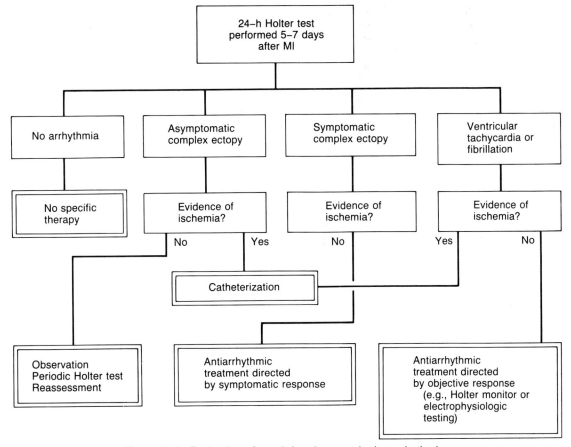

Figure 3–2. Evaluation of postinfarction ventricular arrhythmias.

agement of patients recovering from an infarction. The aim of such testing is to identify those patients who have additional myocardium at risk for recurrent infarction. Patients with evidence of ischemia identified by low level treadmill exercise have a 1-year mortality of approximately 15%. This group of patients will benefit from anti-ischemic therapy. Patients without evidence of ischemia by treadmill testing at the time of discharge constitute a low risk group with an annual mortality of less than 2%.

Exercise testing before discharge is quite safe with appropriate patient selection.[11] Patients who should be excluded from exercise testing are those who have poorly controlled hypertension, evidence of congestive heart failure, or uncontrolled arrhythmias, as well as those who have experienced angina within the preceding few days. Not only are patients with recent angina at increased risk for complications from exercise testing, but also little additional information is likely to be gained in this setting. Postinfarction angina is itself evi-

Table 3–2. Significance of Risk Stratification Measures

Stratification Measure	Level of Risk: % 1-Year Mortality	Approximate % Patients at Risk
Killip classes III and IV	> 30	10
Ejection fraction < 35% at discharge	25	10
Rest ischemia	20	10
Positive submaximal ETT* at discharge	15	10
Positive maximal ETT at 6 wk	10	10
None of the above	2	50

*ETT, exercise tolerance test.

dence that additional myocardium is at ischemic risk. With that fact established a decision must be made as to whether the patient should undergo catheterization directly or first have a trial of medical therapy. The major factors that are considered in making this decision are the risk category of the patient based on ventricular function, the type and size of infarction, and the size of the risk region. If a trial of medical therapy is deemed appropriate, it is of paramount importance to know that the therapy is effective in preventing ischemia. Thus, there remains an important role for subsequent exercise testing and Holter evaluation in such patients to determine the adequacy of therapy. Generally, exercise testing should be delayed at least 24 to 48 hours after a change in a patient's anti-ischemic medical regimen to see if the change is likely to be effective.

The type of exercise study to be performed should depend largely on the ability of the patient to perform exercise and the characteristics of the baseline ECG. If a patient has markedly abnormal ST segments, interpretation of the exercise study becomes difficult and the test less sensitive. In such patients an exercise study with concomitant thallium-201 perfusion scintigraphy or an exercise multigated angiogram will significantly improve diagnostic accuracy. Exercise studies with radioisotopic imaging may also improve the diagnostic accuracy when the patient's exercise capacity is limited.

Approximately 4 to 6 weeks after discharge from the hospital, patients should undergo a second, symptom-limited exercise study. Symptom-limited exercise testing performed approximately 6 weeks after infarction has repeatedly been found to be one of the most useful predictors of 1-year mortality and morbidity.

Integration of Clinical Presentation and Diagnostic Studies

In general, one would expect the clinical presentation to predict many of the results obtained by diagnostic studies. One should be alert to instances where comparison of the clinical presentation and subsequent noninvasive studies yields discrepancies, because additional insights can often be gained from such circumstances. For example, a patient with an anterior myocardial infarction and pulmonary edema (Killip class III) would be expected to have poor ventricular function (ejection fraction < 35%) as seen on a multigated angiogram or echocardiogram. However, if a patient with such a clinical presentation were found to have normal or near normal left ventricular function by these methods, this would suggest that the patient had only a small infarct but has a large region of myocardium at ischemic risk.

Other useful discrepancies can sometimes be found by comparing electrocardiographic findings with the clinical presentation or laboratory findings. An early indication of diffuse coronary disease can sometimes be inferred when the ECG localizes an infarct to one region of the heart, but the echocardiogram or multigated angiogram points to a different region. Many times such discrepancies are merely due to the inaccuracy of the ECG in localizing infarcts; however, in some instances this is an early indicator of diffuse coronary disease.

Medical Therapy

Medical therapy has a definite role in reducing the risk of future infarctions and death in patients who have suffered a myocardial infarction. Randomized prospective clinical trials have demonstrated that beta blockers and aspirin can reduce mortality in some patients after myocardial infarction. Consideration of the risk versus benefit for an individual patient should be considered before initiating therapy with either of these agents.

Beta Blockers

The results of several large randomized trials reported in the early 1980's revealed that beta-adrenergic blockers can substantially lower mortality in postinfarction patients.[12–14] These and other studies have randomized a total of more than 15,000 patients and found an approximate 30% reduction in mortality. It should be noted that approximately 20% of patients screened were excluded for contraindications to beta blockers such as chronic obstructive pulmonary disease, congestive heart failure, and bradycardia. Even so, the reduction in mortality in the treated patients was dramatic. Does this mean that every patient recovering from a myocardial infarction should receive a beta blocker?

Patients in the randomized beta-blocker trials were not stratified according to risk before beta-blocker therapy. Therefore those receiving beta blockers in these studies were high as well as low risk patients. It is known that patients without evidence of ischemia on predischarge treadmill testing have a 1-year mortality of less than 2%, which is approximately the same as those patients treated with beta blockers in these clinical trials. Thus it would be very difficult to demonstrate any benefit of beta-blocker therapy in patients in the low risk group. Furthermore, beta-blocker therapy is not without side effects or expense. In many trials 10 to 20% of patients receiving beta blockers have to stop taking them because of side effects. Subgroup analysis from the Beta Blocker Heart Attack Trial found that the patients with greatest benefit from beta-blocker treatment were those in the highest risk groups.[12] In patients with significant ventricular arrhythmias, the reduction in mortality was approximately 50% greater than that in the untreated group. Clearly there is an important role for beta blockers in postinfarct patients; however, their greatest benefit is probably for patients in high risk groups rather than all postinfarction patients.[15]

Questions regarding the use of beta blockers in this setting remain unanswered. What is the optimum dose? Are all beta blockers equally effective? When should therapy be initiated and how long should it continue? A common practice is to assign the beta-blocker dose according to the response of the heart rate to exercise. If during moderate exercise the heart rate remains low (below 110 beats per minute), beta blockade is said to be adequate. The timing of beta-blocker therapy varies widely. One consideration that may argue for initiation of beta blockers late in the hospital course, when they are used, is the predischarge treadmill study. The predictive value of the predischarge treadmill study may be reduced in patients receiving beta blockers. Thus unless other considerations outweigh this, beta blockers may be best started after the predischarge treadmill study.

In the setting of impaired ventricular function, the decision as to whether a beta blocker can be used safely is often difficult. In such situations the risk of precipitating overt congestive heart failure must be weighed against the expected benefit of the beta blocker. Generally, when the ejection fraction falls below 30 to 35%, the risks may begin to outweigh the benefits. In patients with borderline ventricular function it is often helpful to have a therapeutic trial with a very short-acting

beta blocker such as esmolol, which has a half-life of approximately 10 minutes. If such a short-acting beta blocker is well tolerated, patients can usually tolerate chronic oral therapy.

Aspirin

Several large studies have examined the role of aspirin in preventing recurrent infarction.[16] When the results of these and other trials are analyzed, aspirin is clearly shown to reduce mortality compared with a placebo. In the combined results, aspirin was found to reduce deaths from all causes by approximately 10% and nonfatal infarction by 20%. Aspirin therapy was not entirely benign because an increase in noncardiac mortality with aspirin was noted, although it should be emphasized that overall mortality was reduced. These results do favor the use of low dose aspirin (300 mg/day) when there are no contraindications.

Anticoagulation

Anticoagulants (e.g., heparin) are given routinely to patients with an acute myocardial infarction unless there are specific contraindications. One major benefit of anticoagulation is the reduction of thromboembolic complications: it reduces the rate of postinfarction thromboembolic complications by approximately 50%. Another potential benefit in the immediate postinfarction setting is help in maintaining the patency of the infarct vessel if reperfusion has occurred. One approach to the use of anticoagulants is illustrated in Figure 3–3. The use of anticoagulants, including after myocardial infarction, is discussed in greater detail in Chapter 33.

Cardiac Catheterization and Revascularization

For patients in the convalescent phase of a myocardial infarction the major purpose of coronary angiography is to aid in the management of patients at high risk. The assessment of risk is a clinical judgment made on the basis of the patients' clinical presentation and the results of noninvasive studies. Thus, the various factors that are known to affect prognosis—ventricular function, Q wave versus non–Q wave infarction, evidence of persistent or inducible ischemia, complex ventricular ec-

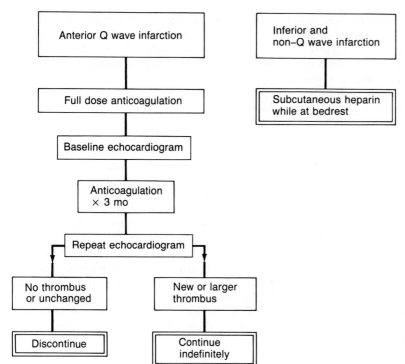

Figure 3–3. *Use of anticoagulation after acute myocardial infarction.*

topy—are the same factors that determine which patients are likely to benefit from coronary angiography. Another factor to be considered in recommending angiography is how suitable a candidate is for a revascularization procedure. With the advent of coronary angioplasty, many patients who might not be suitable candidates for coronary artery surgery may have the option of a nonsurgical revascularization. Patients with uncomplicated infarcts, judged to be at low risk because of the absence of inducible ischemia, generally do not benefit from coronary angiography.

A joint task force of the American College of Cardiology and the American Heart Association recently developed a set of recommendations for the use of diagnostic coronary angiography (Table 3–3).[17] There remains some controversy about whether young patients should routinely undergo catheterization after myocardial infarction. Some believe that coronary angiography is warranted in patients under age 40. It is argued that risk assessment may be less sensitive in young patients, and also that the morbidity that might follow a second infarction would be particularly high. Others have found that in the absence of other indicators of poor prognosis, coronary angi-

ography is a low yield procedure, even in this group.

The use of coronary angioplasty is growing as it proves to be successful in the nonsurgical revascularization of selected patients. Angioplasty can be performed early in the course of hospitalization; however, evidence is accumulating that the procedure is best delayed until at least 48 hours after infarction, particularly in patients who have received a thrombolytic agent.[18, 19]

Patients with refractory ischemia, which makes angioplasty unsuitable, clearly benefit from coronary artery bypass grafting. Definition of the subsets of patients who benefit from coronary artery bypass grafting is constantly being revised. It is clear that bypass surgery decreases mortality of patients with left main coronary artery lesions. Patients with triple vessel coronary artery disease, particularly with impaired left ventricular function, also seem to do better with surgical as opposed to medical treatment.[20]

Risk Factor Modification

The etiology of coronary artery disease is multifactorial. Some factors associated with

Table 3–3. Indications for Catheterization in Myocardial Infarction
(Convalescent Phase)

Major Indications (CONDITIONS FOR WHICH THERE IS GENERAL AGREEMENT THAT CORONARY ANGIOGRAPHY IS JUSTIFIED)	**Other Indications** (CONDITIONS FOR WHICH ANGIOGRAPHY IS FREQUENTLY PERFORMED, BUT WITH DIVERGENCE OF OPINIONS ABOUT ITS UTILITY AND APPROPRIATENESS)
Angina pectoris at rest or with minimal activity	Mild angina
Heart failure	Asymptomatic, < 50 yr of age
Ejection fraction < 45% associated with ischemia or arrhythmias	Need to return to active physical employment
Evidence of ischemia on exercise testing	Past history of myocardial infarction or angina for > 6 mo before current infarction
Non–Q wave myocardial infarction	Thrombolytic therapy during evolving phase of myocardial infarction, especially if evidence of reperfusion

increased risk are modifiable, such as cholesterol level, smoking, obesity, and hypertension, whereas others, including gender and age, are not. There is evidence that modification of risk factors can slow the progression of coronary artery disease. The converse is also true. Smoking, hypertension, and elevated cholesterol levels are associated with a more rapid progression of coronary artery disease. Thus it is important that an effort be made to identify and remove the modifiable risk factors that will lead to an acceleration of coronary artery disease.

Smoking

The association of smoking with coronary artery disease is well established. Patients who have experienced a myocardial infarction and who continue to smoke have approximately twice the risk of reinfarction compared with patients who stop smoking. There are few available interventions that will result in the same degree of risk reduction as will cessation of smoking. An approach to smoking cessation is covered in Chapter 43.

Serum Cholesterol Level

A number of large natural history studies have established the link between elevated serum cholesterol level, particularly low density lipoprotein cholesterol, and the development of coronary artery disease. It has also been firmly established by more than a dozen interventional studies that lowering serum cholesterol level, by either diet modification or drug therapy, decreases the risk for primary coronary events.[21] There is now an increasing body of evidence indicating that reduction in

elevated cholesterol concentration is an important goal in patients with established coronary disease. One recent study found that reductions in elevated serum cholesterol levels reduced the rate of progression of coronary artery disease, and even produced regression of established coronary atherosclerosis, in native vessels as well as bypass grafts.[22] All patients suffering from coronary artery disease should have their cholesterol levels determined. If the levels are elevated, appropriate treatment should be initiated, first by alterations in diet and then if necessary by use of cholesterol level–lowering drugs. Evaluation and management of serum cholesterol levels are covered in Chapter 15.

Progression of Activity after Myocardial Infarction

After myocardial infarction, patients may be confused and apprehensive about resuming many of their previous activities. Family and friends, although well meaning, may express their concern by overly limiting the activity of the patient. A formal program of exercise rehabilitation will often alleviate the anxiety of both the patient and family or friends by providing a monitored, structured environment for progressively increasing activity. Issues of sexual activity and return to work should be discussed with the patient early in the convalescence.

Exercise Rehabilitation

Exercise has been shown to be beneficial in the primary prevention of coronary artery disease. The effectiveness of exercise rehabilitation in the secondary prevention of coronary events remains unproved, even in the wake of several randomized trials that attempted to address this issue. Several studies have reported lower mortality in the group assigned to exercise, although in only one study did this finding reach statistical significance.[23] Most studies, including the one that demonstrated a reduction in mortality with exercise, found no difference in the rate of recurrent nonfatal infarction.

Exercise rehabilitation does have benefits for lifestyle even if its ability to slow the progression of established coronary disease remains uncertain. Exercise has been shown to increase both physical and emotional functional capacity in patients recovering from an infarction. It may even be beneficial to have a spouse observe or participate in the rehabilitation program along with the patient. This helps the spouse understand the patient's work capacity and may prevent the spouse from trying to place undue restrictions on the patient's activities.[24] Cardiac exercise rehabilitation can occur in a variety of settings, even in the patient's home. However, there may be particular advantages to group rehabilitation. In the setting of a formal exercise program and the resulting group reinforcement, it may be easier to modify other risk factors such as smoking, diet, and obesity.

Patients with unstable angina, uncontrolled hypertension, complex ventricular ectopy, high grade heart block, severe pulmonary disease, and significant valvular heart disease should be excluded from exercise rehabilitation programs.

Sexual Activity

Patients who are asymptomatic can usually resume sexual activity 4 to 6 weeks after myocardial infarction. For most individuals the energy expenditure during sexual foreplay approximates 3 METS and rises to approximately 5 METS during orgasm. These levels of work are roughly equivalent to walking briskly for one block and slowly climbing a flight of stairs, respectively. When the patient can achieve these activity levels as an outpatient, without symptoms, then sexual intercourse may resume. Patients should routinely be informed of this, as it may be difficult for them to initiate the discussion of this topic.

Return to Work

Patients who suffer an uncomplicated myocardial infarction during their working years can generally expect to return to work. The type of work and the progress of the patient with cardiac rehabilitation are important factors in determining when a patient will be able to return to work. For instance, a patient who performs clerical work would be expected to be able to return to work more rapidly than someone whose job involves heavy physical labor. Generally after 2 to 3 months, most patients with uncomplicated infarctions can return to work. For patients who have physically demanding or stressful occupations it may be useful to perform stress testing under conditions of simulated work. A Holter study obtained after the patient has returned to work may be useful in the management of some patients who have particularly physical or stressful occupations. If such a study revealed evidence of work-induced ventricular ectopy or ischemia, appropriate diagnostic, therapeutic, or occupational adjustments could be considered.

Summary

Management of patients recovering from a myocardial infarction begins with a clinical assessment of the patient's risk for subsequent untoward events. In addition to left ventricular function, electrical stability and propensity for additional ischemia are key factors in assigning the patient to a prognostic risk group. Many different diagnostic tests are available to aid in making these determinations; it is the task of the physician to select the particular methods that will provide the necessary information for a therapeutic end point.

After the patient leaves the hospital, the focus of management shifts to efforts designed to reduce the risk of recurrent infarction, while periodically reassessing the patient for evidence of disease progression. A symptom-limited exercise test should be performed 4 to 6 weeks after hospital discharge. If this study shows no evidence of ischemia or complex arrhythmias, the patient can be considered at low risk for the near term. However, the long-term outlook will depend on the success of interventions that modify the risk factors that contributed to the development of atherosclerotic disease. In this sense recovery from a myocardial infarction should be viewed not as a single acute event but rather as one episode in a chronic vascular disease.

References

1. Alonso DR, Scheidt S, Post M, et al. Pathophysiology of cardiogenic shock. Quantification of myocardial

necrosis, clinical, pathologic and electrocardiographic correlations. Circulation 48:588–596, 1973.

This clinical pathologic study compares features of patients dying of cardiogenic shock with those of patients dying of other postinfarction complications. Cardiogenic shock generally occurred when approximately 50% of the left ventricle was infarcted.

2. Killip T, Kimball JT. Treatment of myocardial infarction in a coronary care unit: a two year experience with 250 patients. Am J Cardiol 20:457–464, 1967.

This article describes the relationship of clinical presentation to prognosis.

3. Thanvaro S, Kleiger RE, Province MA, et al. Effect of infarct location on the in-hospital prognosis of patients with first transmural myocardial infarction. Circulation 66:742–747, 1982.

Patients with inferior myocardial infarction had lower in-hospital mortality (9.1%) than patients with anterior myocardial infarction (15.5%).

4. Maisel AS, Gilpin E, Hoit B, et al. Survival after hospital discharge in matched populations with inferior or anterior myocardial infarction. J Am Coll Cardiol 6:731–736, 1985.

Among patients with anterior myocardial infarction who died in the first year, 56% of the deaths occurred in the first 60 days compared with 18% for patients with inferior myocardial infarctions and the same time period. One-year mortality was 10% and 7%, respectively.

5. Weisman HF, Healy B. Myocardial infarct expansion, infarct extension, and reinfarction: pathophysiologic concepts. Prog Cardiovasc Dis 30:73–110, 1987.

The pathologic and clinical features of infarct expansion are extensively reviewed.

6. Gibson RS, Beller GA, Gheorghiade M, et al. The prevalence and clinical significance of residual myocardial ischemia 2 weeks after uncomplicated non–Q wave infarction: a prospective natural history study. Circulation 73:1186–1198, 1986.

This detailed natural history study compared Q wave and non–Q wave infarction. Patients with non–Q wave infarction had a higher rate of reinfarction and angina than those with Q wave infarction.

7. Gibson RS, Boden WE, Theroux P, et al. Diltiazem and reinfarction in patients with non-Q-wave myocardial infarction. Results of a double-blind, randomized, multicenter trial. N Engl J Med 315:423–429, 1986.

Diltiazem reduced the rate of reinfarction by 50% in the hospital phase of non–Q wave myocardial infarction.

8. Schuster EH, Bulkley BH. Early post-infarction angina: ischemia at a distance and ischemia in the infarct zone. N Engl J Med 305:1101–1105, 1981.

Patients with ischemia in an area different from the infarct vessel, as identified by a surface ECG, had a worse prognosis than those with ischemia in the same area as the infarct.

9. Josephson ME. Treatment of ventricular arrhythmias after myocardial infarction. Circulation 74:653–658, 1986.

This article is an authoritative review of the current state of antiarrhythmic treatment of ventricular arrhythmias in postinfarction patients.

10. Gottlieb SO, Weisfeldt ML, Ouyang P, et al. Silent ischemia as a marker for early unfavorable outcomes in patients with unstable angina. N Engl J Med 314:1214–1219, 1986.

Silent ischemia, defined as a transient shift in the ST segment of 1 mm or more, identified a high risk subset of patients among those with unstable angina.

11. Theroux P, Waters DD, Halpen C, et al. Prognostic value of exercise testing soon after myocardial infarction. N Engl J Med 301:341–345, 1979.

Patients with a positive low level exercise treadmill are at high risk for early reinfarction.

12. Beta-Blocker Heart Attack Trial Research Group. A randomized trial of propranolol in patients with acute myocardial infarction. I. Mortality results. JAMA 247:1707–1714, 1982.

References 12–15 review the use of beta blockers after acute myocardial infarction.

13. Norwegian Multicenter Study Group. Timolol-induced reduction in mortality and reinfarction in patients surviving acute myocardial infarction. N Engl J Med 304:801–807, 1981.

14. Hjalmarson A, Elmfeldt D, Herlitz F, et al. Effect on mortality of metoprolol in acute myocardial infarction. A double-blind randomized trial. Lancet 1:823–827, 1981.

15. Ahumada GG. Identification of patients who do not require beta antagonists after myocardial infarction. Am J Med 76:900–904, 1984.

16. Aspirin Myocardial Infarction Study Research Group. A randomized controlled trial of aspirin in persons recovered from myocardial infarction. JAMA 243:661–669, 1980.

This is the largest of the recent studies evaluating the utility of aspirin in survivors of acute myocardial infarction. This study also includes an excellent review of several prior studies.

17. Ross J, Fisch C, DeSanctis RW, et al. Guidelines for coronary angiography: a report of the American College of Cardiology/American Heart Association Task Force on assessment of diagnostic and therapeutic cardiovascular procedures (Subcommittee on Coronary Angiography). J Am Coll Cardiol 10:935–950, 1987.

Indications for cardiac catheterization after myocardial infarction as well as other diseases are reviewed.

18. Topol EJ, Califf RM, George BS, et al. A randomized trial of immediate versus delayed elective angioplasty after intravenous tissue plasminogen activator in acute myocardial infarction. N Engl J Med 317:581–588, 1987.

Early angioplasty was associated with a higher incidence of complications than angioplasty performed 48 hours or more after myocardial infarction.

19. Ryan TJ. Angioplasty in acute myocardial infarction: is the balloon leaking? N Engl J Med 317:624–626, 1987.

This is an editorial review of the topic.

20. Killip T, Ryan TJ. Randomized trials in coronary artery bypass surgery. Circulation 71:418–421, 1985.

This is an excellent editorial review of the major coronary artery surgery trials.

21. Lipid Research Clinics Program. The Lipid Research Clinics Coronary Primary Prevention Trial results. I. Reduction in incidence of coronary artery disease. JAMA 251:351–364, 1984.

Reduction in cholesterol was associated with a decrease in risk for coronary artery disease.

22. Blakenhorn DM, Nessim SA, Johnson RL, et al. Beneficial effects of combined colestipol-niacin therapy on coronary atherosclerosis and coronary venous bypass grafts. JAMA 257:3233–3240, 1987.

Reduction in cholesterol was associated with a slowing of the progression of atherosclerotic disease in native vessels and in bypass grafts. In some instances established disease appeared to regress.

23. Kalio V, Hamalainen H, Hakkila J, et al. Reduction

in sudden death by a multifactorial intervention program after acute myocardial infarction. Lancet 2:1091–1094, 1979.

An organized aftercare program reduced the incidence of sudden death by 60% in the first 6 months after acute myocardial infarction.

24. Taylor CB, Bandura A, Ewart CK, et al. Exercise testing to enhance wives' confidence in their husbands' cardiac capability soon after clinically uncomplicated myocardial infarction. Am J Cardiol 55:635–638, 1985.

Wives who observed husbands perform exercise in a supervised setting were more reassured about the recovery of their husbands and less likely to try to overly restrict the patient's activities.

4

Evaluation and Management of Acute Chest Pain

DAVID H. HICKAM, M.D., M.P.H.
GREGORY J. MAGARIAN, M.D.

Introduction

Chest pain is a common symptom for which adults seek the help of a primary care physician. Although there are many different causes of chest pain, systematic evaluation of pain characteristics permits the list of possible etiologies to be narrowed. Although many of the etiologies can have various presentations, it is useful to consider two broad categories of chest pain: acute (or new onset) and recurrent. The evaluation of acute chest pain is reviewed in this chapter, with emphasis on those diagnoses for which hospital admission is often necessary. The following chapter reviews those diagnoses that are typical of recurrent chest pain, including causes of acute pain that do not require hospitalization.

Patients with acute chest pain include those whose pain is of recent onset or who have had a recent increase in the intensity, frequency, or duration of recurrent pain. Such patients frequently seek care in emergency rooms or walk-in clinics but may also visit practitioners' offices. Because several disorders that cause acute chest pain are life-threatening, it is imperative to have a systematic approach to diagnosis and initial management decisions. Many patients with acute chest pain are best managed by admission to the hospital, and it often is not an option to assess a short-term response to therapeutic interventions in these patients. Life-threatening diagnoses must be considered first, before more benign conditions are pursued. A rapid but thorough assessment of the patient's hemodynamic status also should be made during the initial stages of diagnostic pursuit of the etiology of the pain.

Although many disorders can cause acute chest pain, a small number are actually responsible for most cases. Studies of large series of patients evaluated in hospital emergency rooms have found that 25 to 45% of adults with acute chest pain have ischemic heart disease. Nonischemic cardiac disease is the etiology in 5 to 10%. In studies of patients admitted to a hospital for acute chest pain, 60 to 75% had myocardial ischemia. In these studies of hospitalized patients, 5 to 20% had esophageal disease as the confirmed or probable etiology, 3% had pneumonia, and 1 to 2% had pericarditis. In a British study, 13% of patients hospitalized for acute chest pain had no etiologic diagnosis made. These patients had very low morbidity and mortality in the subsequent year.

In this chapter, acute myocardial ischemia, aortic dissection, pericarditis, and acute pulmonary disorders are discussed in detail. Esophageal causes of chest pain are reviewed in the following chapter.

Acute Myocardial Ischemia

In the setting of acute, severe chest pain, the first priority is to estimate the probability that the patient's pain is caused by myocardial ischemia (unstable angina or acute myocardial infarction). These are the most frequent etiologies of acute chest pain and, along with aortic dissection (see later section), require the most urgent management interventions. With rare exceptions these patients should be admitted to the hospital for initiation of interventions to reduce arrhythmic deaths, define coronary anatomy, and reduce infarct size. It is the clinician's task to use the patient's clinical features to minimize the number of patients who are admitted unnecessarily while ensuring that patients who do have cardiac ischemia are admitted for appropriate care.

Myocardial ischemic pain usually has distinguishing features related to its quality, location, radiation patterns, and associated symptoms and signs. Pain caused by myocardial ischemia is most commonly described as being dull, heavy, vise-like, or crushing. Occasionally, the patient describes a pressure or a vague uncomfortable sensation rather than a pain. Pain that is sharp, stabbing, or burning is less typical. Myocardial ischemic pain is usually located substernally or across the anterior chest. It is unusual for it to be located only in the lateral regions of the chest or in the right side of the chest alone. The pain often radiates to the left arm and sometimes to the right arm, neck, or back. If the patient's pain is pleuritic or aggravated by moving the arms or thorax, the etiology is less likely to be myocardial ischemia. Patients with a history of prior myocardial infarction or treatment by a physician for coronary artery disease are more likely to have ischemic heart disease as the cause of acute chest pain. An initial estimate of the probability of acute ischemic heart disease can be made from the patient's initial symptoms (Table 4–1).

Myocardial infarction can be complicated by life-threatening arrhythmias and ventricular failure. Therefore, it requires immediate recognition and medical management. The pain of myocardial infarction is usually more severe and longer lasting than are attacks of angina pectoris. It often occurs without any recognizable inciting factor and is not relieved by sublingual nitroglycerin. Autonomic manifestations are not infrequent during acute myocardial infarction and include nausea, vomiting, and sweating. However, these signs are nonspecific, as they occur in other pain states

as well. Dyspnea, when present, may result from impaired left ventricular contractility or anxiety associated with the pain.

The syndrome of unstable angina pectoris is seen in a diverse group of patients having myocardial ischemic chest pain. The importance of recognizing unstable angina lies in the fact that such patients have a significant short-term risk of acute myocardial infarction and sudden death, and therapeutic interventions have been shown to reduce this risk. Angina can be considered unstable when there has been a significant reduction in the activity level that causes pain (anginal threshold), an increase in intensity or duration of pain, or a poorer response to rest or sublingual nitroglycerin. Of particular concern is the development of spontaneous anginal pain at rest, when it occurs without recognizable factors that increase myocardial oxygen demand. Unlike acute myocardial infarction, unstable angina does improve with sublingual nitroglycerin and rest but often to a lesser degree than previously. The patient's condition should be monitored closely until the pain pattern is clearly established.

Various pathophysiologic mechanisms may be responsible for the development of unstable angina. For patients with a reduction in anginal threshold and increasing frequency of pain, the most likely mechanism is progression of severity of atherosclerotic disease in the coronary arteries. However, for patients with new unprovoked (rest) angina, coronary vasopasm or transient coronary artery occlusions from platelet/fibrin thrombi, or both, may be primarily responsible. Worsening (accelerated) angina may evolve in patients with prior stable angina because of alteration of the patient's medication regimen or because of patient noncompliance. Lack of response to nitroglycerin defines a changing pattern in some patients. However, this may be due only to the loss of pharmacologic effectiveness of nitroglycerin. This is especially likely when the nitroglycerin supply has been previously used infrequently and has become outdated. Loss of a mild burning or stinging sensation under the tongue with sublingual use may be a clue that the nitroglycerin is outdated.

The most important diagnostic test for patients with suspected ischemic heart disease is the electrocardiogram. Large-scale studies of patients presenting to emergency rooms with acute chest pain have provided valuable information on the test performance of the initial electrocardiogram. If the electrocardiogram is

Table 4–1. *Probability of Acute Ischemic Heart Disease in Patients Presenting to an Emergency Room with Chest Pain*

Description of Pain	Probability of Acute Ischemic Heart Disease* (%)
Crushing, pressure, or tightness	54
Burning or indigestion	44
Ache	31
Sharp or stabbing	22

Adapted from Goldman L. Hosp Pract 21(7):94A–94T, 1986, with permission.
*Myocardial infarction or unstable angina.

completely normal, the probability of acute myocardial ischemia or infarction is approximately 5%. The initial electrocardiogram shows new Q waves or ST segment elevations in 60 to 70% of patients with acute myocardial infarction, and approximately two thirds of the remaining patients show ST segment depression or T wave inversion.

Goldman and colleagues have developed an algorithm for using the patient's initial electrocardiogram and characteristics of the clinical history to estimate the probability of acute myocardial infarction (Fig. 4–1). The algorithm is based on electrocardiographic findings and the patient's age, characteristics of pain, and associated symptoms. It classifies patients into a low probability category (approximately 2% probability of acute myocardial infarction) or a high probability category (approximately 32% probability of acute myocardial infarction). These probabilities include only the outcome of acute myocardial infarction. Some patients without an infarction may have unstable angina. This algorithm affirms that the patient's history and initial electrocardiogram provide complementary information for guiding the estimation of the probability of acute myocardial infarction. The electrocardiogram taken in the emergency room can be used to exclude myocardial infarction only in patients who have had pain lasting for 2 days or longer. The algorithm provides a guide for incorporating multiple items from the patient's history to assess the patient. Although Goldman and colleagues caution against routine use of this algorithm to make clinical decisions, it provides a useful scheme for classifying patient data in the emergency room. Careful evaluation of the patient's history and initial electrocardiogram helps avoid the mistake of sending home patients with acute myocardial infarction.

Serum cardiac enzyme levels are of limited value in the assessment of acute chest pain. Initial creatine kinase (CK) levels are elevated in only about 40% of patients presenting to an emergency room with acute myocardial infarction. Thus, the sensitivity of the test is inadequate for excluding myocardial infarction. The sensitivity of the CK level is only slightly better in the subgroup of patients presenting with acute myocardial infarction more than 12 hours after onset of the pain. The false-positive rate of the emergency room CK level is about 20%, whereas the CK-MB isoenzyme level has a false-positive rate of about 12%. However, the limited availability of the isoenzyme test in the emergency room makes it impractical for use as a confirmatory test in deciding whether to admit a patient with an elevated total CK level.

The serum glutamic-oxaloacetic transaminase (SGOT) level is slightly better than the CK level for evaluation of emergency room patients. In patients seen in the emergency room more than 12 hours after onset of chest pain, 67% of those with acute myocardial infarctions had SGOT levels of 60 IU/L or greater. With this same cutoff level for the test, the false-positive rate for these patients was 10%. If on the basis of other clinical information the clinician has estimated that the probability of acute myocardial infarction is less than 30%, an SGOT level less than 60 IU/L more than 12 hours after onset of the pain lowers the probability to below 15%. This information may help the clinician decide whether to admit the patient to an intermediate care unit rather than a coronary care unit.

It is difficult to differentiate clinically between unstable angina and acute myocardial infarction. Hospitalization is often required to clarify the diagnosis and to facilitate treatment interventions. Serial electrocardiograms and cardiac enzyme tests confirm myocardial infarction. If infarction is excluded, intense antianginal therapy with combinations of nitrates, beta blockers, and calcium channel blockers should be given with close monitoring of the patient's response. If the pain episodes do not improve rapidly with bed rest and aggressive titration of antianginal medications, the patient has either refractory coronary artery disease (preinfarction angina) or another etiology of pain. In these patients, imaging studies or coronary arteriography may be necessary for a diagnosis.

In some patients with acute cardiac ischemia, the etiology of chest pain is not apparent at the time of initial evaluation. Approximately 5% of patients with acute myocardial infarction are not admitted after going to an emergency room. The mortality of nonadmitted patients is higher than that of matched patients who are admitted. Thus, it is important to reevaluate within 1 or 2 days those patients with possible myocardial ischemia who are not admitted.

Aortic Dissection

Dissection of the thoracic aorta is a serious and potentially catastrophic cause of acute chest pain. Approximately 70% of patients

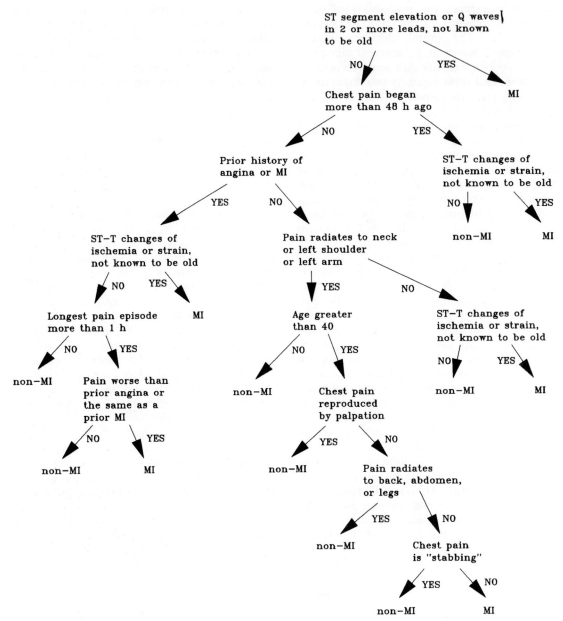

Figure 4–1. Algorithm for estimating probability of acute myocardial infarction in patients with acute chest pain. MI = acute myocardial infarction. In the terminal nodes, non-MI refers to a low (< 5%) probability of acute myocardial infarction, and MI refers to a moderate (> 20%) probability of acute myocardial infarction. Adapted from Goldman et al. Reprinted, by permission of The New England Journal of Medicine (318; 797–803, 1988).

with untreated aortic dissection die within 2 weeks. Because aortic dissection requires immediate, specific treatment, it is important that the clinician exclude this diagnosis at an early stage of the patient's evaluation. There are two primary types of dissection, and these have somewhat different clinical presentations. Proximal dissections arise in the ascending aorta but sometimes extend beyond the aortic arch. Nearly all patients with proximal dissection have sudden onset of severe pain in the anterior chest, and approximately half report radiation to the posterior chest.

The physical examination is extremely important when considering the diagnosis of proximal aortic dissection. In one study of 53 patients with proximal dissection, 68% had a murmur of aortic regurgitation, 51% had pulse deficits, and 36% had neurologic deficits (paraparesis, hemiplegia, or peripheral neuropathy). Thus, the absence of any of these signs makes the diagnosis unlikely. Although only about 10% of patients with proximal dissection have elevated blood pressure on presentation, two thirds have a history of hypertension. Proximal aortic dissection occurs more frequently in patients with congenital connective tissue disorders, particularly Marfan's syndrome. Occasionally, the dissection may damage the ostium of one of the coronary arteries, which results in concomitant acute myocardial ischemia. In such situations, recognition of the ischemia may delay diagnosis of the aortic dissection.

Distal dissection of the thoracic aorta arises in the descending aorta below the great vessels. It occurs predominantly in men over age 40 who have a history of hypertension (a group that is also at significant risk of acute myocardial infarction). Although nearly all patients with acute myocardial infarction have anterior chest pain, 94% of patients with distal dissection have a posterior component of their chest pain (i.e., just 6% have only anterior chest pain). The pain of distal aortic dissection may be described as tearing or ripping and does not improve with nitroglycerin. In one study, 78% of patients with distal dissection had a history of hypertension, and 56% were hypertensive at the time of pain. Physical examination findings are seen less frequently in distal than in proximal aortic dissections.

Few data exist on the prevalence of aortic dissection in patients with chest pain, but it is a relatively rare cause. Furthermore, information from the history and physical examination can help to exclude the diagnosis in most cases. Figure 4–2 is an algorithm for evaluating the possibility of aortic dissection in patients with acute chest pain. Although this algorithm does not provide actual estimates of the probability of aortic dissection, further diagnostic studies should be considered for those patients whom the algorithm identifies as possibly having proximal or distal dissection. Approximately 90% of patients with acute dissection demonstrate widening or other abnormalities of the aorta on good quality posteroanterior, lateral, and oblique chest x-rays. Thus, a completely normal appearance of the aorta on the chest x-ray makes the diagnosis unlikely. However, because abnormalities of the aorta occur in patients without

dissection, plain chest films do not confirm the diagnosis. Although false-negative results occur in approximately 2% of patients with aortic dissection, contrast aortography is the best single test for excluding or confirming the diagnosis. Computed tomography scanning with contrast enhancement may be used as a screening procedure to exclude dissection, but positive computed tomography scans should be confirmed via angiography. Two-dimensional echocardiography also may be used to exclude proximal dissection, but this test is insensitive for distal dissection.

Pericarditis

Pericarditis is a moderately common disorder that frequently causes acute chest pain. There are many etiologies of pericarditis, which can be categorized as infectious, immunologic, metabolic, neoplastic, traumatic, or peri-infarction. The pain is often substernal and may radiate to the left arm, which suggests an ischemic etiology. However, the pain is usually different from that of myocardial ischemia in being sharp and pleuritic or affected by body position. It is often aggravated by lying down and is relieved by sitting up, especially when leaning forward. A pericardial friction rub strongly suggests the diagnosis, but a rub may be absent because of pericardial fluid separating the parietal and visceral pericardial surfaces, thereby preventing them from rubbing together. Occasionally the rub may be mistaken for a systolic ejection murmur.

Diagnostic tests are useful in evaluating patients with suspected pericarditis. The electrocardiogram may show ST segment elevations in multiple leads, which can be confused with acute myocardial infarction. Not all patients with pericarditis have electrocardiographic changes, and uremic pericarditis is particularly notable in this regard. Chest radiographs often show a normal cardiac silhouette. Cardiac echocardiography may assist in defining whether acute chest pain is caused by pericarditis or cardiac ischemia. A pericardial effusion strongly suggests pericarditis as the etiology, whereas regional wall motion abnormalities suggest ischemia.

Because of its diverse presentation, pericarditis is difficult to exclude by routine clinical examination. The diagnosis should be suspected if the patient does not have other likely etiologies of pain and has clinical evidence of one of the precipitating causes of pericarditis.

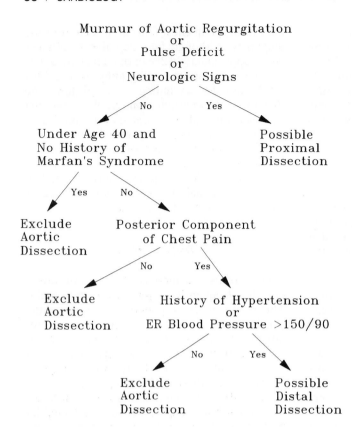

Figure 4–2. Algorithm for estimating likelihood of aortic dissection in patients with acute chest pain.

Hypotension and a pulsus paradoxus suggest cardiac tamponade, which is a medical emergency.

Pulmonary Causes of Acute Chest Pain

Chest pain frequently occurs in acute pulmonary embolism, which requires urgent treatment when present. In about 15% of patients with acute pulmonary embolism, the pain is nonpleuritic and substernal and lasts less than 2 hours. This presentation, thought to be associated with acute pulmonary hypertension, is similar to that of acute myocardial infarction. Nevertheless, pulmonary embolism rarely is the cause of anginal chest pain, and it should be considered only when myocardial ischemia or aortic dissection does not appear to be present. In patients with pleuritic chest pain, pulmonary embolism is relatively frequent. In a recent Canadian study reported by Hull and colleagues, pulmonary embolism was found in 21% of patients presenting to an emergency room with pleuritic chest pain.

Patients with pulmonary embolism typically complain of a sharp pleuritic pain in the lateral chest. Pulmonary embolism can be excluded in patients under age 40 who do not have risk factors for thromboembolic disease (prior pulmonary emboli or deep venous thrombophlebitis, use of oral contraceptives, coexisting malignancy, pregnancy, cardiac failure, or recent surgery or trauma), pleural effusion, or recent swelling of a lower extremity. These clinical criteria have little value for identifying pulmonary embolism in patients age 40 and older. Pulmonary embolism is more likely in patients with an accentuated pulmonary component of the second heart sound, electrocardiographic signs of right-sided heart strain, or chest x-ray changes consistent with pulmonary infarction. However, the sensitivity of any of these findings is low, and their absence does not exclude the diagnosis. Although patients with pulmonary embolism with normal arterial blood gases have been reported, a normal level of arterial oxygen content makes the diagnosis unlikely.

The perfusion lung scan has nearly perfect sensitivity for pulmonary embolism when properly performed. Thus, it is the best test available to exclude the diagnosis. However, its false-positive rate is approximately 30%, and other tests are necessary to confirm emboli in patients with a positive perfusion scan. Ventilation lung scanning and impedance plethysmography can confirm pulmonary embolism in some patients. Both of these tests have high specificity for pulmonary emboli in patients with positive perfusion scans. However, because the sensitivity of these tests is only moderate, pulmonary angiography is often necessary to confirm the diagnosis. Figure 4–3 is an algorithm for the diagnostic evaluation for pulmonary embolism in patients with pleuritic chest pain. On the basis of this algorithm, approximately 25% of patients require pulmonary angiography.

Pneumonias can cause acute dull chest pain that usually is pleuritic. Chest pain also occurs in most cases of acute pneumothorax. The pain of pneumothorax characteristically is uni-

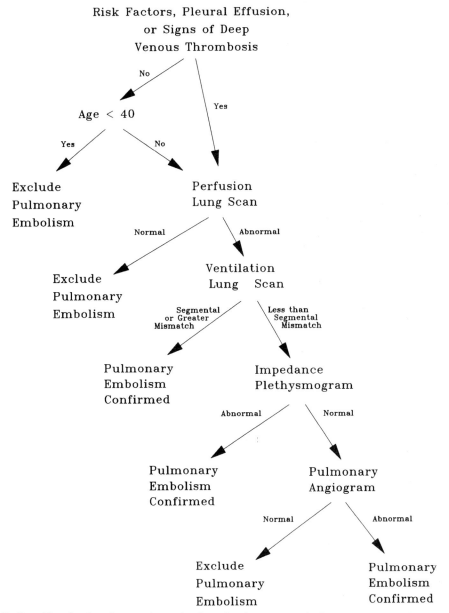

Figure 4–3. Algorithm for the diagnostic evaluation of pulmonary embolism in patients with acute pleuritic chest pain. Risk factors include prior pulmonary emboli or deep venous thrombophlebitis, use of oral contraceptives, coexisting malignancy, pregnancy, cardiac failure, or recent surgery or trauma. Adapted from Hull RD, Raskob GE, Carter CJ, et al. Arch Intern Med 148:838–844, 1988. Copyright 1988, American Medical Association.

lateral, pleuritic, and accompanied by dyspnea. The chest x-ray usually establishes the diagnosis in these cases. Acute chest trauma is a frequent cause of chest pain, but the diagnosis is usually apparent from the patient's history. Traumatic pain is reproduced by chest palpation in most cases, and x-rays sometimes reveal a rib fracture.

Hospital Admission for Acute Chest Pain

Hospital admission is often necessary for patients with acute chest pain. The decision to admit a patient for suspected acute ischemic heart disease depends on the clinician's estimate of the probability of this diagnosis. The patient's history and initial electrocardiogram provide valuable data to estimate the probability of ischemia (Fig. 4–1). However, the physical examination has little usefulness for detecting or excluding ischemia. Although patients whose pain is fully reproduced by chest palpation have a probability of acute ischemia of less than 10%, this assessment should be performed with caution. The sign should be considered positive only if the palpation fully reproduces the pain and the patient has been questioned in a nonleading style. The physical examination has greater usefulness for estimating the probability of nonischemic etiologies of pain such as aortic dissection or pneumonia.

Admission to a coronary care unit or intermediate care unit should be strongly considered in patients having a probability of acute ischemia of greater than 10%. Because acute myocardial infarction can be diagnosed definitively within 24 hours in nearly all cases, time required in a coronary care unit can be short for patients without infarction. Prognosis is good in patients who do not show evidence of cardiac ischemia in the initial period of hospital monitoring. The emergency room electrocardiogram is useful for guiding the decision on admission for patients with possible acute myocardial infarction. Patients whose initial electrocardiogram is normal, is unchanged from previous tracings (without left bundle branch block, left ventricular hypertrophy, or paced rhythm), or shows only minimal ST segment or T wave changes have a low incidence of life-threatening complications, even if an acute infarction occurs. Such patients can be safely managed in an intermediate care unit rather than a coronary care unit.

Immediate therapeutic intervention is sometimes beneficial in patients with acute myocardial infarction or unstable angina. Many cardiologists now prefer to perform immediate coronary arteriography on patients with suspected acute ischemia, followed by administration of intracoronary streptokinase and/or transluminal coronary angioplasty when indicated. If arteriography is not immediately available, short-term high dose intravenous streptokinase may be considered. However, this therapy should be undertaken only in selected patients. Because streptokinase is absolutely contraindicated in aortic dissection and it complicates the treatment of pericarditis, the clinician must be able to exclude these diagnoses before administering streptokinase to the patient with acute chest pain. In most patients, aortic dissection can be excluded by applying the criteria of Figure 4–2. Proximal aortic dissection sometimes occludes a coronary artery, which causes confusion about the principal diagnosis. Echocardiography may be necessary for patients in whom the electrocardiographic changes are consistent with either acute pericarditis or infarction.

Hospital admission is necessary for nearly all patients in whom aortic dissection, pericarditis, pneumothorax, or pulmonary embolism cannot be excluded. Admission is also necessary for the majority of patients with pneumonia, especially the elderly and those with poor home supportive care. Admission is usually not necessary for traumatic chest pain unless breathing is compromised or lung damage is present.

Patients who are not admitted usually should be seen for a follow-up assessment within 3 days. In a recent study of patients sent home after being seen in an urban emergency room for acute chest pain, 4% were subsequently admitted within 3 days. Of these admitted patients, 76% had myocardial infarction or unstable angina.

Bibliography

Brush JE, Brand DA, Acampora D, et al. Use of the initial electrocardiogram to predict in-hospital complications of acute myocardial infarction. N Engl J Med 312:1137–1141, 1985.
Report of 469 patients admitted for suspected myocardial infarction. If the initial electrocardiogram was normal or unchanged from prior tracings or showed only nonspecific changes, the probability of a life-threatening complication was less than 1%.
DeSanctis RW, Doroghazi RM, Austen WG, et al. Aortic dissection. N Engl J Med 317:1060–1067, 1987.

Good recent review of diagnosis and management of aortic dissection.

Fineberg HV, Scadden D, Goldman L. Care of patients with a low probability of acute myocardial infarction. Cost effectiveness of alternatives to coronary-care-unit admission. N Engl J Med 310:1301–1307, 1984.

Formal analysis of costs of admission options for patients with possible myocardial infarction. For patients with a probability of acute infarction of under 20%, admission to an intermediate care unit should be strongly considered as an alternative to the coronary care unit.

Goldman L. Acute chest pain: emergency room evaluation. Hosp Pract 21:94A–94T, 1986.

Good general review of the topic, with emphasis on the diagnosis of acute myocardial infarction.

Goldman L, Cook EF, Brand DA, et al. A computer protocol to predict myocardial infarction in emergency department patients with chest pain. N Engl J Med 318:797–803, 1988.

Report of the development and validation of an algorithm for diagnosis of acute chest pain. The algorithm uses items from the patient's history and initial electrocardiogram.

Hull RD, Raskob GE, Carter CJ, et al. Pulmonary embolism in outpatients with pleuritic chest pain. Arch Intern Med 148:838–844, 1988.

Pulmonary embolism was present in 21% of 173 patients presenting to an emergency room for pleuritic chest pain. Includes useful data on the value of clinical characteristics and diagnostic tests.

Lee TH, Cook F, Weisberg M, et al. Acute chest pain in the emergency room: identification and examination of low-risk patients. Arch Intern Med 145:65–69, 1985.

Report of 596 patients evaluated in an emergency room for acute chest pain. Provides information on the relative usefulness of patient symptoms, electrocardiogram, and serum enzymes for diagnosis of ischemic heart disease.

Lee TH, Rouan GW, Weisberg MC, et al. Clinical characteristics and natural history of patients with acute myocardial infarction sent home from the emergency room. Am J Cardiol 60:219–224, 1987.

Reports clinical characteristics of 35 patients who presented to emergency rooms with acute chest pain caused by myocardial infarction and who were not initially admitted. These patients were compared with 105 patients admitted for acute myocardial infarction. Short-term (within 72 hours) mortality was twice as high for the nonadmitted patients.

Lee TH, Rouan GW, Weisberg MC, et al. Sensitivity of routine clinical criteria for diagnosing myocardial infarction within 24 hours of hospitalization. Ann Intern Med 106:181–186, 1987.

Follow-up study of 1460 patients admitted for acute chest pain. In nearly all with acute myocardial infarction or unstable angina, the diagnosis was made within 24 hours.

Lee TH, Weisberg MC, Cook EF, et al. Evaluation of creatine kinase and creatine kinase-MB for diagnosing myocardial infarction: clinical impact in the emergency room. Arch Intern Med 147:115–121, 1987.

Both the total CK and CK-MB tests have false-positive rates of greater than 10% for emergency room patients with acute chest pain.

Pozen MW, D'Agostino RB, Selker HP, et al. A predictive instrument to improve coronary-care-unit admission practices in acute ischemic heart disease: a prospective multicenter clinical trial. N Engl J Med 310:1273–1278, 1984.

Report of the prospective validation of a calculator-based instrument to estimate probability of acute cardiac ischemia. The instrument is not generally available, but the authors provide the logistic formula from which a patient's probability can be calculated directly. Tables for the formula were published later (N Engl J Med 311:1254–1256, 1984).

Rouan GW, Hedges JR, Toltzis R, et al. A chest pain clinic to improve the follow-up of patients released from an urban university teaching hospital emergency department. Ann Emerg Med 16:1145–1150, 1987.

Four percent of patients initially sent home after emergency room evaluation for acute chest pain were subsequently admitted within 72 hours, most because of suspected cardiac ischemia. Patients discharged from the emergency room should be reassessed within 3 days.

Slater EE, DeSanctis RW. The clinical recognition of dissecting aortic aneurysm. Am J Med 60:625–633, 1976.

Detailed description of the clinical data of patients with aortic dissection.

Slater DK, Hlatky MA, Mark DB, et al. Outcome in suspected acute myocardial infarction with normal or minimally abnormal admission electrocardiographic findings. Am J Cardiol 60:766–770, 1987.

Four percent of patients admitted with an acute myocardial infarction had a normal initial electrocardiogram. Ten percent of patients with a suspected myocardial infarction and a normal electrocardiogram were found subsequently to have an acute infarction. Patients with normal or nonspecific initial electrocardiograms had a low rate of complications requiring intensive care unit intervention.

Spodick DH. Acute pericardial disease. Heart Lung 14:599–604, 1985.

General review of the clinical findings in patients with acute pericarditis.

Stark ME, Vacek JL. The initial electrocardiogram during admission for myocardial infarction: use as a predictor of clinical course and facility utilization. Arch Intern Med 147:843–846, 1987.

Additional report that patients whose initial electrocardiogram is normal or shows minimal changes have a low probability of complications during the subsequent hospitalization.

Wilcox RG, Roland JM, Hampton JR. Prognosis of patients with "chest pain ?cause." Br Med J 282:431–433, 1981.

Twelve-month follow-up data on patients discharged from a coronary care unit with diagnoses of myocardial infarction, unstable angina, and unexplained chest pain. Patients with unexplained chest pain had a low rate of adverse events during the follow-up period.

5

Evaluation and Management of Recurrent Chest Pain

DAVID H. HICKAM, M.D., M.P.H.

Introduction

Chest pain is common and occurs in a variety of clinical syndromes. In Chapter 4, the evaluation of acute chest pain was reviewed. Sometimes, patients may come to the physician with subacute or chronic symptoms rather than acute pain. The pattern of chest pain may be stable, lasting over weeks or even months. Other patients may have been evaluated for acute chest pain and found not to have a life-threatening etiology (i.e., acute myocardial infarction, unstable angina pectoris, aortic dissection, acute pericarditis, or serious pulmonary disease). In these patients, the physician needs to determine the likely etiology of the pain and plan a course of therapeutic intervention to relieve the patient's discomfort.

Many disorders can cause recurrent chest pain. Chest pain may originate from several different structures within the chest, including the skin, ribs, intercostal muscles, pleura, esophagus, heart, aorta, diaphragm, and thoracic vertebrae. The innervations of the deep structures of the thorax follow common pathways to the central nervous system, which makes it difficult to localize the source of pain. Nevertheless, the etiologies of recurrent chest pain can be classified into organ system categories: coronary artery disease, other disorders of the heart, esophageal disease, hyperventilation, and chest wall and musculoskeletal syndromes. Diagnostic evaluation of these patients has traditionally been oriented to determining whether the patient has coronary artery disease. However, if coronary artery disease has been excluded, further evaluation is of value. Identification of the most likely etiology of the patient's symptoms may alleviate the patient's anxieties and enables the physician to plan a specific treatment program.

Identifying the Syndrome of Typical Angina Pectoris

Three categories of chest pain syndrome have been used to describe symptoms in patients with recurrent chest pain: typical angina pectoris, atypical angina pectoris, and nonanginal chest pain. Several studies of coronary arteriography in patients referred for evaluation of recurrent chest pain have found that approximately 90% of patients with typical angina pectoris have significant anatomic coronary disease. Patients with atypical angina have a 50 to 60% prevalence of coronary disease, whereas that in patients with nonanginal chest pain is 20 to 30%. These figures apply to overall populations of patients and should be modified when considering individual patients.

Typical Angina Pectoris

When classifying a patient's symptoms, individual charateristics of the pain are useful as criteria for defining the patient's chest pain syndrome. The best single criterion for classic angina pectoris is precipitation of the pain by exercise. Many studies reporting the results of coronary arteriography have used this criterion to define angina pectoris and have found significant coronary disease to be present in more than 80% of patients meeting this definition. The second most important criterion for defining angina pectoris is relief of the pain by nitroglycerin. Although nitroglycerin also may relieve pain caused by esophageal contraction disorders, it more frequently relieves pain caused by coronary artery disease. In a study of patients undergoing coronary arteriography, it was found that relief by nitroglycerin should be defined specifically as resolution of the pain within 3 minutes of taking a sublingual tablet. The specificity of the pain relief declines if a longer time is used in assessing the response.

In typical angina pectoris, the pain usually is located substernally and is described as being heavy or pressing. Although more difficult to quantify objectively, the severity of the pain also helps to classify the patient's syndrome. Although several different schemes have been used to estimate the severity of anginal chest pain, one useful technique is to ask patients whether they must stop their usual activities when the pain occurs. If they must stop, their pain is more likely to be angina pectoris.

Atypical Angina Pectoris

Criteria for defining the syndrome of atypical angina have not been well defined. There are two circumstances when this label should be used. First, atypical angina is an appropriate classification in patients who have exertional chest pain but have other pain characteristics that are not usually seen in pain caused by coronary artery disease, i.e., the pain has an atypical location (the pain is nonsubsternal), character (the pain is described as sharp or aching), or aggravating factors (the pain is pleuritic or brought on by moving the thorax). Second, the pain should be considered atypical angina when precipitation by exercise and relief by nitroglycerin are not consistent: a well-defined level of exercise unreliably reproduces the pain, or nitroglycerin provides inconsistent relief.

Nonanginal Chest Pain

Nonanginal chest pain has none of the features of atypical angina pectoris. The pain is nonexertional, not reliably relieved by nitroglycerin, and often atypical in its location. It often is aggravated by movement of the chest wall.

Prevalence of Coronary Artery Disease

The probability of coronary artery disease in patients with a particular chest pain syndrome is affected by demographic characteristics. In the Coronary Artery Surgery Study, men with typical angina pectoris had a 93%

incidence of significant coronary disease; the corresponding rate for women was 72%. The prevalence of coronary artery disease also is strongly influenced by age. In men, the risk of coronary disease increases steadily between the ages of 30 and 70, with little further increase above age 70. For women, the risk rises gradually until age 60 and then increases more rapidly between ages 60 and 80. The probability of coronary artery disease is substantially increased in patients with a clinical history of myocardial infarction and is also increased in patients with a history of cigarette smoking, hypertension, elevated serum cholesterol level, or diabetes mellitus. Arteriography studies have reported rates of disease in patients evaluated at referral medical centers, and these selected populations have a higher prevalence of coronary disease than the general population. Clinicians should attempt to estimate the underlying rates of coronary artery disease in their clinical settings when interpreting a patient's complaints.

Diagnostic Tests for Coronary Artery Disease

Coronary arteriography is the definitive test for confirming or excluding coronary artery disease. However, arteriography is expensive and invasive, and the clinician should first use less invasive tests to estimate the patient's probability of coronary artery disease. These other tests include resting electrocardiography and exercise tests.

Resting Electrocardiography

Resting electrocardiography should be part of the routine evaluation of all patients in whom coronary artery disease is suspected. The finding of pathologic Q waves on the electrocardiogram confirms a history of prior myocardial infarction, which makes coronary artery disease more likely to be the cause of the patient's recurrent chest pain. In patients who do not have electrocardiographic evidence of a prior myocardial infarction, the test still has some value. In the Coronary Artery Surgery Study, T wave inversion or ST segment depression of at least 1 mm was used to define a positive resting electrocardiogram result. With this criterion, the test had a sensitivity of 25% in males and 40% in females, and it had a specificity of 83% in males and 71% in females. Thus, a positive resting electrocardiogram increases the probability of coronary artery disease. However, a negative result is not sufficient to exclude coronary artery disease, especially in patients with pain typical of angina pectoris, whose pretest probability is higher than 50%.

Exercise Tests

Exercise tests have greater information value than the resting electrocardiogram for estimating the probability of coronary artery disease. Four different exercise tests have become widely used: exercise electrocardiography, thallium scintigraphy, radionuclide ventriculography, and cardiokymography. The first two of these tests have an established place in the evaluation of patients with recurrent chest pain. Radionuclide ventriculography and cardiokymography have limited usefulness. The former has poor specificity for coronary artery disease, and the latter has no greater informational value than exercise electrocardiography and is uninterpretable in a substantial minority of patients.

Management of coronary artery disease depends on definition of the extent and severity of the disease. The incidence of adverse cardiac events is higher in patients with significant obstruction of the left main coronary artery, obstructions of all three major coronary arteries, or significant left ventricular dysfunction. Thus, some of these patients may have a better prognosis when treated with surgical revascularization. Considerable clinical research has been devoted to determining the informational value of exercise tests for detecting not only the presence of coronary artery disease but also its extent and severity. This research has led to a variety of proposed criteria for defining positive test results.

Ladenheim and colleagues have described a classification scheme for exercise test results to guide the primary care physician in planning the diagnostic evaluation of a patient with recurrent chest pain. Their recommendations are based on the goal of identifying patients with coronary artery disease who will suffer any one of three adverse cardiac events in the subsequent 12 months: cardiac death, acute myocardial infarction, or deterioration of symptoms (progressive angina requiring surgical revascularization). In their research, these investigators found that exercise electrocardiography provided incremental prognostic

information when combined with thallium scintigraphy in patients with an intermediate or high probability of coronary artery disease. Thus, exercise electrocardiography usually should be obtained before a thallium study, unless the resting electrocardiogram is abnormal (ST segment depression, T wave inversion, and/or bundle branch block).

Recommended guidelines for using diagnostic tests in patients with suspected coronary artery disease must be based on assumptions of the acceptable risk of disease in those particular patients. Ladenheim and colleagues have developed algorithms for cardiac tests based on patients being considered at low risk if the probability of an adverse cardiac event during the subsequent 12 months was 5% or less. This criterion is consistent with analytic recommendations based on cost effectiveness of therapeutic options for coronary artery disease.

The algorithms of Ladenheim and colleagues have been adapted in the design of an algorithm for evaluation of patients with recurrent chest pain (Fig. 5–1). The initial node of the algorithm is classification of the patient's resting electrocardiogram because the clinical history is less predictive of coronary anatomy in patients with electrocardiographic changes consistent with coronary artery disease. This definition of an abnormal resting electrocardiogram includes ST segment depression of at least 1 mm in at least one lead, an inverted T wave in any lead other than aV_R, or bundle branch block. Because the prevalence of coronary artery disease is lower in women, patient gender is used to stratify further the initial risk of coronary disease in patients with a normal resting electrocardiogram and typical angina pectoris. Exercise electrocardiography is classified as having either positive, discordant, or negative results (Table 5–1). Thallium scintigraphy is classified as abnormal when there is reversible myocardial hypoperfusion during exercise. The thallium study more frequently provides incremental prognostic information when the resting electrocardiogram is abnormal, and the clinician may choose to perform this test concurrently with exercise electrocardiography in these patients.

The use of thallium scintigraphy can be avoided in many patients, with substantial savings in the cost of testing. Usual charges for the thallium study are approximately three times those for exercise electrocardiography. The algorithm in Figure 5–1 allows classification of approximately 10% of patients as high

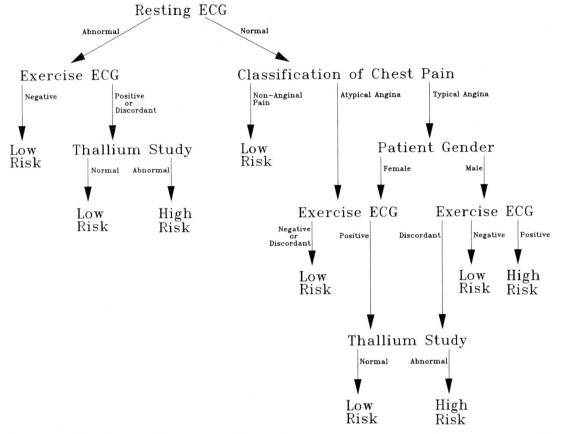

Figure 5–1. Algorithm to guide the use of diagnostic tests for coronary artery disease in patients with recurrent chest pain. Adapted from Ladenheim ML, Kotler TS, Pollock BH, et al. Am J Cardiol 59:270–277, 1987, with permission.

risk (> 5% probability of experiencing an adverse cardiac event during the subsequent 12 months). These patients should be considered for coronary arteriography to define the surgical anatomy or should be supervised closely while being treated with a medication

Table 5–1. Interpretation of Exercise Electrocardiogram*

Classification of Result	Result
Negative	Normal level of stress attained and no ST depression
Discordant	Reduced level of stress attained without ST depression or Normal level of stress attained with ST depression
Positive	Reduced level of stress attained plus ST depression

*Normal level of stress is defined as achieving 85% of age-adjusted predicted heart rate. ST depression is defined as 1 mm or more of ST segment depression.

regimen for coronary artery disease. For patients classified as low risk, the clinician should base management on the estimated probability of coronary artery disease. For example, patients with nonanginal chest pain have a low probability of coronary disease and should be evaluated for other etiologies of the pain. Patients with typical angina pectoris and a negative exercise electrocardiogram have an intermediate probability of coronary disease and should be considered for a therapeutic trial of medications for coronary artery disease.

Other Cardiac Etiologies of Recurrent Chest Pain

Recurrent chest pain may result from myocardial ischemia in the absence of fixed obstructions of the coronary arteries. Obstructive disease of intramural small vessels has been documented in some patients. Although such lesions occur more frequently in diabetics, small vessel disease is a rare cause of chest pain. More likely etiologies of recurrent chest pain should be excluded before pursuing the possibility of small vessel disease. The usefulness of diagnostic tests for small vessel disease has not been documented, but therapeutic trials of beta blockers, nitrates, or calcium channel blockers may be considered. Valvular aortic stenosis, hypertrophic cardiomyopathy, and thyrotoxicosis all can cause myocardial ischemia, but the pattern of pain in these conditions usually is similar to that of coronary artery disease. Because these etiologies nearly always are accompanied by physical examination findings typical of the underlying disease, their detection usually is not difficult.

Coronary vasospasm (in the absence of obstructive coronary disease) is a rare but serious cause of recurrent chest pain. The quality of the pain usually is similar to that of the pain of obstructive coronary disease, but its inducing factors are different. The pain usually is not brought on by exertion, and it sometimes awakens the patient from sleep. Emotional stress may cause the pain of coronary vasospasm. Nitroglycerin usually relieves the pain, and patients often improve after initiation of a therapeutic trial with calcium channel blockers or long-acting nitrates. Approximately 90% of patients with coronary vasospasm have electrocardiographic changes during the pain episodes. The absence of such changes is helpful for excluding this condition as a cause of recurrent chest pain.

Mitral valve prolapse commonly occurs in otherwise healthy adults. In population studies, the incidence of recurrent chest pain was the same in individuals with mitral valve prolapse as in subjects without the disorder. However, many patients have been reported in whom mitral valve prolapse appeared to be the etiology of recurrent chest pain. In these studies, the patients' pain occurred in varying patterns, and an identifiable chest pain syndrome attributable to mitral valve prolapse had not been described. Thus, mitral valve prolapse should be pursued as an etiology of recurrent chest pain only when more likely causes have been excluded. Because there is no specific treatment for mitral valve prolapse, the major value of making this diagnosis is to identify patients who may be at risk for the more serious complications of endocarditis and arrhythmias. Most patients with mitral valve prolapse who develop serious complications have hemodynamically significant mitral regurgitation (see Chap. 1). Echocardiography usually is unnecessary to exclude mitral valve prolapse unless the patient has findings from the physical examination or electrocardiography that suggest a risk of this complication.

Esophageal Etiologies of Recurrent Chest Pain

Other than cardiac disease, esophageal disease is the most frequent cause of recurrent chest pain in adults. Evaluation for esophageal disease should be undertaken only after coronary artery disease has been excluded. In patients with nonanginal chest pain, the clinician may safely exclude coronary artery disease. In patients with atypical or typical angina and a negative exercise electrocardiogram, a therapeutic trial of medications for coronary artery disease should be considered before excluding coronary disease as the cause of pain. Some patients may have both coronary artery disease and esophageal disease and thus respond only partially to beta blockers or other cardiac medications. These patients may benefit from further evaluation for esophageal disease to guide treatment planning.

Two major categories of esophageal disease can cause chest pain: reflux esophagitis and esophageal motor disorders. During the last 5 years, it has become apparent that the prevalence of these disorders is higher than previously suspected. In recent studies of patients who had anginal chest pain but negative evaluations for cardiac disease, the incidence of reflux esophagitis was approximately 10% and that of esophageal motor disorders was approximately 50%. Several different syndromes are included in the category of esophageal motor disorders. Approximately half of patients who have esophageal disease as the cause of their recurrent chest pain have nutcracker esophagus, a syndrome of high amplitude esophageal peristaltic contractions. One third have nonspecific esophageal motor disorders, and 10% have diffuse esophageal spasm. Achalasia and other disorders of the lower esophageal sphincter are common causes of dysphagia but are relatively rare etiologies of chest pain.

Several diagnostic tests are available to evaluate patients with suspected esophageal disease. Barium esophagography is widely available but has little usefulness for the evaluation of chest pain. The barium study is insensitive for nutcracker esophagus, and it cannot be used to exclude this disorder. The test has good sensitivity for achalasia, but achalasia rarely is the cause of unexplained chest pain. The sensitivity of barium esophagography for acid reflux is approximately 80%, but its specificity is less than 70%. Because reflux esophagitis is the etiology of unexplained chest pain in only 10% of patients, the finding of reflux on the barium study is a false-positive result in the majority of cases.

Esophageal manometry is the best single test to exclude or confirm esophageal motor disorders. The cholinergic agonist edrophonium may be given during the procedure to provoke the patient's symptoms. Manometry should be considered positive if the baseline recording shows dysmotility or if edrophonium reproduces the patient's chest pain. Bethanechol and ergonovine have also been used as provocative agents during manometry. However, both can induce coronary artery spasm and so are not as safe as edrophonium. Another test that may be used is radionuclide scintigraphy, recently advocated for the diagnosis of esophageal motor disorders. The patient swallows a labeled sulfur colloid, and transit time and esophageal emptying are measured with a gamma camera. This test has a sensitivity of approximately 80% for esophageal motor disorders, but the false-positive rate in a recent evaluation was 40%. Thus, scintigraphy lacks adequate specificity to confirm esophageal motor disorders in patients with recurrent chest pain.

Patients with positive manometry results should begin a medication trial for symptom relief. Both long-acting nitrates and calcium-blocking agents have been proposed for these disorders. Unfortunately, there have been few studies of the efficacy of medical therapy for esophageal motor disorders. It would be useful to know whether a response to these drugs could be interpreted as a diagnostic test for esophageal disease, but adequate studies have not been conducted. Thus, the usefulness of such a therapeutic trial before manometry is not known.

Patients with reflux esophagitis frequently report a burning pain and aggravation of the pain by certain foods. However, the specificity of these characteristics has not been documented. The definitive test for esophagitis is esophageal endoscopy with biopsy, but this procedure is invasive. Thus, endoscopy usually should not be the initial step in evaluating patients with suspected reflux esophagitis. Acid perfusion of the esophagus, known as the

Bernstein test, can be used as a screening test for reflux esophagitis. The test is performed by placing a nasogastric tube in the midesophagus. Hydrochloric acid (0.1 N at 120 drops per minute) then is instilled into the esophagus. The test is considered positive if this procedure reproduces the patient's chest pain. The sensitivity of the Bernstein test is approximately 80%, but its specificity is only 50% (using esophageal biopsy as the criterion test). Results are more likely to be false positive if there are longer time intervals between the acid infusion and the onset of the induced pain. Some investigators have proposed that a positive Bernstein test sometimes indicates subclinical esophagitis, but truly false-positive Bernstein tests do occur frequently. Thus, a Bernstein test is useful for excluding reflux esophagitis but should not be used to confirm this diagnosis.

Other diagnostic modalities sometimes may be used to evaluate possible reflux esophagitis. Continuous monitoring of the acid content of the lower esophageal lumen has recently been advocated as a test for reflux esophagitis. This test is performed by placing a pH probe in the lower esophagus. With this study, some patients with recurrent chest pain have been found to have elevations of lower esophageal acid content without endoscopic evidence of esophagitis. Whether these patients have false-positive test results or a subclinical esophagitis is uncertain. Further experience with this procedure is necessary. The test is difficult to perform, and it should not yet be considered part of the diagnostic evaluation of unexplained chest pain.

Therapeutic trials probably have greater value for reflux esophagitis than for esophageal motor disorders. However, the usefulness of therapeutic trials has not been studied by clinical investigators. A therapeutic trial (with antacids or histamine blockers) should be considered in patients with a positive Bernstein test and may be used instead of a Bernstein test in patients whose pattern of symptoms suggests reflux esophagitis. Calcium channel blockers and nitrates, which may be used in therapeutic trials for coronary artery disease or esophageal motility disorders, may aggravate symptoms of esophagitis by increasing esophageal reflux.

Chest Wall Disorders

Chest wall syndromes are a well-recognized etiology of recurrent chest pain. In a recent study, 16% of patients with anginal chest pain and normal coronary arteriograms had musculoskeletal disorders established as the cause of pain. However, there is no definitive test for confirming these disorders; the diagnosis is based on clinical inference and reproduction of the pain by chest wall palpation. Several maneuvers used during the physical examination (described in publications given in the Bibliography) are helpful for identifying the disorders, although their sensitivity has not been documented. Chest wall syndromes should be considered when more serious etiologies of the chest pain have been excluded. A therapeutic trial with nonsteroidal anti-inflammatory agents may be useful for evaluation of suspected chest wall conditions.

Bibliography

Cannon RO: Causes of chest pain in patients with normal coronary arteriograms: the eye of the beholder. Am J Cardiol 62:306–308, 1988.
Brief review of the diagnostic approach to identifying cardiac, esophageal, and psychologic etiologies of recurrent chest pain in patients who have normal coronary arteries by arteriography.

Chaitman BR, Bourassa MG, Davis K, et al. Angiographic prevalence of high-risk coronary artery disease in patient subsets (CASS). Circulation 64:360–367, 1981.
Reviews data from more than 8000 patients in the Coronary Artery Surgery Study. Chest pain characteristics and demographic variables are correlated with the extent and severity of coronary artery disease.

Chobanian SJ, Benjamin SB, Curtis DJ, et al. Systematic evaluation of patients with noncardiac chest pain. Arch Intern Med 146:1505–1508, 1986.
Recent evaluation of the informational value of esophageal endoscopy, the Bernstein test, and radionuclide scintigraphy for evaluating patients in whom coronary artery disease has been excluded.

Diamond GA, Forrester JS. Analysis of probability as an aid in the clinical diagnosis of coronary-artery disease. N Engl J Med 300:1350–1358, 1979.
Discusses Bayesian adjustment of the estimated probability of coronary artery disease when patient characteristics and diagnostic test results are serially evaluated.

Epstein SE, Gerber LH, Borer JS. Chest wall syndrome: a common cause of unexplained cardiac pain. JAMA 241:2793–2797, 1979.
Description of physical examintion maneuvers in 12 patients with recurrent chest pain caused by chest wall disorders.

Fam AG, Smythe HA. Musculoskeletal chest wall pain. Can Med Assoc J 133:379–389, 1985.
General review and extensive bibliography of this disorder.

Goldman L, Cook EF, Mitchell N, et al. Incremental value of the exercise test for diagnosing the presence or absence of coronary artery disease. Circulation 66:945–953, 1982.
Study of the informational value of patient characteristics and exercise electrocardiography for predicting coronary artery disease by using data from the Duke University cardiology database. Exercise electrocardiography had limited value in this analysis.

Goldman L, Lee TH. Noninvasive tests for diagnosing the presence and extent of coronary artery disease: exercise electrocardiography, thallium scintigraphy, and radionuclide ventriculography. J Gen Intern Med 1:258–265, 1986.
Discussion of the informational value of exercise tests, including recommendations for testing strategies in patients with different pain syndromes.

Horwitz LD, Herman MV, Gorlin R. Clinical response to nitroglycerin as a diagnostic test for coronary artery disease. AM J Cardiol 29:149–152, 1972.
Report of clinical response to nitroglycerin in 49 patients with ischemic chest pain and 21 patients with noncardiac chest pain. Provides guidelines on how to interpret nitroglycerin response.

Katz PO, Dalton CB, Richter JE, et al. Esophageal testing of patients with noncardiac chest pain or dysphagia: results of three years' experience with 1161 patients. Ann Intern Med 106:593–597, 1987.
Report of systematic evaluation of 910 patients with noncardiac chest pain, providing information on prevalence of esophageal disorders and diagnostic yield of standard tests for these disorders.

Ladenheim ML, Kotler TS, Pollock BH, et al. Incremental prognostic power of clinical history, exercise electrocardiography and myocardial perfusion scintigraphy in suspected coronary artery disease. Am J Cardiol 59:270–277, 1987.
Report of clinical and follow-up data of 1214 patients with recurrent chest pain. Describes algorithm for guiding use of exercise tests to identify patients at risk of complications of coronary artery disease.

Magarian GJ, Hickam DH. Noncardiac causes of angina-like chest pain. Progr Cardiovasc Dis 29:65–80, 1986.
Extensive review of esophageal disorders, chest wall syndromes, and hyperventilation.

Manu P, Runge LA. Testing stable angina: expert opinion versus decision analysis. Med Care 23:1381–1390, 1985.
Describes an expected utility model to guide use of tests for coronary artery disease.

Ott DJ, Richter JE, Wu WC, et al. Radiologic and manometric correlation in "nutcracker esophagus." AJR 147:692–695, 1986.
Recent report of the informational value of barium radiography for esophageal motor disorders.

Richter JE, Castell DO. Esophageal disease as a cause of noncardiac chest pain. Adv Intern Med 33:311–336, 1988.
Up-to-date review of diagnosis and therapeutic approaches to esophageal etiologies of chest pain.

Semble EL, Wise CM. Chest pain: a rheumatologist's perspective. South Med J 81:64–68, 1988.
Overview of chest wall syndromes and methods of physical examination of the chest wall. Includes brief description of a recent study of the prevalence of these disorders in patients with anginal chest pain.

Sox HC Jr. Exercise testing in suspected coronary artery disease. Disease-a-Month 31(12):1–71, 1985.
Detailed review of exercise electrocardiography and thallium scintigraphy, including extensive bibliography.

Waterfall WE, Craven MA, Allen CJ. Gastroesophageal reflux: clinical presentations, diagnosis and management. Can Med Assoc J 135:1101–1109, 1986.
General review of diagnosis and treatment. The described treatment regimen can be used as the basis of a therapeutic trial for this disorder.

Weiner DA, McCabe CH, Ryan TJ. Identification of patients with left main and three vessel coronary disease with clinical and exercise test variables. Am J Cardiol 46:214–217, 1980.

Report of 436 patients who underwent exercise electrocardiography and coronary arteriography. Nineteen percent had an early positive result, 74% of whom had left main or three vessel disease.

Weiner DA, Ryan TJ, McCabe CH, et al. Exercise stress testing: correlations among history of angina, ST-segment response and prevalence of coronary-artery disease in the Coronary Artery Surgery Study (CASS). N Engl J Med 301:230–235, 1979.

Report of test results in 2045 patients, which provides estimates of the informational value of the resting and exercise electrocardiograms for coronary artery disease.

6

Diagnosis and Management of Stable Angina Pectoris

GARY D. PLOTNICK, M.D.

Introduction

The evaluation and management of the patient with stable angina pectoris depend predominantly on the etiology of the chest pain symptoms, an assessment of the pathophysiologic process responsible for the symptoms, and an estimate of the individual patient's prognosis. Evaluation and management must be individualized and depend on the answers to several fundamental questions:

1. Does the patient have pain that reflects myocardial ischemia?

2. What is the likely etiology of the myocardial ischemia?

3. Does the patient fall into a high risk or low risk group?

The answer to the last question will determine the aggressiveness of the diagnostic and therapeutic approaches to the individual patient. Some of the factors that place the patient at high risk of death or future myocardial infarction are listed in Table 6–1.

Evaluation

Patient's History and Classification of Symptoms

The evaluation of the individual should be organized and systematic, and must begin with an evaluation of the patient's history (Fig. 6–1).

The diagnosis of angina pectoris is based solely on the history. Chest pain is often the reason the patient seeks medical attention. The chest pain symptoms can be categorized as one of four types.

1. Typical angina pectoris has three major components. First, typical angina is precipi-

tated by stress, either physical or emotional, and is relieved either by cessation of stress or by sublingual nitroglycerin, usually in less than 5 minutes. Second, the discomfort is central in location, i.e., it touches the sternum. Third, the discomfort is visceral in character, making it very difficult for many patients to describe. Words like squeezing, pressure, vise-like, and indigestion may be used. If all three components are present, the diagnosis of typical angina pectoris is made.

2. The term atypical angina pectoris is used when two of the three components of typical angina are present, for instance, if the patient develops a reproducible visceral discomfort in a noncentral location, such as the jaw or arm, when walking quickly up a flight of stairs (angina-like pain but not in the typical location).

3. Many times, however, the patient's dis-

Table 6–1. Factors Associated with High Risk of Death or Myocardial Infarction

Markedly Positive Functional (Exercise) Test
ST depression ≥ 2 mm at low workloads (< 5 mets)
Prolonged ST depression (> 5 min) in recovery
Multiple ECG leads (≥ 5) with ST depression ≥ 1 mm
Poor exercise tolerance (< 5 mets)
Multiple or extensive thallium-201 perfusion defects
Marked exercise-induced regional left ventricular
   dysfunction or marked fall (> 10%) in ejection
   fraction on radionuclide ventriculography
Fall in systolic blood pressure ≥ 10 mmHg with
   progressive exercise

Abnormal Left Ventricular Systolic Function
Congestive heart failure
Ejection fraction ≤ 30%

Coronary Anatomy
Left main coronary disease
Three-vessel coronary disease
? Combined proximal left anterior descending and
   proximal circumflex coronary disease

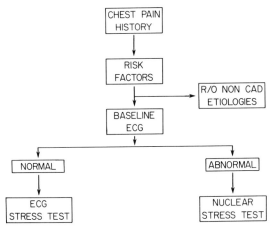

Figure 6–1. Approach to the evaluation of the patient with stable angina. R/O, rule out; CAD, coronary artery disease; ECG, electrocardiogram.

comfort does not fulfill the criteria for either typical or atypical angina, and the patient's symptoms may be labeled chest pain of uncertain etiology (CPUE). This term allows us to admit our uncertainty and reminds us of the need for further evaluation of the patient's complaint.

4. Sometimes the patient may have a chest pain that does not sound ischemic; this can be labeled chest pain–not ischemic (CP-NI). For instance, a sharp pain that starts at rest, travels through the left breast, and lasts seconds can be labeled not ischemic.

One reason why the history is so important is that it helps the physician make an educated guess concerning the underlying anatomy and pathophysiology. Table 6–2 demonstrates the possibility of finding arteriographic coronary artery disease (defined as a narrowing of at least 50% of the intraluminal diameter of one or more major coronary arteries) in males aged 40 to 70. Note that if the chest pain meets the criteria for typical angina, the chance that the patient will have obstructive coronary disease is 90%. If the discomfort is not typical, the odds are reduced, and the anatomic and patho-

Table 6–2. Correlation of Clinical Subgroup with Angiographic Coronary Artery Disease in Males

Subgroup	Coronary Artery Disease* (% of Patients)
Typical angina pectoris	90
Atypical angina pectoris	60
CPUE	30
CP-NI	10

*Coronary artery disease: ≥ 50% stenosis of one or more major coronary arteries.

physiologic diagnoses are less certain. The prevalence of coronary artery disease is dependent on not only the type of chest pain, but also age and gender. For example, women less than 50 years of age with typical angina have a prevalence of coronary artery disease of 59% (compared with 87% for similarly aged men). Women more than 50 years of age with typical angina have a prevalence of coronary artery disease of 72% (compared with 95% for similarly aged men).

Stable angina includes fixed-threshold angina (angina occurring in a highly reproducible pattern provoked by a fixed amount of exertion) and variable-threshold angina (also called mixed angina). Variable-threshold angina may occur with variable amounts of exertion from day to day, and occasionally may occur at rest. The pathogenesis of fixed-threshold angina is related to atherosclerotic lesions within rigid coronary arteries, which limit coronary artery blood flow reserve to a certain level, whereas the pathogenesis of variable-threshold angina is related to alterations in coronary artery tone, usually at the site of an atherosclerotic lesion.

Angina symptoms can be classified by using the Canadian Cardiovascular Society Classification (Table 6–3). Unfortunately there is little correlation between the severity or frequency of angina symptoms and severity of underlying coronary disease or prognosis.

Important in angina classification, however, is the differentiation of stable angina from unstable angina. To be considered stable, unchanging symptoms should have been present for 3 months or longer. Unstable angina can be subdivided into separate categories: angina with symptoms of recent onset (less than 3 months), angina with a crescendo pattern, and rest angina. This chapter will focus on the approach to the patient with stable angina.

Risk Factors

After obtaining the history of the present illness, one should ascertain the presence or absence of cardiovascular risk factors (Table 6–4). Risk factors can be considered as building blocks: the more risk factors present, the greater the chance that the patient will have obstructive coronary artery disease. For example, a 60-year-old male who has symptoms of chest pain of uncertain etiology, but in addition has a family history of premature ischemic disease, is a smoker, and has hypertension, may have an 80% chance of having

Table 6–3. *Canadian Cardiovascular Society Classification for Angina Pectoris*

Class	Characteristics
I	Ordinary physical activity (such as walking or climbing stairs) does not cause angina. Angina may occur with strenuous, rapid, or prolonged exertion (work or recreation).
II	There is slight limitation of ordinary activity. Angina may occur with walking or climbing stairs rapidly; walking uphill; walking or climbing stairs after meals or in the cold, in the wind, or under emotional stress; walking more than two blocks on the level and climbing more than one flight of stairs at a normal pace under normal conditions.
III	There is marked limitation of ordinary physical activity. Angina may occur after walking one or two blocks on the level or climbing one flight of stairs in normal conditions at a normal pace.
IV	There is inability to carry on any physical activity without discomfort; angina may be present at rest.

coronary disease, whereas a 40-year-old male with a similar history of pain but no risk factors may have only a 10% chance of having coronary artery disease. Thus, taking into account both the chest pain history and the presence or absence of cardiovascular risk factors will help determine the pretest likelihood of coronary artery disease.

Physical Examination

The physical examination, chest roentgenogram, and routine blood studies are usually of little help in establishing the diagnosis of coronary artery disease. The physical examination should be performed both to search for findings that increase the likelihood of the presence of coronary artery disease (such as hypertension, xanthelasma, atrial gallop, paradoxical precordial bulge, or peripheral vascular disease) and to determine other disorders that may cause angina or angina-like pain, disorders that may need specific therapy. The latter category includes aortic stenosis, hypertrophic cardiomyopathy, pulmonary hypertension, and mitral valve prolapse. It must be emphasized, however, that the baseline physical examination is often completely normal even in the presence of extensive coronary artery disease. An important finding on physical examination is evidence of left ventricular dysfunction (cardiomegaly, ventricular gallop sound [S_3]) because of its poor prognostic significance. The chest roentgenogram may occasionally reveal calcification in the region of the coronary arteries or demonstrate a bulging cardiac silhouette suggestive of left ventricular aneurysm, but it is usually normal. The history, physical examination, and laboratory tests should be used to identify precipitating or aggravating factors that may alter therapy.

Table 6–4. *Cardiovascular Risk Factors*

Risk Factors Beyond the Control of Physicians and Patients	Risk Factors Controllable by Physician and Patient Effort
Gender (i.e., being male)	Major Risks
Increasing age	Abnormalities of plasma lipids and
Family history of premature ischemic heart disease	lipoproteins
Clinical or ECG evidence of ischemic heart disease	Hypertension
	Cigarette smoking
	Diabetes mellitus
	Minor Risks
	Obesity
	Platelet aggregation and thrombosis
	Oral contraceptive use
	Physical inactivity
	Type A behavior pattern
	Stress and psychosocial factors
	Uric acid levels

Modified from Plotnick GD. Unstable Angina—A Clinical Approach. Mt. Kisco, NY, Futura Publishing Co., 1985, with permission.

These factors include anemia, infection, thyrotoxicosis, hypoxia, hypertension, use of sympathomimetic drugs, arrhythmias, and emotional stress. The electrocardiogram (ECG) may reveal the presence of pathologic Q waves compatible with an antecedent myocardial infarction, but often it is normal or shows only minor nonspecific ST-T abnormalities.

Exercise Stress Testing

The next and extremely valuable step in the evaluation of the patient with suspected or confirmed coronary artery disease is exercise stress testing (Fig. 6–1). This functional testing is helpful from both diagnostic and prognostic standpoints. The diagnosis of important coronary artery disease is more likely if objective evidence of myocardial ischemia can be demonstrated (Table 6–5). The type of stress testing to be performed (electrocardiographic alone or electrocardiographic along with nuclear testing) is dependent on the baseline ECG. If the baseline ECG reveals substantial ST-T abnormalities, left bundle branch block, left ventricular hypertrophy, or Wolff-Parkinson-White syndrome, or if the patient is receiving digitalis (i.e., making it difficult to interpret further ST-T abnormalities during stress), a nuclear test (either a multigated blood pool scan or a thallium-201 nuclear scan) should be performed. The nuclear test chosen depends on the expertise available. Results from stress testing can be used diagnostically along with the pretest evaluation to determine a post-test likelihood of coronary artery disease (Fig. 6–2 *A* to *D*). For diagnostic purposes, the exercise test is most useful for patients with intermediate pretest likelihoods of having coronary artery disease (i.e., men with atypical angina or with chest pain of uncertain etiology and women with atypical or typical angina). Abnormalities suggestive of ischemia include 1 mm or greater of horizontal or downsloping ST segment depression (ECG), less than 0.05 unit of increase in ejection fraction, or new transient wall motion abnormality (multigated blood pool scan) or transient cold spot (thallium-201). The use of immediate postexercise two-dimensional echocardiography to evaluate segmental wall motion and thickening has potential and is being advocated by several investigators, but is not yet widespread.

For patients who cannot undergo a treadmill exercise test, stress testing by using a bicycle, arm cranking, or atrial pacing can be substituted. The use of intravenous dipyridamole along with isometric handgrip has been combined with thallium-201 scintigraphy or two-dimensional echocardiography and shows promise for increasing sensitivity in detecting myocardial ischemia, particularly for patients unable to exercise.

Results from stress testing can also be used prognostically to classify patients for risk and to help determine the aggressiveness of further evaluation and therapy. Factors that place the individual at highest risk are given in Table 6–1. A markedly positive stress test may be used to identify patients most likely to have extensive coronary artery disease and those with the worst prognosis. A markedly positive stress test has a sensitivity of 49 to 92% and a specificity of 58 to 75% in identifying patients with left main or triple vessel disease. The use of antianginal medication may substantially reduce the sensitivity and increase the specificity of an early positive response to predict left main or triple vessel disease. The most important single item for risk stratification is exercise duration. In one study, among patients who developed 2-mm ST segment depression within 3 minutes of treadmill exercise, the likelihood of a future event was 15% per year, whereas it was 8% per year when ST segment depression appeared after 5 minutes and only 4% per year when it appeared after 7 minutes. Left ventricular function at rest is also an extremely powerful independent predictor of prognosis. These factors are probably more important predictors of prognosis than is the angiographically determined extent of coro-

Table 6–5. *Objective Evidence of Myocardial Ischemia*

Electrocardiographic Changes
Transient ST segment depression or elevation
Transient T wave abnormalities
Arrhythmias

Systolic Abnormality of Cardiac Muscle
Segmental wall motion abnormality
Transient paradoxical precordial bulge
Transient regional hypo- or akinesis on multigated blood pool scan or two-dimensional echocardiogram

Diastolic Abnormality of Cardiac Muscle
Transient left ventricular end-diastolic pressure increase
Transient atrial gallop (S₄)
Abnormal diastolic filling on high temporal resolution multigated blood pool scan or two-dimensional echocardiogram

Thallium Scan
Transient cold spot

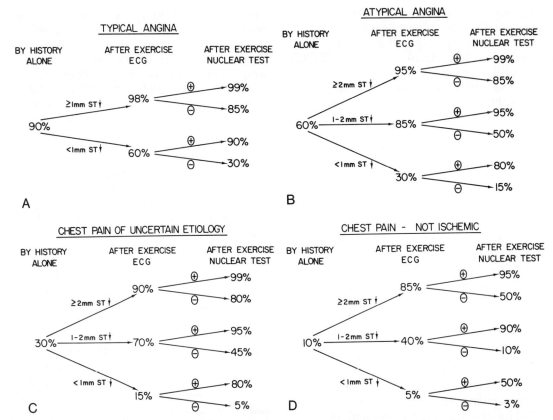

Figure 6–2. *Approximate probabilities of coronary artery disease before and after the sequential use of an exercise ECG and an exercise nuclear test in a male patient with:* A, *typical angina pectoris;* B, *atypical angina pectoris;* C, *chest pain of uncertain etiology;* D, *chest pain–not ischemic. Modified from Goldman L and Lee TH. J Gen Intern Med 1:258–265, 1986, with permission.*

nary artery disease. Functional evaluation (exercise testing) should be performed as part of the initial evaluation of the patient, and the timing of follow-up testing should be individualized depending on the results of the initial study and other clinical variables. A patient with a negative or mildly positive test and a clinically mild stable pattern of angina can be retested at annual or biannual intervals, whereas a patient with a moderately positive test probably should be re-evaluated at 6- to 12-month intervals.

Physiologic Testing and Angiographic Evaluation

There is no universal agreement as to the role of revascularization in patients with stable angina pectoris. Some advocate cardiac catheterization for all patients with suspected coronary artery disease and determine the need

for revascularization based on the anatomic appearance and extent of the coronary artery disease as determined by coronary arteriography.

There are now three large prospective randomized trials comparing the effects of coronary artery bypass surgery with medical therapy in patients with stable angina pectoris. Analysis of the results of these major studies has affected many cardiologists' approach to management. These studies are (1) Veterans Administration Cooperative Study of Stable Angina (VA Coop Study), (2) European Coronary Surgery Study of Coronary Artery Bypass Surgery in Stable Angina (European Coronary Study), and (3) Collaborative Coronary Artery Surgery Study (CASS). The reader is referred to several reviews for details of these important studies. Although performed during somewhat different times (during improvements in both surgical and medical therapies), all three studies confirm that, compared with medical therapy, surgical therapy improves the quality of life as determined by improvement in functional classification, relief of angina, and exercise performance. Although this difference had disappeared at a 10-year follow-up, it was significant when therapies were evaluated at 1 and 5 years.

Although these three large studies have not demonstrated an improvement in survival for the groups as a whole, there has been evidence for prolonged survival after surgical therapy in particular subgroups. Improved survival for the surgical cohort has been shown in patients with left main coronary artery disease and possibly in those with triple vessel disease (European Coronary Study), whereas surgical therapy did not appear to affect survival in other anatomic subgroups.

More recent analysis of these studies has suggested that a number of noninvasive predictors of risk may identify patients who are more likely to have a prolonged life after coronary artery bypass surgery. These noninvasive predictors appear to be more important than the anatomic extent of disease in stratifying risk and in identifying the potential benefit of surgery. Factors that place the patient at low risk of death when treated medically are given in Table 6–6. Recent analysis of a large CASS registry has suggested that even among patients with triple vessel coronary disease one can identify high and low risk groups by using physiologic (exercise) testing, and that the high risk group will have improved survival with surgery whereas the low risk group will not. Among patients with triple vessel disease who fit into a high risk group (developing ≥ 1-mm ST segment depression in stage I of a Bruce protocol), the 7-year survival rate was

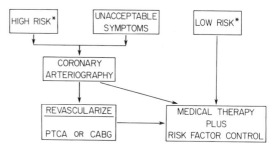

* BASED PREDOMINANTLY ON "FUNCTIONAL" TESTING

Figure 6–3. Approach to the management of the patient with stable angina based on risk stratification. PTCA, percutaneous transluminal coronary angioplasty; CAGB, coronary artery bypass graft.

81% for 278 surgically treated patients and 58% for 120 medically treated patients. Among patients with triple vessel disease who fit into a low risk group (exercising into stage III or higher without ischemic ST segment depression), the surgical cohort did not survive longer than the medical cohort. Based on this and other data, it seems reasonable that physiologic testing precede angiographic evaluation. Patients who are at high risk should undergo anatomic evaluation, whereas patients in stable condition at low risk may be treated medically until serial noninvasive testing suggests a change in risk status or symptoms dictate a change in treatment.

This risk stratification based predominantly on stress testing will determine the therapeutic approach for most patients (Fig. 6–3). Exceptions may occasionally be made and clinical judgment may modify this scheme. Patients who are older and have other life-threatening illness, who are satisfied with their lifestyle, or who are extremely reluctant to undergo invasive procedures may sometimes remain on medical therapy. Those at low risk in whom the "need to know" is a major consideration may undergo catheterization to determine anatomic extent of disease without proceeding to a revascularization procedure. However, catheterization should be performed in the majority of patients at high risk to determine not whether but which revascularization procedure should be performed. Revascularization can be carried out either by percutaneous transluminal coronary angioplasty (PTCA) or by coronary artery bypass graft (CABG). Although the use of PTCA was originally confined to patients with single proximal noncalcified coronary artery lesions, as experience has grown

Table 6–6. Factors Placing the Patient at Low Risk of Death When Treated Medically

Study	Factors
VA Cooperative	Absence of: ST segment depression on baseline ECG, History of myocardial infarction, History of hypertension, New York Heart Association functional class III–IV
European Coronary	Absence of: ≥ 1.5-mm ST segment depression with exercise, Peripheral vascular disease, Abnormal baseline ECG
CASS	Exercising into stage III or greater of Bruce protocol without ischemic ST segment depression

and technical advances have occurred, PTCA is being employed in multivessel and distal disease as well as in patients with previous CABG surgery. Exactly how PTCA will affect the prognosis of patients with stable angina remains to be determined.

Other patients who may undergo catheterization include:

1. Those considered surgical candidates because of "unacceptable" symptoms
2. Those considered surgical candidates because of threatened myocardium:
   a. Markedly positive stress test
   b. Other clinical suspicion of left main or multivessel disease:
      i. Proximal coronary calcification
      ii. Remote myocardial infarction on ECG
3. Those in whom the diagnosis is uncertain:
   a. Arteriographic information needed
   b. Prognostic information needed

Medical Management

General Measures

As previously discussed (Fig. 6–3), a thorough evaluation including history, physical examination, and initial laboratory studies supplemented by an exercise stress test should be obtained not only to determine an accurate diagnosis but also to stratify risk. The importance of modifying remedial risk factors cannot be overemphasized. Counseling about risk factor control should be initiated at the first visit. Evaluation must extend to the offspring of patients with a strong family history of premature coronary artery disease (angina, myocardial infarction, or sudden death in a man less than 55 years of age, or in a woman less than 60 years of age). Most risk factors can be identified by a careful history and physical examination.

Abnormalities of plasma lipids, hypertension, and cigarette smoking are the most significant treatable factors. There is convincing evidence that control of each of these factors will decrease the risk of coronary artery disease complications. The importance of lipid control cannot be overemphasized. Of all the risk factors, it is the one that when controlled will slow the progression of disease after coronary artery bypass surgery. The Lipid Research Clinics Coronary Primary Prevention Trial has demonstrated that reduction of plasma cholesterol and low density lipoprotein cholesterol lowers the mortality and morbidity levels of coronary artery disease. For each 1% reduction in plasma cholesterol there is a 2% reduction in risk. For further information concerning the evaluation and treatment of this important risk factor, the reader is referred to Chapter 15.

Treatment of hypertension and cessation of smoking are also extremely important. The more risk factors present, the more important is control of each individual factor. Cigarette smoking should be thoroughly discouraged, particularly in patients with additional risk factors. Weight reduction and a physical conditioning program can improve an individual's sense of well-being as well as allow the patient to achieve more strenuous exercise at a low heart rate and blood pressure. Education of both the patient and his or her family with regard to work and leisure activities, risk factor control, and prognosis is also extremely important. Cooperation among patient, family, and physician is vital for successful management.

Drug Therapy

The goal of drug therapy is to treat episodes of myocardial ischemia and to prevent recurrent episodes. Although most physicians now aim for a reduction in the patient's episodes of angina, possibly a better end point is a reduction in all ischemic episodes (both symptomatic and asymptomatic). Preventing silent ischemic episodes is rational but as yet of unproven benefit. The drugs used to treat angina are nitrates, beta blockers, and calcium channel blockers (Table 6–7). These drugs have variable effects on the determinants of myocardial oxygen demand and when used in combination usually help decrease the frequency of anginal episodes. Drug therapy must be individualized.

NITRATES

Nitrates have traditionally been the cornerstone of therapy. Their major effect is to cause peripheral venous pooling, thereby decreasing left ventricular wall tension by a reduction in ventricular volume. Nitrates may also decrease arterial pressure by systemic arteriolar dilation, and there is evidence that they may improve the distribution of coronary blood flow to the endocardium and may enhance the

Table 6–7. Antianginal Medication: Nitrates, Beta Blockers, and Calcium Channel Blockers

Drug	Trade Name	Onset of Action (min)	Peak Action (min)	Duration of Action	Dose (mg)	Dosing Interval
			Nitrates*			
Sublingual TNG†	Nitrostat	1–3	4–8	10–30 min	0.15–0.6	As needed
Lingual TNG spray	Nitrolingual	2–5	4–8	10–30 min	0.4	As needed
Buccal TNG	Nitrogard	2–5	4–10	0.5–5 h‡	1–3	3–6 h
Oral isosorbide dinitrate	Isordil, Sorbitrate	15–45	45–120	4–6 h§	10–80	4–6h
TNG ointment (2%)	Nitrostat ointment, Nitrobid ointment	15–60	30–120	3–8 h	0.5–4 in	q 4–8 h
TNG Transderm	Nitro Dur II, Nitro Disc	30–60	60–180	Up to 24 h	2.5–30	Daily

Drug	Trade Name	Half-Life (h)	Usual Dose (mg)	Dosing Interval
		Beta Blockers		
Nonselective				
Propranolol	Inderal	4	40–160	8–12 h
Nadolol	Corgard	20–24	40–240	Daily
Timolol	Blocadren	4–5	10–20	12 h
Pindolol	Visken	3–4	2.5–10	8–12 h
Cardioselective				
Atenolol	Tenormin	6–7	50–100	Daily
Metoprolol	Lopressor	3–7	50–100	8–12 h
Acebutolol	Sectral	3–4	400	8–12 h

Drug	Trade Name	Onset of Action (min)	Usual Dose (mg)	Dosing Interval
		Calcium Channel Blockers		
Nifedipine	Procardia, Adalat	< 20‖	10–40	6–8 h
Verapamil	Calan, Isoptin	< 30	80–160	6–8 h
Diltiazem	Cardizem	< 30	30–90	6–8 h

*Modified from Abrams J. Am J Med 74:85, 1983 with permission.
†TNG, trinitroglycerin.
‡Effect persists as long as tablet is intact.
§Some studies have demonstrated effects to 8 h.
‖Sublingual onset of action is 2–3 min.

electrical stability of acutely ischemic myocardium.

Nitrates are generally well tolerated and, as a rule, inexpensive. In one form or another, nitrates are used early in patients with angina and are often used in combination with other medications. The many different forms of nitrates are given in Table 6–7. The form chosen depends on the onset of action, duration of action, and convenience. To treat individual episodes of angina, sublingual nitroglycerin is usually employed because of its quick onset of action. Rapid onset alternatives used less frequently include lingual spray nitroglycerin or sublingual nifedipine. Although ease of application makes nitroglycerin patches attractive, because of their expense, oral isosorbide dinitrate has been my long-acting nitrate of choice for outpatient therapy. Starting with 10 or 20 mg every 6 hours (omitting the nighttime dose), one can increase each dose by 10 mg every few days to the point of symptom control or intolerable side effects.

A few practical points should be emphasized with respect to nitroglycerin. A number of serious side effects can occur, including postural hypotension and syncope produced by a reduction in preload and afterload. The patient who has never taken nitroglycerin before should take the first dose while observed by the physician. A single tablet of sublingual nitroglycerin (usually 0.3 or 0.4 mg) should be tried in the physician's office after the pharmacologic action of the drug is explained to make the patient aware of the potential for dizziness. The benefit of reclining and of putting the legs upright if dizziness occurs should be explained. The patient should be made aware of the potential deterioration of nitroglycerin tablets with time and exposure to light. Nitroglycerin tablets should be routinely replaced every 6 months, or sooner if the patient notices no peppermint taste or burning under the tongue. The patient should be cautioned that if three nitroglycerin tablets (one every 5 minutes) are taken in succession without relief of a prolonged episode of pain, he or she should go immediately to the nearest emergency facility. The prophylactic use of nitroglycerin should also be emphasized. A long-acting form of nitroglycerin is usually chosen in an attempt to prevent further episodes of angina. Nitrate tolerance may develop in a significant percentage of patients, necessitating an increase in dosage. Recent studies suggest that the development of nitrate tolerance may be delayed by a nitrate-free interval. Because most patients experience angina during the day, omitting the nighttime dose of nitrate is reasonable. Patients with predominately nocturnal angina may have their nitrate-free interval during the day.

BETA BLOCKERS

Beta blockers are commonly employed in patients with stable angina. They exert their beneficial effect by blunting heart rate, arterial blood pressure, and contractility responses to stress, thereby decreasing myocardial oxygen demand at each level of stress. Beta blockers have additive effects when combined with nitrates in controlling the determinants of myocardial oxygen demand. Nitrates decrease preload whereas appropriate doses of beta blockers may prevent the reflex tachycardia that may occur with the nitrates. There are many forms of beta blockers from which to choose (Table 6–7). The beta blocker chosen depends on which side effects one is trying to avoid, duration of action (convenience), and expense. The relatively cardioselective drugs atenolol, metoprolol, and acebutolol antagonize catecholamine effects more at the $beta_1$ receptor than the $beta_2$ receptor. Although these cardioselective beta blockers may be preferable in patients with asthma, chronic reactive airway disease, insulin-requiring diabetes, or peripheral vascular disease, it should be appreciated that cardioselectivity is apparent only at lower doses. As higher doses are needed, cardioselectivity may be lost. The water-soluble beta blockers nadolol and atenolol do not readily cross the blood–brain barrier, thus producing fewer central nervous system side effects such as depression and fatigue; are metabolized slowly by the liver; and are long-lasting. Pindolol is the beta blocker that has "intrinsic sympathomimetic activity" or partial beta agonist activity. This effect may be advantageous in patients with resting bradycardia, atrioventricular conduction disturbances, or peripheral vascular disease, but not in the majority of patients with angina.

Therapy with beta blockers must be individualized. These drugs should be carefully titrated in each patient to a dosage that will achieve adequate beta blockage (ideally judged by a blunting of heart rate response to light exercise [< 90 beats per minute]). Because of the hepatic first-pass metabolism effect, there is tremendous variability in the dose necessary for different patients; for example, the propranolol dose ranges between 60 and 1000 mg.

Side effects of beta blockers include fatigue, bronchoconstriction, exacerbation of heart failure, mental depression, symptomatic bradycardia, impaired sexual function, and coolness of the extremities. Contraindications, absolute and relative, to beta blockers include bronchospasm, insulin-requiring diabetes mellitus, severe congestive heart failure, advanced heart block, symptomatic bradycardia, peripheral vascular disease, and psychiatric disease, particularly depression.

If there are no contraindications, these drugs are usually started early in therapy for several reasons. First, beta blockers are among the few drugs in cardiology for which there is some proof that life may be prolonged by their use. Although the data suggesting prolongation of life have so far been confined to patients after a myocardial infarction, it is hoped that this protective benefit extends to other patients with coronary artery disease. Second, beta blockers, at doses high enough to substantially blunt the rapid heart rate response to exercise, almost always reduce the frequency of future episodes of effort angina. (This benefit is seen especially in patients whose angina occurs only at a rapid [> 120 beats per minute] heart rate.) Unfortunately not all patients can achieve this benefit without experiencing side effects sufficient to warrant a reduction in dose. Use of a beta blocker is especially helpful in patients with hypertension in addition to angina.

CALCIUM CHANNEL BLOCKERS

The calcium channel blockers (Table 6–7) are a heterogeneous group of drugs that share the ability to modify the transmembrane transport of calcium ions in a variety of tissues. They differ from each other in their chemical structure, their mechanisms of action at the cellular level, and their pharmacologic effects. The calcium blockers have powerful but different effects on various subcomponents in the cardiovascular system. The net effect seen with each drug is dependent on the results of a

Table 6–8. Side Effects of Antianginal Drugs*

Drug	Frequency of Side Effects†	Flushing Headache, Hypotension	CHF‡	Bradycardia, Heart Block	Constipation	Peripheral Edema
Nitrates	—§	+ + +‖	0	0	0	0
Beta blockers	—§	0	+ + +	+ + +‖	+	0
Nifedipine	9–39	+ + +	0	0	+	+ + +
Verapamil	10–14	+	+ +	+ +	+ + +	+
Diltiazem	0–3	+	+	+	+	+

*The number of + signs indicates the relative magnitude of the effect.
†Percentage of patients developing side effects.
‡CHF, congestive heart failure.
‖In patients with sick sinus or conduction system disease.
§Often pushed to tolerance.

complex interaction between its peripheral and central effects. These drugs have contributed substantially to the management of patients with angina. They may be used either in combination with nitrates and beta blockers or as substitutes for beta blockers when the patient is unable to tolerate beta blockers or nitrates. Nifedipine may be employed to decrease blood pressure. Verapamil may be used to decrease contractility as well as blood pressure and heart rate. When combined with a beta blocker, diltiazem may be the drug of choice because of the low incidence of adverse effects. Side effects of the antianginal drugs are summarized in Table 6–8. Medical therapy must be tailored to the individual patient. Because of side ef-

fects, the choice of beta blocker or calcium channel blocker must take into account underlying medical conditions (Table 6–9). In patients with mixed angina, calcium blockers are usually preferred to beta blockers, but often patients receive triple therapy (combination of nitrates, beta blockers, and calcium blockers). The advantage to triple therapy is that additive effects may cause better relief of symptoms than less aggressive therapy. The obvious disadvantages are the difficulty in taking multiple medications, the potential for adverse effects, and the expense.

Either medical or surgical therapy of patients with stable angina is costly. Although revascularization procedures are expensive,

Table 6–9. Selection of Beta Blocker or Calcium Channel Blocker in Patients with Angina and Other Conditions*

Clinical Condition	Beta Blocker			Calcium Channel Blocker		
	Nonselective	Selective	ISA	Nifedipine	Verapamil	Diltiazem
Systemic hypertension	+	+	+	A	A	A
Asthma/bronchospasm		A†	A†	+	+	+
Claudication		A	A	+	A	A
Insulin-requiring diabetes		A†	A†	+	+	+
Mental depression				+	+	+
Arrhythmias and conduction abnormalities						
Sinus bradycardia			A	+		
Sinus tachycardia	+	+				
Supraventricular tachycardia			A		+	
Rapid atrial fibrillation	+	+			+	
Ventricular arrhythmias	+	+	+			
Atrioventricular conduction delay			A	+		
Left ventricular dysfunction						
No overt heart failure						
Mild to moderate	+ †	+ †	+ †	+ †	+ †	
Severe				+ †		
Overt heart failure				+ †		
Aortic/mitral regurgitation				+		

*Symbols: + = drug of choice; A = alternative; † = low dose with caution. ISA = intrinsic sympathomimetic activity.

long-term medical therapy, particularly when numerous laboratory tests are added, take a tremendous toll on societal and personal resources. It must be emphasized that even when patients undergo revascularization procedures, risk factor control and medical therapy may continue to be necessary because these procedures are palliative and not curative. Antiplatelet therapy, particularly aspirin, is highly recommended after revascularization. With appropriately aggressive management, which includes risk factor modification, multiple medications (short- and long-acting nitrates, beta blockers, and calcium blockers), and revascularization procedures (PTCA and CABG) when indicated, the majority of individuals with stable angina may enjoy productive and relatively angina-free lives.

Bibliography

Abrams J. Nitroglycerin and long-acting nitrates in clinical practice. Am J Med 74:85–94, 1983.
Gives insights into the use of nitrates in patients with ischemic heart disease.

CASS Principal Investigators and Their Associates. Coronary Artery Surgery Study (CASS): a randomized trial of coronary artery bypass surgery. Comparability of entry characteristics and survival in randomized patients and non-randomized patients meeting randomization criteria. J Am Coll Cardiol 3:114–128, 1984.
Presents data from a large prospective randomized trial comparing medical with surgical therapy in patients with stable angina.

European Coronary Surgery Study Group. Long-term results of prospective randomized study of coronary artery bypass surgery in stable angina pectoris. Lancet 2:1173–1180, 1982.
Presents results from one of three large prospective randomized trials comparing medical with surgical therapy in patients with stable angina.

Friesinger GC. The reasonable workup before recommending medical or surgical therapy: an overall strategy. Circulation 65(Suppl II):21–26, 1982.
Gives a rational approach to the work-up of patients, dependent on multiple factors including symptoms, extent of anatomic disease, objective evidence of ischemia, extent of left ventricular dysfunction, and recent intercurrent ischemic events.

Frishman WH. Multifactorial actions of beta-adrenergic blocking drugs in ischemic heart disease: current concepts. Circulation 67(Suppl I):11–18, 1983.
Provides insights into the use of beta blockers in patients with ischemic heart disease.

Froelicher VF. Exercise testing as part of the reasonable workup before recommending medical or surgical therapy for coronary heart disease. Circulation 65(Suppl II):15–20, 1982.
Emphasizes the role of exercise testing in decision-making.

Goldman L, Lee TH. Noninvasive tests for diagnosing the presence and extent of coronary artery disease: exercise electrocardiography, thallium scintigraphy, and radionuclide ventriculography. J Gen Intern Med 1:258–265, 1986.
Concentrates on the use of noninvasive testing for diagnosis and prognosis.

Goldschlager N, Sox H. The diagnostic and prognostic value of the treadmill exercise test in the evaluation of chest pain, in patients with recent myocardial infarction, and in asymptomatic individuals. Am Heart J 116:523–535, 1988.
Includes a useful table on the prognosis in patients with particular exercise test results as part of a well-written review.

Mark DB, Hlatky MD, Harrell FE, et al. Exercise treadmill score for predicting prognosis in coronary artery disease. Ann Intern Med 106:793–800, 1987.
Emphasizes the role of exercise testing in decision-making.

Peduzzi P, Hultgren H, Thomsen J, et al. Ten-year effect of medical and surgical therapy on quality of life: Veterans Administration Cooperative Study of Coronary Artery Surgery. Am J Cardiol 59:1017–1023, 1987.
Provides data from one of the three large prospective randomized trials comparing medical with surgical therapy in patients with stable angina.

Plotnick GD. Approach to the management of unstable angina. Am Heart J 98:243–255, 1979.
Summarizes a rational approach to the management of the patient with unstable angina.

Plotnick GD. Unstable Angina—A Clinical Approach. Mt. Kisco, NY, Futura Publishing Company, 1985.
Describes a rational approach to the management of the patient with unstable angina.

Plotnick GD. Coronary artery bypass to prolong life? Less anatomy/more physiology. J Am Coll Cardiol 8:749–751, 1986.
Summarizes results from the three major large prospective randomized trials comparing medical with surgical therapy that document the value of noninvasive predictors of risk in identifying patients most likely to have life prolonged with coronary artery bypass surgery.

Robertson WS, Feigenbaum H, Armstrong WF, et al. Exercise echocardiography: a clinically practical addition in the evaluation of coronary artery disease. J Am Coll Cardiol 2:1085–1091, 1983.
Evaluates newer methods of exercise testing in an attempt to improve diagostic capability.

Silverman KJ, Grossman W. Angina pectoris. Natural history and strategies for evaluation and management. N Engl J Med 310:1712–1717, 1984.
Outlines strategies for evaluation of patients with chronic angina, unstable angina, and variant angina.

Zelis RF. Calcium entry blockers in cardiologic therapy. Hosp Pract 16:49–56, 1981.
Describes the use of calcium channel blockers in patients with ischemic heart disease.

7

Management of Ventricular Premature Complexes

STEVEN P. KUTALEK, M.D.
JOEL MORGANROTH, M.D.

The problem of sudden death is one of profound social, personal, and economic impact. It remains the most common cause of death in the population group from 20 to 64 years of age and continues to account for more than 400,000 deaths per year in the United States.

Mobile medical intensive care units have had some impact in improving chances for survival at the time of a sudden death episode. The most successful programs can resuscitate one third of all patients whose cardiac arrest is witnessed; however, this group constitutes only half of all patients who die suddenly. In the best of circumstances, therefore, 80 to 90% of patients die before reaching the hospital, even with community-wide dedication to a rescue squad program that supplies care rapidly.

Although such resources provide some degree of protection against sudden death, they cannot be relied on to produce a major decrease in mortality. Identification of patients likely to succumb to sudden death episodes, coupled with effective prophylactic measures directed toward those individuals, seems to be a more reasonable course.

Compiled studies of patients who fortuitously wore Holter monitors at the time of their sudden death episodes demonstrate that at least 80% succumb to a ventricular tachyarrhythmia, which leads to terminal ventricular fibrillation. The remaining 20% succumb to bradyarrhythmia, usually a heart block or sinus arrest with an associated junctional or idioventricular escape rhythm, leading to asystole. These episodes may be due to coronary ischemia; the frequency of ST segment changes is higher in this group of patients than in those who develop tachyarrhythmias. Attempts to resuscitate the individuals with bradyarrhythmias are frequently unsuccessful.

The Patient at Risk of Sudden Death

Before prophylactic measures can be applied in attempts to diminish the risk of sudden death for individual patients, groups at highest risk must be identified. For a large number of patients, this involves determining who is prone to myocardial infarction, with its attendant sudden death risk. These patients manifest electric disease secondary to acute *ischemic* myocardial injury.

An equally large group of patients dies suddenly as the result of ventricular tachyarrhythmia in a chronic, *nonischemic* setting. This group comprises individuals with myocardial scarring from prior infarction as well as those with dilated and hypertrophic cardiomyopathies from a number of etiologies. Although anatomic studies demonstrate that, even in this group, significant coronary artery disease is present in up to 80% of sudden death victims, it is important to recognize that ventricular arrhythmias in these patients are not acutely ischemic in origin. Rather, they originate in areas of previously scarred myocardium.

Individuals with dilated cardiomyopathies and congestive heart failure have high mortality rates; 40 to 50% die of ventricular tachyarrhythmias. Likewise, of patients who have survived a myocardial infarction, half of the 10% who succumb in the first year die suddenly. The unifying trait in all of these patients with cardiac arrhythmias is the existence of multicellular islands of myocardial fibrosis that enable the formation of slowly conducting pathways; in the appropriate metabolic and electric settings, these situations lead to micro–re-entry and ventricular tachycardia or fibrillation.

Not all individuals with chronic ventricular premature complexes (VPCs) are at equal risk for sudden death (Table 7–1). Identifying those at increased risk involves a determination of the degree of electric instability by using a 24-hour Holter monitor, as well as an elucidation of the extent of myocardial dysfunction via echocardiography or radionuclide angiography.

It is important to understand available data describing the manner in which VPCs relate to sudden death in various population groups.

Approach to the Patient

A large number of patients arrive at the physician's office with palpitations. Although the patient's medical history (rate, regularity, and duration of palpitations) and physical examination (premature beats or other abnormalities seen during cardiac examination) may suggest particular arrhythmias, 24-hour ambulatory monitoring remains the best noninvasive technique for diagnosing the frequency, type, and severity of cardiac arrhythmias. In patients with infrequent symptoms, event monitors may also be useful.

Rare, brief palpitations in patients who are otherwise healthy and have a normal cardiovascular physical examination may be dismissed without further diagnostic work-up. Patients with more significant symptoms potentially related to arrhythmia, such as frequent or prolonged palpitations, associated lightheadedness, syncope, shortness of breath, or chest pain, should be approached more aggressively and have ambulatory 24-hour monitoring. Patients with symptoms suggesting arrhythmia concomitant with a family history of sudden death require a thorough work-up, especially if these patients have mitral valve prolapse or hypertrophic cardiomyopathy. In these two last groups, studies should begin with ambulatory monitoring plus an assessment of left ventricular (LV) function and may proceed to electrophysiologic testing if symptoms or documented arrhythmias are especially severe.

In patients with asymptomatic or minimally symptomatic ventricular ectopy, the most important factor to consider is the extent of LV contractile abnormality. Those who have clinical evidence of ventricular dysfunction should have ambulatory 24-hour monitoring. Clinical indicators of LV dysfunction include dyspnea, heart failure, murmurs, or evidence of cardiomyopathy at the physical examination. Resting electrocardiographic abnormalities may also be associated with LV contractile disorders; such electrocardiographic findings include left ventricular hypertrophy, intraventricular conduction defects, bundle branch blocks, infarctions, or ST-T abnormalities. Patients with resting electrocardiographic ST-T wave abnormalities, frequent VPCs, and mitral valve prolapse, for example, are at increased risk of sudden death.

Clinical evidence for LV dysfunction can easily be substantiated by two-dimensional echocardiography or radionuclide angiography. The nuclear study has the advantage of providing a quantitative determination of LV ejection fraction (LVEF).

Ambulatory 24-hour monitoring of patients with documented LV dysfunction and evidence of VPCs or symptoms suggestive of ventricular arrhythmias allows stratification of risk for sudden arrhythmic death. After myocardial infarction, all patients should have Holter monitoring when they are not administered antiarrhythmic agents (at least 10 to 14 days after infarction) and an assessment of LV function, because risk stratification by these techniques has its greatest validity in this population group. Diuretic-induced hypokalemia and theophylline derivatives may exacerbate ventricular ectopy; these factors should be considered before using a basal 24-hour monitor for risk stratification.

Frequent VPCs and LV dysfunction are independent predictors of sudden death, apart from the presence of ischemia. The presence of coronary artery disease per se does not increase the risk from VPCs unless associated with active ischemia, significant wall motion abnormalities, or a depressed LVEF. Active ischemia, manifested by angina or ST depression, may itself generate arrhythmias; the clinical approach in these patients should be to lessen the frequency and intensity of ischemia rather than to administer antiarrhythmic agents.

Exercise testing should be considered for chronic ventricular arrhythmia patients with clinical evidence of coronary artery disease and active ischemia, whether detected by history, physical examination, or electrocardiogram (ECG). Exercise testing should be cautiously performed in patients with frequent nonsus-

Table 7-1. Classification of Ventricular Arrhythmias*

	Benign	Potentially Lethal	Lethal
Sudden death risk	Very low	Moderate	High
VPC frequency	≤ 5/h (normal population) > 5/h and/or NSVT (primary electrical disease)	≥ 10 VPC/h and/or NSVT	SUVT, VF, or hemodynamically compromising NSVT
LV function	Normal†	Moderately depressed‡	Severely depressed‡
Symptoms	None or palpitations (usually none)	None or palpitations (usually none)	Syncope, CHF, or angina
Need for therapy	No (unless symptomatic)	Unknown (unless symptomatic)	Yes (to prevent SCD)
Therapeutic guide	Holter	Holter	EPS
Antiarrhythmic agents§	II → IC (if symptomatic)	IC → IA → IB → IA + IB	IA → IA + IB → IC → III

*Abbreviations: CHF, congestive heart failure; EPS, electrophysiologic study; LVEF, left ventricular ejection fraction; NSVT, nonsustained ventricular tachycardia; SCD, sudden cardiac death; SUVT, sustained ventricular tachycardia; VF, ventricular fibrillation; VPC, ventricular premature complex.
†Includes patients with chronic arrhythmias and no LV dysfunction. Patients may have coronary artery disease with no active ischemia.
‡Depressed LV function may be on the basis of prior myocardial infarction or cardiomyopathy from other etiologies.
§By modified Vaughan-Williams classification.

tained ventricular tachycardia (NSVT). The use of thallium imaging will improve the predictive accuracy of exercise testing for the diagnosis of atherosclerotic disease.

Patients who have symptoms suggesting exercise-induced arrhythmia should undergo stress testing. This can often provide a diagnosis of abnormal rhythm and can guide antiarrhythmic therapy. Suppression of exercise-induced ventricular tachycardia or symptomatic NSVT suggests an improved prognosis.

Ventricular Arrhythmias: Risk Stratification for Sudden Death

Benign Ventricular Arrhythmias

Patients with no underlying structural cardiac disease but who have VPCs (Fig. 7–1) with or without ventricular couplets or NSVT (less than 30 seconds long) (Fig. 7–2) are considered to have benign ventricular arrhythmias provided that the ectopy does not compromise the patient hemodynamically.

The patients with benign arrhythmias can be categorized into two groups, the normal population and those with benign primary electric disease. In the normal group, the frequency of VPCs, as detected by 24-hour ambulatory (Holter) monitoring, remains very low, i.e., less than 100 VPCs in 24 hours, or fewer than 5 VPCs per hour. Complex forms, namely, ventricular couplets or short episodes of NSVT, are absent. VPC frequency tends to increase gradually with age. The risk of sudden

death in these individuals is exceedingly small; no definitive antiarrhythmic therapy is required.

Other patients with no evident structural heart disease have more than five VPCs per hour and may have complex forms shown by the 24-hour Holter monitor, including ventricular couplets and NSVT without hemodynamic compromise. These patients may be considered to have benign ventricular arrhythmias or primary electrical heart disease. Although VPC frequency remains higher than that anticipated in the normal population, these individuals also have a very low incidence of sudden death. In one study, 73 asymptomatic, healthy patients were followed for a mean of 6.5 years. All had frequent VPCs (a mean of 566 per hour), 60% had ventricular couplets, and 26% had NSVT. The prognosis for the group was similar to that for the "normal" population.

Lethal Ventricular Arrhythmias

Lethal ventricular arrhythmias include those with distinct malignant potential, such as sustained ventricular tachycardia or ventricular fibrillation. Ventricular tachycardia may be recurrent and monomorphic or may progress and degenerate to ventricular fibrillation. The principal characteristic of these arrhythmias involves the potential for hemodynamic compromise or collapse, leading to syncope, exacerbation of angina or congestive heart failure, or outright sudden death. NSVTs (less than 30 seconds long), which compromise the

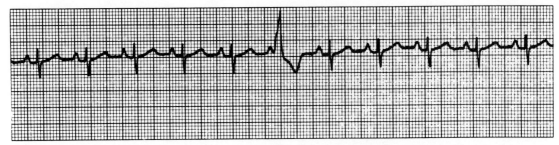

Figure 7–1. *Sinus rhythm punctuated by a single VPC. The surface electrocardiographic characteristics of VPCs may be variable, but VPCs are usually wider than normally conducted QRS complexes and have a different morphology. Because VPCs often do not conduct in a retrograde manner through the atrioventricular node, they are frequently followed by a compensatory pause; the RR interval between the QRS complexes before and after a VPC is equal to twice that during sinus rhythm.*

patient hemodynamically, must also be considered lethal arrhythmias.

Lethal arrhythmias are the most likely to result in sudden death. Survivors of these arrhythmias who remain untreated, when the arrhythmias are not associated with acute myocardial ischemia or infarction, have a 1-year sudden death recurrence rate of 25 to 30%.

It is important to distinguish malignant arrhythmic events that occur in association with acute myocardial infarction or cardiac surgery (within 72 hours) from those that occur in a chronic setting. Although suppression of sustained arrhythmias is justified in the immediate postinfarction or perioperative period to maintain hemodynamic stability, the occurrence of such arrhythmias in the acute setting bears little relation to subsequent cardiac arrests in the chronic state.

The onset of hemodynamically compromising ventricular arrhythmias in patients in the chronic setting, however, either long after infarction or in association with congestive cardiomyopathy, is particularly serious. Most of these individuals have significant basal depression of LVEF, often to less than 30%. This itself may lead to complicating factors of increased end diastolic pressure, congestive heart failure, recurrent ischemia, and metabolic abnormalities (particularly hypokalemia associated with diuretic therapy). Basal catecholamine levels are generally elevated. Each of these factors may exacerbate the tendency to re-entrant sustained arrhythmias and must be controlled diligently to minimize the propensity for recurrent sudden death episodes. Nevertheless, even with careful management of congestive heart failure and angina, patients who have once developed a sustained ventricular arrhythmia in the chronic setting are likely to have a recurrence if antiarrhythmic therapy is not initiated.

These patients are best managed by using invasive cardiac electrophysiologic testing. Because sudden death episodes may occur infrequently (and only one is necessary to cause a patient's demise) and because the absolute frequency of VPCs and NSVT discovered by ambulatory monitoring does not necessarily correlate with the likelihood of sudden death recurrence, provocative testing through endocardial programmed electrical stimulation remains the preferred technique to guide therapy for patients with lethal ventricular arrhythmias.

Electrophysiologic Testing

Because this procedure involves special equipment and expertise, its use has generally

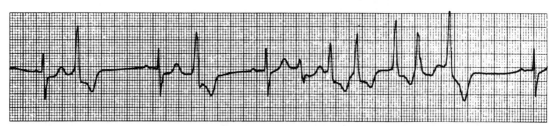

Figure 7–2. *Underlying sinus rhythm with VPCs in a bigeminal pattern, followed by polymorphic NSVT of six complexes in duration. NSVT on an ambulatory ECG is defined as three sequential ventricular complexes at a rate greater than 120 per minute.*

been confined to tertiary care referral centers having a relatively high number of patients with malignant arrhythmias. A basal electrophysiologic examination is performed after stabilization of congestive heart failure, angina, and electrolyte and metabolic disturbances, and after stopping all antiarrhythmic agents for at least five half-lives. Antiarrhythmic drugs are discontinued before the study, first so that induced arrhythmias may be contrasted to those subsequently initiated (or not initiated) during medical therapy, and second because some sustained arrhythmias occur as the result of proarrhythmic (arrhythmia-exacerbating) effects from agents initially administered for NSVT or frequent isolated VPCs.

Ventricular stimulation includes rapid ventricular pacing and the introduction of ventricular extrastimuli (one, two, or three) during sinus rhythm and with ventricular pacing at various right and left ventricular sites. The goal is to reproduce the patient's clinical arrhythmia in terms of heart rate and morphology with as specific an induction mode as possible (Fig. 7–3). In 3 to 5% of patients with recurrent sustained ventricular tachycardia, the basal arrhythmia cannot be initiated by programmed stimulation, which necessitates empiric therapy.

After initiation and termination of the basal arrhythmia in the electrophysiology laboratory, oral antiarrhythmic agents may be administered, either singly or in combination, and programmed stimulation may be repeated after achieving a steady state. Effective suppression of induction by medication has a predictive value of over 90% for preventing sustained monomorphic ventricular tachycardia and is clearly the preferred technique for guiding therapy in these patients. Although electrophysiologically directed medical therapy has not been as successful for polymorphic ventricular tachycardia or for ventricular fibrillation, serial drug testing can reduce the incidence of recurrent sudden cardiac death even in these groups. In individuals in whom adequate suppression cannot be achieved with antiarrhythmic agents, electrophysiologic testing can guide the use of alternative modes of therapy, including antitachycardia pacing, endocardial mapping for surgical resection of the ventricular tachycardia focus, ablative techniques, or implantation of a defibrillator.

Potentially Lethal Ventricular Arrhythmias

Sustained ventricular tachyarrhythmias and hemodynamically compromising NSVT, despite their malignant potential, constitute only about 5% of all ventricular arrhythmias seen in the general population. By far the largest group of patients with ventricular ectopy, about two thirds, falls into the category of potentially lethal arrhythmias. These individuals have some degree of basal myocardial dysfunction, either because of ischemic cardio-

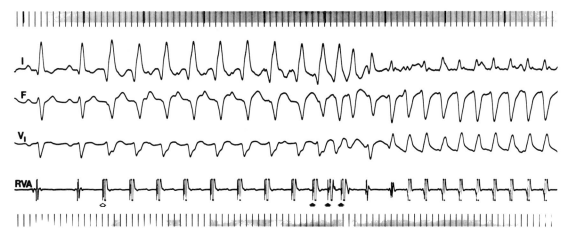

Figure 7–3. Induction of sustained ventricular tachycardia through programmed ventricular stimulation. Two sinus complexes are followed by an eight-beat drive train of ventricular pacing, the first pacing complex indicated by the open arrow. Three premature extrastimuli (filled arrows) are introduced, which initiates rapid, sustained, monomorphic ventricular tachycardia. Surface electrocardiographic leads I, aVF, and V₁ are depicted, as is an intracardiac endocardial right ventricular apical recording (RVA). Major time line divisions represent 1 second; intermediate time line divisions each represent 100 ms.

vascular disease and prior myocardial infarction or because of congestive cardiomyopathy. LVEF is reduced, but generally to a lesser degree than in patients with lethal arrhythmias. Most of these patients have angiographically demonstrable coronary artery disease.

In untreated patients with a depressed LVEF of less than 40%, the presence of 10 or more VPCs per hour or even a single ventricular triplet recorded by a 24-hour Holter monitor (Fig. 7–2) correlates with a three-fold increase in risk of sudden death (from about 8 to 25%) in the first year after myocardial infarction. Rates of sudden death are similar for those with congestive cardiomyopathy but increase as LVEF diminishes. Thus, such arrhythmias in these patient groups may be termed potentially lethal because they predict an increased incidence of sudden death in the group as a whole.

Although VPC frequency is increased in this group, patients remain hemodynamically stable. They may be aware of frequent VPCs or episodes of NSVT by the occurrence of palpitations or occasional dizziness, but they have no associated syncope. Most individuals are in fact unaware of the presence of ventricular ectopy even if it is very frequent.

It is currently not possible to identify which patients within this group will develop a sustained arrhythmia. No controlled trials have yet established the validity of electrophysiologic testing in predicting sudden death in these patients. Thus, to ensure treatment of potential sudden death victims, many physicians advocate directing therapy toward the entire group of patients with potentially lethal arrhythmias despite the attendant potential toxicities of antiarrhythmic agents. Medical therapy for these individuals is best guided by the use of noninvasive Holter monitoring.

Overall ventricular ectopy is more common in patients with mitral valve prolapse than in those with normal mitral valve function. Fifty to 60% of patients with prolapse manifest frequent VPCs on ambulatory monitoring, many with associated ventricular couplets or NSVT. Arrhythmia complexity does not appear to correlate with the degree of regurgitation or mitral prolapse. The likelihood of sudden death, although somewhat increased in this population, remains low. Identifying patients at increased risk is nevertheless difficult. Those with the most frequent VPCs and NSVT seem to be at highest risk for the development of a sustained ventricular arrhythmia, especially if they have associated ST-T wave abnormalities on their resting ECG. The predictive role of electrophysiologic testing is not well defined in this group, although such testing can be useful to direct antiarrhythmic therapy in patients with a prolapse who have symptomatic or sustained arrhythmias.

Ambulatory ECG Monitoring

Twenty-four-hour Holter monitoring provides an accurate and reproducible method of quantifying basal ventricular ectopy, in terms of both the number of VPCs and the presence of NSVT. It should be performed in patients with structural heart disease, particularly after myocardial infarction, to enable risk stratification into benign and potentially lethal groups. A single 24-hour monitoring period is generally sufficient to exclude or demonstrate the presence of significant ventricular ectopy. VPC frequency is determined as the mean number of complexes per hour. Forty-eight-hour monitoring increases sensitivity for the detection of infrequent arrhythmias but is rarely clinically necessary.

If VPC frequency is low (fewer than 10 per hour) and there is no NSVT, no antiarrhythmic therapy is indicated, even in the presence of depressed LV function.

On the other hand, with a VPC frequency of 10 or more per hour or with NSVT, the decision to proceed with treatment is based on the presence of LV dysfunction. Those *with* LV dysfunction (LVEF <40% or significant regional wall motion abnormalities) *and* such arrhythmias have a significantly increased risk of sudden death. However, it is unknown whether antiarrhythmic therapy will decrease the risk of sudden death. No firm recommendations on treatment can be given until clinical trials have demonstrated conclusively that such treatment does in fact prevent sudden arrhythmic death.

Finally, those patients with NSVT and/or frequent VPCs in the absence of significant LV dysfunction (i.e., LVEF > 40% and no significant regional wall motion abnormalities) should not be treated unless they are symptomatic. Attempts at antiarrhythmic therapy in these individuals are likely to result in a low benefit/risk ratio because their sudden death rates are quite low.

The presence of multiformed VPCs does not itself increase the risk of sustained arrhythmia; VPC frequency and NSVT remain the more important variables. Similarly, R-on-T VPCs

Table 7–2. Definitions of Proarrhythmia for Ventricular Arrhythmias

1. A new arrhythmia
   a. NSVT
   b. Sustained ventricular tachycardia
   c. Torsades de pointes
   d. Ventricular fibrillation
2. Increase in VPC frequency (by Holter monitor)
   a. VPCs:

MEAN VPC/H AT BASELINE	INCREASE REQUIRED FOR PROARRHYTHMIA
1–50	10×
51–100	5×
101–300	4×
>301	3×

   b. NSVT: ≥ 10× increase in mean hourly frequency of NSVT beats
3. Significantly more difficult termination of ventricular tachyarrhythmia

These events are considered proarrhythmic if they occur:
1. More than 72 h after myocardial infarction and
2. Within 30 days of receiving the same daily dosage of antiarrhythmic medication and
3. Unrelated to inciting events such as hypokalemia or acute myocardial ischemia

Adapted from Morganroth J, Borland M, Chao G. Am J Cardiol 59:97, 1987, with permission.

add little to the risk of sudden death except in patients with a significantly prolonged basal QT interval. Multiformed and R-on-T VPCs are often present when overall VPC frequency is high.

After a decision is made to treat the patient with potentially lethal arrhythmias, a 75 to 80% reduction in total VPC count is required on a 24-hour Holter monitor before drug efficacy can be assumed because of spontaneous day-to-day variability in VPC frequency. Also required to define drug efficacy is a 90 to 100% reduction in NSVT. If therapy with one agent fails to effect these changes, a change to an entirely new agent is necessary or another antiarrhythmic medication should be added to the first for combination therapy.

Because proarrhythmic effects of antiarrhythmic drugs may be asymptomatic, Holter monitoring should be repeated after achieving steady-state to be certain that such adverse proarrhythmic events have not occurred, even if the patient is otherwise apparently doing well on the therapy (Table 7–2).

Practical Considerations Regarding Therapy

The benefit of antiarrhythmic therapy must be weighed against its potential toxicity. Any antiarrhythmic medication (Table 7–3) may result in substantial side effects and could produce a significant systemic adverse reaction. Moreover, some 10% of patients administered any antiarrhythmic agent experience a worsening of their basal arrhythmia (proarrhythmia). This effect may range from an increase in VPC frequency to the development of a new sustained ventricular tachyarrhythmia.

Decisions regarding antiarrhythmic therapy involve two aspects: (1) whether to treat the patient and (2) which agent to use. Deciding whether treatment is indicated for an individual patient should be based on risk stratification for sudden death, i.e., how likely will the underlying ventricular ectopy lead to the development of a malignant ventricular arrhythmia?

Patients with benign arrhythmias do not require therapy because they are at minimal risk for sudden death. Reassurance or anxiolytic agents may be useful; however, individuals with frequent palpitations may feel more comfortable if VPC frequency is substantially reduced. This can often be accomplished by titrating doses of beta-adrenergic blockers or by initiating therapy with a class IC antiarrhythmic medication such as flecainide or encainide. These IC drugs are potent agents for the suppression of VPCs and NSVT (Table 7–4) and rarely cause organ toxicity with prolonged use. Proarrhythmic effects are not increased in patients with normal ventricles, nor is the negative inotropic effect of flecainide significant in these individuals.

Patients with potentially lethal arrhythmias manifest some degree of LV dysfunction. The indication for antiarrhythmic therapy in this group of patients is currently unclear; the Cardiac Arrhythmic Suppression Trial (CAST) being conducted by the National Institutes of Health intends to define whether suppression of VPCs and NSVT in this group of patients will indeed prevent sudden death. We prefer to follow an algorithm for selecting drugs that maximize VPC suppression with a minimal risk of toxicity, usually beginning therapy with a IC antiarrhythmic agent such as flecainide or encainide because most of these patients have already received a beta-blocking agent. If these drugs fail to suppress VPCs or NSVT adequately, we then consider the use of a class IA medication, or combinations of IA + IB drugs, with the understanding that these IA and IB agents carry a higher risk of organ toxicity than do the IC drugs, as well as a lower likelihood of successful arrhythmia

Table 7–3. *Antiarrhythmic Drug Classification (Modified Vaughan-Williams)*

Class	Description		Examples
I	Sodium channel blockers **Phase 0 Depression**	**Repolarization Effects**	
IA	Moderate	Lengthen	Procainamide, quinidine, disopyramide
IB	Weak	Shorten	Lidocaine, tocainide, mexiletine
IC	Strong	Minimal	Flecainide, encainide, indecainide
I (unclassified)			Propafenone,* moricizine, pirmenol, cibenzoline
II	Beta blockers		Propranolol, acebutalol
III	Prolong repolarization		Amiodarone, sotalol,* bretylium
IV	Calcium channel blockers		Diltiazem, verapamil

*Also has beta-blocking effects.

suppression. Until the results of CAST are available, it is unknown whether one should treat patients who have potentially lethal arrhythmias in the hope that some sudden death episodes could be averted. Nevertheless, one should not hesitate to discontinue therapy if intolerable side effects or organ toxicity occurs.

Flecainide and disopyramide should be used cautiously in patients with significant reduction in LVEF ($< 30\%$) and are best avoided entirely in patients with ejection fractions less than 20% or in association with class III or IV congestive heart failure symptoms because of the drugs' negative inotropic effects.

Patients with severe or symptomatic LV dysfunction should have any antiarrhythmic therapy initiated on an inpatient basis, as should those with bifascicular block, pronounced intraventricular conduction delay (QRS > 0.16 seconds), or significant atrioventricular nodal dysfunction such as recurrent Mobitz I atrioventricular block. Persons with atrial fibrillation who are to receive quinidine should also have the drug started as inpatients.

Table 7–4. *Efficacy of Antiarrhythmic Agents for Ventricular Arrhythmias (% of Patients Responding)*

Class of Drug	Benign or Potentially Lethal Arrhythmias (Holter Monitoring)*	Lethal Arrhythmias (Electrophysiologic Testing)†
IA	50–70	20–25
IB	40–50	10–20
IC	80–90	20–30
II	40–60	5–10
III	N/A‡	20–30

*≥ 75% reduction in VPC frequency.
†Prevention of the induction of sustained ventricular tachycardia.
‡N/A, not applicable.

Patients without significant congestive heart failure, baseline conduction defects, or sick sinus syndrome can usually safely start the drug as outpatients.

In patients with lethal ventricular arrhythmias, management is best guided by an electrophysiologic approach. These individuals are often concomitantly receiving many potentially toxic agents and, because little differential efficacy exists among the antiarrhythmic drug classes, we tend to use first the traditional class IA drugs followed by combinations of class IA + IB medications for this group. We reserve the class IC agents for later use because they are more likely to be proarrhythmic in these patients and cause significant LV dysfunction and lethal arrhythmias (proarrhythmia rates of 15 to 20% are expected in this group). We use amiodarone last because it is an effective but highly toxic agent that is indicated for the treatment of lethal ventricular arrhythmias only when all other agents have failed.

Therapy for lethal arrhythmias guided by electrophysiologic testing improves survival and decreases the recurrence of arrhythmia. For patients who do not respond to all reasonable antiarrhythmia agents, options of implantable defibrillators and investigational antitachycardia pacemakers are now available.

Summary

Despite their frequent occurrence, VPCs require therapy only when LV dysfunction is present. Ventricular arrhythmias need to be classified into benign, potentially lethal, and lethal categories to guide the decisions about whether treatment is indicated and which antiarrhythmic agent should be administered. Although patients with benign arrhythmias should be treated only if symptomatic (Fig. 7–4A), therapy is mandatory for patients with lethal ventricular arrhythmias (Fig. 7–4B). Indications for treatment among patients with potentially lethal arrhythmias remain unclear (Fig. 7–4A).

Decisions regarding the choice of antiarrhythmic drugs must be based on a risk/benefit assessment of the utility of therapy with respect to the type of arrhythmia and the degree of LV dysfunction, i.e., how likely is the arrhythmia a marker for the occurrence for sudden death and how toxic are the available medications? Therapy for benign and potentially lethal arrhythmias should begin with class IC or II drugs, which have low toxicity, and should proceed to class IA or IB agents if necessary. Patients with lethal arrhythmias may be initially approached with class IA medications or combinations of class IA and IB drugs, with progression to class IC agents if the other drugs are not successful. Class III medications should be reserved for patients with lethal arrhythmias when other agents have failed.

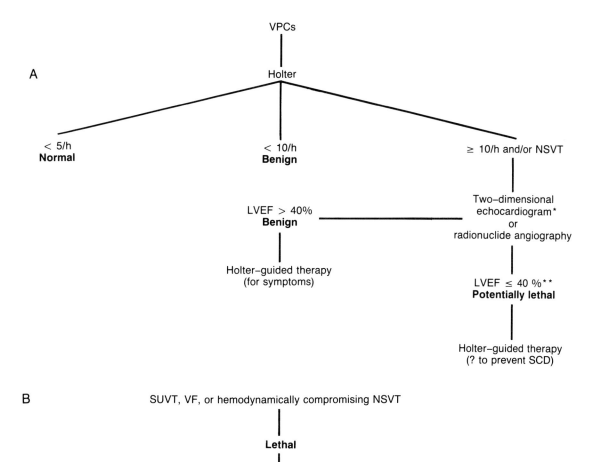

Figure 7–4. Schematic representation of the approach to ventricular arrhythmias. EPS, electrophysiologic testing; LVEF, left ventricular ejection fraction; NSVT, nonsustained ventricular tachycardia; VF, ventricular fibrillation; VPC, ventricular premature complexes; SUVT, sustained ventricular tachycardia; SCD, sudden cardiac death. *Assessment may begin with two-dimensional echocardiography or radionuclide angiography in patients with asymptomatic or minimally symptomatic VPCs and then may proceed to Holter monitoring if LVEF is less than 40% or if significant regional LV wall motion abnormalities are present. **Depressed LVEF may be due to prior myocardial infarction or cardiomyopathy of other etiologies. Patients with coronary artery disease, no active ischemia, and normal LV function with chronic arrhythmias remain in the benign category.

The potentially lethal subset of patients comprises the largest population of individuals with ventricular arrhythmias, yet indications for antiarrhythmic therapy in this group are the least well defined. Prospective trials are under way to establish common protocols for the use of antiarrhythmic agents in these patients.

References

Bigger JT Jr, Weld FM, Rolinitsky MS. Prevalence of characteristics and significance of ventricular tachycardia (three or more complexes) detected with ambulatory electrocardiographic recordings in the late hospital phase of acute myocardial infarction. Am J Cardiol 48:815–823, 1981.

NSVT recorded on a Holter monitor after myocardial infarction before hospital discharge was associated with a 1-year mortality rate of 38% compared with a 1-year mortality rate of 11.6% in patients without ventricular tachycardia.

Horowitz LN, Josephson ME, Kastor JA. Intracardiac electrophysiologic studies as a method for the optimization of drug therapy in chronic ventricular arrhythmia. Prog Cardiovasc Dis 23:81–98, 1980.

Programmed ventricular stimulation can initiate lethal ventricular arrhythmias and guide therapy.

Kennedy HL, Whitlock JA, Sprague MK, et al. Long-term follow-up of asymptomatic healthy subjects with frequent and complex ventricular ectopy. N Engl J Med 312:193–197, 1985.

A six-year follow up of normal patients with frequent ventricular ectopy showed no increase in mortality.

Kostis JB, McCrone K, Moreyra AE, et al. Premature ventricular complexes in the absence of identifiable heart disease. Circulation 63:1351–1356, 1981.

VPC frequency is low in the absence of identifiable heart disease, with 95% of patients exhibiting fewer than 100 VPCs per 24 hours.

Morganroth J, Michelson EL, Horowitz LN, et al. Limitations of routine long-term electrocardiographic monitoring to assess ventricular ectopic frequency. Circulation 58:408–414, 1978.

A 75 to 80% reduction in VPC frequency is necessary on serial 24-hour Holter monitors to define drug efficacy.

Morganroth J. Ambulatory "Holter" electrocardiography: choice of technologies and clinical uses. Ann Intern Med 102:73–81, 1985.

This discussion provides an analysis of available Holter monitoring systems, their features, detection accuracies, and reliabilities.

Morganroth J. Ambulatory ECG monitoring in the evaluation of new antiarrhythmic drugs. Circulation 73(Suppl II):92–97, 1986.

Holter monitoring can define relative potencies of antiarrhythmic agents for the suppression of potentially lethal arrhythmias.

Morganroth J. Risk factors for the development of proarrhythmic events. Am J Cardiol 59:32E–37E, 1987.

The primary risk factors for proarrhythmia from flecainide and encainide include structural cardiac disease, sustained ventricular tachycardia, and large-dose escalations.

Morganroth J, Borland M, Chao G. Application of a frequency definition of ventricular proarrhythmia. Am J Cardiol 59:97–99, 1987.

A simple algorithm is defined that can delineate proarrhythmic responses despite spontaneous variability in VPC frequency.

Morganroth J, Horowitz LN: Antiarrhythmic drug therapy, 1988: for whom, how, and where? Am J Cardiol 62:461–465, 1988.

This concise editorial review contains guidelines for the treatment of ventricular arrhythmias.

Panidis I, Morganroth J. Sudden death in hospitalized patients: cardiac rhythm disturbances detected by ambulatory electrocardiographic monitoring. J Am Coll Cardiol 2:798–805, 1983.

Most episodes of sudden cardiac death are the result of ventricular tachyarrhythmias.

Vaughan Williams EM. A classification of antiarrhythmic actions reassessed after a decade of new drugs. Clin J Pharmacol 24:129–147, 1984.

This treatise provides a pragmatic classification of antiarrhythmic medications.

8

Management of Patients after Coronary Artery Bypass Surgery

NANETTE K. WENGER, M.D., F.A.C.P., F.A.C.C.

Introduction

Currently, 175,000 to 200,000 patients undergo coronary artery bypass surgery in the United States each year, with a resultant substantial improvement in prognosis, morbidity, and symptomatic status.[1-3] These patients return to their primary care physicians for long-term surveillance and management. Because successful coronary bypass surgery neither cures the underlying coronary atherosclerosis nor significantly alters its progression, the follow-up care of these patients should include (1) identification of individuals at increased risk of recurrent coronary events because of graft narrowing or closure or because of progression of disease in the native circulation; as well as those at increased risk because of ventricular dysfunction or ventricular arrhythmias; and subsequent use of appropriate interventions; (2) modification of the conventional coronary risk factors, designed to limit the progression or induce regression of the residual coronary atherosclerotic lesions; and (3) restoration and maintenance of cardiovascular functional status, with encouragement to resume an active and satisfying lifestyle, including return to work when appropriate.[4, 5]

Assessment of Risk Status and Appropriate Interventions

Evaluation for Ischemia

Patients may be at increased risk of recurrent coronary events owing to recurrent myocardial ischemia related either to narrowing or closure of the bypass graft vessel or to progression of atherosclerosis in the native circulation. Symptoms of chest discomfort, often comparable to those initiating the surgery, may signal the recurrence of myocardial ischemia. Serial exercise testing,[6] with and without radionuclide studies, is indicated even for asymptomatic patients; it can identify earlier the recurrence of myocardial ischemia and define the extent of myocardium in jeopardy. The timing of serial exercise testing should be guided both by the completeness of myocardial revascularization and by the severity of atherosclerotic narrowing of the nonbypassed coronary arteries.

Angina recurred or progressed in about 5% of patients per year after coronary bypass surgery in the Coronary Artery Surgery Study.[7] In that study, although 67% of patients were pain-free 1 year postoperatively, only 54% remained pain-free at 5 years. The most pronounced graft attrition occurs between 6 and 11 years after surgery. A better outcome is described for internal mammary artery bypass grafting,[8, 9] with far less prominent atherosclerosis in these arterial conduits. The characteristics of the ischemic abnormalities at exercise testing—the time of onset, the severity, and the duration of ischemic electrocardiogram (ECG) abnormalities; the association of ECG evidence of ischemia with symptomatic or hemodynamic concomitants of ischemia (inappropriate heart rate or blood pressure response, angina, or arrhythmia at low exercise intensities); and the extent of myocardial ischemia at thallium scintigraphy—help guide the recommendation for medical therapy or the decision to perform coronary arteriography as evaluation for additional myocardial revascularization, either coronary angioplasty or repeat coronary bypass surgery. The latter procedures are indicated for patients with a significant ischemic burden or with failure to respond to medical therapy with nitrate drugs, calcium channel blockers, or beta blockers.

It remains uncertain whether beta-blocker therapy should be continued in patients without clinical evidence of residual ischemia who have had complete myocardial revascularization, when this procedure was performed after myocardial infarction. The improvement in survival after infarction associated with beta-blocker therapy has not been specifically assessed in patients who have had subsequent myocardial revascularization.

A number of therapies have been employed in an attempt to enhance late saphenous vein graft patency and limit or obviate recurrent myocardial ischemia. The predominant drugs used have been the cyclo-oxygenase inhibitors, aspirin and sulfinpyrazone, and the phosphodiesterase inhibitor dipyridamole.[10–12] There has also been interest in using thromboxane A_2 synthetase inhibitors as well as beta adrenergic blocking drugs and calcium channel blockers to limit graft closure.[13–16] In animal models, calcium channel blockers appear to limit coronary atherosclerosis; diltiazem decreased recurrent nonfatal infarctions in patients who had non–Q wave myocardial infarction,[17–20] but studies with postoperative patients are needed. Aspirin at a dosage of 325 mg daily is currently approved by the U.S. Food and Drug Administration (FDA) for the reduction of death and nonfatal reinfarction after unstable angina or myocardial infarction; the FDA has not approved aspirin or dipyridamole after coronary bypass surgery, although variable-dose combinations of both are commonly used.

Evaluation of Left Ventricular Dysfunction and Ventricular Arrhythmias

Patients with significant left ventricular dysfunction are also at increased risk of recurrent coronary events; this feature is more encountered with a prior or perioperative myocardial infarction and, at times, with a history of serious or prolonged elevation of systemic arterial pressure. In patients with clinical evidence of heart failure or with cardiac enlargement on chest x-ray, left ventricular dysfunction can be identified and quantified noninvasively by using rest and exercise radionuclide ventriculography or exercise echocardiography. Patients with left ventricular aneurysm may be considered candidates for aneurysmectomy with or without coronary vascular surgery if there is associated serious arrhythmia, evidence of ischemia, or resulting arterial embolism. The therapy of left ventricular systolic dysfunction involves vasodilator and/or inotropic drugs; anticoagulation should be considered in patients with severe ventricular dysfunction.

Ventricular arrhythmias are more likely to be life-threatening in patients with ischemia or ventricular dysfunction. Diagnostic ambulatory electrocardiography (Holter monitoring) is indicated for patients with residual myocardial ischemia or heart failure; decisions about subsequent antiarrhythmic therapy depend both on the complexity and frequency of the arrhythmias and on the severity of the myocardial ischemia and dysfunction. Although no studies identify an improvement in outcome related to treatment of arrhythmias, i.e., no data document therapeutic benefit, there has been considerable interest in the control of ventricular arrhythmias because they impart increased risk. There is also no evidence that successful coronary bypass surgery (or other myocardial revascularization procedures) decreases the occurrence of arrhythmias that were not precipitated by episodic ischemia.[21–24] Beta-blocker therapy of arrhythmia may worsen the serum lipid levels, whereas lessening of atherosclerosis has been described with calcium-blocker therapy in experimental animals.[18–20] Holter monitoring is not indicated when there is no evidence of myocardial ischemia or dysfunction, or no history of prior serious ventricular arrhythmias.

Alteration of Conventional Coronary Risk Factors

This approach is designed to limit the progression of coronary atherosclerosis or potentially induce regression of the atherosclerotic lesions, both in the bypass graft vessels and in the native circulation. This progression of atherosclerosis limits the benefits of coronary bypass surgery. Progression of coronary atherosclerosis has been documented in about 50% of the nonbypassed coronary arteries in the first decade after surgery, and this process appears to be accentuated in the saphenous vein grafts.[25–27] Only about 60% of the saphenous vein grafts remain patent at repeat angiography 10 to 12 years after coronary bypass surgery[25]; there is less prominent graft closure when the internal mammary artery is used.[28]

A variable relationship has been described

between conventional coronary risk factors and progression or accleration of atherosclerosis in coronary bypass graft vessels.[29–31] The more prominent risk factors that correlate with accelerated atherosclerosis include an elevated serum cholesterol level, cigarette smoking, increased blood pressure, physical inactivity, and elevated blood glucose concentrations.[32, 33] Although an adverse effect of elevated blood lipid levels has not been consistently demonstrated, recent data suggest that lowering an elevated serum cholesterol level by a combination of dietary and drug therapy can decrease atherosclerotic progression in patients with moderate to severe hypercholesterolemia; this has been associated with regression of some atherosclerotic lesions.[34–39]

Recommendations for risk reduction include advice to discontinue cigarette smoking. Hypercholesterolemia should be treated with dietary measures and pharmacotherapy; among the drugs that appear effective are bile acid sequestrants,[38, 39] niacin,[40] fibric acid derivatives,[41] probucol, and the hydroxymethylglutaryl coenzyme A reductase inhibitors.[42] Control of elevated blood pressure is also advised, initially with lifestyle alterations including weight control, sodium restriction, moderate exercise, and the avoidance of excessive alcohol intake, and subsequently with pharmacotherapy. There is concern that thiazide diuretics and beta-blocker drugs used to control hypertension may elevate serum cholesterol levels and negate the beneficial effects of blood pressure control. Weight control or weight reduction, if appropriate, is recommended for risk reduction, as is the institution of a regular exercise regimen; the latter intervention improves functional capacity, enhances weight control, and can increase the high density lipoprotein cholesterol concentration.[5]

Although there is no definitive experimental evidence that any of these interventions can decrease morbidity and mortality, broad-based coronary risk reduction was recommended by the U.S. Consensus Conference. Also, there is no evidence that these components are harmful, their use is rational, and they entail only limited expense and inconvenience.[43]

There is also no evidence that coronary bypass surgery per se encourages modification of coronary risk factors, either as instituted by patients or as recommended by their physicians.[44] For example, in the Coronary Artery Surgery Study,[45, 46] there was a 39% preoperative incidence of cigarette smoking, a 32% incidence of hypercholesterolemia, and a 21%

incidence of obesity. Postoperatively, 32% of patients continued cigarette smoking at 1 year, and this percentage did not change at 5 years. The prevalence of postoperative hypercholesterolemia increased, being present in 40% of patients, as did that of obesity, which was present in 25% of patients postoperatively.

The initial approach to risk intervention should be the provision of appropriate information, followed by encouragement and motivation to adopt healthy behaviors. Training should be provided for the skills needed to implement these favorable behaviors, which must be reinforced by both social support and environmental modification.[5] The primary care physician must continue to be vigilant to ensure maintenance of a favorable risk profile in patients after coronary bypass surgery.

Restoration and Maintenance of Residual Cardiovascular Function, Psychosocial Enhancement, and Motivation for Return to Work

In the European Coronary Surgery Study, exercise training improved the functional capacity of postoperative patients over and above the improvement that occurred as a result of coronary bypass surgery.[2] In general, exercise training is associated with an improvement in functional capacity and psychosocial status, and it appears to aid patients in renouncing the sick role and to encourage a return to work.[5] Control of hypertension, as well as weight reduction, may also improve the capacity for physical work.

The prescription of exercise for the patient who has undergone coronary artery bypass surgery, as for other patients with coronary disease, is based on the results of exercise testing. Sign- or symptom-limited bicycle or treadmill exercise testing can be safely performed as soon as the leg sites of saphenous vein removal are sufficiently healed so that local discomfort does not limit the exercise test; this is often possible before hospital discharge. Exercise testing that is done to determine an exercise prescription or to evaluate the patient for return to work should be performed with the patient receiving all medications that will be taken long term; this recommendation differs markedly from the practice of limiting medications as much as possible during diagnostic exercise testing.

Patients with a good exercise capacity, at

least 6 to 8 mets, and no evidence of myocardial ischemia at exercise testing can be encouraged to return rapidly to preillness activity levels, including sexual activity and remunerative work. The small subset of patients whose occupations require high level physical activity may require exercise training before return to work.

Traditional exercise regimens for coronary patients have included recommendations for physical activity to be performed two or three times weekly on nonsuccessive days, for 30- to 45-minute sessions that include warm-up and cool-down periods, at an exercise intensity (target heart rate range) of 70 to 85% of the highest heart rate safely achieved at exercise testing. More recent evidence suggests that a training effect can be anticipated with exercise of somewhat lower intensity, a 60 to 75% heart rate range, with the decrease in intensity compensated for by an increase in exercise duration or frequency, or both. A decrease in exercise intensity may enhance the safety of unsupervised exercise and encourage compliance because of reduced discomfort and increased enjoyment of the exercise.

In the early years of exercise training of coronary patients (with most patients recovering from myocardial infarction rather than having undergone coronary bypass surgery), supervised and ECG-monitored exercise was thought to decrease cardiovascular complication rates and increase the safety of exercise. More recent information suggests that ECG monitoring does not improve the safety of exercise regimens for low risk coronary patients; unsupervised exercise was not addressed in the study documenting the safety of non–ECG-monitored exercise. Patients at increased risk of cardiovascular complications of exercise—individuals who should exercise in a supervised setting, often with ECG monitoring, as recommended by the American College of Sports Medicine—include those with a markedly reduced exercise capacity, severely depressed left ventricular function, or complex ventricular rhythm disturbances; those who develop angina pectoris, marked ST segment depression, QT internal prolongation, or exercise-induced hypotension (as evidence of ischemia-induced ventricular dysfunction) at low levels of exercise; or those who are unable to effectively monitor their exercise heart rate.[5] Also at risk are patients who have an above normal exercise capacity without exercise-induced angina but who typically exceed their recommended training heart rate and have

markedly ischemic T segment responses at exercise testing. The increased risk of cardiovascular complications in these individuals persists long after an acute coronary episode, but the relationship to coronary bypass surgery is not known.[5] Ideally, exercise supervision should be available for the initial few sessions to enable education about exercise techniques; the proper shoes, clothing, and equipment for exercise; signs of overexertion; and to enable the institution of education about coronary risk modification.

An exercise regimen generally includes 5 to 15 minutes of stretching and range of motion warm-up exercise, 20 to 30 minutes of therapeutic exercise, and 5 to 15 minutes of cool-down activities. Dynamic or aerobic exercise training is preferred to stimulate the oxygen transport system. The therapeutic component of exercise initially involves walk-jog or bicycle exercise, modalities in which skill only minimally influences the work demand. Both arm and leg muscles should be included in the exercise training regimen, as the benefits of exercise training are in part muscle-specific. Subsequent aerobic endurance activities may include rope jumping, bicycling, skating, rowing, swimming, or aerobic dancing. Combined dynamic and isometric exercise can be introduced later.

However, the decrease in symptoms and improvement in functional capacity subsequent to coronary bypass surgery correlate poorly with favorable psychosocial outcomes, with resumption of the preillness lifestyle, and with return to remunerative employment. Individual counseling is often needed to facilitate resumption of a normal or near normal lifestyle.[47–49] Specific items to be addressed for suitable patients include the appropriateness and timing of return to work, and the recommended return to leisure and recreational activities, to sexual activity, and to preoperative and preillness family and social roles. Data from predischarge exercise testing can guide the physician's recommendation for the timing of return to work. It can also favorably influence the perception of patients and their families of the level of activity that can be undertaken without adverse effects and of the patients' ability to safely resume employment.

The return to work remains limited after coronary bypass surgery, and is often less than that occurring after uncomplicated myocardial infarction, despite the lessening of symptoms, the improvement in functional status, the improvement in perceived health status, and the increase in leisure time activities among these patients.[50] There was no significant increase in employment in surgically treated patients in the Coronary Artery Surgery Study,[46] and only 51% of patients returned to their preoperative levels of household activities.[46] Other studies also described a decrease in postoperative employment of previously working patients.[49, 50]

Psychosocial components of care may favorably influence three aspects of rehabilitation[49]; they may aid in (1) decreasing the psychosocial consequences of the illness, (2) improving compliance with recommendations for care, and (3) encouraging the behavior modification needed for the implementation of secondary preventive measures.

A risk profile can delineate those patients unlikely to return to work after coronary bypass surgery. These include individuals who have been unemployed preoperatively for more than 3 to 6 months, older persons, and those having jobs requiring high levels of phys-

Table 8–1. Perioperative Care: Coronary Artery Bypass Surgery

---

1. Exercise testing with or without radionuclide procedures
   a. Functional status
   b. Prognosis
   c. Exercise prescription
   d. Recommendations for return to preillness activities, including sexual activity, and for return to work

2. Additional testing for patients with complications of coronary bypass surgery or prior coronary episodes
   a. Suspected congestive heart failure: rest and exercise echocardiogram or radionuclide ventriculogram
   b. Congestive heart failure/ischemia/prior serious ventricular arrhythmias: ambulatory electrocardiography

3. Needed therapy
   a. Antiplatelet drugs: aspirin, persantin
   b. Anti-ischemic drugs when appropriate for residual myocardial ischemia: nitrates, calcium blockers, beta blockers
   c. Drugs to manage congestive heart failure when appropriate: digitalis and other positive inotropic agents, vasodilators, ? anticoagulant therapy
   d. Antiarrhythmic drugs if appropriate

4. Coronary risk assessment and reduction
   a. Detection and management of hypertension
   b. Detection and management of hyperlipidemia (based on preoperative lipid levels)
      i. Diet
      ii. Drugs
   c. Cigarette smoking cessation
   d. Weight reduction if appropriate
   e. Exercise training
   f. Psychosocial assessment and counseling

---

ical activity. The attitudes of the family and the employer also seem important, but the advice given by the primary care physician[51] appears to play a major role; patients who failed to return to work often defined as their reason for not working the lack of assurance from the primary care physician that they could appropriately and safely do so.

Greater preoperative job satisfaction, greater satisfaction with other important life aspects, and higher personal well-being scores characterize patients more likely to return to work.[52] One of the best predictors of postoperative employment is the patient's preoperative perception that he or she would be able to resume work.[52] This feature can be favorably altered by preoperative education and counseling and can be reinforced postoperatively as well.

In addition to presenting coronary bypass surgery as a restorative procedure designed to enhance the patient's postoperative functional capabilities, physicians can work with industry and with community services and resources to provide a favorable milieu for postoperative coronary patients to resume the positive aspects of their preillness lifestyle.[53]

Summary

A multifactorial approach to the long-term surveillance and management of patients after coronary bypass surgery has been described (Table 8–1). It is designed to enhance and maintain the improvements achieved by this procedure.

References

1. Detre KM, Takaro T, Hultgren H, et al. Long-term mortality and morbidity results of the Veterans Administration randomized trial of coronary artery bypass surgery. Circulation 72 (Suppl V): 84–89, 1985.
2. European Coronary Surgery Study Group. Long-term results of prospective randomized study of coronary artery bypass surgery in stable angina pectoris. Lancet 2:1173–1180, 1982.
3. Principal Investigators of CASS and Their Associates. The National Heart, Lung, and Blood Institute Coronary Artery Surgery Study (CASS). Circulation 63 (Suppl I): 1–81, 1985.
4. Varnauskas E, European Coronary Surgery Study Group. Survival, myocardial infarction, and employment status in a prospective randomized study of coronary bypass surgery. Circulation 72 (Suppl V):90–101, 1985.
5. Wenger NK. Rehabilitation of the coronary patient. Status 1986. Prog Cardiovasc Dis 29:181–204, 1986.

6. Weiner DA, Chaitman BR. Role of exercise testing in relationship to coronary artery bypass surgery and percutaneous transluminal coronary angioplasty. Cardiology 73:242–258, 1986.
7. Frye RL, Frommer PL. Consensus development conference on coronary artery bypass surgery: medical and scientific aspects. Circulation 65(Suppl II):1–129, 1982.
8. Singh RN, Sosa JA, Green GE. Long-term fate of the internal mammary artery and saphenous vein grafts. J Thorac Cardiovasc Surg 86:359–363, 1983.
9. Tector AJ, Schmahl TM, Canino VR. The internal mammary artery graft: the best choice for bypass of the diseased left anterior descending coronary artery. Circulation 68(Suppl II):214–217, 1983.
10. Chesebro JH, Fuster V, Elvebach LR, et al. Effect of dipyridamole and aspirin in late vein graft patency after coronary bypass operations. N Engl J Med 310:209–214, 1984.
11. Brown BG, Cukingnan RA, De Rouen T, et al. Improved graft patency in patients treated with platelet-inhibiting therapy after coronary bypass surgery. Circulation 72:138–146, 1985.
12. Boerboom LE, Olinger GN, Bonchek LI, et al. Aspirin and dipyridamole individually prevent lipid accumulation in primate vein bypass grafts. Am J Cardiol 55:556–559, 1985.
13. Chesebro JH, Fuster V. Platelet-inhibitor drugs before and after coronary artery bypass surgery and coronary angioplasty: the basis of their use, data from animal studies, clinical trial data, and current recommendations. Cardiology 73:292–305, 1986.
14. Chesebro JH, Clements IP, Fuster V, et al. A platelet-inhibitor drug trial in coronary artery bypass operations: benefit of perioperative dipyridamole and aspirin therapy on early postoperative vein-graft patency. N Engl J Med 307:73–78, 1982.
15. Fuster V, Chesebro JH. Aortocoronary artery vein-graft disease: experimental and clinical approach for the understanding of the role of platelets and platelet inhibitors. Circulation 72(Suppl V):65–70, 1982.
16. Lorenz RL, Schacky CV, Weber M, et al. Improved aortocoronary bypass patency by low-dose aspirin (100 mg daily). Lancet 1:1261–1267, 1984.
17. Gibson RS, Boden WE, Theroux P, et al. and Diltiazem Reinfarction Study Group. Diltiazem and reinfarction in patients with non–Q-wave myocardial infarction. N Engl J Med 315:423–429, 1986.
18. Henry PD, Bentley KI. Suppression of atherogenesis in cholesterol-fed rabbits treated with nifedipine. J Clin Invest 68:1366–1369, 1981.
19. Rouleau J-L, Parmley WW, Stevens J, et al. Verapamil suppresses atherosclerosis in cholesterol-fed rabbits. J Am Coll Cardiol 1:1453–1460, 1983.
20. Ginsburg R, Davis K, Bristow MR, et al. Calcium antagonists suppress atherogenesis in aorta but not in the intramural coronary arteries of cholesterol-fed rabbits. Lab Invest 49:154–158, 1983.
21. Sami M, Chaitman BR, Bourassa MG, et al. Long-term follow-up of aneurysmectomy for recurrent ventricular tachycardia or fibrillation. Am Heart J 96:303–308, 1978.
22. Molajo AO, Summers GD, Bennett DH. Effect of percutaneous transluminal coronary angioplasty on arrhythmias complicating angina. Br Heart J 54:375–377, 1985.
23. Bryson AL, Parisi A, Schechter E, et al. Life-threatening ventricular arrhythmias induced by exercise. Cessation after coronary bypass surgery. Am J Cardiol 32:995–999, 1973.
24. Tommaso C, Kehoe R, Zheutlin T. Survivors of ischemic mediated sudden death. Clinical, angiographic and electrophysiologic features and response to therapy. Circulation 66(Suppl II):25, 1982 (abstract).
25. Campeau L, Engelbert M, Lesperance J, et al. Atherosclerosis and later graft closure of aortocoronary saphenous vein grafts: sequential angiographic studies at 2 weeks, 1 year, 5 to 7 years, and 10 to 12 years after surgery. Circulation 68(Suppl II):1–7, 1983.
26. Cashin WL, SanMarco ME, Nessim SA, et al. Accelerated progression of atherosclerosis in coronary vessels with minimal lesions that are bypassed. N Engl J Med 311:824–828, 1984.
27. Loop FD, Lytle BW, Cosgrove DM, et al. Influence of the internal mammary artery graft on 10-year survival and other cardiac events. N Engl J Med 314:1–6, 1986.
28. Lytle BW, Loop FD, Cosgrove DM, et al. Long-term (5 to 12 years) serial studies of internal mammary artery and saphenous vein coronary bypass grafts. J Thorac Cardiovasc Surg 89:248–258, 1985.
29. Campeau L, Engelbert M, Lesperance J, et al. The relation of risk factors to the development of atherosclerosis in saphenous-vein bypass grafts and the progression of disease in the native circulation. N Engl J Med 311:1329–1332, 1984.
30. Bourassa MG, Campeau L, Lesperance J, et al. Atherosclerosis after coronary artery bypass surgery: results of recent studies and recommendations regarding prevention. Cardiology 73:259–268, 1986.
31. Gibson CF, Loop FD. Choice of internal mammary artery or saphenous vein graft for myocardial revascularization. Cardiology 73:235–241, 1986.
32. Palac RT, Meadows WR, Hwang MH, et al. Risk factors related to progressive narrowing in aortocoronary vein grafts studied 1 and 5 years after surgery. Circulation 68(Suppl I):40–44, 1982.
33. Raichlen JS, Healy B, Achuff SC, et al. Importance of risk factors in the angiographic progression of coronary artery disease. Am J Cardiol 57:66–70, 1986.
34. Lipid Research Clinics Program. The Lipid Research Clinics Coronary Primary Prevention Trial results. 1. Reduction in incidence of coronary heart disease. JAMA 251:351–354, 1984.
35. Lipid Research Clinics Program. The Lipid Research Clinics Coronary Primary Prevention Trial results. 2. The relationship of reduction in incidence of coronary heart disease to cholesterol lowering. JAMA 251:365–374, 1984.
36. Grondin CM, Campeau L, Lesperance J, et al. Comparison of late changes in internal mammary artery and saphenous vein grafts in two consecutive series of patients 10 years after operation. Circulation 70(Suppl I):208–212, 1984.
37. Levy RI, Brensike JF, Epstein SE, et al. The influence of changes in lipid values induced by cholestyramine and diet on progression of coronary artery disease: results of the NHLBI Type II Coronary Intervention Study. Circulation 69:325–337, 1984.
38. NHLBI Type II Coronary Intervention Study. The influence of cholestyramine-induced lipid changes on coronary artery disease progression. Circulation 68(Suppl III):188, 1983 (abstract).
39. Blakenhorn DH, Nessim SA, Johnson RL, et al. Beneficial effects of combined colestipol-niacin therapy on coronary atherosclerosis and coronary venous bypass grafts. JAMA 257:3233–3240, 1987.
40. Canner PL, Berge KG, Wenger NK, et al., for the Coronary Drug Project Research Group. Fifteen year

mortality in Coronary Drug Project patients: long-term benefit with niacin. J Am Coll Cardiol 8:1245–1255, 1986.

41. Frick MH, Elo O, Haapa K, et al. Helsinki Heart Study: primary-prevention trial with gemfibrozil in middle-aged men with dyslipidemia. Safety of treatment, changes in risk factors, and incidence of coronary heart disease. N Engl J Med 317:1237–1245, 1987.

42. Havel RJ, Hunninghake DB, Illingworth R, et al. Lovastatin (Mevinolin) in the treatment of heterozygous familial hypercholesterolemia. A multicenter study. Ann Intern Med 107:609–615, 1987.

43. Proceedings of the Conference on the Decline in the Coronary Heart Disease Mortality, Bethesda 1978. U.S. Department of Health, Education and Welfare, Public Health Service, NIH Publication No. 79-1610, 1979.

44. Leaman DM, Brower RW, Meester GT. Coronary artery bypass surgery. A stimulus to modify existing risk factors? Chest 81:16–19, 1982.

45. CASS Principal Investigators and Their Associates. Coronary Artery Surgery Study (CASS): a randomized trial of coronary artery bypass surgery. Survival data. Circulation 68:939–950, 1983.

46. CASS Principal Investigators and Their Associates. Coronary Artery Surgery Study (CASS): a random-ized trial of coronary artery bypass surgery. Quality of life in patients randomly assigned to treatment groups. Circulation 68:951–960, 1983.

47. Eliastam M, Gastel B. Technology assessment forum on coronary artery bypass surgery: economic, ethical, and social issues. Circulation 66(Suppl III):1–101, 1982.

48. Jenkins CD, Stanton B-A, Savageau JA, et al. Coronary artery bypass surgery. Physical, psychological, social, and economic outcomes six months later. JAMA 250:782–788, 1983.

49. Walter PJ. Return to Work after Coronary Artery Bypass Surgery. Psychosocial and Economic Aspects. Berlin, Springer-Verlag, 1985.

50. Russell RO Jr, Abi-Mansour P, Wenger NK. Return to work after coronary bypass surgery and percutaneous transluminal angioplasty: issues and potential solutions. Cardiology 73:306–322, 1986.

51. Almeida D, Bradford JM, Wenger NK, et al. Return to work after coronary bypass surgery. Circulation 68(Suppl II): 205–213, 1983.

52. Stanton BA, Jenkins CD, Denlinger P, et al. Prediction of employment status after cardiac surgery. JAMA 249:907–921, 1983.

53. Russell RO Jr, Wayne JB, Oberman A, et al. Return to work after treatment for coronary artery disease: role of the physician. Primary Cardiol 7:12–23, 1981.

PART TWO

Dermatology

9

Management of Acne

STEPHEN V. TANG, M.D.
PETER E. POCHI, M.D.

Acne is one of the most common dermatologic disorders with an incidence of 70 per 1000 community members. It affects more than 17 million people in the United States, and the estimated cost of care for this disorder exceeds $300 million annually. The peak incidence and severity of acne occur during the teenage years, but acne can first occur in children before the age of 10 or in adults in their third to fourth decades.

Until the advent of oral isotretinoin, the treatment of acne involved the suppression of its clinical signs without affecting the natural course of the disease. Because of the high incidence of side effects of isotretinoin, we must still rely on less potent therapies in the treatment of the vast majority of acne patients. These therapies are usually tailored to the particular patient, sometimes in a trial-and-error manner, which reflects the multifaceted pathophysiology and clinical presentation of this disorder.

Pathogenesis

Research on acne has brought to light a complex cascade of interrelated events (Fig. 9–1) focused on the specialized pilosebaceous unit of the face and upper trunk. Research has not yet elucidated how this process begins or why it normalizes with time.

The clinician sees acne as a folliculitis that results from the rupture of the follicular epithelium of susceptible pilosebaceous units. The first step in this process is an abnormal follicular retention hyperkeratosis resulting in the clinically invisible microcomedo. Sebum production driven by androgens provides the substrate for the resident anaerobic bacterium *Propionibacterium acnes,* which in turn elaborates chemotactic substances. This process may end harmlessly with the formation of an open or closed comedo. However, the follicular epithelium may allow chemotactic substances to diffuse and to generate a neutrophilic response leading to the eventual physical rupture of the follicular wall. This rupture results in an intense, perifollicular inflammatory response to the follicular contents composed not only of neutrophilic enzymes but also of skin cells, hair fragments, sebum, and irritating free fatty acids (sebum by-products). The clinical reflection of this follicular wall breakdown is an inflamed papule, pustule, or nodule.

Individual inflammatory lesions last 2 to 3 weeks and usually heal without residual defects. Occasionally a pronounced erythema or hyperpigmentation, or both, may persist for many weeks. A small percentage of patients have scarring, usually atrophic, with either abrupt margins ("ice pick" scars) or rounded margins. Less frequently, patients suffer hypertrophic scarring, usually on the upper trunk. Once formed, atrophic scars do not change, whereas hypertrophic scars tend to decrease in thickness with time.

Treatment Principles

The treatment of acne attempts to correct the three major abnormalities associated with this disorder: abnormal follicular keratinization, resident *P. acnes* population, and increased sebum production. The interaction of these processes leads to inflammation. The relative contribution of each of these factors to acne varies from patient to patient. Therefore, combination therapy is best to increase the chance for a successful outcome.

Before developing a treatment plan, the physician must exclude the possibility of acne "look-alikes" (Table 9–1) that may go unrec-

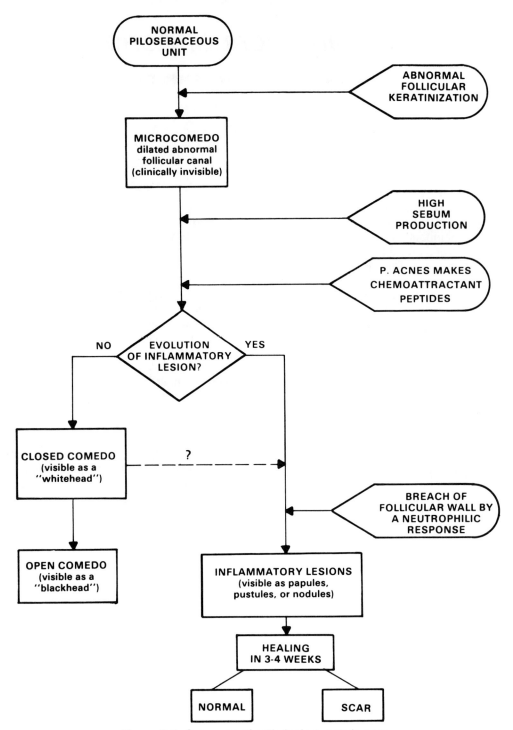

Figure 9–1. Sequence of pathologic events in acne.

Table 9–1. Differential Diagnosis of Acne Vulgaris

Diagnosis	Age of Onset	Important Factors	Location	Clinical Appearance
Acne rosacea	30 to 50 yr	Slow onset; aggravated by cold, ethyl alcohol, hot foods, stress; unknown etiology	Central face	Erythema, telangiectasias, papules/pustules; can present with rhinophyma or chronic eye inflammation
Perioral dermatitis	Primarily adult women	Sometimes associated with prolonged use of high potency topical steroids	Chin, perioral, and nasolabial folds	Erythematous, sometimes scaly 1- to 2-mm papules; may progress to diffuse, scaly, yellow-red plaques
Gram-negative folliculitis	Any age	Can be seen with long-term antibiotic therapy	A. Nose and mouth areas (common) B. Neck (uncommon)	A. Superficial pustules B. Large nodules
Steroid acne	Teenage to adult years	Associated with oral corticosteroid therapy	Chest, upper arms, and scalp	Small, monomorphic papules, pustules, or closed comedones

ognized because of a partial response to acne therapy. A history may similarly disclose drug causes of acne such as lithium or systemic steroids. Women should be questioned about abnormal menstrual cycles as well as other evidence for androgen excess (hirsutism or scalp hair loss). A history of acne therapy and clinical response will increase the chance of correct initial therapy for the patient.

At this point, the nature of this disorder should be explained to the patient in such a way as to maximize the correct use of the acne regimen and to encourage realistic expectations for treatment outcome. In particular, the physician should make clear that:

1. Treatments are generally suppressive and therefore must be maintained until the skin condition reverts to normal. Because this may take months to years, patients should receive maintenance therapy for several months before stopping therapy.

2. Most treatments work by preventing new lesions and do not generally expedite the healing of existing lesions; this preventive effect is not clinically apparent much before 3 to 6 weeks.

3. Topical medication should therefore be applied to the entire affected area, not just to existing lesions.

4. Truncal acne appears to be less responsive than facial acne to treatment, particularly with topical agents.

With this background, we can now consider specific treatment modalities, each of which may have varying degrees of impact on the three major acne factors (Table 9–2). Selection of the treatment mix must be tailored to each patient and may be helped by a simplified algorithm (Fig. 9–2).

Topical Treatment

Most cases of mild to moderate acne can be managed successfully by topical medications, which are usually directed at reducing the *P. acnes* population or being comedolytic, or both. To a certain degree, their utility is limited by their irritant effect. Few generate an allergic response, and they do so infrequently. Most are used in combination for increased efficacy. During tapering of topical medication, there should be 2 to 3 months between dosage changes for assessing the efficacy of the new lower level. Usually, topical antibiotics are tapered first and topical tretinoin last, especially for acne with a prominent comedonal component.

Benzoyl Peroxide

Benzoyl peroxide is the most frequently used topical acne medication and has a significant antibacterial effect and a mild comedolytic effect. It is available in concentrations between 2.5 and 10% and in many formulations as a soap, wash, liquid, and cream, and by prescription as a gel. Benzoyl peroxide may make the skin dry, erythematous, or scaly. These effects are dose-dependent, can improve despite continued use, and can be seen more often with

Table 9–2. Relative Efficacy of Acne Treatments on Pathogenic Factors

Therapy	Decreases Abnormal Follicular Keratinization	Reduces Sebum Production	Decreases P. acnes	Reduces Inflammation
Benzoyl peroxide	+	−	+ +	−
Topical tretinoin	+ + +	−	−	−
Topical antibiotics	+/−	−	+	+/−
Oral antibiotics	+/−	−	+ +	+
Oral isotretinoin	+ +	+ + +	+ + +	+
Oral hormone(s)	−	+ +	−	−

gels, which tend to offer greater penetration. For these reasons, a lower starting concentration is preferred, especially for patients with sensitive skin. Typically, it is used once or twice a day after washing. If adequate control is not achieved, topical tretinoin (see next section) may be added for greater effect. Flare-ups of acne while the patient is using benzoyl peroxide are interpreted as quantitative worsening of the disorder and not *P. acnes* resistance, which does not develop with benzoyl peroxide.

Topical Tretinoin

Topical tretinoin is probably the most effective of the externally applied acne medications because it can reverse, at least partially, the abnormal follicular keratinization. Its effect can be enhanced by combination with benzoyl peroxide or a topical antibiotic. This drug would be the ideal topical treatment if it were not for its potent primary irritant effect, which limits the maximum usable concentration to 0.1%. Some patients cannot tolerate it even at a low concentration. It is available in creams (0.05 and 0.1%) and in the more potent gels (0.01 and 0.025%) and liquid (0.05%).

Greater patient acceptance can be achieved if it is introduced slowly (every other day), used in the lowest concentration in a cream base, and applied no sooner than 20 to 30 minutes after washing and in the evening. Also, if patients are informed of the possible self-limited flare-up of the acne during the early weeks of treatment, they are less apt to terminate the treatment prematurely.

Topical Antibiotics

Topical antibiotics are widely used for acne but as a rule are clinically somewhat less effective than benzoyl peroxide. These preparations include tetracycline, clindamycin, erythromycin, or meclocycline sulfosalicylate (a tetracycline derivative), usually in hydroalcoholic vehicles but also in gel, cream, or ointment bases. Their low allergic potential and ease of application result in high patient acceptability.

The most frequently prescribed formulations contain either clindamycin or erythromycin, although topical antibiotics are usually of equal efficacy. Switching to another topical antibiotic may prove helpful, especially in cases of drug resistance. Combination with tretinoin or benzoyl peroxide yields a more effective treatment than does each agent alone. Combination therapy should be introduced carefully, with each agent started one at at time and used at different times of the day, especially benzoyl peroxide, which is a potent oxidizing agent. Topical antibiotics have proved safe for use. Early concern about the possible development of pseudomembranous colitis from the topical use of clindamycin has been shown to be unwarranted.

Oral Therapy

Several circumstances make systemic therapy preferable to topical treatment:

1. Severe nodular (cystic) acne, resistant to topical therapy
2. Progressive acne scarring despite adequate topical therapy
3. Prominent, persistent, and progressive hyperpigmentation despite topical therapy
4. Poor tolerance to topical therapy because of sensitive skin

The systemic therapies include antibiotics, isotretinoin, hormonal agents, and anti-inflammatory medications. Just as with topical therapy, each agent may have a different impact on the pathogenic factors of acne (Table 9–2). The patient may therefore benefit from combination therapy, including use of concomitant topical agents.

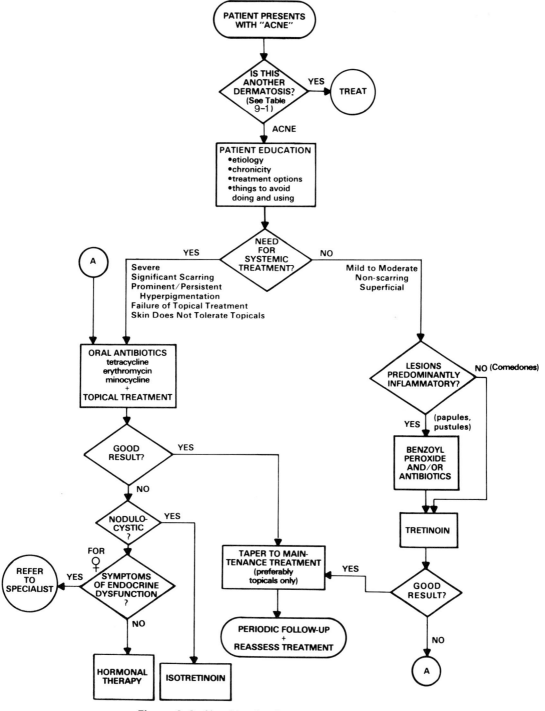

Figure 9–2. *Algorithm for the management of acne.*

Oral Antibiotics

Tetracycline is the most frequently prescribed oral antibiotic and is administered in doses ranging from 500 to 2000 mg/day. Typical treatment is begun with 1000 mg/day, and the dose is adjusted depending on the severity of the acne. Maximum efficacy is usually achieved after several weeks, at which time the dose can be tapered to a maintenance level, often as little as 250 mg/day. Intervals between dose changes should be 2 to 3 months to accurately assess treatment efficacy. The chief side effects are vaginal candidiasis and a mild phototoxicity (minimal with minocycline and severe with demeclocycline).

Minocycline has been effective in treating tetracycline-resistant acne probably because of its more efficient absorption from the gastrointestinal tract and high lipophilicity. Its disadvantages are ototoxicity (dizziness) at the higher doses of 150 to 200 mg/day, and the occasional but reversible skin pigment changes. We usually start with 100 mg/day except for severe acne, for which we start with 200 mg/day. A major drawback is its very high cost.

Erythromycin is a reasonable alternative to tetracycline, is less affected by food, is associated with a lower incidence of candidal vaginitis and no phototoxicity, and is helpful against tetracycline-resistant *P. acnes*. Drawbacks include more frequent gastrointestinal intolerance and greater cost than tetracycline. The usual dose is 750 to 1000 mg/day in divided doses.

Clindamycin has proved to be a highly effective antibiotic for acne but is rarely used now because of the risk, albeit small, of development of pseudomembranous colitis and because of the availability of isotretinoin for severe, resistant cases of acne.

Prolonged oral antibiotic therapy can sometimes lead to the development of a gram-negative folliculitis, which clinically mimics acne (Table 9–1) but is poorly controlled with the above oral antibiotics and rapidly flares up just days after stopping the antibiotic. Bacterial cultures of the nares and skin lesions and appropriate antibacterial therapy are indicated for this complication.

Isotretinoin

This synthetic vitamin A analogue was introduced into clinical practice in 1982 and has proved to be a superior treatment for severe acne resistant to other modes of therapy. It reduces sebum production profoundly and, in turn, the growth of *P. acnes* organisms for which sebum is the growth substrate. Follicular hyperkeratosis is also reduced. The net result of these actions is the quenching of the perifollicular inflammatory response. Since 1982, three quarters of a million people in the United States have been treated with oral isotretinoin, with sustained clearing for many months or longer after stopping therapy and with no recurrence in some patients.

Isotretinoin's usefulness is limited by a host of side effects, most of which are innocuous and involve inflammation and dryness of the skin and mucous membranes (80 to 90%). More serious side effects, although uncommon, include pseudotumor cerebri; abnormal adaptation to darkness; and small, asymptomatic, nonprogressive hyperostoses of the vertebral column (all so rare that actual frequencies have not been established). The most frequent systemic side effect is an elevation in serum cholesterol (mild) and serum triglyceride (moderate to marked) levels. The U.S. Food and Drug Administration requires monitoring of blood lipids during therapy. We obtain a base line and blood lipid levels at 2 and 4 weeks, and repeat measurements until the rise in values begins to level off. Consideration should be given to stopping treatment if the fasting triglyceride blood level exceeds 500 mg/dl to avoid the risk of acute pancreatitis.

The most critical side effect is the drug's teratogenicity, which involves a 25-fold increase in development of major fetal abnormalities in women who are or become pregnant while being treated with isotretinoin for acne. Women should be using adequate birth control before starting therapy and for 1 month after stopping therapy. They should also be fully informed of the risks to the fetus if they conceive while taking isotretinoin. On the other hand, they can be assured that the drug is not mutagenic.

A dosage of 1 mg/kg per day for 16 to 20 weeks is usually required; a second treatment is usually unnecessary. Smaller dosages, e.g., 0.1 to 0.5 mg/kg per day, may be nearly as effective, but relapses are more frequent at these amounts than at the higher dosage.

Antisebum (Hormonal) Therapy

Endocrine therapy may be considered for women who have not responded to standard treatment, even if there are no symptoms of hormonal dysfunction. The goal of such treatment is to reduce sebum production by reducing androgens, the stimulus for sebaceous activity. Levels of testosterone and dehydro-epiandrosterone sulfate (DHEAS) may be helpful in determining whether to suppress ovarian or adrenal androgens. An elevated testosterone level with normal DHEAS suggests the need to suppress ovarian androgen with daily estrogen (at least 50 µg/day). Conversely, an elevated DHEAS level suggests the need to suppress adrenal androgen with low doses of glucocorticoids (dexamethasone 0.25 to 0.5 mg/day or prednisone 5.0 to 7.5 mg/day). Maximal androgen suppression can be achieved by combined therapy with estrogen and glucocorticoid.

When hormone levels are normal, the problem may be with androgen receptors. Spironolactone, with antiandrogen receptor activity at high dosages, will help some patients with chronic treatment-resistant acne. Dosages of 150 to 200 mg/day are usually required, and menstrual irregularities are a frequent side effect.

The response of acne to any hormonal intervention is slow, taking 3 to 4 months before improvement is noted. This therapy is preventive, and improvement remains only while the patient is taking these drugs.

Oral Anti-Inflammatory Drugs

Corticosteroids at dosages of 20 to 40 mg/day are effective in suppressing acne inflammation. Once the dosage is reduced to 10 to 15 mg/day, the acne will usually begin to flare up. The potential side effects of this form of therapy limit its use to special circumstances, such as in patients who have infrequent but severe flare-ups of their acne, for example

1. A patient with mild acne that infrequently becomes explosively active for short periods
2. A woman with severe, premenstrual flare-ups of acne but with little or no acne during the remainder of the menstrual cycle (in this case the steroid may be needed only a few days each month)
3. A patient with a severe flare-up in association with isotretinoin treatment
Nonsteroidal anti-inflammatory drugs are not generally helpful for acne, except that ibuprofen (at 2.4 g/day) can enhance the effect of tetracycline (at 1.0 g/day).

Lesional Therapy

The majority of treatments considered so far are preventive and do not materially shorten the time for resolution of existing lesions. Other local treatments are helpful for the treatment of existing acne lesions that are tender or cosmetically unacceptable.

Intralesional steroid injections (e.g., 2.5 mg/ml triamcinolone acetonide) are usually adequate to reduce inflammation rapidly. Larger nodular lesions may require 5 to 10 mg/ml. These higher concentrations can lead to atrophy, but this is almost always temporary.

Cryotherapy with liquid nitrogen, carbon dioxide slush, or even ice can reduce the inflammatory response of a lesion.

Extraction of comedonal contents can result in significant cosmetic improvement, particularly if comedones are numerous and prominent. No prevention of inflammatory lesions can be expected, however, because these open and closed comedones rarely evolve into inflammatory lesions.

Miscellaneous Treatments

Cleansing does not improve acne but may temporarily improve the patient's appearance by degreasing the oily skin surface. Diet, too, does not appear to benefit acne. Ultraviolet light is only minimally helpful in reducing acne but can improve cosmesis by darkening and reddening background skin to make existing acne lesions less apparent. Good animal models are lacking for comedogenicity assays of cosmetics. If, however, a patient has many closed comedones in an area where heavy, oil-based make-up is applied, it is advisable for the patient to change to water-based make-up.

Scar Modification

A variety of procedures are used to improve the appearance of scars that can result from healing acne lesions. Hypertrophic scars more rapidly decrease in size in response to injection with triamcinolone acetonide suspension (10 to 40 mg/ml). Hypertrophic scars usually decrease in size spontaneously, but very slowly.

Atrophic scars are permanent. A range of surgical or cosmetic techniques are available to improve these lesions. Depending on the number of lesions, their location, and the degree of severity, the following techniques may be appropriate: bovine collagen injection, dermabrasion, simple excisions, and excisions plus punch-graft. No technique is perfect, and the patient should be helped to have reasonable expectations before corrective treatment.

Conclusion

Mild acne can usually be controlled with a combination of topical benzoyl peroxide, tretinoin, and topical antibiotics. If this treatment fails or is not tolerated by the patient's skin, an oral antibiotic should be tried while adjunctive topical therapy is continued if possible. In difficult, severe cases, oral isotretinoin is the drug of choice.

Bibliography

Cunliffe WJ. Evolution of a strategy for the treatment of acne. J Am Acad Dermatol 16:591–599, 1987.
  Pragmatic exposition of acne therapies with comparative data on relative efficacy.
Marynick SP, Chakmakjian ZH, McCaffree DL, et al. Androgen excess in cystic acne. N Engl J Med 308:981–986, 1983.
  Recent findings on the role of androgen levels in acne patients as a guide to diagnostic and pathologic considerations.
Olsen TG. Therapy of acne. Med Clin North Am 66:851–871, 1982.
  A comprehensive review of acne treatment through 1982.
Pochi PE. Acne vulgaris, in Dermis DJ, Dobson RL, McGuire JL (eds). Dermatology. Philadelphia, Harper & Row, 1985, unit 10–12, vol 2, pp 1–25.
  Excellent, comprehensive review of pathologic, clinical, and therapeutic aspects of acne.
Pochi PE. Endocrinology of acne. J Invest Dermatol 81:1, 1983 (editorial).
  Recent findings on the role of androgen levels in acne patients as a guide to diagnostic and pathologic considerations.
Shalita AR, Cunningham WJ, Leyden JJ, et al. Isotretinoin treatment of acne and related disorders: an update. J Am Acad Dermatol 9:629–638, 1983.
  Summary of current thinking about treatment with isotretinoin of acne, acne rosacea, and gram-negative folliculitis; more recently documented side effects such as hyperostoses not found.
Strauss JS, Rapini RP, Shalita AR, et al. Isotretinoin therapy for acne: results of a multicenter dose-response study. J Am Acad Dermatol 10:490–496, 1984.
  Summary of current thinking about treatment with isotretinoin of acne, acne rosacea, and gram-negative folliculitis; more recently documented side effects such as hyperostoses not found.
Tolman EL. Acne and acneiform dermatoses, in Moschella SL, Hurley HJ (eds). Dermatology, ed 2. Philadelphia, WB Saunders, 1985, pp 1306–1322.
  Excellent, comprehensive review of pathologic, clinical, and therapeutic aspects of acne.

10

✓ *Topical Corticosteroids*

JOHN L. BEZZANT, M.D.

Introduction

Dr. Albert Szent-Gyorgyi's reflections make one realize the remarkable boon of standardized, commercial topical corticosteroids (*The Crazy Ape,* p. 45):

This information is like the medical recipes we used to write in Hungary in my student days. We had no end of entirely useless drugs and we prescribed them in the most complex recipes, all in Latin, so that our patients would not understand them, and would thus be kept in the dark about our business, which we tried to keep a mystery.

When I was in medical school, I asked Dr. Louis S. Goodman how much one should know about a drug before prescribing it? He took the ever-present cigar out of his mouth and emphatically said, "A lot! And you can quote me on that!" I wrote this chapter to provide "a lot" of information regarding the following points:
1. When to use topical corticosteroids
2. Which drug to use
3. How much drug to use
4. How long to use topical corticosteroids
5. Cost of treatment
6. Complications of corticosteroid use
May his wish find fulfillment in the author and reader.

Diagnosis of Corticosteroid-Responsive Dermatoses

Procedures

To evaluate an inflammatory skin eruption properly, one must have the facilities and ability to do the following procedures:

Potassium Hydroxide Mount. Scrape scale or blister roofs off the skin, place them on a microscope slide, immerse the scale in 20% potassium hydroxide, cover this with a coverslip, and gently heat the slide over an open flame for about 5 seconds. Examine the slide under a microscope with about a $10\times$ objective: fungal hyphae are tubular, often branching, and sometimes septate.

Mineral Oil Mount. Rub a thin layer of mineral oil on the eruption, scrape those areas firmly with a no. 10 or 15 scalpel blade, place the scrapings on a microscope slide, apply a coverslip, and examine the slide microscopically with a $10\times$ objective to identify mites or other small insects.

Gram's Stain. Place any fluid from the eruption on a slide, gently heat the slide for 3 to 5 seconds, and then cool the slide. Stain the material with the four standard solutions for Gram's stain. Apply immersion oil and scan the slide with a $100\times$ objective. Note: Yeast are gram positive and much larger than bacteria. If yeast are infecting the tissue, one should see not only the oval budding form but also the mycelial (tubular) form, which develops when yeast grow in the less than optimal environment of tissue.

Wright's Stain. If blisters are present, scrape the bases of several blisters, smear this material on a microscope slide, fix it in methyl alcohol (do not heat-fix the slide because heating destroys cell morphology), and stain the slide with the three solutions of Wright's Giemsa quick stain. After staining, do not rinse the slide or dry it but immediately examine it with a $40\times$ objective (high dry).

Multinucleated giant cells, which are usually present in the blistering stage of a herpes infection, measure about 40μ in diameter (roughly four times the diameter of a leukocyte) and have two or more nuclei.

Three-Millimeter Punch Biopsy. Using a 3-mm-diameter punch, obtain a biopsy specimen of full-thickness skin, which usually is 1 to 4 mm thick. Sample the red area if the eruption is red, the edge of a blister if the eruption is vesicular. Biopsies are routinely stained with hematoxylin and eosin. If special immunofluorescent studies may be required, consult a dermatologist or pathologist regarding the choice of biopsy site and the type of holding medium needed for tissue transport.

Diagnostic Aids

PROCEDURAL ALGORITHM (Fig. 10–1)

Inflammatory skin diseases, such as eczema, may have superimposed yeast, fungal, bacterial, or viral infections; if such secondary infections are not diagnosed initially, the red-ness, scaling, or blistering caused by infection will persist in spite of otherwise proper topical corticosteroid therapy. Obviously, a delay in diagnosing certain infections can be disastrous.

Anatomic Distribution

Common anatomic distributions of steroid-responsive dermatoses are provided here. Stippled areas are those commonly involved.

ATOPIC DERMATITIS (ECZEMA) (Fig. 10–2)

Lesions are red and scaly; sometimes pinhead-sized blisters appear, especially on the hands and feet.

Areas of distribution include scalp (occasionally), postauricular area, neck, nipples,

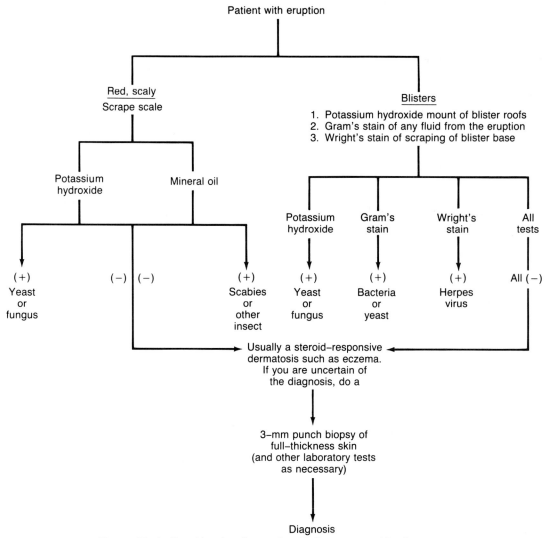

Figure 10–1. Algorithm for diagnosis of inflammatory skin diseases.

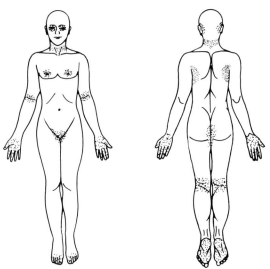

Figure 10–2. *Anatomic distribution of atopic dermatitis (eczema).*

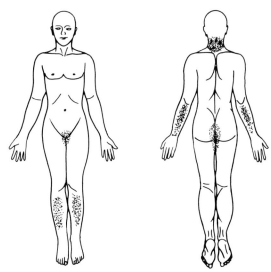

Figure 10–4. *Anatomic distribution of lichen simplex chronicus.*

antecubital and popliteal fossae, posterior axillary fossae, hands, groin, perianal area, and feet.

NUMMULAR ECZEMA (Fig. 10–3)

In the acute form, lesions are round or oval, 1- to 2-cm-diameter clusters of pinhead-sized blisters and exudate. In the chronic form, lesions are round or oval, 1- to 2-cm-diameter areas of redness and scaling.

The extremities and trunk are involved. If the eczema has been present for several weeks or longer, there is a relatively symmetric distribution on the body.

LICHEN SIMPLEX CHRONICUS (Fig. 10–4)

Lesions are red, scaly areas. Often there is thickening of the skin secondary to scratching.

Lesions are seen on the nape of the neck, forearms, genitals and perianal area, and shins.

PSORIASIS (Fig. 10–5)

Beefy-red plaques with thick silvery scale, usually 1 to 2 cm in diameter or greater, are found on the scalp, elbows, umbilicus, natal cleft, knees, and occasionally hands and feet. Pitted or thickened nails are also seen.

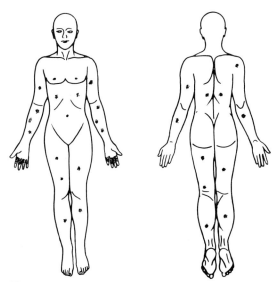

Figure 10–3. *Anatomic distribution of nummular eczema.*

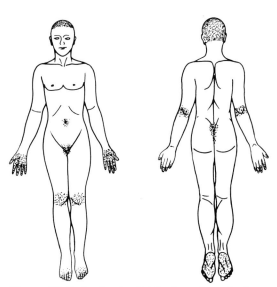

Figure 10–5. *Anatomic distribution of psoriasis.*

SEBORRHEIC DERMATITIS (Fig. 10–6)

Lesions include redness and scaling, occasional exudate, and crust formation in the more severe cases, especially in the ear canals.

The scalp (especially the margin), postauricular area, ear canals, brows, nasolabial folds, beard (cheeks), central chest, and occasionally axillae and groin in the most severe cases are locations where lesions are found.

Topical Corticosteroids

Definition

Corticosteroids are anti-inflammatory agents that are synthesized from cholesterol; cholesterol has been modified to form cortisol and other more potent corticosteroids. In the United States, at least 87 topical corticosteroid preparations are available by prescription.

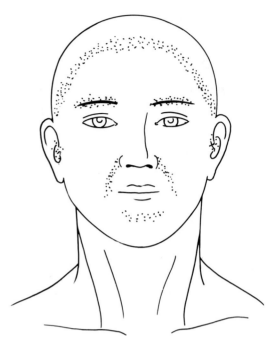

Figure 10–6. Anatomic distribution of seborrheic dermatitis.

Potency

The potency of a topical corticosteroid is a function of the inherent anti-inflammatory effect of the corticosteroid *molecule,* and the efficiency with which the *vehicle* transports the steroid through the epidermis to the dermis.

Molecular Potency. The vasoconstrictor assay of McKenzie and Stoughton indicates the degree of biological activity of a topical corticosteroid and is generally believed to be predictive of therapeutic efficacy. Table 10–1 presents selected examples.

Vehicles. There are no legally mandated definitions of the various topical vehicles used for corticosteroids and other medications; however, those shown in Figure 10–7 are generally accurate.

Note: Many vehicles contain propylene glycol, acetone, or alcohol to enhance penetration of the steroid; however, these products cause moderate to severe stinging when applied to broken skin.

Relative Potency. The relative anti-inflammatory potency of topical corticosteroids in specific vehicles is shown in Table 10–2.

Note: Current nonprescription topical corticosteroids contain only 0.5% hydrocortisone; hence, they are effective in controlling only very mild inflammation of the skin.

✓ Choice of Potency and Vehicle
(Fig. 10–8)

Intensity of Eruption

The general rule is to match the potency of the corticosteroid to the intensity of the eruption (Table 10–3).

Note: In severe, widespread dermatitis it is generally better to use oral corticosteroids, e.g., prednisone at 1 mg/kg per day, and taper (if given for 3 weeks or more) or stop as soon as possible. Do *not* treat psoriasis with oral steroids because patients may develop a severe pustular flare on withdrawal, or the psoriasis can become resistant to topical therapy.

Location of Eruption

SPECIAL CONSIDERATIONS

Age. Because of the high ratio of surface to mass in children (sometimes greater than 2) and the resultant danger of significant systemic concentrations, only low or medium potency corticosteroids should be used to treat them. Furthermore, preterm infants have increased skin permeability, and only low potency corticosteroids should be used on them. If it appears that high potency corticosteroids may

Table 10–1. *Vasoconstrictor Index of Ethanolic Extracts of Topical Corticosteroids*

Generic Name	Sample Brand Name	Relative Vasoconstriction
Hydrocortisone	Hytone	1
Triamcinolone acetonide	Kenalog	75
Fluocinolone acetonide	Synalar	100
Halcinonide	Halog	160
Fluocinonide	Lidex	220
Betamethasone valerate	Valisone	360
Betamethasone dipropionate	Diprolene	1660
Clobetasol propionate	Temovate	1869

Data courtesy of Glaxo Dermatology Products, Glaxo Inc.

be required for an infant or child, the child should be referred to a dermatologist.

Pregnancy. Almost without exception, corticosteroids are teratogens in laboratory animals. The primary defect induced in all species is cleft lip/palate. There are no adequate, well-controlled studies of the teratogenic effects of topically applied corticosteroids in pregnant women. As a group, topical corticosteroids have not been associated with congenital malformations. Nevertheless, if the patient is a pregnant woman, use the least potent corticosteroid for the briefest time necessary to control the eruption.

Fluorination of Corticosteroids. Fluorinated corticosteroids should not be applied to the face; if they are applied thereon for more than 2 or 3 months, they may cause an acneiform eruption, erythema around the mouth

(perioral dermatitis), and thinning of the skin. Nonfluorinated corticosteroids rarely cause these complications. The skin of the eyelids, axillae, and groin is comparatively thin. If fluorinated corticosteroids are used on these areas, the skin may develop visible atrophy within 2 to 6 weeks, and eventually irreversible striae may form. Most of the atrophy, but not striae, resolves, usually in 2 to 8 months. Again, *non*fluorinated corticosteroids rarely cause these problems. Current *non*fluorinated corticosteroids include:

- Medium potency
  - Hydrocortisone valerate (Westcort)
  - Hydrocortisone butyrate (Locoid)
- Low potency
  - Hydrocortisone (Hytone)
  - Desonide (DesOwen)

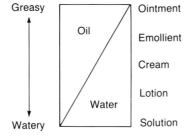

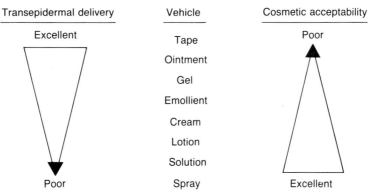

Figure 10–7. *Characteristics and efficacy of vehicles for topical corticosteroids.*

Table 10–2. *Potency Ranking of Some Commonly Used Topical Steroids*

Potency	Group	Brand Name (U.S.)	Size	Generic Name
Ultra potent		Temovate Ointment 0.05%	15, 30 g	Clobetasol propionate
		Temovate Cream 0.05%	15, 30 g	Clobetasol propionate
	1	Diprolene Ointment 0.05%	15, 45 g	Betamethasone dipropionate in
		Diprolene Cream 0.05%	15, 45 g	optimized vehicle
	2	Cyclocort Ointment 0.1%	15, 30 g	Amcinonide
		Diprosone Ointment 0.05%	15, 45 g	Betamethasone dipropionate
		Florone Ointment 0.05%	15, 30, 60 g	Diflorasone diacetate
		Halog Cream 0.1%	15, 30, 60, 240 g	Halcinonide
		Lidex Cream 0.05%	15, 30, 60, 120 g	Fluocinonide
		Lidex Gel 0.05%	15, 30, 60, 120 g	Fluocinonide
		Lidex Ointment 0.05%	15, 30, 60, 120 g	Fluocinonide
		Maxiflor Ointment 0.05%	15, 30, 60 g	Diflorasone diacetate
High		Maxivate Ointment 0.05%	15, 45 g	Betamethasone dipropionate*
		Maxivate Cream 0.05%	15, 45 g	Betamethasone dipropionate*
		Maxivate Lotion 0.05%	60 ml	Betamethasone dipropionate
		Topicort Cream 0.25%	15, 60, 120 g	Desoximethasone*
		Topicort Ointment 0.25%	15, 60 g	Desoximethasone*
	3	Aristocort Ointment 0.1%	15, 60, 240 g	Triamcinolone acetonide
		Diprosone Cream 0.05%	15, 45 g	Betamethasone dipropionate
		Florone Cream 0.05%	15, 30, 60 g	Diflorasone diacetate
		Maxiflor Cream 0.05%	15, 30, 60 g	Diflorasone diacetate
		Valisone Ointment 0.1%	15, 45 g	Betamethasone valerate
	4	Benisone Ointment 0.025%	15, 60 g	Betamethasone benzoate
		Cordran Ointment 0.05%	15, 30, 60, 225 g	Flurandrenolide
		Kenalog Ointment 0.1%	15, 60, 80 g	Triamcinolone acetonide
		Synalar Cream (HP) 0.2%	12 g	Fluocinolone acetonide
		Synalar Ointment 0.025%	15, 30, 60, 120 g	Fluocinolone acetonide
		Topicort LP Cream 0.05%	15, 60 g	Desoximethasone
Medium	5	Locoid Cream 0.1%†	15, 45 g	Hydrocortisone butyrate†
		Locoid Ointment 0.1%†	15, 45 g	Hydrocortisone butyrate†
		Benisone Cream 0.025%	15, 60 g	Betamethasone benzoate
		Cordran Cream 0.05%	15, 30, 60, 225 g	Flurandrenolide
		Diprosone Lotion 0.02%	20, 60 ml	Betamethasone dipropionate
		Kenalog Cream 0.1%	15, 60, 80, 240 g	Triamcinolone acetonide
		Kenalog Lotion 0.1%	15, 60 ml	Triamcinolone acetonide
		Synalar Cream 0.025%	15, 30, 60, 120 g	Fluocinolone acetonide
		Valisone Cream 0.1%	15, 45, 110 g	Betamethasone valerate
		Valisone Lotion 0.1%	20, 60 ml	Betamethasone valerate
		Westcort Ointment 0.2%	15, 45, 60 g	Betamethasone valerate
		Westcort Cream 0.2%	15, 45, 60, 120 g	Hydrocortisone valerate†
	6	Hytone Cream 1 and 2.5%	30, 120 g	Hydrocortisone†
		DesOwen Cream 0.05%†	15, 60 g	Desonide†
		Locorten Cream 0.03%	15, 60 g	Flumethasone pivalate
		Synalar Solution 0.01%	20, 60 ml	Fluocinolone acetonide
		Tridesilon Cream 0.05%†	15, 60 g	Desonide†
Low	7	Hytone Ointment 2.5%†	30, 120 g	Hydrocortisone†
		Nutracort Cream 1%†	30, 60, 120 g	Hydrocortisone†
		Nutracort Lotion 1%†	60, 120 ml	Hydrocortisone†
		and other topicals with hydrocortisone, dexamethasone, flumethalone, prednisolone, and methyl prednisolone		

Courtesy of Owen Laboratories and Dr. Richard Stoughton. From Cornell RC, Stoughton RB. The use of topical steroids in psoriasis. Dermatol Clin 2:397–409, 1984.
*Indicates no propylene glycol in the vehicle.
†Indicates a nonfluorinated corticosteroid.

Table 10–3. *Potency of Topical Steroid as Related to Intensity of Eruption*

Intensity of Eruption	Potency of Topical Steroid
Severe (intense redness, scaling, often blistering)	High
Moderate (moderate redness and scaling)	Medium
Mild (mild redness and scaling)	Low

Amount, Frequency, and Time of Application

Amount (Fig. 10–9)

Frequency of Application

Generally, topical corticosteroids should be applied twice a day. If tachyphylaxis occurs, intermittent application (called pulse dosing) may restore skin responsiveness. For example, the corticosteroid is applied twice a day for 2 days, and then a bland lubricant (Vaseline or Moisturel) is used for 2 days; continuing that sequence has reversed tachyphylaxis and has restored control of the eruption for several years. More recently, it has been shown that as little as thrice weekly application of a corticosteroid produced excellent control for some patients. Apparently the epidermis acts as a drug reservoir and is thought to be the reason for the success of intermittent-dosing programs.

Time of Application

Water is one of the most important "drugs" used on the skin. The penetration of a topical corticosteroid is generally enhanced by hydrating (and heating) the skin. The patient can utilize these facts by bathing or showering for about 10 minutes and immediately thereafter applying the medication to damp skin. To help retain water and heat in the skin, a very thin layer of petrolatum (e.g., Vaseline) or cream (e.g., Moisturel) should be applied on top of the medication. This continues to enhance drug penetration and also helps prevent drying of the skin and possible worsening of the eruption.

Cost

The average retail cost of brand name corticosteroids, as of September 1988, is shown in Table 10–4.

Follow-up Evaluation, Expected Results, and Duration of Treatment

After the initial evaluation, the patient should be seen again within 1 or 2 weeks. If

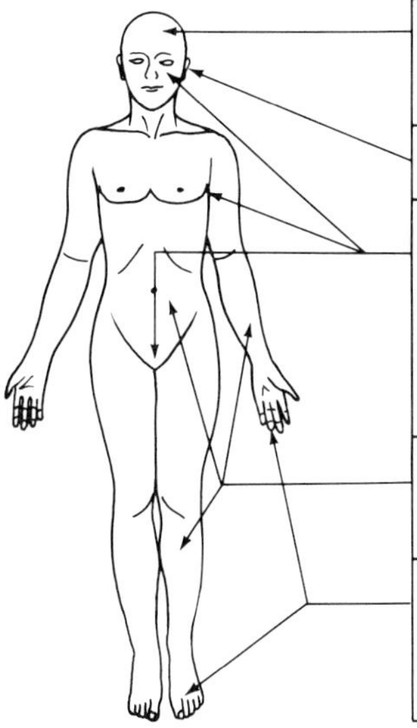

Area	Potency	Vehicles	Examples
Scalp	Medium or high	Solutions Sprays Gels	Valisone lotion Kenalog spray Topicort gel
Ear canals	Low	Solutions	Penecort solution
Face, axillae, groin	Low or medium (*non*fluorinated)	Creams or lotions	DesOwen cream LactiCare HC 1 or 2.5% lotion Westcort cream Locoid cream
Trunk extremities	Medium or high	Ointments Emollients Creams	Topicort ointment Synemol (emollient) Lidex–Cream
Hands, feet	High	Ointments Emollients Creams Gels	Diprolene ointment Lidex–E Diprolene AF cream Lidex gel

Figure 10–8. *Corticosteroid potency, vehicles, and examples of medications related to specific locations of eruption.*

	Hands, head, face, anogenital area	One arm, front or back of trunk	One leg	Whole body
Amount of medication needed per application	2 g	3 g	4 g	30–60 g
Twice a day for 1 wk	28 g	42 g	56 g	420–840 g

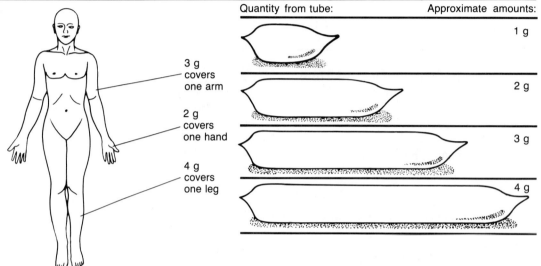

3 g covers one arm

2 g covers one hand

4 g covers one leg

Quantity from tube: Approximate amounts:

1 g

2 g

3 g

4 g

Figure 10–9. *Amounts of corticosteroid medications needed for specific areas of the body. From Drug information handout from Syntex Laboratories, Inc., Palo Alto, CA, 1985, with permission.*

the diagnosis and treatment are correct (and the patient is compliant), there should be a significant decrease in redness, scaling or blistering, and itching; if there is no improvement, both diagnosis and treatment should be re-evaluated.

Severe, acute dermatitis, such as poison ivy dermatitis, generally requires about 3 weeks to resolve. Lichenification (thickening of the epidermis secondary to scratching) requires 1 to 2 months to resolve after the patient stops scratching.

Significant Side Effects

Suppression of Hypophyseal-Pituitary-Adrenal Axis

Suppression of the hypophyseal-pituitary-adrenal (HPA) axis may occur when ultrapotent topical steroids are used for 5 days or longer on inflamed skin. Suppression has been repeatedly reported when use of the ultrapo-

tent corticosteroid clobetasol (Temovate) has exceeded 50 g/week (7 g/day), and in some patients using as little as 2 g/day.

Atrophy

Epidermal and dermal atrophy occasionally occurs when potent or ultrapotent corticosteroids are applied for 3 weeks or more, especially if used under occlusion (e.g., Saran wrap), or if applied on the thin skin of the eyelids, axillae, or groin. There are even reports of underlying fat and muscle atrophy when medium or high potency corticosteroids are used in excessive amounts—especially under occlusion. Atrophic skin looks and feels thinner than the normal surrounding skin and tends to look wrinkled; the dermal and sub-dermal blood vessels become more visible. Eventually the vessels can lose their surrounding connective tissue support and become permanently dilated and fragile. Skin atrophy is almost always reversible and takes from 1 to 9 months to resolve.

Table 10–4. Average Retail Cost of Topical Corticosteroids, September 1988

Amount	Vehicle	Cost (U.S. Dollars)
15-g tube	Ointment, cream, gel, or emollient	13.00
30-g tube	Ointment, cream, gel, or emollient	20.00
60-g tube	Ointment, cream, gel, or emollient	28.00
120-g tube	Ointment, cream, gel, or emollient	46.00
23-g canister	Spray	14.00
60 × 7.5 cm roll	Tape	15.00
200 × 7.5 cm roll	Tape	26.00

Striae

Atrophy can progress to the point that striae form. Striae are the result of corticosteroid-induced diminution of dermal collagen and ground substance; both are so reduced that the dermis is about half its normal thickness histologically. Striae are *not* reversible, although their purple-red coloration diminishes with time.

Acne

After roughly 3 months of continuous therapy, fluorinated (and rarely nonfluorinated) corticosteroids can induce an acneiform eruption on the face, chest, and back. It resolves with cessation of corticosteroid use; however, resolution can be accelerated by treating the patient with 1 g/day of either tetracycline or erythromycin.

Perioral Dermatitis

Fluorinated (and rarely nonfluorinated) corticosteroids applied to the face can induce a redness on the chin and nasolabial folds called perioral dermatitis. Some experts maintain that inducement of the eruption is related to the potency of the corticosteroid, and not to fluorination per se. This eruption usually resolves several weeks after corticosteroid treatment is stopped; if it does not resolve, it can be successfully treated with 1 g/day of oral tetracycline or erythromycin given for 2 to 4 weeks. The patient must be warned that after the causative corticosteroid is stopped, the involved areas may develop an intense, rebound erythema for a week or two before improvement begins.

Teratogenicity

Use the least potent corticosteroid necessary for the least time necessary to control a skin eruption on a pregnant woman (see earlier section on pregnancy).

Folliculitis

Folliculitis occurs occasionally, usually with the use of corticosteroid-impregnated tapes or when a plastic wrap covers the steroid application. The folliculitis resolves about 2 to 3 weeks after stopping therapy.

Hypopigmentation

Lightening of skin color may occur as early as 2 weeks after beginning therapy if the corticosteroid is applied under occlusion. Hypopigmentation resolves, as does atrophy, within about 2 to 9 months.

Summary

Diagnosis

Be as certain of the diagnosis as you can; at the least use the algorithm provided. If you are uncertain of the diagnosis, seek the assistance of a dermatologist.

Corticosteroid Potency and Vehicle

If you are uncertain about which corticosteroid and vehicle to use, giving a medium potency, nonfluorinated topical corticosteroid ointment (e.g., Locoid or Westcort) helps control most types of inflammatory dermatoses; this type of drug does not itself worsen the patient's condition. However, if a secondary viral or bacterial infection is present, a delay in diagnosis and treatment can lead to serious complications. Remember: Inflamed skin can generally be more easily infected than normal skin.

Method and Frequency of Application

Heat and hydration enhance topical penetration. Twice daily application is usually sufficient. Topical penetrations should be applied with the direction of hair growth, i.e., downward.

Morning and evening:

1. Bathe or shower in lukewarm water for 10 minutes.

2. Pat off excess water, and immediately apply the corticosteroid to the eruption.

3. Apply a thin layer of ointment (Vaseline) or cream (Moisturel) on top of the medication and to any areas of dry skin.

Amount

Prescribing a 30- or 60-g tube generally (1) provides adequate medication for a week and (2) prevents abuse and serious side effects if the patient incorrectly uses the medication or gives the medication to someone else.

Cost

Most patients spend between $20 and $30 for the amount of drug needed for 1 to 2 weeks of therapy.

Duration of Treatment

The patient should be seen again within 1 or 2 weeks. If there is improvement, treatment is usually continued until the eruption clears or until significant side effects supervene. If within 1 or 2 weeks there is no improvement or a worsening of the eruption, re-evaluate the diagnosis and therapy. If there is still uncertainty about diagnosis or treatment, refer the patient to a dermatologist when possible. The patient should not be subjected to the bother and expense of therapeutic experimentation if it can be avoided.

Bibliography

Blank H, et al. Topical corticoid therapy; a round table discussion. Cutis 24:446–448, 633–638, 1979.
Experts sharing their experiences and experimental information.

Bucks DAW, et al. Bioavailability of topically administered steroids: a "mass balance" technique. J Invest Dermatol 90:29–33, 1988.

Carruthers JA, et al. Observations on the systemic effect of topical clobetasol propionate. Br Med J 4:203–204, 1975.

Clobetasol—a potent new topical corticosteroid. Med Lett 28:57–59, 1986.

Discussion and a long, comprehensive list of comparative wholesale prices.

Fisher AA. Steroid rosacea: a friendly pharmacist syndrome. Cutis 40:209–211, 1987.
Dramatic photographs of steroid-induced rosacea.

Frosch PJ, et al. The Duhring chamber assay for corticosteroid atrophy. Br J Dermatol 104:57–65, 1981.

Gallant C, Kenny P. Oral glucocorticoids and their complications. J Am Acad Dermatol 14:161–177, 1986.
Excellent.

Gomez EC, Kaminester L, Frost P. Topical halcinonide and betamethasone valerate effects on plasma cortisol. Arch Dermatol 113:1196–1202, 1977.

Guin JD. Complications of topical hydrocortisone. J Am Acad Dermatol 4:417–422, 1981.

Hendrikse JCM, Moolenaar AJ. Adrenal suppression with topical hydrocortisone butyrate. Dermatologica 147: 191–197, 1973.

Katz HI, et al. Betamethasone dipropionate in optimized vehicle: intermittent pulse dosing for extended maintenance treatment of psoriasis. Arch Dermatol 123:1308–1311, 1987.
Less may be more—or the same—in some cases.

Lee SS. Topical steroids. Int J Dermatol 20:632–641, 1981.
Details of chemical structure and potency.

Maibach HI, Boisits EK. Neonatal Skin, Structure and Function. New York, Marcel Dekker, 1982.
Best book on skin of infants and children.

Maibach HI, Bronaugh RL. Percutaneous Absorption: Mechanisms—Methodology—Drug Delivery. New York, Marcel Dekker, 1985.
Excellent, comprehensive.

Mecham RP. Regulation of Matrix Accumulation. Orlando, Academic Press, 1986.
Excellent information on the action of corticosteroids on collagen, elastin, and extracellular matrix.

Mometasone—a new topical steroid. Med Lett 29:96–98, 1987.
An abbreviated, comparative list of wholesale costs.

Orentreich N, et al. Local injection of steroids and hair regrowth in alopecias. Arch Dermatol 82:898–899, 1960.
Atrophy and resolution from injected steroids.

Parrish JA. Are we applying topical corticosteroids too frequently? Dermatol Capsule Comment 4:1–2, 1982.
Interesting and helpful suggestions for reversing tachyphylaxis.

Ponec M. Effects of glucocorticoids on cultured skin fibroblasts and keratinocytes. Int J Dermatol 23:11–24, 1984.
Very helpful summary charts of data.

Rasmussen JE. Percutaneous absorption of topically applied triamcinolone in children. Arch Dermatol 114:1165–1167, 1978.
Gives proper perspective on use of medium potency steroids in children.

Rasmussen JE. Childhood eczema and topical corticosteroid therapy. JAMA 248:3029–3030, 1982.
Rational, helpful information on corticosteroid use on children.

Robertson DB, Maibach HI. Topical corticosteroids. Int J Dermatol 21:59–67, 1982.
A good, brief review.

Schardein, JL. Chemically Induced Birth Defects. New York, Marcel Dekker, 1985, pp 306–313.
Superb presentation of animal and human data—very helpful comparative tables.

Storrs FJ. Use and abuse of systemic corticosteroid therapy. J Am Acad Dermatol 1:95–104, 1979.
Excellent.

Stoughton, RB. Are generic formulations equivalent to trade name topical glucocorticoids? Arch Dermatol 123:1312–1314, 1987.

Sometimes yes and sometimes no.

Streck WF, Lockwood DH. Pituitary adrenal recovery following short-term suppression with corticosteroids. Am J Med 66:910–914, 1979.

Simulated dose and duration often used in outpatient dermatology.

Sudilovsky A, Muir JG, Bocobo FC. A comparison of single and multiple applications of halcinonide cream. Int J Dermatol 20:609–613, 1981.

Sudilovsky A, Muir JG, Bocobo FC. Topical corticosteroids: the need (?) for frequent applications. Int J Dermatol 20:594–596, 1981.

Tan PL, et al. Current topical corticosteroid preparations. J Am Acad Dermatol 14:79–98, 1986.

A comprehensive list of available topical corticosteroids and their vehicles.

Weston WL, et al.: Comparison of hypothalamus-pituitary-adrenal axis suppression from superpotent topical steroids by standard endocrine function testing and gas chromatographic mass spectrometry. J Invest Dermatol 90:532–535, 1988.

Wilkinson DS, et al. Perioral dermatitis: a 12-year review. Br J Dermatol 101:245–257, 1979.

11

Urticaria and Angioedema

KENNETH P. MATHEWS, M.D.
BRUCE L. ZURAW, M.D.

Multiple, circumscribed, slightly elevated, pruritic swellings are so commonplace that patients themselves frequently make a correct diagnosis of hives or urticaria. In less obvious cases, the fact that the *individual* lesions seldom last longer than 24 to 48 hours is almost diagnostic of urticaria, although new hives frequently develop as the older ones fade. Lack of pruritus almost excludes the diagnosis. About 50% of adult urticaria patients also experience angioedema, which occurs especially on the eyelids and lips. The angioedematous swellings, however, are associated with little or no itching, and in contrast to most other forms of edema they do not characteristically occur in dependent areas, they are often asymmetric, they are transient (but often recurrent), and they are associated with urticaria in about 85% of adult patients (less commonly in children).

It has been estimated that about one fifth of the populace of the U.S. has urticaria at some time during their lifetime. It occurs at all ages, but chronic urticaria or angioedema—defined as the continuous or frequent occurrence of lesions for longer than about 6 weeks—develops more commonly in middle-aged persons, especially women. As noted later, certain types of urticaria occur more often in atopic persons, but the majority of afflicted individuals are not atopic. Mild urticaria may be scarcely more than a slight annoyance, but severe, chronic urticaria can be disabling, and hereditary angioedema may be fatal.

Pathophysiology

Histamine has been suspected to play a pathogenic role because intracutaneous injec-tions grossly reproduce the pruritic wheal-and-flare reaction typical of urtication. Furthermore, if the distal extremity of a patient with cold urticaria is submerged in cold water for 5 minutes, a significant but transient rise in plasma histamine is frequently observed in blood taken from that extremity as it is rewarmed. Similar occurrences have been observed after an appropriate challenge of some patients with solar urticaria, dermographism, cholinergic urticaria, localized heat urticaria, vibratory angioedema, and aquagenic urticaria. However, other mast cell–derived mediators can also be found in these venous effluents, such as eosinophil chemotactic factors and a high molecular weight neutrophil chemotactic factor.

It is likely that immunoglobulin E (IgE)–mediated histamine release by allergens from cutaneous mast cells is responsible for many cases of *acute* urticaria or angioedema. However, it has become increasingly apparent that no IgE-mediated allergy can be found to account for the vast majority of cases of *chronic* urticaria or angioedema. One possibility is that nonimmunologic mechanisms or immune processes not involving IgE may also feed into a final common pathway of mast cell stimulation, histamine release, and urticaria (Fig. 11–1). Trauma and cholinergic urticaria exemplify nonimmunologic histamine-releasing processes. Patients with the latter disorder exhibit tiny wheals surrounded by large areas of erythema after exercise, emotional stress, or exposure to heat. It also is clear that many drugs can cause histamine release by mechanisms other than immunologic ones. Narcotics, *d*-tubocurarine, and polymyxin antibiotics exemplify this property.

Complement activation can also lead to urticaria, probably through the generation of the C5a, C3a, and C4a anaphylatoxins, which are

This is publication no. 4876-BCR from the Research Institute of Scripps Clinic.

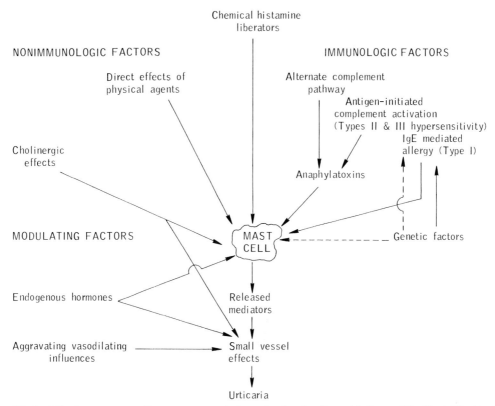

Figure 11–1. *A final common pathway representation of urticaria. From Mathews KP. Med Clin North Am 58:188, 1974, with permission.*

extremely potent histamine releasers from human mast cells. Clinical examples include some cases of cryoglobulinemia, systemic lupus erythematosus (SLE), Sjögren's syndrome, leukocytoclastic vasculitis, hives associated with transfusion reactions or, very rarely, with drug reactions and chronic idiopathic urticaria. Kinins and protease inhibitor deficiencies may also play a role in some cases, but these have been studied more extensively in hereditary angioedema (discussed later in this chapter). The frequent exacerbations of chronic urticaria by aspirin also suggest the possible involvement of arachidonate metabolites. Substance P, a neuropeptide, is a histamine liberator that may be responsible for the flare surrounding urticarial wheals.

Relatively recent studies of chronic urticaria provide some clues as to why some individuals develop this problem: these persons have increased numbers of cutaneous mast cells and an increased content of histamine in the skin. In addition, they exhibit enhanced histamine release as shown by increased reactivity to intracutaneous histamine-releasing drugs. Most of these patients also have a mononuclear

cell infiltrate around lesional venules, and the majority of these cells are helper T cells. These patients should be distinguished from those with the much rarer urticarial leukocytoclastic vasculitis featuring polymorphonuclear neutrophil infiltration, leukocytoclasis with nuclear dust, endothelial cell proliferation, fibrinoid deposits, and/or erythrocyte extravasation. Immunofluorescent staining often shows deposition of immunoglobulin and complement.

Clinically, certain modulating factors appear to exacerbate hives. These include agents producing vascular dilatation in the skin, such as heat, exertion, emotional factors, alcoholic drinks, fever, and hyperthyroidism. Catecholamines may play a role both by a direct vascular effect and by modulation of mediator release. Premenstrual exacerbations suggest that ovarian hormones may also play a role.

Clinical Assessment

The diagnosis of urticaria or angioedema is obvious in many instances. Determining its cause, however, may lead to a challenging exercise in medical detective work in patients with acute or sporadic disease. A cause for chronic urticaria cannot be found in the vast majority of cases, but a restricted effort along these lines is appropriate for patient and professional reassurance and especially to rule out significant underlying disease.

The patient history is particularly important because it determines which if any of the large number of etiologic possibilities should be pursued. From the previous discussion, it is apparent that one first should determine whether the urticaria or angioedema is acute or chronic, the duration of the individual lesions, and the presence of pruritus. Obtaining clues about pathogenesis can be aided by the types of questions used to assess patients with other types of potentially allergic disease. *When* do hives and angioedema occur (time of year, month, week, and day)? *Where* do lesions occur (effect of travel, onset in specific locales)? *What* has the patient suspected? Although patients are often misleading, astute patients can be correct. Specific inquiry then should be made about the agents that have most frequently been implicated in causing urticaria or angioedema; these causes include:

- Drugs and foreign sera
- Foods and food additives
- Infection
- Psychic factors
- Inhalants
- Bites and stings
- Direct contact of skin with various agents
- Connective tissue diseases
- Neoplasms
- Physical agents
- Genetics
- Miscellaneous

Drugs

A thorough, searching inquiry is necessary to avoid important omissions. Common sources of error are: the patient forgets to indicate *all* drugs taken, including those taken without prescription; the patient or physician fails to consider all routes of administration; or the patient thinks that the physician is inquiring about illicit drugs. Relatively common offenders include penicillin, other antibiotics, and narcotics. Remember that the onset of serum sickness reactions is delayed about 7 to 21 days, and the cutaneous manifestations commonly are accompanied by fever, arthral-

gias, and lymphadenopathy. Aspirin causes exacerbations of chronic urticaria or angioedema in up to 30 to 40% of patients, but hives generally continue even when it is assiduously avoided. Other cyclo-oxygenase inhibitors (e.g., the nonsteroidal anti-inflammatory agents) have a similar effect. Angioedema occurring during the treatment of hypertension by angiotensin-converting enzyme inhibitors may be related to the kininase activity of this enzyme.

Foods

These are a common cause of *acute* urticaria in the community at large. Fish, seafood, nuts, peanuts, and eggs are common offenders, but numerous other foods can cause trouble. Atopic persons are more likely to have this type of urticaria.

Food additives also have received much attention with emphasis on tartrazine yellow dye, other azo dyes, benzoic acid, and 4-hydroxybenzoic acid. However, many critical observers doubt that these are frequently important. Various vegetable gums have long been known to be rare offenders, and more recently aspartame has been well documented to cause hives or angioedema. The well-known sulfite intolerance is related largely to asthma and anaphylactic reactions, but urticaria and angioedema may be a feature of the latter.

Infection

In pediatric practice, acute transient urticaria often seems to be associated with infections, especially common viral types. During the prodromal phase of hepatitis B virus infections there may be a transient vasculitis that occasionally features urticaria. Parasitic infestations can also be associated with urticaria and angioedema, its prevalence obviously varying with geographic locale. On the other hand, many older claims about focal, chronic, pyogenic infection as a cause of chronic urticaria have not withstood critical appraisal. Likewise, claims about an etiologic role for *Candida* in the gastrointestinal tract require substantiation, but immediate-type hypersensitivity to *Trichophyton* may be relevant in some cases.

Psychic Factors

Although it is common clinical experience to observe exacerbations of urticaria or angioedema during periods of emotional stress, these can be accounted for to a substantial extent by the documented increase in cutaneous blood flow that accompanies such stress. However, to regard psychologic factors as the primary cause of urticaria does not explain why some patients develop these lesions rather than a variety of other psychosomatic complaints. Psychiatrists have also not been able to agree on a characteristic personality profile of these patients.

Inhalants

Urticaria sometimes develops in atopic persons on exposure to inhalant allergens such as animal emanations (dander, saliva, urine) or (rarely) pollen, but it seldom occurs in the absence of respiratory symptoms.

Bites and Stings

Urticaria or angioedema is a common feature of anaphylactic reactions to the stings of Hymenoptera or other insects such as fire ants and *Triatoma*. Quite different are the lesions of papular urticaria caused by insects such as bedbugs, fleas, or mites. These most often are seen on the legs of children, and they are less evanescent than most hives.

Contact Urticaria

These lesions are often produced by agents that actually penetrate the skin, such as nettles, Portuguese man-of-war, other forms of sea life, moth and butterfly scales, tarantula hairs, and caterpillar foot processes. Other substances, however, can produce urticaria on contact with intact skin. Examples include drugs, foods, chemicals used on the job, benzoic acid, sorbic acid, and numerous other agents that can produce either nonimmunologic or immunologically mediated reactions.

Connective Tissue Disease

There is a documented increase in the prevalence of urticaria associated with SLE, and of course urticaria or angioedema is a cardinal feature of serum sickness. These lesions have also been reported in association with Sjögren's syndrome, polymyositis, hypersensitiv-

ity or leukocytoclastic vasculitis, essential mixed cryoglobulinemia, and hypocomplementemic urticarial vasculitis. The pathology often shows a leukocytoclastic vasculitis, and clinically the lesions tend to be more persistent than in most other forms of urticaria, the lower extremities are primarily involved, residual bruising may be evident, and the patients often have symptoms in the joints or other hints of systemic disease.

Neoplasms

There are a number of reports of urticaria associated with neoplasms, especially lymphomas, but because both types of lesions are common, the relationship at times may be coincidental. In patients without a known neoplasm, prudence calls for a thorough history, physical examination, and screening laboratory studies (discussed later in this chapter). In the absence of any suggestion of a malignancy, however, an exhaustive study of every patient with hives is not warranted. On the other hand, the possibility of malignancy warrants strong consideration in patients with chronic angioedema without urticaria. As discussed later, this can be due to an acquired C1 inhibitor deficiency.

Genetic Types

These include hereditary angioedema; the syndrome of urticaria, deafness, and amyloidosis (Muckle-Wells syndrome); vibratory angioedema; familial cold "urticaria"; delayed cold-induced urticaria; familial localized heat urticaria of delayed type; erythropoietic protoporphyria with solar urticaria; C3 inactivator deficiency with urticaria; and serum carboxypeptidase N deficiency with angioedema. With the exception of hereditary angioedema, which is discussed later, all are very rare and are transmitted as autosomal dominant traits.

Physical Agents

As mentioned previously, the physical urticarias (Table 11-1) have provided valuable models for studying the mechanisms of urticaria. In addition to demonstrating mediator release, dermographism, cold urticaria, and solar urticaria can sometimes be transferred to normal skin by the Prausnitz-Kustner test. IgE

Table 11–1. *Physical Agents Producing Urticaria*

Type of Agent	Type of Urticaria
Mechanical	Dermographism
	Primary
	Idiopathic
	Allergic
	Secondary
	Cutaneous mastocytosis
	Transient forms
	Delayed dermographism
	Delayed-pressure urticaria
	Immediate-pressure urticaria
Thermal	Cold
	Acquired
	Idiopathic
	Associated with
	cryoglobulinemia,
	cryofibrinogenemia, or cold
	hemolysins
	Transient forms associated with
	drugs or infection
	Delayed cold-induced urticaria
	Familial cold "urticaria"
	Cold-induced cholinergic urticaria
	Cold-dependent dermographism
	Heat
	Cholinergic urticaria
	Localized heat urticaria
	Familial localized heat urticaria of
	delayed type
Light	Solar urticaria
	Probably allergic types
	Associated with abnormal
	protoporphyrin metabolism
	Idiopathic types

Modified from Mathews KP. Med Clin North Am 58:194, 1974, with permission.

usually is responsible for this passive transfer. It also is intriguing that a number of patients have been found to have more than one type of physical urticaria, such as combined cholinergic and cold urticaria or dermographism and cold allergy.

Dermographism is present in about 2 to 5% of the populace. It is more readily elicited by stroking the back than the forearm and should be routinely tested for in cases of urticaria. It is likely to be present in patients with increased numbers of cutaneous mast cells, as in diffuse cutaneous mastocytosis. Sometimes symptomatic dermographism provides an explanation for all of the patient's difficulty with itching wheals, whereas in other cases it may be coincidental or only a minor aspect of the problem.

With *delayed pressure urticaria,* patients develop deep, painful swellings about 4 to 6 hours after pressure is applied to the skin, with the palms, soles, and buttocks being most often involved. Frequently there are associated constitutional symptoms such as malaise, fever,

arthralgia, and headache. The swelling may occur alone but more often is associated with severe chronic idiopathic urticaria and angioedema. The diagnosis is confirmed by attaching two sandbags or jugs of fluid with a combined weight of 15 lb to the ends of a strap that is applied over the shoulder or thigh for 10 to 15 minutes; the site is then observed for a number of hours for the development of a linear wheal.

The genetic forms of *cold urticaria* are quite rare, but idiopathic cold urticaria is a relatively common problem. The diagnosis involves excluding an associated cryoglobulinemia, cryofibrinogenemia, luetic cold hemolysin disease, or relationship to drugs (rarely) or infections such as infectious mononucleosis. Recognition of cold urticaria is important because it has been responsible for deaths from swimming in cool water, which caused massive mediator release, syncope, and drowning. Often the diagnosis can be confirmed by the simple ice cube test: place an ice cube on an extremity for 3 to 5 minutes and then observe the area for the development of a pruritic wheal, surrounded by erythema, as the skin rewarms over the following 5 to 15 minutes. However, this test is not invariably positive; some patients require exposure of the entire body to cold air.

Localized *heat urticaria* mimics cold urticaria but is much less common. *Cholinergic urticaria* was described earlier. The diagnosis can be confirmed by having the patient reproduce the lesions by exercising, ideally in a warm environment or while wearing a wet suit or plastic occlusive suit. The diagnosis of *solar urticaria* is usually evident from the history and distribution of the skin lesions and can be confirmed by controlled exposure to light. Solar urticaria can be divided into several groups depending on the wavelength of light eliciting the lesions. One type results from a genetic abnormality in protoporphyrin IX metabolism, and others appear to be immunologically mediated in that they can be passively transferred by the Prausnitz-Kustner technique.

Miscellaneous Types

Aquagenic urticaria consists of tiny, perifollicular urticarial lesions developing after contact with water of any temperature. The diagnosis is confirmed by the "tepid towel test," wherein a towel soaked in 37°C water is applied to the skin for 30 minutes. Urticaria or angioedema has also been reported from implanted materials such as Vitallium cups or nails and retained myelographic contrast medium; it can be associated with hyperthyroidism, chronic thyroiditis, hyperparathyroidism, polycythemia vera, the hemolytic-uremic syndrome, pregnancy, direct electric current stimulation, and ultraviolet irradiation. Urtication also occurs when the lesions of urticaria pigmentosa (benign mast cell tumors) are rubbed (Darier's sign). Rare cases have also recently been described of episodic angioedema associated with an extreme degree of eosinophilic leukocytosis, fever, and transient weight gain.

In summary, numerous possible etiologic agents need to be considered in evaluating these patients. Food, drugs, and childhood infections are the most common offenders in acute urticaria and angioedema. As noted previously, no discernible cause, aside from physical agents, can be ascertained in the vast majority of chronic cases. As implied by this discussion, a *complete physical examination* is important, especially in cases of chronic urticaria and angioedema, to rule out an underlying condition such as a connective tissue, infectious, neoplastic, or endocrine disease. Unfortunately the appearance of the lesions is usually not helpful, but Table 11–2 provides some clues. Remember to test for dermographism.

Diagnostic Procedures

If the history or complete physical examination gives any clues to the cause of the patient's urticaria or angioedema, these should be pursued by using the appropriate tests. These might include a trial of dietary restriction, tests for SLE, exercise test for cholinergic urticaria, ice cube test, delayed pressure test and so on. Skin tests with atopic allergens are likely to be helpful only in exceptional patients with inhalant allergy or in some patients with suspected food allergy when the history is not diagnostic. When the skin problem has been present for only a few hours or days, one generally postpones a relatively extensive evaluation until it becomes clear that there will not be an early spontaneous remission. In sporadic cases it is simple enough to have patients keep a retroactive diary of food intake and activities before their attacks. In the many cases of chronic urticaria or angioedema when the history provides no clues to etiology, a major objective is to exclude important underlying disease. Accordingly it is appropriate to supplement the history and complete physical examination with the tests given in Table 11–3.

Because the cause of *chronic* urticaria or angioedema is unknown in the large majority of cases, further routine testing is *not* cost effective and yields primarily increasing frustration of both the patient and physician. Indeed, in cases of chronic disease it generally is wise to tell patients at the outset that no specific cause is likely to be found, and in fact one hopes that no serious underlying condition will be revealed.

Treatment

Obviously the preferred treatment is avoidance of causative agents when these can be identified and when avoidance is feasible. This generally is the case when allergy to drugs, foods, inhalants, insects, or contactants is involved. An explanation of the disease process and its triggers should be helpful for patients with dermographism, cholinergic urticaria, and delayed pressure urticaria. Common sense avoidance measures should be reviewed with patients afflicted with cold or solar urticaria, and the former should be forewarned about

Table 11–2. Appearance of Urticarial Lesions as a Clue to Etiology

Appearance	Type of Urticaria
Small wheals surrounded by large areas of erythema	Cholinergic urticaria
Linear wheals	Dermographism
Lesions limited to exposed areas	Possible solar or cold urticaria
Hives mainly on lower extremities	Urticarial vasculitis or papular urticaria
Small perifollicular hives	Aquagenic urticaria or follicular dermographism
Persistent pigmented macules, papules, or nodules that urticate when rubbed (Darier's sign)	Urticaria pigmentosa
Occurrence on the abdomen (and sometimes elsewhere) of women in the third trimester of pregnancy	Pruritic urticarial papules and plaques of pregnancy (PUPP)

Table 11–3. Suggested Tests for Chronic Urticaria or Angioedema When the History Gives No Clues Regarding Etiology

Total and differential white blood cell count
Urinalysis
Sedimentation rate
Chemistry panel
Antinuclear antibody
Elimination diet, 5- to 7-day trial
Possible tartrazine challenge
If sedimentation rate is elevated and/or systemic or
   rheumatic symptoms are present:
  Skin biopsy
  CH_{50}, C3, C4
  Cryoglobulins
  ?Hepatitis B antigen and antibody tests
  ?Tests for immune complexes

the dangers of swimming in cool water and of swimming alone. Sun screens containing *p*-aminobenzoic acid help to protect against light of 285 to 320-nm wavelength. Treatment of any discovered underlying disease is of course imperative, and genetic counseling should be provided to families with hereditary forms of these conditions. In addition, patients should avoid, to the extent feasible, the previously mentioned potentiating factors such as alcoholic drinks, heat, exertion, and aspirin.

Reassurance is another significant aspect of therapy because the skin lesions are often more frightening in appearance than the generally favorable prognosis warrants. When no cause can be found, patients can also be encouraged that a variety of medications are available to maintain them in reasonable comfort until a spontaneous remission occurs. However, they should be made aware of the need for an emergency room visit if laryngeal edema oc-

curs. If the patient has experienced laryngeal edema, many physicians would prescribe and instruct the patient in the use of an ANA-KIT or Epi-Pen for the self-administration of epinephrine. However, one should avoid generating undue anxiety about laryngeal edema because the only known fatalities from this cause have been in patients with hereditary angioedema or Hymenoptera anaphylaxis.

Drugs used for the symptomatic treatment of more persistent urticaria or angioedema are outlined in Table 11–4. Most H_1-type antihistamines have some degrees of effectiveness in mild urticaria, but among the commonly employed drugs of this type, hydroxyzine and doxepin have greater potency. Side effects, especially drowsiness, are substantial problems but can be reduced by using the drugs initially only at half strength; side effects usually diminish with continued use. Cyproheptadine provides another option and has been recommended particularly for cold urticaria, but its side effects also may include substantial weight gain because of stimulated appetite. Problems with most side effects are largely eliminated with the newer generation of H_1 antagonists, such as terfenadine, mequitazine, and astemizole. The latter has an especially potent and prolonged H_1-blocking effect and should be commercially available in the United States soon. A disadvantage of these newer drugs is their high cost. In general, H_1 antihistamines show their beneficial effects after just a few doses (astemizole may take a few days), and failure to achieve a fairly prompt therapeutic response thus calls for trying another drug. When one or more potent H_1 blockers have

Table 11–4. Drugs for Symptomatic Treatment of Persistent Urticaria

H_1-type antihistamines; any type may help in some mild cases
  Hydroxyzine (initially 100 mg daily but increasing dose as required and tolerated, up to 400 mg daily)
  Doxepin (initially 75 mg H.S. and increasing as necessary)
  Cyproheptadine (initially 4 mg q.i.d. but double dose if required)
  Astemizole 10 mg H.S. (if available)
  Terfenadine (60 mg b.i.d. or more)

If inadequate response, add an H_2-type antihistamine
  Cimetidine (300 mg q.i.d.) or ranitidine (150 mg b.i.d.)
  Ephedrine sulfate (25 mg q.i.d.; not very potent)

If available, ketotifen

If necessary, corticosteroids for severe, acute serum sickness (e.g., prednisone 60 mg daily with rapid
  taper) or severe delayed pressure urticaria (e.g., 10–15 mg prednisone q.o.d. after initial daily
  administration of higher doses)

Nonsteroidal anti-inflammatory drug trial (e.g., ibuprofen 600 mg q.i.d.) in refractory delayed pressure
  urticaria or urticarial vasculitis

Hydroxychloroquine, colchicine, dapsone, and doxantrazole should be considered in urticarial vasculitis
  or urticaria associated with SLE

Danazol or stanazolol for refractory cholinergic urticaria

proved to be ineffective, an H_2 antihistamine (e.g., cimetidine or ranitidine) may be added. H_2-blocking agents generally should not be used alone for treating urticaria and angioedema, but in some cases they significantly enhance the therapeutic efficacy of H_1 antihistamines.

Unless specifically contraindicated, epinephrine remains the drug of choice for very severe, acute urticaria (an intravenous antihistamine would be an option). Ephedrine and related drugs occasionally are helpful, particularly when used in combination with antihistamines, but they are not very potent.

Corticosteroids are the drugs of choice in severe delayed pressure urticaria and in severe serum sickness not responding to other medications. Prolonged daily administration of high doses involves an unacceptable risk/benefit ratio for most urticaria patients, but occasionally small alternate day doses, in combination with other drugs, are reasonable in severe cases not responding to other forms of treatment.

Newer drugs inhibiting mediator release from mast cells (along with other actions) should provide therapeutic benefit in urticaria, and this has been substantiated by recent investigations. It is hoped that ketotifin will become commercially available in the United States soon. Nonsteroidal anti-inflammatory drugs have been reported to be of some benefit in delayed pressure urticaria and urticarial vasculitis, but care should be taken in initiating therapy in view of their capacity to exacerbate urticaria. Doxantrazole and dapsone sometimes help urticaria associated with SLE, and hydroxychloroquine and colchicine have improved urticarial vasculitis. Innumerable other

Table 11–5. Differentiation between Hereditary Angioedema and Acquired C1INH Deficiency

Parameter	Hereditary Angioedema	Acquired Angioedema
Most frequent age at onset	6–20 yr	> 50 yr
Family history	Yes	No
Underlying disease	No	Yes
C1INH function	Low	Low
C1q antigen	Normal	Low

suggested treatments have not withstood the test of time.

C1 Inhibitor Deficiency and Angioedema

Recurrent angioedema without urticaria should suggest a possible C1 inhibitor (C1INH) deficiency. This is particularly important to recognize and treat because of its potential morbidity and mortality—as high as 33%. The angioedematous swelling seen in C1INH-deficient patients is poorly circumscribed, nonpitting, nonpruritic, and not associated with concomitant urticaria. Unlike idiopathic angioedema, this swelling generally increases over 12 to 24 hours and slowly subsides over the subsequent 48 to 72 hours. The swelling may affect the extremities, face, gastrointestinal tract, or upper airway.

Two major types of hereditary angioedema have been described, both of which are inherited in an autosomal dominant pattern. The classic type (or type I), found in 85% of the patients with hereditary angioedema, has a low serum concentration of C1INH. The remaining

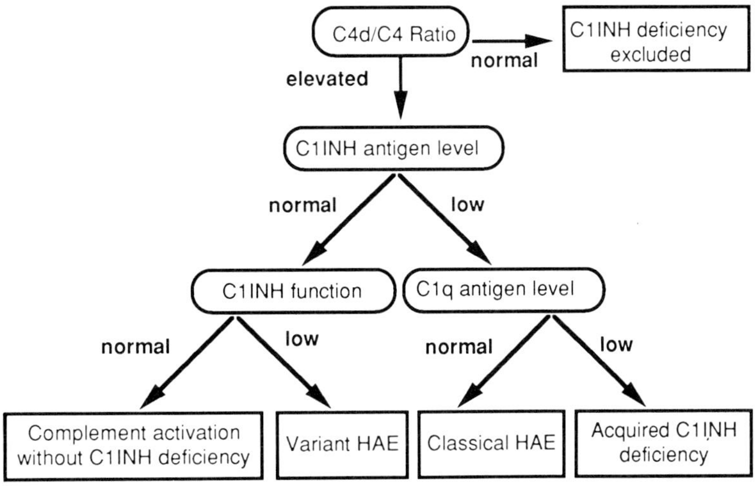

Figure 11–2. Complement evaluation of the patient with recurrent angioedema without associated urticaria. HAE, hereditary angioedema.

15% of the patients have variant hereditary angioedema (or type II) and have C1INH levels that are normal or elevated immunologically, but their C1INH shows little or no activity in functional tests. There is an increased incidence of autoimmune or immunoregulatory disorders in hereditary angioedema patients. C1INH deficiency may also be acquired. This was initially described in patients with lymphoreticular malignancies, and it has now also been described in association with a variety of conditions including paraproteinemia, anti-idiotypic antibody reactions, autoimmune diseases, other types of malignancies, and autoantibodies to C1INH itself. The angioedema may precede the emergence of the underlying disease by 5 years or more, and successful treatment of the underlying disease has been associated with resolution of the angioedema and C1INH deficiency.

C1INH deficiency should be considered for all patients with recurrent angioedema without associated urticaria. Table 11-5 presents the salient clinical features of hereditary and acquired C1INH deficiencies. Angioedema that worsens in a woman taking estrogens suggests C1INH deficiency. Similarly, recurrent absences from school because of abdominal pain may be the presenting symptom of hereditary angioedema. Figure 11–2 shows an algorithm designed to efficiently evaluate patients suspected of having a C1INH deficiency. The C4d/C4 ratio is 100% sensitive in identifying patients with a C1INH deficiency irrespective of whether they have an active swelling or are already being treated; this test is available through SmithKline Bioscience or the Scripps Clinic Immunology Reference Laboratory. Alternatively, the total C4 level is always low in C1INH-deficient patients during an attack of angioedema and almost always between attacks.

Many patients with C1INH deficiency do not require long-term prophylactic therapy. However, patients with frequent severe attacks or with attacks involving the upper airway should be treated with either attenuated androgens (stanazolol or danazol) or ϵ-aminocaproic acid to decrease the frequency and severity of their attacks. Short-term prophylaxis with one of these agents or with freshly frozen plasma is indicated before expected trauma such as surgery and especially dental procedures, which have a high likelihood of precipitating laryngeal swelling. Acute angioedema of the oropharynx is potentially life-threatening in C1INH-deficient patients, and these patients should be hospitalized so that they can be intubated if the swelling progresses.

Bibliography

Elias J, Boss E, Kaplan AP: Studies of the cellular infiltrate of chronic idiopathic urticaria: prominence of T-lymphocytes, monocytes, and mast cells. J Allergy Clin Immunol 78:914–918, 1986.
> *The immunopathology of typical chronic idiopathic urticaria is assessed with the aid of monoclonal antibodies and enzyme histochemistry to identify the infiltrating cells.*

Frank MM, Gelfand JA, Atkinson JP. Hereditary angioedema: the clinical syndrome and its management. Ann Intern Med 84:580–593, 1976.
> *Excellent review of the pathophysiology, diagnosis, and management of HAE is presented.*

Hentges F, Humbel R, Dicato M, et al. Acquired C1 esterase inhibitor deficiency: case report with emphasis on complement and kallikrein activation during two patterns of clinical manifestations. J Allergy Clin Immunol 78:860–867, 1986.
> *Unusual case of acquired C1INH deficiency is described. The accompanying editorial by Dr. Frank is an up-to-date review of this syndrome.*

Jorizzo JL, Smith EB. The physical urticarias. An update and review. Arch Dermatol 118:194–201, 1982.
> *This article encompasses both clinical aspects of the subject and a review of mechanisms.*

Kaplan AP. Chronic urticaria. Possible causes, suggested treatment alternatives. Postgrad Med 74:209–215, 218–222, 1983.
> *A review.*

Mathews KP. Urticaria and angioedema. J Allergy Clin Immunol 72:1–14, 1983.
> *A review.*

Rosenstreich DL. Chronic urticaria, activated T cells and mast cell releasability. J Allergy Clin Immunol 78:1099–1102, 1986.
> *The pathogenesis of chronic idiopathic urticaria is discussed in the light of its microscopic pathology and enhanced mediator releasability by the cutaneous mast cells.*

Soter NA, Wasserman SI. Physical urticaria/angioedema: an experimental model of mast cell activation in humans. J Allergy Clin Immunol 66:358–365, 1980.
> *This is an authoritative review of mast cell activation in physical urticaria/angioedema.*

Symposium on urticaria and the reactive inflammatory vascular dermatoses. Derm Clin 3:1–193, 1985.
> *Most of this issue is devoted to a series of papers on various aspects of urticaria. The article on the contact urticaria syndrome by Burdick and Mathias (p 71) is especially comprehensive and includes 171 references.*

Zuraw BL, Sugimoto S, Curd JG. The value of rocket immunoelectrophoresis for C4 activation in the evaluation of patients with angioedema or C1-inhibitor deficiency. J Allergy Clin Immunol 78:1115–1120, 1986.
> *Comparison of alternative complement tests that can be used to make the diagnosis of C1INH deficiency.*

PART THREE

Endocrinology/ Metabolism

12

Self-Monitoring in Diabetes Mellitus

MARGARET F. ODELL, M.S.N.
JEREMY M. GLEESON, M.B., Ch.B.
DANA E. WILSON, M.D.

Because the signs and symptoms of diabetes mellitus are such poor markers of glycemic control, some other means of estimating blood glucose concentration is essential. Blood glucose concentrations can be estimated directly by using venous or capillary blood, or they can be inferred from urinary glucose measurements. Self-monitoring of blood glucose (SMBG) has become the preferred method of assessing glycemic control for most patients; it provides direct measurements of blood glucose concentrations as opposed to the indirect, insensitive, and frequently misleading estimates provided by tests for glucose in the urine.

Several studies have established the accuracy and precision of SMBG when performed by trained personnel or closely supervised patients. When integrated into a comprehensive treatment plan, SMBG may improve glycemic control; this has been shown in short-term studies with selected patients. The use of SMBG and the attainment of near normal glucose concentrations in pregnant women have resulted in improved clinical outcome with fewer perinatal complications. Most diabetologists encourage SMBG in the belief that it results in improved glycemic control and reduces the incidence of long-term diabetic complications. Although there is no proof of these effects, available evidence supports the use of SMBG in most patients.

A major concern about SMBG is the possibility that inaccurate results will be obtained and lead to inappropriate treatment. Errors in technique are the main source of inaccuracy, and adequate patient education with frequent review of technique is essential to ensure valid results. The high cost of SMBG may restrict or even preclude its use by some patients.

In this chapter we review the indications for and techniques of SMBG and urinary glucose testing, and we include recommendations about patient education and equipment selection.

Indications for SMBG

The decision to use SMBG should be tied to the therapeutic goals for each patient. Candidates for SMBG include patients following intensive insulin regimens in whom tight diabetic control is being attempted, patients undergoing frequent changes in therapy, and patients whose diabetes is unstable, such as those at risk for ketoacidosis or hypoglycemia. In particular, patients who do not have an adrenergic response to hypoglycemia and who might be unaware of it need to perform SMBG (Table 12–1). Most patients with type I (insulin-dependent) diabetes fall into one or more of these categories. SMBG is mandatory in pregnant diabetic patients in whom euglycemia is the goal of treatment.

For many patients with type II (non–insulin-dependent) diabetes, the indications for

Table 12–1. Indications for SMBG

Patients attempting tight control of diabetes
    Undergoing insulin pump therapy
    Taking multiple daily doses of insulin
    Pregnant or planning pregnancy
Patients with unstable diabetes
    Experiencing frequent episodes of hypoglycemia
    Unaware of/unresponsive to hypoglycemia
    Ketosis prone
Patients with non–insulin-dependent diabetes
    Being stabilized and adjusting to insulin
    Experiencing intercurrent illness or emergencies
    Using SMBG as an adjunct to urine testing
    Undergoing patient education
Patients who cannot use urine testing
Patients who prefer SMBG

SMBG are less well defined. Regular SMBG is appropriate in many of these patients, particularly those who have unstable glucose control, those with intercurrent illness, and those undergoing adjustment of therapy or diabetes education. However, patients with stable type II diabetes whose treatment is unchanged over long periods or those in whom tight control is not a therapeutic goal (such as older patients with other significant disease and limited life expectancy) may not need to perform regular SMBG. Such patients can perform occasional SMBG as an adjunct to regular urine testing. Some patients cannot perform urine testing (for example, anephric patients and those with bladder neuropathy) and must use SMBG.

SMBG techniques are not acceptable for the diagnosis of diabetes. Frequent determinations of glucose levels at the bedside by using SMBG techniques are useful in the management of diabetic ketoacidosis and other emergencies but should not be used in life-threatening situations without confirmatory laboratory measurements.

Use of SMBG

The SMBG program should be individualized for each patient. In type I diabetes, monitoring four to seven times daily has been recommended. This is appropriate for well-motivated type I patients and is essential for pregnant patients and patients using an insulin pump. For other patients this may be too demanding, and a more flexible routine can be used. Because the blood glucose concentration is affected by food and insulin, SMBG should be performed at specified times in relation to meals and insulin injections. A common schedule for patients taking two or more doses of insulin daily involves testing four times daily, before meals and at bedtime. Two-hour postprandial testing, in addition to premeal testing, is important if tight control is being attempted. Insulin doses are adjusted according to the results. For example, for patients taking a twice daily mixture of intermediate-acting (e.g., isophane insulin suspension) and regular insulin:

- The prebreakfast blood glucose value can be used to adjust the p.m. dose of intermediate-acting insulin.
- The prelunch blood glucose level can be used to adjust the a.m. dose of regular insulin.
- The predinner blood glucose value can be used to adjust the a.m. dose of intermediate-acting insulin.
- The bedtime blood glucose level can be used to adjust the p.m. dose of regular insulin.

Whether patients are advised to change their own insulin doses according to a prescribed algorithm or only after consultation with a health professional is determined individually.

Similar intensive monitoring is appropriate in patients with type II diabetes who are being educated about their diabetes or whose diabetes is unstable (i.e., during adjustment of insulin dose or during intercurrent illness). On achieving glycemic control, these patients can usually perform the test less often. The appropriate frequency of testing in type II patients is quite variable; for some patients as few as two tests per week suffice, for others two or more each day are required. Testing at several different times on selected days gives more useful information than testing at a single time every day.

Intercurrent illness causes deterioration in glucose control, and all patients should intensify their usual schedule of monitoring when they are ill. Testing every 4 to 6 hours is usually recommended. SMBG is useful to document hypoglycemic rections and should be performed in hypoglycemia-prone patients before, during, and after exercise (the effects of which can last up to 24 hours). Occasional testing at 2 to 4 a.m. in all patients is helpful to exclude nocturnal hypoglycemia.

Excessive SMBG data collection should be avoided; the number of tests should not exceed that likely to be useful in patient management. If too demanding a schedule is insisted on without perceived benefit to the patient, discouragement, frustration, and ultimately noncompliance often result. Patients can easily lose enthusiasm for SMBG when the results obtained are ignored by the clinician.

Patients doing SMBG should keep permanent diaries of their blood glucose values and bring them to each clinic visit (Fig. 12–1). Patients are instructed to indicate events that may affect blood glucose, such as symptomatic hypoglycemia, exercise, and variations in food intake, in addition to recording blood glucose data. To facilitate identification of trends and patterns in the data, we favor a vertical format in which numbers that are to be compared (e.g., prebreakfast values) are arranged in columns.

Name: _____									
	Blood Glucose				Insulin Dose				
Date	Breakfast	Lunch	Dinner	Bedtime	a.m.	a.m.	p.m.	p.m.	Comments

Figure 12–1. *Sample SMBG data sheet.*

An adequate set of data must be examined before deciding that a consistent pattern exists. Often this will require data from a week or more of testing, particularly with patients whose glycemic control is labile. Trends suggested by data from only a few days often disappear with longer observation. The practitioner should review the patient's diary for evidence of noncompliance; such clues include

- The SMBG logbook is too neat. All entries appear to have been made at the same time with the same pen or pencil.
- The numerical values are too similar and fail to show expected biologic variation.
- The values are inconsistent with the glycosylated hemoglobin.
- The values are inconsistent with the clinical picture.

When inaccurate results are suspected, the patient's equipment and technique should be checked carefully.

Technique of SMBG

Blood Collection

SMBG requires obtaining a drop of capillary blood from a finger (usually the lateral border of the distal phalanx) and placing the blood on a glucose oxidase reagent strip, which changes color according to the amount of glucose present. The strip is then read visually or with a reflectance meter.

Accuracy depends on obtaining a drop of blood large enough to cover the reagent pad on the strip completely; this is facilitated by the use of an automatic puncturing device and a fine-pointed lancet. A number of devices are available, and the price of lancets used for each device varies considerably (Table 12–2). These devices ensure uniform wound depth and minimize pain. Devices are available to allow deeper skin penetration in patients with thickened skin. Pain can be further minimized by site rotation. Cold hands should be warmed in warm (not hot) water before attempting to prick a finger. Hand washing with soap and water provides adequate skin cleanliness. Infection of the fingertips is not a problem in patients who use a good handwashing technique and a new lancet for each test. However, SMBG must be used with caution by immunosuppressed patients.

Tremor, hand deformities, poor blood flow, toughened skin, and visual impairment may all interfere with satisfactory blood collection, especially in older patients.

The drop of blood is placed on the strip, covering the entire reagent pad, without rubbing, smearing, or adding additional blood. The amount of time the blood is left on the strip and the method of removal (wiping, blotting, or washing) are critical, and the manufacturer's instructions must be followed exactly.

Visual Reading of Strips

This involves comparison of colors with a chart and has the advantage of not requiring the added cost of a meter. A good light source, either daylight or incandescent, must be used. Fluorescent light can alter the perception of some hues. Hue discrimination and interpolation are skills that may have to be learned and that may improve with pratice. Decreased hue

Table 12–2. *Automatic Finger-Puncturing Devices and Their Cost*

Device	Cost*	Compatible Lancets	Cost*
Autolet	$20–30	Monolet	$8–12 per 200
		Autoclix	$8–12 per 200
		Unilet	$8–12 per 200
Autoclix	$10–20	Monolet	
		Autoclix	
Penlet	$15	Monolet	
		Autoclix	
		Unilet	
Autolance	$15	Microfine	$8 per 100

*Approximate cost only.

discrimination occurs with normal aging as well as in diabetic retinopathy.

Before attempting to read strips visually, patients should be tested for visual acuity and color vision. The standard color blindness screening charts are not satisfactory for this purpose because they do not exclude subtle abnormalities in hue discrimination sufficient to impair reading of strips. The Farnsworth D-15 test is recommended as a simple and sensitive way to exclude such deficits; however, the equipment for this test costs about $250. A cheap and practical alternative is to obtain color chips from a paint store that match those used by the Farnsworth test. The examiner selects a card at one end of the range, and the patient is asked to progressively match the closest color. Patients who fail this test cannot read strips accurately by visual comparison and must use a meter.

Some strips are more accurate and easier to read visually than others. We find that Chemstrips bG are satisfactory for this purpose. This strip has two color-impregnated pads; the top color panel (beige to green) is more accurate in the range of 80 to 240 mg/dl, whereas the lower panel (blue) is useful for values outside this range. When interpolating, most patients tend to underestimate blood glucose concentration. Patient accuracy should be documented by comparison with simultaneous laboratory measurements. However, the accuracy of visual comparison is limited, and results within 20% of simultaneous laboratory determinations are considered acceptable.

For many patients, performing SMBG by visual comparison alone is sufficient. This is true for patients with adequate color vision who do not make small changes in insulin doses according to SMBG results. For others, such as pregnant patients in whom meticulous glycemic control is mandatory and patients using insulin pumps, the more accurate measurements provided by a meter are necessary.

It should be remembered that the real improvement in accuracy provided by a meter is often much less than it appears, and meters are not necessary for clinical management in many patients.

Meters

Reflectance meters are used to obtain more quantitative estimates of glucose concentration than are possible by visual comparison alone. They give a numerical read-out in proportion to the color change of a test strip. Currently available meters are portable, battery operated, and have a useful range from 40 to 400 mg/dl. At the extremes of this range (e.g., < 60 or > 300 mg/dl), accuracy diminishes.

Numerous meters made by various manufacturers are available. At the time of writing, studies documenting meter accuracy and precision are not available for all products on the market. Three major manufacturers of reflectance meters and reagent strips whose products have been found to be generally reliable are Ames, Boehringer Mannheim, and Lifescan (Table 12–3). As previously mentioned, accuracy is user dependent: failure to obtain an adequate drop of blood or to follow the manufacturer's instructions about timing and blood removal causes inaccurate results. Periodic cleaning of the meter and changing of the batteries are essential for accuracy. Because of lot-to-lot variability in reagent strips, periodic recalibration of the meter is necessary. This process is more complicated with the older meters. Values from meters should be within 15% of simultaneous laboratory determinations.

There are a number of factors to consider when choosing a meter. Some meters are more reliable and easier to calibrate and use than others. Some companies' supplies are widely available at drugstores and pharmacies,

Table 12–3. *Characteristics of Selected Reflectance Meters*

Manufacturer and Products	Cost*	Strips	Strip Cost*	Strips Widely Available	Reliability	Ease of Use	Visual Reading
Ames							
Glucometer		Dextristix	$25/50	Yes	+	−	±
Glucometer II	$150	Glucostix	$44/100	Yes	+	+	+
Boehringer Mannheim							
Accuchek BG		Chemstrips bG	$40/100	Yes	+	+	+
Accuchek II	$140	Chemstrips bG II	$40/100	Yes	+	+	+
Tracer	$130	Tracer bG	$40/100	No	?	+	−
Lifescan							
Glucoscan Plus		Glucoscan	$45/100	No	+	+	−
Glucoscan 2000	$150	Glucoscan	$45/100	No	+	+	−
One Touch	$210	One Touch	$25/50	No	?	+	−

*Approximate cost only, e.g., $25 per 50 strips.

whereas others can be purchased only through medical supply houses. A meter whose strips can also be read visually is convenient and provides a check for gross meter inaccuracy. (Strips designed for some meters give only a crude estimate when read visually.) Selection of a meter should also take into account the manufacturer's reputation for honesty, service, and concern for its customers.

Talking meters for the visually impaired are available; however, blind patients have other difficulties with SMBG technique (in particular, obtaining a satisfactory drop of blood) and ideally should perform SMBG with the assistance of a sighted person.

Whenever possible, advice should be sought from a health professional familiar with the products currently available. Because of rapidly changing technology, products recommended here may soon become obsolete. Diabetes Care, a bimonthly published by the American Diabetes Association, is a good source of up-to-date scientific information on diabetes monitoring. Patient-oriented magazines such as Diabetes Forecast also provide useful practical information.

Memory Chips and Computers in SMBG

Meters are now available with built-in memory chips that store glucose concentration results and allow them to be recalled later. With some meters, the stored values can be transferred to a computer for analysis. Calculations can then be performed easily to determine values such as the average glucose or range of glucose values at a particular time of day. Computers can display glucose values graphi-

cally, making trends easier to discern. Software packages for analyzing the recordings are provided with some meters, whereas others permit the user to develop individualized methods of analysis.

Periodic computer analysis of glucose recordings in the physician's office or clinic can provide useful information and make interpretation of the results easier. Microcomputer systems for this purpose are likely to become widespread in the next few years. However, for most patients the hand recording of blood glucose data will remain essential to ensure that the information is immediately available.

Precautions and Complications

Hematocrit

Changes in hematocrit can affect the results obtained by SMBG. If there is an elevated hematocrit, SMBG may underestimate plasma glucose values; conversely, SMBG may overestimate blood glucose levels in the presence of anemia. This effect depends on the extent to which red cells can penetrate the woven matrix of the reagent strip, and the magnitude of the effect depends on the brand of strip used. With Chemstrips bG (used for visual comparison and in the Accuchek meters), the effect of differences in hematocrit is minimal. Other brands of strips (e.g., Glucoscan strips and Glucostix strips for the Glucometer II) may overestimate the blood glucose concentration by up to 30% in the presence of severe anemic (hematocrit $\leq 25\%$) or underestimate the glucose concentration by a similar amount in the presence of polycythemia (hematocrit $\geq 60\%$). Because of their potential failure to detect hypoglycemia, these products must be used with extreme caution in anemic patients. In general, all strips provide reliable results when the hematocrit is between 40 and 50%.

Hypoglycemia

Paradoxically, an increased incidence of hypoglycemia has been observed in patients doing SMBG, presumably related to their attempts at tighter control of the diabetes.

Psychologic Considerations

Rare individuals have an intense fear of doing the necessary finger pricks and may be unable to perform SMBG. Others have an obsessive desire to maintain euglycemia and do an excessive number of tests. Correctly recorded measurements are obviously crucial to effective use of SMBG data in patient management. We and others using meters with memory chips have observed patients who falsify many of their SMBG recordings. Lesser degrees of inaccurate recording appear to be common. Patients will admit to adding "good" measurements that have not been performed and deleting "bad" measurements. No set of physiologic or behavioral characteristics that consistently predicts this behavior has been identified. The extent to which pressure perceived by the patient to achieve good control results in alteration of the records is unclear. These considerations illustrate the need to negotiate reasonable goals for glycemic control with the patient and to use testing strategies that the patient perceives to be beneficial.

Cost of SMBG

In the United States a basic meter can be purchased for $150 (Table 12–3); talking meters for the blind and meters with memory chips cost from $200 to $400. Automatic finger-puncturing devices cost from $15 to $30 (Table 12–2). However, the initial outlay is not the major expense. With the present price of approximately $0.50 per reagent strip, a patient monitoring four times daily spends about $700 per year for reagent strips alone. It is possible to economize by splitting strips in half lengthwise. This can be done when strips are read by visual comparison, or when the meter has a special adaptor for split strips (currently available only for the Glucochek). Splitting strips, however, leads to inaccurate results when read in a meter without an adaptor and may make reading by visual comparison more difficult.

Third-party payment for meters and reagent strips is inconsistent, with frequent changes occurring in reimbursement policies. In general, health insurers are accepting an increasing responsibility for covering the provision of SMBG supplies. Some insurers pay for SMBG supplies for hospital inpatients more readily than for outpatients. Medicare currently pays 80% of the cost of a meter and 100% of the cost of the strips if a physician certifies a need for these items.

Patient Education

Patient education is the most important factor determining the accuracy of SMBG. Without adequate patient education, SMBG may result in grossly inaccurate test results that are misleading and can be worse than none at all. Certified American Diabetes Association diabetic educators and clinical nurse specialists in diabetes are trained specifically to teach patients the necessary skills. However, such expertise is not always available. Medical supply houses and company representatives are often eager to give demonstrations and provide teaching materials; many have certification programs for persons teaching SMBG.

There are certain basic principles of SMBG that must be learned whether or not a meter is used. *The importance of obtaining an adequate drop of blood and following the strip manufacturer's instructions exactly cannot be overemphasized.* Patients learning SMBG need several instruction sessions with ample time for practice. Numerous potential sources of error exist in SMBG and require careful assessment of the patient's technique (Table 12–4). Strategies to ensure good technique include having patients save their strips to evaluate whether the blood covers the strip completely, having patients demonstrate their technique with their own equipment, and correlating SMBG values with simultaneous laboratory determinations of venous plasma glucose. *Frequent follow-up sessions with evaluation of accuracy and reinstruction on technique are often required.*

Testing for Ketones

In addition to SMBG, urine testing for ketones in patients with ketosis-prone (type I)

Table 12–4. *Points to Check for Correct SMBG Technique*

1. The meter is clean and calibrated, and the proper reagent strips are used. Strips are not outdated or contaminated.
2. Hands are clean and dry.
3. A large hanging drop of blood is obtained.
4. The blood is dropped on the reagent strip without rubbing, smearing, or adding additional blood.
5. Blood is left on the strip the for the time recommended by the manufacturer.
6. The blood is removed from the strip without excessive washing, wiping, or blotting.
7. Visual comparison and interpolation are performed accurately.
8. The value obtained is recorded promptly and correctly.

diabetes remains important during periods of illness or in the presence of persistent hyperglycemia (blood glucose concentration > 250 mg/dl). This allows early recognition of impending diabetic ketoacidosis.

Urine Testing

For patients who cannot or will not use SMBG, urine testing is the only practical method of assessing glycemic control on a day-to-day basis. In the presence of a normal renal threshold for glucose, glycosuria will occur when the blood glucose reaches 180 to 200 mg/dl. Urine testing provides no information whatsoever when the blood glucose concentration is below the renal threshold, that is, when a patient is euglycemic or hypoglycemic. Urine testing provides only an index of gross hyperglycemia and is inappropriate when tight control of diabetes is attempted. Other disadvantages of urine testing are individual variability in the renal threshold, which should be determined for each patient, and inconvenience. On the positive side, urine testing is relatively cheap, painless, and does not require cumbersome equipment. As in SMBG, visual acuity and hue discrimination are prerequisites for using urine glucose strips.

Use of Urine Testing

Three premeal tests and a bedtime test used to be the standard recommendation for diabetic patients. Most patients testing this frequently now use SMBG, and urine testing is usually reserved for stable patients who need to test less often. Such patients should be asked to perform the test at various times on selected days rather than at the same time every day. Urine testing 2 hours after meals is useful in patients with high renal thresholds who usually have a negative test result before meals. Patients should intensify urine testing (to four or six tests per day) or preferably use SMBG when they are ill or unable to eat. Changes in insulin doses in sick patients should be made only on the basis of blood glucose measurements.

Double voiding of urine in the morning has been advocated to minimize the mixture of old and fresh urine. This technique requires the patient to empty the bladder, drink, and test a second specimen voided 30 minutes later. Patient compliance with this technique is limited, and low urine osmolality may result in overestimation of glycosuria. Double voiding is required when the renal threshold is being estimated; otherwise the procedure is now rarely used.

Urinary glucose measurements have traditionally been recorded in terms of pluses, however, different testing methods give different numbers of pluses for the same glucose concentration. To avoid potential confusion, recording the absolute glucose concentration (expressed as a percentage) is recommended.

Products Available for Urine Testing

At present three products are commonly used: Clinitest, Testape, and Chemstrips uG (Table 12–5). Clinitest uses a copper reduction method that detects all reducing substances; as a result the method lacks specificity and is subject to false-positive reactions in the presence of a number of drugs. In addition the test is inhibited by proteinuria, it is cumbersome, and the reagent tablets are toxic, which makes a child-resistant cap essential.

Testape and Chemistrips uG both have the advantage of using a specific glucose oxidase method. Testape is inexpensive, easy to use, and readily portable. However, its use is limited by the difficulty of distinguishing the color change between 0.25 and 2%. In our view the most satisfactory product available is Chemstrips uG. There are two color-impregnated pads, which help accuracy. The range is wide, from 0.1 to 5%; however, the color change takes 2 minutes to develop. Vitamin C inhibits the glucose oxidase reaction, and thus a modest vitamin C supplement, 350 to 1000 mg/a day, can give falsely lowered readings. Nitrofurantoin may also interfere with this reaction.

Table 12–5. Products for Urine Testing

Product	Method	Cost*	Range (%)
Clinitest	Copper reduction	$7.60 per 100	0–2+
Testape	Glucose oxidase	$4.70 per roll	0–2+
Chemstrips uG	Glucose oxidase	$5.80 per 100	0–5+

*Approximate cost only.

Conclusion

In deciding to use SMBG rather than urine testing, consideration must be given to the cost to the patient, the amount of time required for teaching and follow-up, and whether the more accurate information obtained will actually be useful in patient management. SMBG has resulted in more accurate monitoring of diabetic control and has allowed intensive insulin regimens to be used safely. It has allowed patients to have much greater control over their disease and their daily lives. It is clearly the preferred monitoring method for many patients. However, for some stable patients (particularly older persons with type II diabetes) it may be equally effective and cheaper to use urine testing most of the time and to reserve SMBG for spot checks, sick days, and emergency situations.

References

Belmonte MM, Schiffrin A, Dufresne J, et al. Impact of SMBG on control of diabetes as measured by HbA₁: 3-yr. survey of a juvenile IDDM clinic. Diabetes Care 11:484–488, 1988.
   A study of 219 unselected type 1 diabetic children demonstrating that simple teaching of SMBG and a physician's recommendation to use it do not improve glycemic control. Patients must be taught to adjust insulin and diet according to SMBG results and must be motivated to comply with a comprehensive regimen.
Bresnick GH, Groo A, Palta M, et al. Urinary glucose testing inaccuracies among diabetic patients. Effect of acquired color vision deficiency caused by diabetic retinopathy. Arch Ophthalmol 102:1489–1496, 1984.
   A description of the acquired color vision deficits most likely found in patients with diabetes and the tests available to screen for these deficits.
Consensus statement on self-monitoring of blood glucose. Diabetes Care 10:95–99, 1987.
   The policy of the American Diabetes Association on the use of SMBG, including its use in the hospital setting and quality assurance issues.
Gander-Frederick L, Julian D, Cox D, et al. Self-measurement of blood glucose: accuracy of self-reported data and adherence to recommended regimen. Diabetes Care 11:579–585, 1988.
   By using reflectance meters containing memory chips, this study found that 53% of patients' self-recorded glucose diaries were clinically inaccurate, with frequent omissions of values contained in meter memory and additions of values not contained in meter memory.
McCall AL, Mullin CJ. Home blood glucose monitoring: keystone for modern diabetes care. Med Clin North Am 71:763–787, 1987.
   Available products for SMBG and urinary glucose testing, including a table of substances interfering with urine testing.
North DS, Steiner JF, Woodhouse KM, et al.: Home monitors of blood glucose: comparison of precision and accuracy. Diabetes Care 10: 360–366, 1987.
   The most recent study examining the precision and accuracy of available meters. Eight meters are compared to a reference method. This article does not give information regarding ease of use or cost, however.
Orzeck E. Blood-glucose monitoring: technology for taking control. Diabetes Forecast May: 8–13, 1986.
   A patient-oriented description of available SMBG products including meters, reagent strips, and puncturing devices. Costs and special features of products are described.
Pernick NL, Rodbard D. Personal computer programs to assist with self-monitoring of blood glucose and self-adjustment of insulin dosage. Diabetes Care 9:61–69, 1986.
   Description of computer programs for storage, analysis, and display of glucose measurements and other relevant data. Insulin doses are suggested by using a customized algorithm.
Skyler JS, Skyler DL, Seigler DE, et al. Algorithms for adjustment of insulin dosage by patients who monitor blood glucose. Diabetes Care 4:311–318, 1981.
   Algorithms that allow patients following various insulin regimens to adjust their own insulin doses according to blood glucose levels and other factors.
Wilson DE. High-tech diabetes care: present and future. Diabetes Care 9:87–88, 1986.
   A perspective on the future of computerized diabetes management.

13

Osteoporosis

RICHARD J. HABER, M.D.

Introduction

Osteoporosis is a reduction in bone mass that predisposes to fractures, especially in the hip, vertebrae, distal forearm (Colles' fracture), humerus, and pelvis. In the fourth or fifth decade of life, all people begin to lose bone. Women have less bone mass than men and have accelerated loss of bone for many years after menopause. With advancing age, a large number of elderly persons, especially white women, are likely to sustain a fracture as a result of minimal trauma such as a fall. These osteoporotic fractures, particularly of the hip, can cause disability and premature death. Because measures to substantially increase bone mass are still experimental, current strategies to prevent osteoporotic fractures are directed at preventing bone loss and the falls causing these fractures.

Osteoporotic Fractures

Hip fractures account for more deaths and disability than all other osteoporotic fractures combined. More than 200,000 hip fractures occur in the United States each year; 75% of these occur in women and 50% after age 80. Those who sustain a hip fracture have a 5 to 20% greater risk of dying within 1 year of the fracture than patients of similar age, although some of this excess mortality may be due to concomitant medical conditions that predispose to falls. Of those who lived independently at the time of their hip fracture, 10 to 25% remain in chronic care institutions and about half who return home need assistance to care for themselves. In the United States, hip fractures cost more than 7 billion dollars a year for medical and nursing services.

Colles' fractures are the most common type of fracture among adults before age 75, after which hip fractures are more frequent. These fractures rarely require hospital admission and almost never cause deaths.

The incidence of vertebral fractures is unknown, but by age 70 approximately 5% of white women have at least one vertebral compression and by age 80 approximately 40% have at least one vertebral deformity seen on an x-ray of the spine. These fractures appear to occur most often spontaneously or after minimal trauma. Although some fractures may result in severe back pain, many cause no symptoms. In some women these vertebral fractures and the resultant deformities may cause loss of height, a kyphotic "dowager's hump," and occasionally chronic back pain.

Pathophysiology and Differential Diagnosis

Osteoporosis is characterized by bone resorption in excess of formation. Bone mineral content and matrix are lost in equal proportion, in contrast to osteomalacia, in which a lack of mineral content is the primary disorder. The pathophysiology of osteoporosis is incompletely understood. Loss of bone mass appears to result from a complex interaction of multiple factors including gonadal hormones, parathyroid hormone, calcitonin, the vitamin D metabolites, calcium intake, hereditary factors, and perhaps physical activity. Bone loss begins in the fourth or fifth decade of life, in women appears to accelerate at the time of menopause, and then slows again in the eighth and ninth decades.

Age-related osteoporosis is by far the most common cause of chronic bone loss. However, several endocrinopathies, including hypercorticolism (endogenous or exogenous), hyperparathyroidism (primary or secondary), hyperthyroidism, hypogonadism, and hyperprolactinemia, can also result in decreased bone mass. Other conditions such as malignancy (e.g., metastatic disease, multiple myeloma, lymphoma, leukemia), drug use (e.g., alcoholism, long-term heparin or phenytoin administration), osteomalacia, prolonged immobilization, and certain uncommon inherited disorders of collagen synthesis may mimic osteoporosis. A directed history and physical examination combined with selected bone x-rays and laboratory measurements are usually sufficient to exclude these entities in persons with osteopenia (radiographic evidence of decreased bone mass) and fractures. The laboratory features of age-related osteoporosis include normal calcium, phosphorus, and alkaline phosphatase levels, although the alkaline phosphatase concentration may be elevated if there is a healing fracture. The more atypical the patient profile for age-related osteoporosis (see below), the more appropriate it is to initiate an extensive search for a secondary cause.

Identification of Those at Risk for Fractures

It would be advantageous to prospectively identify those most likely to suffer a fracture so that treatment can be directed to persons at highest risk. At the present time, decisions regarding the likelihood of fractures must be made primarily on epidemiologic grounds (Table 13–1).

Table 13–1. Factors Altering Risk for Osteoporotic Fractures*

Risk Factors	Protective Factors
Advanced age	Male gender
Female gender	Black/Latino
White	Obesity
Premature surgical menopause	Postmenopausal estrogen use
Thin body build	
Alcoholism	? Active lifestyle
Chronic corticosteroid use	? Calcium supplementation
Factors that predispose to falls (relevant to hip fractures)	
? Asian	
? Cigarette smoking	
? Sedentary lifestyle	
? Low calcium intake	
? Northern European origin	

*? indicates factors that are not well established.

Osteoporotic fractures occur most commonly in postmenopausal white women. Black women and white or black men, perhaps because of a greater initial bone mass, have a much lower incidence of hip and other osteoporotic fractures. The risk of fractures for Asians, Latinos, and other racial and ethnic groups is less well known. Recent data indicate that fracture rates for Asians are closer to those for whites, and that those for Latinos are closer to those for black persons. Women who have undergone premature surgical menopause (bilateral oophorectomy before age 50) are at high risk for osteoporosis. Thin women, persons with alcoholism, smokers, and perhaps women of northern European origin or persons with a history of gastrectomy or a sedentary lifestyle may also be at increased risk. Patients treated with corticosteroids, especially at doses higher than 15 mg of prednisone per day (or its equivalent) for more than 2 years, are more likely to fracture their vertebrae and ribs than nonusers of corticosteroids. Women who have disorders or take medications that predispose them to fall may also be considered to be at additional risk.

Although the technology to measure bone mass noninvasively is currently available (e.g., single- or dual-photon absorptiometry, computed tomography), such measurements have not yet been proved to identify those who will later sustain fractures, especially of the hip. Until their predictive ability is validated, measures of bone mass remain expensive tests of uncertain value. Further study is required before they can be recommended for routine screening.

Prevention of Bone Loss

Estrogen Therapy

Estrogen therapy prevents loss of bone mass and decreases the risk of osteoporotic fractures. No other therapeutic strategy results in preservation of bone to the same degree. The mechanism of action of estrogen on bone is unclear. Because estrogen therapy prevents further bone loss but does not substantially increase bone mass, it is best begun in the perimenopausal period and should be regarded primarily as prophylactic.

Estrogen therapy appears to prevent postmenopausal bone loss for as long as a woman continues to take it. Treatment is effective whether begun in the perimenopausal period or as late as age 70 and after natural or surgical menopause. When estrogen therapy is used for at least 5 years, the risk of hip fracture appears to be reduced by about 50%. The risk of Colles' and vertebral fractures is also decreased. There is accelerated bone loss when estrogen therapy is discontinued, and protection against fractures might be lost as soon as 5 years after stopping therapy.

The postmenopausal use of estrogen does not appear to increase the risk of breast cancer. Nonetheless, because breast cancer is a hormone-sensitive tumor, a history of breast cancer precludes routine estrogen therapy, as may a maternal family history of the disease. Attention to routine breast cancer screening in women receiving estrogen is important, although there is no evidence that screening must be more frequent or different from that recommended for the general population. An increased risk of thromboembolic disease, similar to that experienced by younger women using oral contraceptives, has not been observed with estrogen use in the postmenopausal period, possibly because of the lower postmenopausal estrogen dose. A history of thromboembolic disease, however, remains a relative contraindication to estrogen use. An approximately two-fold increase in gallbladder disease has been observed with estrogen therapy.

Postmenopausal estrogen use is associated with an approximately three- to five-fold increased risk of endometrial cancer. Such cancers are almost always detected at an early stage. The risk of endometrial cancer can probably be reduced by the periodic administration of a progestin. Potential disadvantages of progestin use include undesirable alterations in serum lipid levels (e.g., reduction of high density lipoprotein cholesterol and elevation of low density lipoprotein cholesterol) and resumption or continuation of periodic uterine bleeding. The long-term safety of combined estrogen and progestin treatment in postmenopausal women is unknown.

Most studies indicate that postmenopausal estrogen therapy reduces the incidence of coronary heart disease and lowers overall mortality rates, possibly because of the favorable effects of estrogen on serum lipids. If proved by additional data, this benefit would be more important than all the other risks and benefits of estrogen therapy combined. Because a combined estrogen and progestin regimen has adverse effects on lipids compared with estrogen alone, there is concern that the addition of a progestin might negate the cardiovascular benefits of estrogen therapy. Premenopausal women receiving progestins in oral contraceptives experienced an increased risk of cardiovascular disease, which was directly related to the progestin content of the contraceptive used. Because coronary heart disease is more common than endometrial cancer in the postmenopausal period, even small increases in cardiovascular risk could outweigh endometrial benefits.

Generic conjugated estrogens and medroxyprogesterone acetate are the least expensive estrogen and progestin preparations (Table 13–2). Transdermal estradiol patches are the most costly; they also have less favorable effects on lipids than oral preparations and the dose required to prevent loss of bone mass is uncertain.

Calcium Supplementation

White women require about 1 g of elemental calcium per day before menopause and 1.5 g/day after menopause to prevent a net loss of body calcium. In the United States, women consume an average of only 475 to 575 mg of elemental calcium per day. Postmenopausal women treated with supplemental calcium generally, but not always, lose bone more slowly than untreated women. However, calcium supplementation is not as effective as estrogen therapy in preventing bone loss, and there is little evidence that increases in calcium intake can reduce the risk of osteoporotic fractures.

Generic calcium carbonate is the least expensive form of calcium supplementation (Table 13–3). Calcium carbonate is 40% elemental calcium; therefore, to obtain 1 g of elemental calcium a person must take 2.5 g of calcium carbonate—from two to five tablets a day, depending on the preparation used. To enhance absorption, the tablets should be taken with meals and in divided doses. A similar quantity of calcium can be obtained from 3 cups of milk or yogurt per day.

Persons with renal failure, hyperparathyroidism, or a history of calcium-containing renal stones should not increase calcium intake except under unusual circumstances and then only when carefully monitored. In other individuals, an increase in dietary calcium of 2 to 3 g of calcium per day appears to be safe and without side effects. Measurement of calcium concentration in the serum or urine is not routinely necessary.

Table 13–2. Content and Costs of Commonly Used Hormone Preparations

Drug	Daily Dose (mg)	Approximate Cost Per Daily Dose
Estrogen		
Conjugated estrogens (generic)	0.625	$0.10
Conjugated estrogens (Premarin)	0.625	$0.19
Estradiol-17β, oral (Estrace)	2.0	$0.29
Estradiol-17β, transdermal patch (Estroderm)	0.1	$0.57
Progestin		
Medroxyprogesterone acetate (generic)	10.0	$0.27
Medroxyprogesterone acetate (Provera)	10.0	$0.39

Exercise

Women who perform regular weight-bearing exercise in the premenopausal period appear to have greater bone mass than women not performing equivalent physical activity, provided the degree of exercise is not so extreme as to be associated with amenorrhea. Whether this leads to less osteoporosis and osteoporotic fractures in the postmenopausal period is uncertain. The results of a few small trials have suggested that postmenopausal women may reduce their bone loss by performing weight-bearing exercise 30 to 60 minutes three times a week. Whether regular exercise reduces the risk of fractures is not yet known. A further potential benefit of exercise is the preservation of neuromuscular conditioning, which might lead to a decreased risk of falling.

Other Therapies

Vitamin D supplementation does not appear to prevent fractures or loss of bone in postmenopausal women. Low doses of vitamin D (400 to 1000 units per day) may be useful in preventing osteomalacia in elderly patients who have no exposure to sunlight and whose diets are deficient in vitamin D. Vitamin D supplementation may also be of value in pa-

tients using chronic corticosteroid therapy. Steroid use may decrease intestinal absorption of calcium by interfering with the effect of vitamin D metabolites on the gut. The majority of postmenopausal women do not need supplementation. Serum concentrations of calcitriol (1,25-dihydroxycholecalciferol) decline with age, and some studies suggest that the use of calcitriol may preserve bone mass in women with vertebral fractures. Because vitamin D and its metabolites can cause hypercalcemia and because their efficacy is unproved, their use should generally be reserved for women with recurrent vertebral fractures refractory to more standard therapy.

In pharmacologic doses, sodium fluoride induces formation of new but histologically abnormal trabecular bone and appears to reduce the incidence of new vertebral fractures in postmenopausal women who already have had such fractures. However, these doses of fluoride may cause gastritis, gastrointestinal bleeding, or synovitis, and there is concern that fluoride may paradoxically weaken the outer cortical layer of bone and possibly increase the risk of hip fracture. The proper role for fluoride therapy in the prevention and treatment of osteoporosis is currently unclear. Use should be reserved for postmenopausal women with vertebral fractures refractory to initial therapy.

Calcitonin therapy may increase total body

Table 13–3. Content and Costs of Calcium in Food and Supplements

	Approximate Serving Per Gram of Elemental Calcium	Approximate Cost Per Gram of Elemental Calcium
Foods		
Milk	3 c	$0.50
Cheese	5 oz	$1.00
Yogurt	3 c	$1.50
Green vegetables	2–3 c	$1.00
Supplements (generic)		
Calcium carbonate	2.5 g (2–5 tablets)	$0.05
Calcium phosphate	2.7 g (4–8 tablets)	$0.15
Calcium lactate	7.7 g (12–24 tablets)	$0.15
Calcium gluconate	11.0 g (12–20 tablets)	$0.25

calcium and, by inference, skeletal mass. However, whether this effect is sustained is uncertain and whether such therapy will prevent osteoporotic fractures is unknown. Calcitonin is expensive and cannot be taken orally. Until further data are available, calcitonin therapy should also be reserved for those with recurrent fractures refractory to other treatments.

Some studies have indicated that women using thiazide diuretics long term may have greater bone mass than nonusers. Whether thiazide use prevents osteoporosis and osteoporotic fractures remains to be demonstrated. Further study is required before they can be recommended for this purpose.

The use of low dose parathyroid hormone and the administration of diphosphonates have also been suggested as possible therapies for osteoporosis. The efficacy and safety of such treatments have yet to be established.

Prevention of Falls

In women over age 70, most bone loss has already occurred; many such women already have osteoporosis. Measures to prevent falls may be more beneficial in this group than therapies to prevent further loss of bone mass.

Some patients may have correctable impairments of visual acuity; a few have disorders such as Parkinson's disease, recurrent arrhythmias, or seizures that can be specifically treated. The use of alcohol, long-acting sedative hypnotics, and major tranquilizers, which predispose to falls especially at night, should be avoided or minimized. Walking aids (canes or walkers) may be of value for some patients. Because most falls occur at home, attempts to reduce environmental hazards should be focused on the home, and a home inspection may be invaluable. Hazards such as loose rugs, wires, or obstructions on the floor should be removed; nonslip surfaces and railings on stairs and in bathrooms should be installed; and rooms should be adequately lit. (For a more complete discussion of strategies to prevent falls, see Chapter 29.)

Recommendations

Age-based clinical strategies to prevent osteoporosis and osteoporotic fractures are summarized in Table 13–4. Although these recommendations are most applicable to white women, they may also benefit nonwhite

Table 13–4. Age-Based Clinical Strategies to Prevent Osteoporotic Fractures

Population Group	Strategies
Premenopausal women and men	Maintain adequate calcium intake (1 g elemental calcium per day) Exercise regularly (30 min three times a week) Avoid smoking and excessive alcohol use
Perimenopausal and early postmenopausal women	Consider estrogen therapy (0.625 mg conjugated estrogen per day or equivalent) Maintain adequate calcium intake (1 g elemental calcium per day with estrogen therapy, 1.5 g/day without estrogen therapy) Exercise regularly (30 min three times a week) Avoid smoking and excessive alcohol use
Elderly women and men	Treat medical disorders and disabilities that may cause falls Correct home hazards that may cause falls Avoid smoking, excessive alcohol use, and sedative drugs Maintain adequate calcium intake (1.5 g elemental calcium per day) Exercise regularly

women and men. In the premenopausal period, avoidance of smoking and excess alcohol consumption, encouragement of regular exercise, and maintenance of adequate calcium intake are the foci of management. Although these recommendations have little associated risk and other potential health benefits, their efficacy in preventing osteoporotic fractures is unproved. In the perimenopausal and early postmenopausal periods, the mainstays of prevention and management are estrogen therapy and adequate calcium intake. In the elderly, strategies to prevent falls may be the most important intervention.

An algorithm to help structure the decision-making process as to which perimenopausal and postmenopausal women should be given estrogen is presented in Figure 13–1. If postmenopausal osteoporosis has resulted in symptomatic vertebral fractures, estrogen therapy is indicated to reduce further morbidity. For women who have not sustained osteoporotic fractures, the major goal of long-term estrogen therapy is prevention of fractures. Because the risk of osteoporotic fractures in black persons

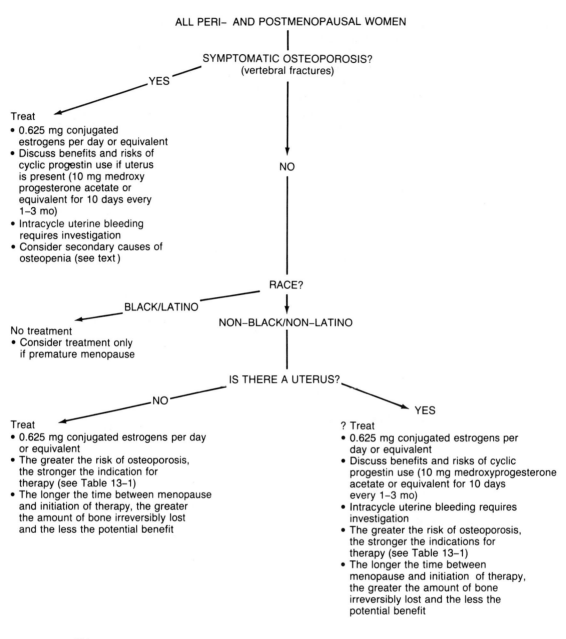

Figure 13–1. *Algorithm for the use of estrogen therapy to prevent osteoporotic fractures in perimenopausal and postmenopausal women.*

and probably in Latinos is low, it is difficult to recommend estrogen treatment except perhaps in those who have undergone premature surgical menopause. If estrogen therapy is proved to lower coronary heart disease risk, this racial and ethnic differentiation should be re-evaluated. Approximately 30% of women in the

postmenopausal age group in the United States have undergone a hysterectomy. Because such women are no longer at risk for endometrial cancer, the relative indication for estrogen therapy is stronger. For the majority of women who have not undergone a hysterectomy, estrogen therapy is still reasonable if they are at risk for osteoporosis (Table 13–1) and understand the benefits and risks of such therapy.

Effective preservation of bone mass appears to require 0.625 mg of conjugated estrogen per day or its equivalent (e.g., estradiol valerate [2 mg], ethinyl estradiol [15 μg], mestranol [25 μg], or estradiol-17β [2 mg] orally or [3 mg] transdermal gel). The required dose for the long-acting estradiol patch system has not yet been determined. Although one recent study suggests that lower doses of estrogen (0.3 mg conjugated estrogens) may prevent bone loss if combined with 1.5 g of elemental calcium per day, this requires confirmation before being accepted for widespread use. Most recommendations suggest that estrogen should be cycled for 21 to 25 days each month, although there is no convincing evidence that this is superior to continuous use. Bone loss slows and may stop after age 70, and there is no strong evidence that estrogen therapy is beneficial for preventing fractures when started after that age.

Women with an intact uterus should be advised of the risks of endometrial cancer associated with use of estrogen alone and the cardiovascular risks of the cyclic addition of a progestin. If progestins are used, protection of the endometrium appears to require 10 mg of medroxyprogesterone acetate or its equivalent (e.g., DL-norgestrel [0.15 mg], norethindrone [1 mg], or micronized progesterone [300 mg]) for at least 10 days every 1 to 3 months. Whether lower doses of progestin would be equally effective if used continuously is not known. There is no convincing evidence that progestins should be routinely used for women who have undergone a hysterectomy and are no longer at risk for endometrial cancer.

Intracycle uterine bleeding requires investigation to rule out endometrial cancer. The role of routine endometrial sampling remains unclear, and this procedure requires further study before it can be recommended for screening. The optimal duration of estrogen therapy is unknown. Because there is accelerated bone loss when estrogen therapy is discontinued and fracture protection may be lost as early as 5 years after stopping therapy, the ideal duration of therapy may be lifelong. Estrogen therapy should be combined with adequate calcium intake, at least 1 g of elemental calcium per day.

Because the decision to use hormones requires long-term compliance and balancing of risks and benefits and because hormones may produce side effects such as resumption of uterine bleeding, each woman should actively participate in the decision. Choices should be based on current medical knowledge and patient preferences.

For women at risk for osteoporosis who are unwilling or unable to use estrogens, there are no demonstrated therapeutic strategies that have equivalent bone-preserving properties. Supplemental calcium therapy seems to be the best alternative, although studies have not always shown it to be better than a placebo. Because postmenopausal women require a higher daily calcium intake than premenopausal women or postmenopausal women using estrogen, the sum of dietary and supplemental calcium should be 1.5 g of elemental calcium per day if estrogen therapy is omitted. Fluoride, calcitonin, and vitamin D and its active metabolites may have a role in the secondary prevention of vertebral fractures or in primary prevention when estrogen therapy is not used, but such therapy is of unproven value, is associated with complications, and should be regarded as experimental.

Summary

Osteoporosis is an age-related reduction in bone mass that predisposes to fractures of the hip, vertebrae, distal forearm, humerus, and pelvis. Thin, postmenopausal white women, especially those who have undergone premature menopause, appear to be at greatest risk. Current strategies to prevent osteoporotic fractures are directed at preventing bone loss and the falls that precipitate these fractures. Estrogen therapy is the most effective means of preserving bone mass and preventing fractures, but it is associated with an increased risk of endometrial cancer. This risk can probably be reduced by the periodic administration of a progestin; however, this addition may increase cardiovascular risk and could outweigh endometrial benefits. Calcium supplementation, exercise, and avoidance of smoking and excessive alcohol use may also help preserve bone mass. Treatment with fluoride, calcitonin, and vitamin D and its active metabolites should be reserved for women with recurrent vertebral fractures refractory to initial therapy. In the elderly, measures to prevent falls such as correction of medical disorders that predispose to falling, proper use of sedative hypnotics and tranquilizers, availability of walking aids, and reduction of home hazards may be more beneficial than therapies to reduce further bone loss.

Bibliography

Bush TL, Barrett-Connor E. Noncontraceptive estrogen use and cardiovascular disease. Epidemiol Rev 7:80–104, 1985.

A comprehensive review of the effects of postmenopausal hormone use on the risk of cardiovascular disease (220 references).

Canadian Task Force on the Periodic Health Examination. The periodic health examination: 2. 1987 update. Can Med Assoc J 138:618–626, 1988.

Statement on postmenopausal osteoporosis and related fractures; recommends that estrogen therapy should not be routinely used but that the decision be made on an individual basis; concludes that measures of bone mass do not reliably identify those at risk for osteoporotic fractures and should be excluded from the periodic health examination (54 references).

Cummings SR, Kelsey JL, Nevitt MC, et al. Epidemiology of osteoporosis and osteoporotic fractures. Epidemiol Rev 7:178–208, 1985.

A comprehensive review of the epidemiology of osteoporosis and osteoporotic fractures (323 references).

Haber RJ. Should postmenopausal women be given estrogen? West J Med 142:672–677, 1985.

A concise review of the benefits and risks of postmenopausal estrogen therapy (34 references).

Health and Public Policy Committee, American College of Physicians. Bone mineral densitometry. Ann Intern Med 107:932–936, 1987

Statement of the Clinical Efficacy Assessment Project of the American College of Physicians; concludes that densitometry is still a research tool and should not be used for routine screening until its predictive accuracy is validated (43 references).

Hillner BE, Hollenberg JP, Pauker SG. Postmenopausal estrogens in prevention of osteoporosis: benefit virtually without risk if cardiovascular effects are considered. Am J Med 80:1115–1127, 1986.

A decision analysis model of postmenopausal estrogen therapy that includes the potential impact of changes in cardiovascular risk; has references for other published analyses of overall benefit and risk (61 references).

MacDonald PC. Estrogen plus progestin in postmenopausal women: act II. N Engl J Med 315:959–961, 1986.

Editorial identifying the major issues of benefit and risk in deciding whether to add a progestin to postmenopausal estrogen therapy; urges a conservative approach (3 references).

Martin AD, Houston CS. Osteoporosis, calcium and physical activity. Can Med Assoc J 136:587–593, 1987.

Review of the relationship of calcium intake, exercise, and osteoporosis; includes summary of trials addressing the effect of calcium supplementation and exercise on bone loss in postmenopausal women (94 references).

Office of Medical Applications of Research, National Institutes of Health. Osteoporosis: Consensus Conference. JAMA 252:799–802, 1984.

Summary statement from the NIH Consensus Conference on osteoporosis; a succinct review of current knowledge and recommendations for prevention and treatment (no references).

Riggs BL, Melton LJ. Involutional osteoporosis. N Engl J Med 314:1676–1686, 1986.

In depth, well-referenced review of age-related osteoporosis; argues for division of osteoporosis into early (postmenopausal) and late (senile) forms, although whether the pathophysiology of each is different remains uncertain (124 references).

Riggs BL, Seeman E, Hodgson SF, et al. Effect of the fluoride/calcium regimen on vertebral fracture occurrences in postmenopausal osteoporosis: a comparison with conventional therapy. N Engl J Med 306:446–450, 1982.

A nonrandomized study of the effect of calcium, estrogen, vitamin D, and fluoride therapy, used individually or in combination, on the rate of new fractures in women with recurrent vertebral fractures (18 references).

Weiss NS, Ure CL, Ballard JH, et al. Decreased risk of fractures of the hip and lower forearm with postmenopausal use of estrogen. N Engl J Med 303:1195–1198, 1980.

One of multiple case-control studies indicating postmenopausal estrogen use results in a decreased risk of hip and forearm fractures; includes an assessment of the effect of dose and duration of therapy on fracture risk (12 references).

14

Diagnostic Evaluation and Management of Impotence

MOLLY COOKE, M.D.

Introduction

Impotence, defined as the failure to achieve penile turgidity adequate for intercourse in 25% or more of attempts, is the second most common cause of sexual dysfunction (after premature ejaculation) in healthy men. Impotence is more common in chronically ill than in healthy men and is estimated to affect as many as 25% of male outpatients over age 40. An identifiable cause may be discovered in 80 to 90% of cases; this fact is important because etiology determines the appropriate therapy and is closely linked to the probability of successful intervention. Mixed etiologies are common, however, and psychosexual difficulties typically accompany erectile dysfunction even when the primary etiology is organic. The physician must vigorously attempt to understand the pathogenesis of impotence and should be flexible in its categorization.

Physiology and Pathophysiology of Male Sexual Performance

A knowledge of the physiology of normal male sexual performance provides the best framework for proper assessment and management of male sexual dysfunction. Table 14–1 summarizes the physiology and pathophysiology of male sexual response. Normal libido, defined as a healthy enthusiasm for intercourse, is an important component of normal performance. Although poorly understood, the genesis of libido is presumed to involve cortical phenomena for which testosterone exerts a permissive effect. Adequate alertness and both physical and psychologic well-being are also required. A number of conditions,

including sedation, general medical illnesses that reduce stamina or cause exertional discomfort, certain endocrine conditions that depress testosterone or elevate prolactin, and various psychologic disturbances, can depress libido. Our culture places such importance on sexual interest that many men do not recognize a decrease in their libido and complain instead of erectile dysfunction. Therefore, the stated presence of a normal libido does not necessarily exclude these cortically mediated problems.

Normal erectile functioning requires the integrity of at least one of two neural control mechanisms, an adequate arterial blood supply, intact control of venous drainage, and anatomically normal erectile structures in the penis. The cortical erectile center, a limbic dopaminergic center with sympathetic spinal efferents at T12 through L2, controls erections in response to visual and mental sexual stimulation. The sacral erectile center coordinates reflex erections in response to tactile stimulation and is the more important of the two centers. For example, 90% of patients with thoracic cord injuries but only 20% of patients with sacral cord injuries eventually recover erectile function. This sacral center is part of a parasympathetic spinal cord reflex loop. Either anatomic (e.g., radical prostatectomy, abdominoperineal resection of the rectum) or pharmacologic (e.g., anticholinergic effects from drugs) parasympathectomies may cause impotence.

Normal erectile function requires adequate arterial perfusion. Atherosclerosis is the most common cause of arteriogenic impotence and results in either partial tumescence inadequate for intromission or a partial erection sufficient for penetration followed by prompt detumescence (gluteal steal). Diabetic impotence likely reflects both vascular disease and autonomic

Table 14–1. Components of Male Sexual Response and Mechanisms of Impotence

Response	Physiology	Disorders Causing Impotence
Libido	Cortical phenomenon, testosterone required	*Psychic:* fatigue, stress, performance anxiety, depression, relationship disturbance, profound psychiatric disorders *Sedation* and sedative abuse *Endocrine* disease: testosterone deficiency, elevated prolactin, thyroid disease *Poor general health*
Erection	Cortical erectile center, sympathetic outflow at T12 to L2	Diseases of limbic system *Cord injuries* and diseases: transection above T11, multiple sclerosis, tabes dorsalis *Sympathetic* neuropathies: surgical—aortoiliac bypass, lumbar sympathectomy, node dissection, abdominoperineal resection of rectum, radical prostatectomy; pharmacologic—sympatholytic antihypertensives, alpha blockers including phenothiazines
	Reflexogenic erectile center, parasympathetic spinal reflex S-1 to S-4	*Cord injuries* and diseases involving sacral cord *Parasympathetic* neuropathies: surgical—abdominoperineal resection of the rectum, radical prostatectomy; pharmacologic—anticholinergics, antidepressants, antihistamines, antipsychotics
	Vascular supply and normal erectile tissue	*Vascular diseases:* atherosclerosis, trauma *Penile diseases:* Peyronie's disease, chordee, microphallus, priapism
Emission and ejaculation	Sympathetic thoracolumbar reflex	*Sympathetic* neuropathies: surgical, as in cortical erectile center dysfunction; pharmacologic, especially guanethidine, thioridazine hydrochloride
Orgasm	Cortically mediated, independent of erection and ejaculation	

Modified by permission of the Western Journal of Medicine (Cooke M, Evaluation of impotence, 1986, July, vol 145, pp 106–110).

neuropathy. Recent evidence suggests that the arterial vasoconstrictor effects of cigarette smoking may predispose smokers to impotence. Venous leakage is a second vascular mechanism of impotence. Abnormally rapid efflux of blood from the corpora cavernosa prevents the development of a rigid erection even when the arterial supply is normal. Venous leakage is a common sequela of recurrent priapism, but the leak may also develop without antecedents. More rigid erections in the upright position than in the prone position is a common feature.

Finally, erection requires anatomically normal tissues. Peyronie's disease, an acquired condition characterized by the development of fibrous plaques on the dorsal penile shaft and distortion of the erect phallus, is a relatively common structural cause of impotence. Phimosis and balanitis are also associated with erectile dysfunction.

Emission—the delivery of semen into the proximal urethra and closure of the internal vesical sphincter—and ejaculation are primarily sympathetically controlled through a thoracolumbar reflex. Retrograde ejaculation is a clinical manifestation of decreased alpha-adrenergic input. Erectile disturbances may also occur with sympathectomies, however. The physiologic basis of orgasm appears to be cortically mediated but is not well understood.

Causes and Relative Prevalence of Impotence

It is difficult to ascertain the relative prevalence of various causes of impotence for three reasons. First, critical investigation has been hampered by the myth that 90% of impotence is psychogenic. Second, our understanding of the physiology of erection is still developing. Third, referral bias has distorted most study samples. Table 14–2 presents some commonly cited prevalence figures, but prospective data on unselected samples do not exist. Primary

Table 14–2. Effect of Study Population on Relative Prevalence of Various Causes of Impotence

Cause of Impotence	% of Study Population with Specific Cause		
	105 Patients in Whom Serum Testosterone Level Was Measured*	188 General Medical Patients Undergoing Evaluation†	165 Patients Referred to Urology Clinic‡
Psychogenic	14	14	51
Organic	66	80	47
Medication	7	25	2
Alcohol	3	0	1
Neurologic (excluding diabetes)	0	7	4
Vascular/penile	0	6	15
Endocrine	51	38	25
Primary and secondary hypogonadism	26	19	25
Diabetes	7	9	—
Other: thyroid, prolactin	18	10	—
Miscellaneous	5	4	9
Mixed or unknown	19	7	2

Modified by permission of the Western Journal of Medicine (Cooke M, Evaluation of impotence, 1986, July, vol 145, pp 106–110).
*Spark RF, et al. (JAMA 243:750–755, 1980).
†Slag MF, et al. (JAMA 249:1756–1740, 1983).
‡Montague DK, et al. (Urology 14:545–548, 1979).

care physicians should particularly note that at least 50% of impotence is organic. Prescription drugs are an important cause of dysfunction; in a study of patients seen in a medical clinic, 25% of all impotence was caused by medication. Table 14–3 gives drugs associated with sexual dysfunction and their putative mechanism of action. Table 14–4 presents the estimated prevalence of impotence associated with antihypertensive medications.

Evaluation of the Impotent Patient

Diagnostic evaluation of impotence by the primary care physician is complicated by a large number of potential diagnostic tests, conflicting information about the diagnostic accuracy of these tests, and the lack of "gold standard" techniques. Fortunately, during the past 5 years, increasing effort has been devoted to the formal evaluation and comparison of various diagnostic strategies.

There is no controversy about the utility of the history and physical examination in the evaluation of the impotent patient. The history should clarify the nature of the sexual dysfunction, uncover any clues regarding pathogenesis, and determine the impact on the patient and his partners. Nonspecialists often feel uneasy when discussing sexual dysfunction and fear that the interview will take an inordinate amount of time, that personal or interpersonal

Table 14–3. Commonly Used Drugs Associated with Impotence and Their Postulated Mechanism of Action

Sexual Response	Mechanism of Action	Drugs
Libido	Sedation	Antihypertensives (methyldopa, reserpine, clonidine, beta antagonists), alcohol, narcotics, minor tranquilizers, barbiturates, phenothiazines, baclofen
	Testosterone antagonism	Alcohol, marijuana, spironolactone, cimetidine, estrogen, digoxin
	Elevation of prolactin	Narcotics, phenothiazines, methyldopa
Erection	Parasympatholysis	Atropine, benztropine, propantheline, disopyramide, metoclopramide, antidepressants (especially amitriptyline), antipsychotics (especially chlorpromazine and thioridazine), antiparkinsonian drugs/antihistamines
Ejaculation	Sympatholysis	Antihypertensives (guanethidine, phenoxybenzamine, prazosin, monoamine oxidase inhibitors), antipsychotics (especially thioridazine)

Modified by permission of the Western Journal of Medicine (Cooke M, Evaluation of impotence, 1986, July, vol 145, pp 106–110).

Table 14-4. Estimated Prevalence of Impotence Associated with Antihypertensive Therapy*

Antihypertensive Therapy	%
Untreated (receiving placebo)	10
Diuretics (thiazide)	19
Beta blocker (propranolol)	15
Centrally acting agents	
Guanethidine	60
Reserpine	30
Clonidine	24
Methyldopa	30
Prazosin	†
Vasodilators	
Hydralazine	Occasional
Minoxidil	Rare
Captopril	Occasional

Modified by permission of the Western Journal of Medicine (Cooke M, Evaluation of impotence, 1986, July, vol 145, pp 106–110).
*Prevalence is expressed as a percentage for convenience, although the number of subjects on whom these percentages is based is often quite small.
†Rarely reported but common in clinical practice, especially at higher doses.

material may be uncovered that is beyond the expertise of the nonspecialist, and that there is little chance of benefit. None of these concerns are well founded, however. A comprehensive exploration of sexual dysfunction can be accomplished in less than an hour. It may be not only acceptable but helpful to divide the interview into two or more visits. Patients often feel significantly relieved after an opportunity to discuss problems that they have viewed with anxiety and embarrassment. The probability of uncovering the cause of impotence is excellent.

Several questions are particularly useful. The patient should describe the onset of the dysfunction. An onset of impotence that is temporally associated with stressful events or depression suggests a psychogenic derivation. Patients with organic impotence may initially have difficulty in maintaining an erection, followed by difficulty in achieving an erection. The patient should give a concrete, graphic description of attempts at intercourse characterizing both his interest in sex and the turgidity and duration of erection. The clinician should elicit information clarifying the frequency and context of opportunities for sexual intercourse, the number of partners, differences in erectile dysfunction with different partners, and the percentage of unsuccessful attempts. Finally, a history of potentially offending drugs, chronic medical illnesses including atherosclerotic diseases, or previous pelvic trauma or surgery should be obtained. Differentiation between primary impotence (dys-

function from the onset of sexual activity) and secondary impotence (dysfunction developing after a period of normal function) is not particularly useful because the vast majority of men fall into the secondary category and may have either a psychologic or an acquired organic pathogenesis. Likewise, the observation that morning erections are preserved has minimal diagnostic utility because incompletely turgid morning erections inadequate for intercourse are commonly seen when there is organic erectile dysfunction.

The clinician should perform a complete physical examination. Particular emphasis should be placed on clinical evidence of endocrinopathies (decreased visual fields from a pituitary adenoma, gynecomastia, testicular atrophy), vascular insufficiency (diminished peripheral pulses, abdominal or femoral bruits), and autonomic neuropathies (irregular pupillary responses, orthostatic hypotension, resting tachycardia). The genital examination must be complete. Examination of the phallus should note the presence or absence of microphallus, the corporeal plaques of Peyronie's disease, chordee, hypospadias, phimosis, or balanitis. The prostate gland should be examined, and the anal wink (contraction of the anal sphincter when stroked by a tongue blade) and anal sphincter tone should be assessed. The bulbocavernosus reflex tests the sacral reflex arc and can be performed by squeezing the glans penis and observing contraction of the scrotum. Peripheral neuropathies associated with diabetes mellitus, alcoholism, and vitamin B_{12} deficiency can cause abnormalities in this particular reflex.

Discussion of the sexual dysfunction with the patient and his partner is the third central element in the assessment of impotence. There are many impediments to this interview, including awkwardness on the part of the clinician, the casual sexual lifestyles of some patients who do not have a single preferred partner, and the patient's refusal to include the partner. However, when the sexual dysfunction occurs within an established relationship, the diagnostic and therapeutic value of an interview with the patient's partner is great. The practitioner gains insight into the psychodynamics of the relationship, the couple's level of sophistication about sexual physiology, and their comfort and skill in communication within the relationship. Furthermore, this particular interview allows time for reassurance and counseling. It should be noted that sexual dysfunction often produces considerable anxiety in the patient's partner and may lead to misunderstandings that exacerbate the initial problem.

Use of Diagnostic Tests in the Evaluation of Impotence

The role of diagnostic testing in the evaluation of erectile dysfunction is controversial. Paradoxically, research clarifying the importance of organic etiologies in the pathogenesis of impotence has intensified the dilemma about the proper use of diagnostic tests. The primary care clinician may be uncertain about whether invasive and expensive research methodologies are appropriate for the less highly selected patients seen in general practice (Fig. 14–1).

The prevalence of primary and secondary gonadal failure in relatively unselected series of men with erectile dysfunction justifies determination of serum testosterone, prolactin, thyroid, and fasting glucose levels if impotence persists after withdrawal of suspect drugs. Testosterone secretion in normal individuals is pulsatile; therefore a single determination in the low or low normal range is consistent with either normal function or hypogonadism. To avoid this problem of interpretation, three separate samples may be collected at 20- to 40-minute intervals in the morning, and equal aliquots may be mixed for one testosterone measurement. The range of normal serum testosterone levels is quite wide, but there is no evidence that patients whose values consistently fall above the low end of normal range have partial hypogonadism or benefit from treatment designed to augment their serum testosterone level. Free testosterone levels measure unbound (or free) hormone levels and are theoretically better for diagnosing testosterone deficiency. Unfortunately these assays are expensive and infrequently available. Either hypo- or hyperthyroidism can cause impotence. Erectile dysfunction may be seen with hyperprolactinemia despite normal serum testosterone levels. Finally, impotence may rarely be the presenting clinical manifestation of diabetes mellitus.

The role of nocturnal penile tumescence (NPT) testing in the evaluation of the unselected impotent patient is highly controversial. Research using formal NPT with observation in a sleep laboratory for 2 consecutive nights coupled with additional techniques designed to assess rigidity has helped to eradicate the myth that 90% of impotence is psychogenic. However, the unselected use of this expensive and intrusive technology for a condition that may affect millions of men seems neither logical nor feasible.

Several techniques have been promoted to obtained NPT data without using a sleep laboratory. The postage stamp test is performed by having the patient place a strip of postage stamps around his flaccid penis and checking in the morning to see if the strip has been broken, presumably by penile tumescence during sleep. However, this test is limited by poor patient compliance and the failure to assess rigidity necessary for intercourse. The preferred approach for obtaining NPT information without using the sleep laboratory involves the use of Snap-Gauge testing. Snap-Gauges are circumferential bands with three overlapping plastic snaps that break with different degrees of penile pressure, thus providing indirect data on rigidity. Patients who break all three bands on one night and at least two on the second night of observation are presumed to have psychogenic impotence, whereas patients who fail to break more than one band on either night are likely to have organic impotence. The sensitivity of the Snap-Gauge for detecting psychogenic impotence is lowered if the bands are placed too loosely around the penis or if rapid eye movement sleep is disturbed. The specificity of the test is affected when the bands break on patients with rigid but excessively brief erections. Although the Snap-Gauge technique may produce indeterminate results, the economy of the test justifies its use when there is a high degree of uncertainty about etiology or when documentation of organic impotence is necessary before referral to a urologist.

Several techniques for demonstrating an arteriogenic basis of impotence have been developed. Penile systolic pressure can be measured by using a Doppler probe and can be compared to brachial systolic pressures. The normal penile/brachial systolic pressure ratio (penile brachial index or PBI) is greater than 0.9, whereas values less than 0.6 suggest penile vascular insufficiency. Values between 0.6 and 0.9 are indeterminant. There are conflicting reports about the correlation of the PBI with penile arteriography, and use of the PBI is being superseded by pharmacologic maneuvers that are more sensitive for diagnosing penile arterial insufficiency. Papaverine injected into the corpora cavernosum causes normal erections in men with psychogenic and neurogenic impotence, whereas men with penile arterial disease do not have a full erection. The recognition of vascular impotence is improved by using Doppler duplex scanning to document dilatation of the dorsal penile arteries and increased blood flow. Proponents of pharma-

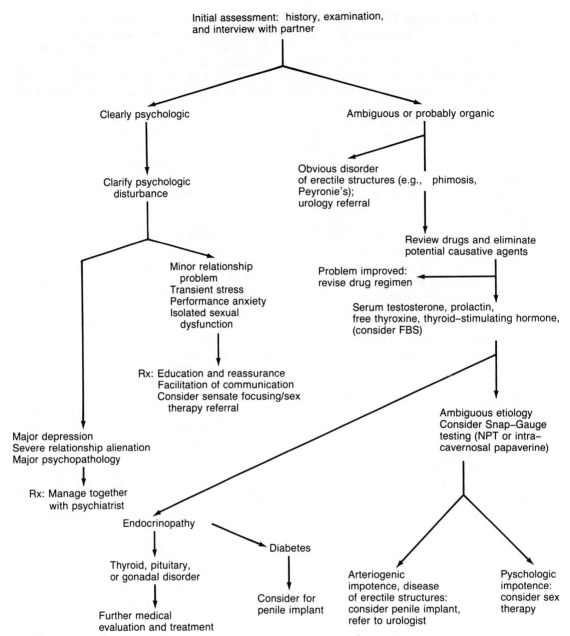

Figure 14–1. A diagnostic strategy in impotence.

cologic testing argue that this method provides as much information about the patient's physiology as NPT testing in a sleep laboratory and is cheaper and more convenient. To the extent that these tests are useful, it is likely that the papaverine Doppler technique will predominate because it is simple and can be performed in a urologist's office. At the present time, however, all of these methods of vascular evaluation are research techniques that are limited by the absence of distinct and specific management interventions.

Despite the importance of vascular disease as a cause of impotence, conventional angiography has not been useful in the evaluation of erectile dysfunction. Selective pudendal catheterization and angiography result in better visualization of the penile circulation, particularly when blood flow is augmented by papaverine or nitroglycerin. Cavernosography, the injection of radiopaque material into the corpora cavernosum, has been used effectively to demonstrate venous incompetence. A high suspicion of venous leakage, which is occasionally correctable by surgery, is probably the best justification for invasive vascular evaluation. Table 14–5 gives the costs of commonly advocated testing techniques used in evaluating erectile dysfunction.

Management of the Impotent Patient

Sexual dysfunction is invariably associated with psychologic reactions including anxiety, depression, and relationship tension. Performance anxiety, an anticipatory apprehension about the success of an attempt at intercourse, may exacerbate organic erectile dysfunction of all types as well as cause psychogenic impotence. The primary care practitioner is capable of managing patients with performance anxiety, particularly if the problem has had a recent onset. Education and reassurance are the primary therapeutic modalities; in addition, participation of the patient's partner in the treatment process is very useful.

Sensate focusing exercises may help patients who do not benefit from education and reassurance; this modality is particularly useful if sexual dysfunction has had a recent onset and is not associated with major relationship disturbances or psychopathology. With this technique, the couple is instructed to avoid sexual intercourse and to substitute a graded series of activities from romantic dinners through massage to masturbation. These exercises are intended to de-emphasize vaginal penetration as the sine qua non of sexual pleasure and to break the association among sexual activity, anxiety, and erectile failure. When performance anxiety complicates organic impotence, the primary care clinician may help the couple find other ways to achieve mutual sexual gratification and eliminate the component of dysfunction related to performance anxiety. When

Table 14–5. Typical Cost of Diagnostic Tests for Impotence

Test	Cost ($)
Serum testosterone level	40
Serum prolactin level	50
Thyroid testing (free thyroxine, total triiodothyronine, thyroid-stimulating hormone)	90
Snap-Gauge testing or screening device, 2 cuffs	40
Intracavernosal papaverine with Doppler flow studies	150–300
NPT in a sleep laboratory, 2 nights	1000

impotence related to performance anxiety is refractory to sensate focusing instruction or when it occurs as a complication of more fundamental relationship disturbance, referral to a sexual therapist or counselor is appropriate.

Discontinuation of offending drugs frequently restores potency. Impotence associated with heavy alcohol use has an excellent prognosis for recovery if the physical examination does not reveal testicular atrophy, spider angioma, or other signs of estrogenization. Patients should also be counseled to avoid cigarettes and recreational drugs. A common clinical scenario involves an impotent patient taking antihypertensive medications. Although a drug-free trial is ideal, impotence may improve with a lower dose of medication or after substituting a drug with less potential for causing sexual dysfunction. Furosemide, angiotensin-converting enzyme inhibitors, and calcium channel blockers are not yet reported to cause impotence. The management of patients with severe hypertension, especially that associated with diabetes, requires a good therapeutic alliance and the recognition on the part of doctor and patient that it may not be possible to control blood pressure and maintain full potency. The cooperation of the patient in identifying the least troublesome combination of drugs is important.

Patients who have low levels of serum testosterone should have gonadotropin levels measured. The preferred method is to take three samples at 20- to 40-minute intervals; luteinizing hormone and follicle-stimulating hormone values may be determined by using a single pooled specimen. Elevated gonadotropin levels suggest primary testicular failure, whereas normal or low levels are associated with hypothalamic-pituitary disease. Testosterone enanthate or cypionate, 200 mg intramuscularly every 2 to 3 weeks, should restore potency in primary hypogonadism. Androgen therapy will stimulate both normal and neoplastic prostatic tissue; therefore it is imperative to evaluate and monitor the prostate gland carefully, especially in an older male. Secondary hypogonadism requires further evaluation by an endocrinologist. Hyperprolactinemia, an uncommon cause of impotence in males, may be due to certain drugs, hypothyroidism, or hypothalamic-pituitary disease; further evaluation should be directed to these causes.

Patients who have normal potency as assessed by Snap-Gauge testing or NPT may benefit from sex therapy as well as the explanation and support of their primary clinician. Patients who have vascular or neurogenic impotence occasionally respond to oral vasodilators including yohimbine (5 mg three times a day) or isoxsuprine hydrochloride (10 mg three times a day). However, studies with these agents are uncontrolled and short. Hypertension and coronary artery disease are contraindications to a trial of either agents. Implantation of a penile prosthesis is the only generally accepted therapy for severe arteriogenic or neuropathic impotence. The primary care provider has a role in the selection of candidates for a penile prosthesis. Patients and their partners referred to a urologist for penile prostheses should recognize that the prosthesis will not restore penile sensation or the ability to ejaculate. Prostheses are made in two basic types: semirigid and inflatable. Semirigid prostheses have the advantage of low cost, ease of placement, and a low rate of complications; however, they do not mimic the process of erection and present a problem in concealment. The inflatable devices address the deficiencies of the semirigid devices but have a much higher rate of mechanical failure and are two to three times as expensive. Hinged and malleable semirigid prostheses attempt to improve concealment without significantly increasing cost. A semirigid device costs approximately $1,000, whereas the inflatable prostheses cost from $2,000 to $3,000. These devices are variably acceptable to patients, and disappointment with penile prostheses is common.

Bibliography

Abber JC, Lue TF, Orvis BR, et al. Diagnostic tests for impotence: a comparison of papaverine injection with the penile-brachial index and nocturnal penile tumescence monitoring. J Urol 135:923–925, 1986.
This useful paper compares intracavernosal papaverine to Snap-Gauge testing in the classification of impotence. Concordance was poor with Snap-Gauge testing, which resulted in the apparent over-diagnosis of organic impotence.

Anders EK, Bradley WE, Krane RJ. Nocturnal penile rigidity measured by the Snap-Gauge band. J Urol 129:964–966, 1983.
Snap-Gauges and their performance are described in 66 patients with impotence of various etiologies.

Buffum J. Pharmacosexology: the effect of drugs on sexual function—a review. J Psychoactive Drugs 14:5–41, 1982.
This is a definitive review of the effect of drugs on sexual function.

Condra M, Morales A, Owen JA, et al. Prevalence and significance of tobacco smoking in impotence. Urology 27:495–498, 1986.
Cigarette smokers and ex-smokers are over-represented among impotent men. The deleterious effects of smoking on erectile function may be mediated through effects on the small vasculature.

Davis SS, Viosca SP, Guralnik M, et al. Evaluation of impotence in older men. West J Med 142:499–505, 1985.
Intensive evaluation of impotent men over age 50 revealed organic etiologies in the overwhelming majority. Intercurrent general medical problems, medications, endocrinopathies, and vascular disorders were especially important.

Elist J, Jarman WD, Edson M. Evaluating medical treatment of impotence. Urology 28:374–375, 1984.
In a preliminary uncontrolled study of 60 men whose treatment included smoking cessation and oral vasodilator therapy, 38% showed improved NPT activity and erections adequate for intercourse.

Gregory JG, Purcell MH. Penile prostheses: review of current models, mechanical reliability, and product cost. Urology 24:150–152, 1987.
This article is a good brief overview of both penile prostheses (semirigid and inflatable), describing performance, cost, and patient satisfaction.

Krane RJ (ed). Urol Clin North Am 15:1–137, 1988.
This entire issue is devoted to the pathophysiology, diagnosis, and treatment of impotence.

Levine SB. Marital sexual dysfunction: introductory concepts. Ann Intern Med 84:448–453, 1976.
A helpful, basic discussion is given of the psychological components of good sexual function, characteristics of dysfunctional couples, and an introduction to sex therapy.

Maatman TJ, Montague DK, Martin LM. Cost-effective evaluation of impotence. Urology 27:132–135, 1986.
In a study from the perspective of primary care, 200 men were evaluated as outpatients at a cost of $250–$450 each, with 55% organic, 28% functional, and 17% indeterminant etiologies being found.

Master WH. Sex and aging—expectations and reality. Hosp Pract 21:175–198, 1986.
This review of age-related changes in sexual physiology provides useful information for clinicians counseling older patients.

Montague DK, James RE Jr, DeWolfe VG, et al. Diagnostic evaluation, classification, and treatment of men with sexual dysfunction. Urology 14:545–548, 1979.
A study of 165 impotent men evaluated by urologists and psychiatrists refutes the assertion that impotence is usually psychogenic. The discussion of the work-up is helpful.

Mulligan T, Katz PG. Erectile failure in the aged: evaluation and treatment. J Am Geriatr Soc 36:54–62, 1988.
This is a recent review of the pathophysiology, diagnosis, and treatment of impotence.

Nickel JC, Morales A, Condra M, et al. Endocrine dysfunction in impotence: incidence, significance and cost-effective screening. J Urol 132:40–43, 1984.
This study by urologists questions the utility of hormonal testing beyond that for serum testosterone levels.

Schiavi R. Male erectile disorders. Annu Rev Med 32:509–520, 1981.
This review article covers the physiology of male sexual function and the pathogenesis of erectile disorders.

Sidi AA, Cameron JS, Duffy LM, et al. Intracavernous drug-induced erections in the management of male erectile dysfunction: experience with 100 patients. J Urol 22:704–706, 1986.
The use of intracavernosal papaverine in the evaluation of impotence is described. Self-injection of papaverine as a long-term management technique is also described.

Slag MF, Morley JE, Elson MK, et al. Impotence in medical clinic outpatients. JAMA 249:1736–1740, 1983.

Unselected medical patients at a VA hospital were screened by history for impotence. One third were impotent, although the dysfunction had rarely been identified by the patient's own physician. Impotence was organic in 80% of patients, with medication side effects and endocrinopathy being the most important causes.

Spark RF, White RA, Connolly PE. Impotence is not always psychogenic. JAMA 243:750–755, 1980.

Evaluation of 105 men with impotence revealed an organic etiology in 66%, but the paper is flawed by a prominent ascertainment bias.

Van Thiel DH, Gavaler JS, Sanghvi A. Recovery of sexual function in abstinent alcoholic men. Gastroenterology 84:677–682, 1982.

The response of 60 impotent alcoholic men, mean age 36, to a period of abstinence was evaluated. Of those with normal testicular volume, 68% recovered normal potency, whereas no men with atrophy regained normal erectile function.

15

Hyperlipidemia: Practical Diagnosis and Management

JEFFREY M. HOEG, M.D., F.A.C.P.

The management of hyperlipidemia has long been one of the more controversial issues facing the medical community. Epidemiologic studies, animal investigations, and detailed analyses of rare inborn errors in cholesterol and lipoprotein metabolism have supported the view that blood cholesterol and, more specifically, plasma lipoproteins can play a central role in the atherosclerotic process. However, the implications of these various studies on the routine evaluation and treatment of patients with hyperlipidemia were not well defined until recently. Several large, multicenter clinical trials were instituted in the late 1960's and early 1970's that were designed to assess the benefit of a reduction of blood cholesterol concentrations on cardiovascular morbidity and mortality. The results of these studies have become available during the past 4 years. It is now clear that reducing the concentrations of total cholesterol and low density lipoprotein (LDL) cholesterol in the blood by combined diet and drug therapy can reduce the risk of developing symptomatic cardiovascular disease. A 1% reduction in the blood cholesterol concentration in a hypercholesterolemic patient leads to a 2% reduction in risk of developing cardiovascular morbidity and mortality. Therefore, the evaluation and treatment of hyperlipidemia have entered the mainstream of patient care for reducing the risk of cardiovascular disease.

The diagnosis and management of hyperlipidemia have similarities to the management of hypertension. Many patients are entirely asymptomatic and encounter the health care system for the first time. The use of diets and drugs in the management of both hypertension and hyperlipidemia requires constant surveillance and encouragement because the rewards for therapeutic intervention, for both the pa-

tient and the physician, are not as apparent as are those for care of symptomatic illnesses. Consistency in a supportive system is therefore necessary to manage both of these cardiovascular risk factors effectively.

However, there are also marked differences in the management of hypertension and hyperlipidemia. This is partly because of the complexity of the metabolic pathways involved in lipoprotein transport. A single number and an easily remembered goal for therapy are therefore not as available for hyperlipidemia treatment as for hypertension therapy. An understanding of the plasma lipoproteins and their metabolism is important for the effective treatment of hyperlipidemia.

Plasma Lipoproteins

Energy is derived from the diet and from energy stores within the body primarily via glucose and triglycerides. Unlike glucose, which is water-soluble, triglycerides are not miscible with the aqueous environment of the blood. In addition, other hydrophobic substances such as cholesterol, which are needed by all body tissues, require a lipid transport system. The plasma lipoproteins are particles that subserve this function of lipid transport. These particles are aggregations of noncovalently associated molecules of cholesterol, cholesteryl esters, phospholipids, triglycerides, and proteins. The proteins associated with these particles are termed apolipoproteins, and they direct the metabolism and transport of the fats present in each particle.

The plasma lipoproteins are heterogeneous with respect to their size, composition, origin, and physiologic roles (Table 15–1). The tri-

Table 15–1. Summary of Characteristics of Plasma Lipoproteins

Lipoprotein Class	Origin	Primary Lipid	Primary Apolipoprotein	Function
Chylomicrons	Intestine	Triglycerides	Apo B, Apo E, Apo C's	Transport triglycerides in food to the tissues
Very low density lipoproteins (VLDLs)	Intestine and liver	Triglycerides	Apo B, Apo E, Apo C's	Transport triglycerides from the liver to the tissues
Low density lipoproteins (LDLs)	Derived from VLDLs	Cholesterol	Apo B	Transport cholesterol to the tissues
High density lipoproteins (HDLs)	Liver and intestine	Cholesterol	Apo A-I, Apo A-II	Transport cholesterol to the liver for biliary excretion

glyceride-rich chylomicrons and very low density lipoproteins (VLDLs) primarily transport triglycerides to the tissues utilizing fatty acids for energy use or storage. After the triglycerides have been removed from these particles, the cholesterol-rich LDL particles are formed. When the total blood cholesterol level is determined, most of the cholesterol measured reflects cholesterol in the LDL form. LDL delivers the cholesterol necessary for cell membrane integrity and for hormone synthesis in steroidogenic tissues, but it is also involved in the atherosclerotic process. Therefore, dietary and drug therapy is directed to the reduction of LDL cholesterol levels.

The high density lipoproteins (HDLs), which are synthesized in the liver and intestine, are involved in reverse cholesterol transport. Cells cannot degrade cholesterol. Excess cellular cholesterol is adsorbed from cells and transported to the liver, where cholesterol can be either directly secreted into the bile or converted to bile acids. Increased levels of HDL cholesterol may represent efficient reverse cholesterol transport because there is an *inverse* relationship between HDL cholesterol and atherosclerotic cardiovascular disease. Therefore, total cholesterol concentrations reflect the cholesterol present in a variety of particles that may have a direct role in atherosclerosis, no effect on the process, or even an inhibiting role in atherogenesis. By using a few simple measurements and calculations, it is possible to define more precisely which lipoprotein species is elevated, and this process can lead to specific treatment guidelines.

Screening for Hyperlipidemia

All patients seeing a physician should be screened for hyperlipidemia. A random, non-fasting total cholesterol concentration is sufficient for the initial evaluation. Screening for hypertriglyceridemia by using a fasting triglyceride determination should be considered in patients with xanthomas, symptomatic cardiovascular disease, or recurrent pancreatitis. A screening triglyceride determination, however, is not necessary for the initial evaluation of cardiovascular disease risk in asymptomatic individuals. Patients with a strong personal or family history of atherosclerotic cardiovascular disease should be particularly targeted for cholesterol screening. The American Heart Association currently recommends that plasma lipid determinations should be performed every 5 years in patients between the ages of 20 and 60.

Patients at moderate and high risk of cardiovascular disease can be stratified according to their age. The values in Table 15–2 were recommended as screening cutoff values by the NIH Consensus Development Conference. Individuals with levels in the high risk category and those with levels in the moderate risk category who have cardiovascular disease or a strong family history of premature cardiovascular disease (parents and siblings with cardiovascular disease before age 60) should undergo further diagnostic testing.

Lipoprotein Evaluation

Positive results from the initial screening for hypercholesterolemia are further evaluated by

Table 15–2. Blood Cholesterol Concentrations Leading to Further Evaluation and Treatment

Age (Years)	Cholesterol Concentrations (mg/dl)	
	Moderate Risk	High Risk
20–29	> 200 (5.17 mM)	> 220 (5.69 mM)
30–39	> 220 (5.69 mM)	> 240 (6.21 mM)
> 40	> 240 (6.21 mM)	> 260 (6.72 mM)

Adapted from the NIH Consensus Development Conference statement, JAMA 253:2080–2086, 1985.

obtaining fasting cholesterol and triglyceride concentrations. A fasting triglyceride level less than 250 mg/dl and a normal cholesterol reading end the evaluation. Individuals with borderline elevated blood lipid levels should be rescreened within 1 to 2 years. If, however, the fasting values are elevated, a calculated LDL cholesterol concentration should be determined. This is accomplished by obtaining an HDL cholesterol level at the time that another fasting cholesterol and triglyceride sample is determined. Because the cholesterol concentration of VLDL is about one fifth of the total triglyceride concentration, dividing the triglyceride concentration by 5 leads to the VLDL cholesterol value. The LDL cholesterol concentration can then be calculated as outlined in Figure 15–1. The subsequent treatment algorithms utilize these calculated VLDL and LDL cholesterol values to guide further diagnostic and therapeutic steps. The data from the Framingham studies indicate that the ratio of total cholesterol to HDL cholesterol is one of the most powerful predictors of cardiovascular disease risk. Basing treatment decisions on the LDL cholesterol concentration is intimately related to this ratio because LDL cholesterol represents most of the total cholesterol used in this ratio. In addition, most of the currently recommended treatment strategies result in reductions in total and LDL cholesterol levels with either a neutral or a beneficial impact on HDL cholesterol concentration. Therefore, strategies designed to reduce LDL cholesterol levels have a direct effect on this ratio.

Plasma HDL levels should be determined for other reasons as well. An elevated HDL cholesterol concentration could be the principal cause of a high total cholesterol level. This is often observed in premenopausal women. Because HDL cholesterol concentrations are inversely related to cardiovascular disease, no further evaluation would be necessary. In addition, some patients with clinically apparent cardiovascular disease may have low HDL concentrations with or without alterations in the other lipoprotein subfractions. Although

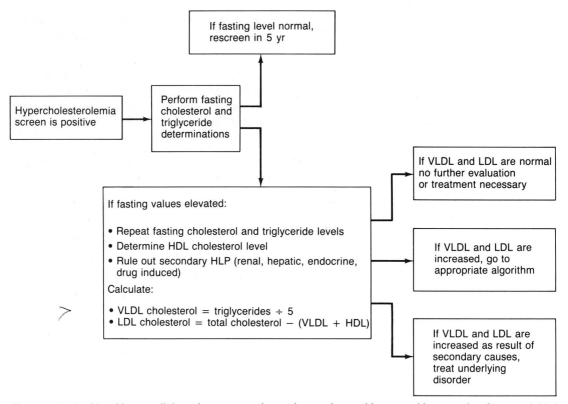

Figure 15–1. *Algorithm outlining the approach to the patient with a positive result after an initial hypercholesterolemia screening. HLP, hyperlipoproteinemia; HDL, high density lipoprotein; VLDL, very low density lipoprotein; LDL, low density lipoprotein.*

Table 15–3. Cardiovascular Disease Risk Based on LDL Cholesterol Concentration Stratified by Age and Gender*

Gender and Risk	Age-Adjusted LDL Cholesterol Level					
	0–14	15–19	20–29	30–39	40–49	50
Men						
Moderate risk	106	109	128	149	160	166
High risk	120	123	148	171	180	188
Women						
Moderate risk	113	115	127	143	155	170
High risk	126	135	148	163	177	195

*LDL cholesterol concentration was measured as mg/dl.
Values represent the 75th percentile (moderate risk) and 90th percentile (high risk) values obtained by the Lipid Research Clinics.

no data are available that address this issue directly, many experts believe that patients with low HDL concentrations may also benefit from treatment directed toward increasing the HDL cholesterol concentration.

At the time that the LDL cholesterol is calculated, secondary causes for hyperlipidemia should be sought. Underlying renal and hepatic disorders can be detected by using routine serum chemistry panels. Hypothyroidism (levels of thyroxine and thyroid-stimulating hormone), hypercorticalism (morning cortisol value), gammopathies (serum protein electrophoresis), and nephrosis (urinalysis) should also be ruled out because treatment of these underlying disorders also leads to normalization of the plasma lipoprotein concentrations. However, an evaluation of the Lipid Research Clinics study by Wallace and coworkers indicates that the vast majority of hyperlipidemic patients have primary hyperlipoproteinemias.

A variety of medications can also affect the plasma cholesterol and lipoprotein concentrations. Medications that have been shown to increase total plasma cholesterol from 5 to 25 mg/dl include estrogens, androgens, tricyclic antidepressants, thiazide diuretics, loop diuretics, allopurinol, coumarins, and the beta blockers propranolol, nadolol, metoprolol, and timolol. However, beta blockers with intrinsic sympathomimetic activity such as pindolol and acebutolol and the calcium channel blockers (nifedipine, diltiazem, verapamil), angiotensin-converting enzyme inhibitors (captopril and enalapril), hydralazine, and minoxidil are without adverse effects on plasma lipoprotein concentrations. Therefore, decisions concerning the relative importance of specific antihypertensive therapies as well as other medications must be made to determine the optimal pharmacologic regimen for the hypercholesterolemic patient.

Dietary Therapy

The risk of developing atherosclerosis related to the LDL cholesterol concentration can be stratified by age and gender (Table 15–3). Individuals with LDL cholesterol concentrations above the 90th percentile have a 2- to 4-fold increased (high) risk of developing cardiovascular disease. Patients with LDL cholesterol concentrations in the 75th to 90th percentile range have a 1.5- to 2-fold (moderate) risk. High risk patients as well as moderate risk patients who have symptomatic atherosclerosis or a strong family history of atherosclerotic cardiovascular disease should start dietary therapy (Table 15–4). Physicians should strongly encourage a modification of the patient's diet and provide some concrete guidance such as the recommendations outlined in the American Heart Association patient information brochures. These materials can be obtained from the local chapters of the American Heart Association, which are located in all 50 states. All hyperlipidemic patients should attain and maintain the ideal body weight and enhance their fiber intake. In addition, patients with elevated LDL cholesterol levels either with or without an increase in VLDL cholesterol levels should reduce their fat intake to less than 30% of total calories. In addition, the dietary cholesterol intake should be reduced to less than 250 mg/day, and mono- and polyunsaturated fats should be substituted for saturated fats such as palm and coconut oils. Substitution of deep sea fish for red meat is also desirable because it increases the intake of omega-3 fatty acids. (However, fish oil supplements cannot be recommended at this time, because the safety and efficacy of such treatment are not yet established.)

Converting these abstract dietary prescriptions, especially the modifications necessary for the high risk patient, into a realistic and

Table 15–4. Dietary Management of Hyperlipoproteinemia

Diet Constituent	VLDL Cholesterol > 200 mg/dl (Triglycerides > 1000 mg/dl) and LDL Normal	VLDL Cholesterol 100–200 mg/dl (Triglycerides 500–1000 mg/dl) and LDL Normal	LDL Cholesterol Elevated and VLDL Normal	*Both* VLDL and LDL Cholesterol Increased
Total fat (% energy)	10–20	20–30	25–30	20–30
Dietary cholesterol (mg/dl)	ND*	< 300	150–250	150–250
Polyunsaturated/saturated fatty acid ratio	ND	1–1.5	1.5–2.0	1.5–2.0

*ND, not specifically defined.

palatable diet requires collaboration with a registered dietitian (R.D.). Dietary therapy is the cornerstone of all treatment. A 5 to 15% reduction in total and LDL cholesterol concentrations is generally achieved, and there is normalization of plasma lipid levels in many patients. Also, drug therapy is much less effective if it is not associated with a well-designed diet.

Patients with an elevated VLDL cholesterol (fasting triglyceride concentrations > than 500 mg/dl) *without* an associated increase in LDL cholesterol levels are at risk of pancreatitis, eruptive xanthomas, and (for some) cardiovascular disease (Fig. 15–2). Patients with triglyceride concentrations higher than 1000 mg/dl are at very high risk of pancreatitis, xanthomas, and intermittent abdominal pain. Because of this high risk, they should be referred to a center specializing in lipid disorders if dietary therapy does not reduce the triglyceride concentrations to less than 1000 mg/dl within 6 to 8 weeks. These patients should be placed on a *very* low fat diet (< 20% calories from fat) and must abstain completely from alcohol intake. Patients with triglyceride levels greater than 500 mg/dl are also at increased risk of pancreatitis. In addition, all patients with fasting triglyceride concentrations higher than 250 mg/dl should be carefully questioned about familial hyperlipidemia and a familial history of premature cardiovascular disease. A subset of hypertriglyceridemic patients suffers from inborn errors in apolipoprotein metabolism. These patients should be considered for drug therapy if dietary treatment does not normalize their plasma lipoprotein concentrations. Although the diagnostic tools for identifying these patients (such as apolipoprotein B determinations) are not yet routinely available, the family history should guide the necessary therapeutic decisions.

Drug Therapy for Hyperlipidemia

If diet-only treatment does not reduce the LDL cholesterol concentration to less than the target value of 160 mg/dl, drug therapy should be considered. The principal drugs available in the United States for the treatment of hypercholesterolemia are outlined in Table 15–5. These agents vary as to their efficacy, cost, and adverse effects. Three drugs that have been demonstrated both to lower LDL cholesterol concentrations and to reduce cardiovascular morbidity and mortality are the bile acid sequestrant cholestyramine, the B complex vi-

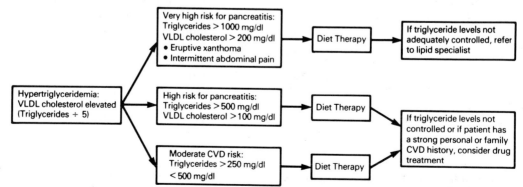

Figure 15–2. Algorithm summarizing the stratification of patients with hypertriglyceridemia. The treatment of all hypertriglyceridemic patients begins with dietary therapy. CVD, cardiovascular disease.

Table 15–5. Summary of Medications Used to Lower LDL Cholesterol Concentrations

Drug	Dose	LDL % Cholesterol Reduction (%)	Cost/month ($)	Contraindications	Side Effects	Useful Tips
Bile acid seques-trants*				Use of coumarins Hypertriglycerid-emia	Constipation Abdominal pain	Prescribe stool softeners Prepare entire dose in liquid 1 day in ad-vance
Cholestyra-mine Packet Powder	4–24 g/day	27	155.28 38.39		Drug interaction (coumarins, thiazides, digoxin, thyroxine)	Start at half dose Build to full dose over 3 wk
Colestipol Packet Powder	5–30 g/day	23	95.46 82.19			
Niacin* plain Sustained release	1–3 g/day	31	5.04 19.01	Diabetes Gout Peptic ulcer Asthma Hepatic diseases	Skin flushing Headache Pruritis Glucose intoler-ance	Start at low dose (100 mg t.i.d.) Increase to 1 g t.i.d. over 3–5 wk 325 mg acetyl-salicylic acid 1 h before dose Take with meals Avoid hot drinks Sustained re-lease form better toler-ated
Lovastatin	20–80 mg/day	31	187.50	Should not be used for women who may become pregnant	Gastrointestinal upset	Take with meals
Neomycin	1 g b.i.d.	16	16.80	Renal disease Hepatic disease Intestinal disease	Nausea Diarrhea	Take with meals Diarrhea self-limited to < 3 wk
Fibric acid derivatives Gemfibrozil Clofibrate	0.6 g b.i.d. 1.0 g b.i.d.	11 14	39.56 38.76	Cholelithiasis Coumarin treat-ment	Abdominal pain Nausea Diarrhea Myalgias	
Probucol	0.5 g b.i.d.	12	42.46	Cardiac arrhythmia Prolonged QT in-terval	Diarrhea Nausea Flatulence Eosinophilia Prolonged QT interval	

*Indicates current drugs of choice in 1988. Average wholesale price to pharmacist based on Blue Book Values for a maximum dose for 1988–1989.

tamin niacin, and gemfibrozil. In addition, these drugs have been found to be relatively safe over an extended period and in a large number of patients. Therefore, the bile acid sequestrants and niacin are the drugs of choice for the treatment of elevated LDL cholesterol concentrations. However, both the bile acid sequestrants and niacin frequently lead to troubling adverse side effects (Table 15–5). Fore-

warning the patient of these side effects and taking steps to prevent or minimize them greatly improve patient compliance.

A new class of cholesterol-lowering compounds, the hydroxymethylglutaryl coenzyme A (HMG-CoA) reductase inhibitors, offers hope for effective as well as easily tolerated hypolipidemic drug therapy. The first of these compounds that is available for use in the

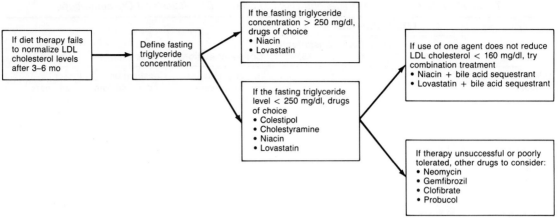

Figure 15–3. Algorithm outlining the use of drugs in the management of elevated LDL cholesterol concentrations.

United States is lovastatin. This drug is as effective as any other compound that has been tried and is extremely well tolerated by patients. Lovastatin should be used if attempts to reduce the LDL cholesterol level to less than 160 mg/dl with the bile acid sequestrants or niacin fail. The starting dose is 20 mg/day, and this can be increased to 80 mg/day. A twice daily regimen is slightly more effective than administration once a day. Compared with conventional agents, lovastatin is very well tolerated. However, because it is a newly released compound, close observation for potential adverse side effects is necessary. Monitoring for myositis, hepatitis, and cataract formation, as well as for mild gastrointestinal symptoms, is recommended. Liver function studies should be performed every 4 to 6 weeks, and the drug should be stopped if the transaminase levels exceed twice the upper limit of normal. Creatine kinase levels should be determined if myalgia develops. Rhabdomyolysis and acute renal tubular necrosis have occurred in patients also receiving cyclosporine after heart transplantation. Finally, a slit lamp examination should be performed before instituting therapy and yearly thereafter to assess cataract formation. It should be pointed out that less than 5% of patients receiving lovastatin have experienced any of these adverse effects. If lovastatin and its analogues can also be shown to reduce cardiovascular morbidity and mortality and if long-term safety can be established, this compound will greatly facilitate the management of hypercholesterolemia.

The drug treatment algorithm for an elevated LDL cholesterol concentration refractory to dietary therapy is outlined in Figure 15–3. The treatment decision is based on whether there is hypertriglyceridemia in addition to an elevated LDL cholesterol concentration. If hypertriglyceridemia is present, niacin and lovastatin should be considered. In the absence of hypertriglyceridemia, the bile acid sequestrants colestipol and cholestyramine should be considered as the drugs of choice in addition to niacin and lovastatin. If after 3 to 6 months of drug treatment with a single agent the plasma LDL cholesterol level is not sufficiently affected, combination therapy with a second drug can result in an additive cholesterol-lowering effect. The other drugs that could be used to treat hypercholesterolemia include neomycin, gemfibrozil, clofibrate, and probucol. However, not all of these have been approved as cholesterol-lowering agents by the U.S. Food and Drug Administration, and they are less effective in reducing LDL cholesterol concentrations.

In hypertriglyceridemic patients (with normal LDL levels) at risk of developing pancreatitis or in patients with a strong personal or family history of cardiovascular disease, drug treatment should be considered if dietary therapy fails to control their lipid concentrations. The drug of choice is niacin. If contraindications to niacin treatment exist or if niacin is not tolerated, the fibric acid derivatives gemfibrozil and clofibrate should be used. Patients with profound hypertriglyceridemia (> 1000 mg/dl) are often very difficult to treat, and referral to a center specializing in lipid disorders should be considered if a 6- to 12-month attempt with diet and drug treatment does not successfully reduce the plasma VLDL and triglyceride concentrations.

Summary

Recent evidence indicates that diet and drug treatment of hyperlipidemia prevents not only pancreatitis and eruptive exanthoma but also the development of symptomatic cardiovascular disease. By identifying which of the plasma lipoproteins is increased in concentration, a rational and effective approach in managing these patients is readily available. Eventually, the management of hyperlipidemia will become as commonplace as the treatment of hypertension. Combined risk factor modification will undoubtedly reduce the cardiovascular morbidity and mortality that have been so prevalent in developed countries.

Bibliography

Blankenhorn D, Nessim S, Johnson R, et al. Beneficial effects of combined colestipol-niacin therapy on coronary atherosclerosis and coronary venous bypass grafts. JAMA 257:3233–3240, 1987.
> *This well-designed, prospective clinical trial demonstrates that combined drug treatment directly affects the progression of atherosclerosis in patients after aortocoronary bypass grafting. The data strongly support intervention in patients with symtomatic coronary artery disease with cholesterol concentrations between 200 and 240 mg/dl.*

Canner PL, Berge KG, Wenger NK, et al. 15 year mortality in coronary drug project patients: long term benefit with niacin. J Am Coll Cardiol 8:1245–1255, 1986.
> *This study indicates that niacin therapy reduces the risk of death in patients who have already experienced a myocardial infarction. Therefore, both bile acid sequestrants and niacin have been demonstrated to favorably affect cardiovascular morbidity and mortality.*

Frick MH, Elo O, Haapa K, et al. Helsinki Heart Study: primary-prevention trial with gemfibrozil in middle-aged men with dyslipidemia. N Engl J Med 317:1237–1245, 1987.
> *This clinical trial demonstrated that the fibric acid derivative gemfibrozil can also reduce cardiovascular disease risk. In addition, the data from this study indicate that intervention to raise HDL cholesterol levels may be of clinical value.*

Gotto AM, Bierman EL, Conner WE, et al. Recommendations for treatment of hyperlipidemia in adults. The Nutrition Committee of the American Heart Association. Circulation 69:1067A–1090A, 1984.
> *This is an excellent summary of the cornerstone of hyperlipidemia management—diet.*

Grundy SM, Greenland P, Herd A, et al. Cardiovascular and risk factor evaluation of healthy Americans: a statement for physicians by an ad hoc committee appointed by the steering committee, American Heart Association. Circulation 75:1340A–1362A, 1987.
> *This excellent summary of cardiovascular disease prevention strategies outlines the approach to prevention recommended by the American Heart Association.*

Hoeg JM, Brewer HB Jr. 3-Hydroxy-3-methylglutaryl-coenzyme A reductase inhibitors in the treatment of hypercholesterolemia. JAMA 258:3532–3536, 1987.
> *This article is a concise review of this new class of hypolipidemic agents.*

Hoeg JM, Gregg RE, Brewer HB Jr. An approach to the management of hyperlipoproteinemia. JAMA 255:512–521, 1986.
> *In addition to treatment guidelines being outlined, plasma lipoprotein metabolism is summarized in detail.*

Hoeg JM, Maher MB, Bou E, et al. Combination use of neomycin and niacin normalizes the plasma-lipoprotein concentrations in type II hyperlipoproteinemia. Circulation 70:1004–1011, 1984.
> *This article indicates that several drug combinations lead to enhanced efficacy in reducing total and LDL cholesterol concentrations.*

Hoeg JM, Maher MB, Zech LA, et al. Effectiveness of mevinolin on plasma lipoprotein concentrations in type II hyperlipoproteinemia. Am J Cardiol 57:933–939, 1986.
> *This article summarizes the experience with the new HMG-CoA reductase inhibitor lovastatin (formerly called mevinolin). This drug is very effective, is easily tolerated, and has just been approved for use in the United States by the U.S. Food and Drug Administration.*

Illingworth DR. Mevinolin plus colestipol in therapy for severe heterozygous familial hypercholesterolemia. Ann Intern Med 101:598–604, 1984.
> *This article indicates that several drug combinations lead to enhanced efficacy in reducing total and LDL cholesterol concentrations.*

Kane JP, Malloy MJ, Tun P, et al. Normalization of low density lipoprotein levels in heterozygous familial hypercholesterolemia with a combined drug regimen. N Engl J Med 304:251–258, 1981.
> *This article indicates that several drug combinations lead to enhanced efficacy in reducing total and LDL cholesterol contentrations.*

National Institutes of Health Consensus Development Conference statement: lowering blood cholesterol to prevent heart disease. JAMA 253:2080–2086, 1985.
> *This statement summarizes the various lines of evidence supporting the conclusion that hypercholesterolemic patients should have their blood cholesterol concentrations reduced.*

The expert panel: report of the National Cholesterol Education Program Expert Panel on detection, evaluation, and treatment of high blood cholesterol in adults. Arch Intern Med 148:36–69, 1988.
> *This is a comprehensive review of the management of hyperlipidemia from the National Heart, Lung, and Blood Institute.*

The Lipid Research Clinics Coronary Primary Prevention Trial results I. Reduction in incidence of coronary heart disease. JAMA 251:351–364, 1984.
> *This paper summarizes the results of the large, multicenter study demonstrating that the treatment of patients with hypercholesterolemia reduced cardiovascular morbidity and mortality. The data from this trial indicated that a 1% reduction in the plasma cholesterol concentration leads to a 2% decline in the cardiovascular disease.*

The Lipid Research Clinics Coronary Primary Prevention

Trial results II. The relationship of reduction in incidence of coronary heart disease to cholesterol lowering. JAMA 251:365–374, 1984.

This paper summarizes the results of the large, multicenter study demonstrating that the treatment of patients with hypercholesterolemia reduced cardiovascular morbidity and mortality. The data from this trial indicated that a 1% reduction in the plasma cholesterol concentration leads to a 2% decline in the cardiovascular disease.

The Lovastatin Study Group II: therapeutic response to lovastatin (mevinolin) in nonfamilial hypercholesterolemia. JAMA 256:2829–2834, 1986.

This article summarizes the experience with the new HMG-CoA reductase inhibitor lovastatin (formerly called mevinolin). This drug is very effective, is easily tolerated, and has just been approved for use in the United States by the U.S. Food and Drug Administration.

16

Oral Contraceptives: Prescription and Monitoring by Internists

NICHOLS VORYS, M.D., M.M.Sc.

Introduction

Family planning dates back to the early 19th century, but effective birth control was not attained until the 1960's with the availability of oral synthetic sex steroids and the intrauterine device (IUD). It is estimated that 60 million women worldwide use oral contraceptives and another 60 million (40 million in China) use the IUD (Table 16–1). The purpose of this chapter is to review the pharmacology, physiologic and adverse effects, and clinical use of oral contraceptives.

Pharmacology

Most oral contraceptives combine a synthetic estrogen with a progestin component.

The synthetic estrogens, ethinyl estradiol and mestranol, also have slightly different biologic activities: it is estimated that ethinyl estradiol is about 1.7 times as potent as an equivalent weight of mestranol. Mestranol is biologically inert and must undergo demethylation to the biologically active estradiol. The synthetic progestins are formed by the removal of the 19-carbon atom from testosterone and are called 19-nor compounds. There are five different progestins marketed in the United States: norethynodrel, norethindrone, norethindrone acetate, ethynodiol diacetate, and norgestrel. Molecular structural differences give these progestins variable combinations of progestogenic, estrogenic, antiestrogenic, and androgenic activity. As noted in Figure 16–1, norgestrel has the greatest progestogenic and androgenic effect of the progestins.

Table 16–1. *Effectiveness of and Mortality Related to Contraceptive Methods*

Method	Pregnancies Per 100 Women-Years, All Ages	Estimated Annual Deaths Resulting from Contraceptive Method and/or Pregnancy Per 100,000 Women-Years by Age					
		15–19	*20–24*	*25–29*	*30–34*	*35–39*	*40–44*
No contraception	60–80	6	5	7	14	19	22
Surgical sterilization (tubal ligation)	0.2–0.6	4	4	4	4	4	4
Combination oral contraceptives	0.3–1.2						
Nonsmokers		1	1	1	2	4	3
Smokers		2	2	2	11	13	59
Progestin-only oral contraceptives	2–3	1	1	1	1	1	1
Intrauterine devices	1–6	1	1	1	1	2	1
Barrier methods	2–36	1	1	2	4	5	4
Diaphragm with spermicide	2–20	1–2	1–2	1–2	1–4	1–6	1–7
Aerosol foams	2–29	1–2	1–2	1–3	1–6	1–8	1–9
Condoms	3–36	1–3	1–3	1–4	1–7	1–11	1–12
Jellies, creams, tablets	4–36	1–3	1–3	1–4	1–7	1–11	1–12
Periodic abstinence (rhythm)	1–47	1–4	1–4	1–5	1–9	1–14	1–15
Mucus and temperature chart	1–25	1–2	1–2	1–3	1–5	1–7	1–8
Calendar method	4–47	1–4	1–4	1–5	3–9	4–14	5–15

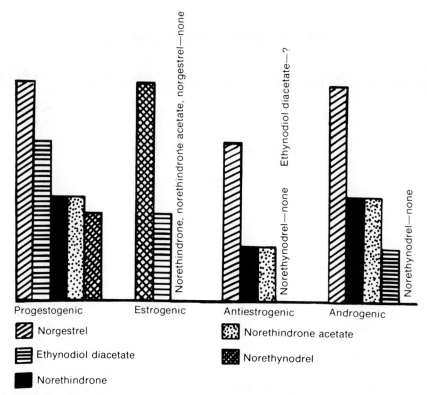

Figure 16–1. *Inherent biologic effects of the synthetic progestins. From Vorys N, Scommegna A, Givens JR. Therapy of menstrual dysfunction, in Gold JJ, Josimovich JB (eds). Gynecologic Endocrinology, ed 3. New York, Harper & Row, 1980, p 388, with permission.*

Anatomic and Pathophysiologic Changes Induced by Oral Contraceptives

The anatomic, physiologic, and pathophysiologic changes in the reproductive tract induced by the combination of estrogens and progestins are outlined in Table 16–2. Oral contraceptives work mainly in the central nervous system to inhibit ovulation but have additional inhibitory effects in the genital tract.

Many of the side effects of oral contraceptive therapy are due to changes in the enterohepatic circulation and to changes in protein synthesis by the hepatic cells. The excretion of bilirubin and bile salts is a major hepatic function. The capacity of the liver to excrete organic anions (bile salts or organic dyes) is consistently decreased by steroid hormones. Gross clinical tests, such as serum bilirubin concentration and the standard Bromsulphalein (BSP) test, do not detect these changes, but a decrease in excretory function is readily identifiable by kinetic studies. Combination oral contraceptives appear to impair the final transport of bilirubin or BSP from the liver cell to the bile canaliculi. Continuous use of synthetic progestins and estrogens may be associated with jaundice, pruritus, and laboratory and pathologic evidence of intrahepatic cholestasis. Oral contraceptive patients with cholestasis are also prone to jaundice in pregnancy.

Many plasma proteins are synthesized by the hepatocyte. Estrogen can influence the synthesis, distribution, degradation, and function of RNA, which has a central role in the control of protein synthesis. Estrogen may activate genes and allow transcription of new species of mRNA, which then code the synthesis of specific plasma proteins by the hepatocyte. Oral contraceptives alter the synthesis of a wide variety of hepatic proteins. Albumin and cholinesterase levels decrease during oral contraceptive use. The $alpha_1$, $alpha_2$, and beta globulins are increased, and the albumin/globulin ratio is further decreased. Oral contraceptives increase the synthesis of many carrier proteins such as thyroxine-binding globulin (TBG), steroid-binding globulin, and vitamin K–dependent coagulation factors. Cortisol-binding globulin shows the best cor-

Table 16–2. *Effects of Combination Oral Contraceptives on Reproductive Tract**

Organ/Tissue	Anatomy and Pathophysiology
Central nervous system/ hypothalamus and pituitary axis	Estrogen suppresses FSH; progestins supress LH; low dose oral contraceptives (< 0.35 mg estrogen) suppress midcycle LH peak but not base-line FSH and LH
Ovary	Morphology: ovaries are small, inactive, with no loss of germ cells
	Steroid production: estradiol and estrone decrease to < 50 pg/ml; serum testosterone decreases by 50%; serum androstenedione decreases by 50%
Oviducts	Endosalpinx lining, cilia, and muscular activity are impaired
Uterus	Endometrium becomes atrophic; glandular secretion and prostaglandin synthesis decrease
	Myometrium shows cellular hypertrophy, dilated sinusoids, and uterine congestion
	Cervix: squamocolumnar junction is advanced, becomes congested with erosion of external portion; cervical gland secretions become inspissated and thick and provide a barrier to sperm and vaginal pathogens
Vagina	Vaginal secretions are scanty, multicellular, and contain large numbers of leukocytes and bacteria; glycogen deposits are heavy, number of Döderlein's bacilli is reduced
Breast	Contraceptives may increase breast size and nipple tenderness, decrease milk volume, shorten lactation, and alter milk constituents; mastodynia may occur and may be associated with breast lumps, but most fibrocystic disease improves with oral contraceptive administration, especially with Lo/Ovral and Ovral

*FSH, follicle-stimulating hormone; LH, luteinizing hormone.

relation between estrogen dose and hepatocyte protein synthesis because estrogen is the only factor known to increase this globulin. Table 16–3 indicates changes in laboratory tests caused by oral contraceptives; some of these changes are attributed to alterations in serum proteins.

Preparations

Two oral contraceptive formulations—combinations and daily progestin—are available.

The most widely used combination pills contain fixed doses of estrogen and progestins that are taken daily for 21 consecutive days. Withdrawal bleeding occurs 3 to 5 days after the last pill is taken, and the routine is started again on the fifth day of the new cycle. Biphasic preparations, introduced in 1983, attempt to mimic physiologic steroid levels during the menstrual cycle. During the first 10 days of treatment, lower progestin doses mimic the follicular phase levels of progesterone and during the second 11 days, higher progestin doses mimic the luteal phase; synthetic estrogen doses remain fixed. In 1984, triphasic preparations consisting of a fixed estrogen dose with various amounts of progestins attempted to lower the dose of progestins and minimize breakthrough bleeding. However, there is no evidence that either biphasic or triphasic combinations have any particular advantage compared with the fixed dose combination tablets.

The second type of oral contraceptive consists of a progestin taken daily without any estrogen or steroid-free interval. Use of this type of pill is associated with overall fewer side effects but there is a higher incidence of breakthrough bleeding and a slightly higher pregnancy rate because of inconsistent ovarian suppression.

Benefits

The health benefits of contraceptives include decreased incidences of ovarian carcinoma (two- to three-fold), ovarian cysts, endometrial carcinoma, and benign breast cystic disease (two- to three-fold). Thickened cervical secretions appear to be responsible for the 50% reduction in pelvic inflammatory disease seen in contraceptive users. The diminished menstrual flow caused by synthetic steroids decreases the incidence of iron deficiency anemia. It has been estimated that these positive effects from oral contraceptives prevent 50,000 women from being hospitalized in the United States each year.

Clinical Complications

Patient Concerns and Side Effects

There are many potential adverse reactions seen with oral contraceptive use in otherwise healthy patients. Table 16–4 outlines these side effects and describes the likely etiology and

Table 16–3. Effects of Oral Contraceptives on Laboratory Tests

Laboratory Test	Effect	Probable Mechanism
Serum, Plasma, Blood		
Albumin	Slightly decreased	Decreased hepatic synthesis
Aldosterone	Increased	Activates renin-angiotensin system
Amylase	Slightly increased (common)	Not established
	Markedly increased (rare)	Pancreatitis
Antinuclear antibodies	Become detectable	Not established
Bilirubin	Increased (rare)	Reduced secretion into bile
Ceruloplasmin	Increased	Increased hepatic synthesis
Cholinesterase	Decreased	Decreased hepatic synthesis
Coagulation factors	Increased (II, VII, IX, X)	Increased synthesis
Cortisol	Increased	Increased cortisol-binding globulin
Fibrinogen	Increased	Increased hepatic synthesis
Folate	Decreased or no change	Decreased folate absorption
Glucose tolerance tests	Small decrease in tolerance	Several mechanisms proposed
Gamma-glutamyltransferase	Increased	Altered secretion in bile
Haptoglobin	Decreased	Decreased hepatic synthesis
High density lipoprotein cholesterol	Increased with estrogens and decreased with progestins	Not established
Iron-binding capacity	Increased	Increased transferrin levels
Magnesium	Decreased or no change	Decreased bone resorption
Phosphatase, alkaline	Increased (rare)	Altered secretion in bile
Plasminogen	Increased	Increased hepatic synthesis
Platelets	Slightly increased	Not established
Prolactin	Increased	Not established
Renin activity	Increased	Increased synthesis of renin substrate
Thyroxine (total)	Increased	Increased thyroxine-binding globulin
Transaminases	Slightly increased	Not established
Transferrin	Increased	Increased hepatic synthesis
Triglycerides	Increased	Increased synthesis
Triiodothyronine resin uptake	Decreased	Increased thyroxine-binding globulin
Vitamin A	Increased	Increased retinol-binding protein
Vitamin B_{12}	Decreased	Not established
Zinc	Decreased	Shift of zinc into erythrocyte
Urine		
Delta aminolevulinic acid	Increased	Increased hepatic synthesis
Ascorbic acid	Decreased or no change	Not established
Bacteria	Increased incidence of bacteriuria	Not established
Calcium	Decreased	Decreased bone resorption
Cortisol (free)	Unchanged	
Porphyrins	Increased (may precipitate porphyria in susceptible patients)	Increased aminolevulinic acid synthetase
17-Hydroxycorticosteroid	Slightly decreased or no change	Increased binding proteins
17-Ketosteroid	Slightly decreased or no change	Increased binding proteins

recommended management. The majority of these effects occur in the first 3 months, and two thirds of users discontinue taking the pill in 1 year. Many physiologic changes may be managed by reassurance alone or by changing the preparation to a different estrogen and/or progestin component. Symptoms similar to those seen premenstrually (nausea, nervousness, irritability, edema, headaches) are likely from estrogen excess; symptoms similar to those occurring during pregnancy (fatigue, lassitude, depression, increased appetite, weight gain) are primarily from progestin excess. An organic etiology must always be considered, especially when side effects are severe or persist after the medication is either changed or discontinued.

Interactions with Other Drugs. The interaction between oral contraceptives and other drugs (Table 16–5) may be significant in one of two ways: (1) the activity of the oral contraceptive may be lowered, resulting in breakthrough bleeding or pregnancy; or (2) the oral contraceptive may impair the metabolism of the other compound. Decreased absorption because of diarrhea (especially with penicillins or magnesium-containing compounds) or more rapid metabolism lowers circulating steroid levels and decreases desired activity. Rifampin, anticonvulsants, and barbiturates induce microsomal enzymes, resulting in the breakdown of oral contraceptives into less biologically active metabolites. Oral contraceptives competitively inhibit certain microsomal en-

Table 16–4. Patient Concerns About and Side Effects of Oral Contraceptives*

Problem	Etiology	Recommendations
Hyperandrogenism Acne Hirsutism Weight gain	1. Ovral decreases steroid hormone–binding globulin and serum albumin. 2. Norgestrel in Ovral is anabolic and androgenic. 3. Norethindrone and norethindrone acetate may be anabolic at > 1 mg dose. 4. Estrogen promotes fluid retention.	1. For acne and hirsutism, cycle with Ovulen, Demulen Ortho 2 mg or Ortho 1/80, which increases steroid hormone–binding globulin. 2. For weight gain, minimize estrogen/progestin (i.e., Ovcon).
Breast Mastodynia Cystitis-mastitis Enlarged breasts	1. Estrogens increase ductal proliferation. 2. Progestins increase alveolar proliferation.	1. Use lower dose estrogen/progestin (progestin should be androgenic; i.e., Lo/Ovral or Ovral).
Amenorrhea	1. Endometrium is inadequately primed. 2. Progestin/estrogen ratio is excessive.	1. Rule out pregnancy. 2. Discontinue OCs for 3 mo. 3. Recycle with triphasic OCs.
Postpill amenorrhea	1. Hypothalamus-pituitary malfunction. 2. Hypoestrogenism. 3. Prolactin level is elevated.	1. Do hormone profile. 2. Cycle with natural estrogen (Premarin 1.25 µg) one days 1–25, and Provera 10 mg on days 15–25. 3. Stimulate ovulation after hormone profile if pregnancy desired.
Amenorrhea-galactorrhea	1. Hypothalamus-pituitary malfunction.	1. Check serum prolactin level. 2. Rule out tumor. 3. Do Pap smear of any unilateral breast discharge. 4. Discontinue OCs if annoying.
Premenstrual tensionlike symptoms Fluid retention Nervousness Irritability Headache	1. Estrogen is associated with fluid retention. 2. Estrogen/progestins have an effect on renin-angiotensin-aldosterone system. 3. Estrogen/progestins are associated with pelvic congestion and cerebral edema and lowered albumin/globulin ratio affecting osmolarity.	1. Use minimal dose estrogen/progestin. 2. Suggest sodium-restricted diet. 3. Minimize use of diuretics.
BTB	1. Estrogen priming is inadequate 2. Progestin level is inadequate. 3. Estrogen/progestin ratio is inappropriate.	1. Use higher dose estrogen/progestin preparation. 2. If BTB continues, discontinue OCs.
Chloasma	1. Estrogen stimulates melanocyte-stimulating hormone secretion.	1. Use minimal effective dose estrogen/progestin. 2. Avoid exposure to sunlight.
CNS symptoms Fatigue Lassitude Decreased libido Mild depression	1. Changes are similar to first trimester of pregnancy changes. 2. Vitamin B_{12} level is altered. 3. Pyridoxine is relatively deficient.	1. Use minimal effective dose estrogen/progestin. 2. Use multiple vitamin replacement. 3. Use pyridoxine 30 mg q.i.d.
GI disturbances Nausea Vomiting Epigastric distress Bloating Pruritus	1. GI symptoms are like those of pregnancy. 2. Oral synthetic estrogen induces cholestasis. 3. Progestin relaxes smooth muscle and GI motility. 4. Cholelithiasis and pancreatitis.	1. Use minimal effective dose estrogen/progestin. 2. Pruritus is associated with BSP retention and occasional peripheral bile salts; therapy with oral cholestyramine and discontinue OC.
Monilial vaginitis	1. Glycogen level in vagina is increased. 2. Vaginal pH, flora are altered.	1. Treat monilial.

*OCs, oral contraceptives; BTB, breakthrough bleeding; CNS, central nervous system; GI, gastrointestinal.

Table 16–5. Drugs That Interact with Oral Contraceptives*

Class of Compound	Drug	Supposed Method of Action	Suggested Management
Drugs That May Reduce OC Efficacy			
Anticonvulsant drugs	Barbiturates; phenobarbital, primidone, phenytoin, ethosuximide	Microsomal liver enzymes are induced; fluid retention caused by OCs may precipitate seizures.	20–35 μg combination OCs or progestin-only pills or another method.
Antibiotics	Rifampin, penicillin V	Enzymes are induced; estrogen in liver is broken down rapidly; intestinal motility is increased with penicillins.	Higher dose OCs during short course of antibiotics or additional contraceptives; for a long course use another method.
Sedatives and hypnotics	Benzodiazepines	Plasma benzodiazepine is elevated.	
	Barbiturates	OC metabolism is increased.	
Modification of Other Drug Activities by OCs			
Anticoagulants	All	Efficacy is impaired, as OCs increase clotting factors.	Do not use OCs with anticoagulant therapy.
Antidiabetic agents	Insulin and oral hypoglycemic agents	High dose estrogen pills cause impaired glucose tolerance.	Use 20–35 μg OCs or progestin only; consider other methods.
Antihypertensive agents	Guanethidine and occasionally methyldopa	Estrogen component is involved with Na++ retention and increased angiotensinogen.	Use progestin-only pill or another method.
Phenothiazine	All phenothiazides: reserpine, tricyclic antidepressants	Serum prolactin may be elevated; combination OCs are associated with increased response of serum prolactin to TRH.	Use alternative method.

*OCs, oral contraceptives; THR, thyrotropin-releasing hormone.

zymes and may actually increase the circulating levels of corticosteroids, certain benzodiazepines (diazepam, nitrazepam, chlordiazepoxide, alprazolam, triazolam), imipramine, and metoprolol.

Gallstone Formation. Combination agents increase the lithogenicity of bile by raising cholesterol saturation, whereas progestins decrease bile excretion. The incidence of chole-

lithiasis is approximately doubled in women who take oral contraceptives for 4 years or less, but after 4 years of use, the incidence decreases to below normal. Thus, women prone to develop gallstones show manifestations earlier with oral contraceptive use, but the overall incidence is generally unchanged.

Hepatic Tumors. The development of benign liver tumors is an uncommon but poten-

Table 16–6. Cardiovascular Disease Mortality* for Oral Contraceptive Users, Former Users, and Controls

Cause	Current Users	Former Users	Controls	Current Users vs Controls	Former Users vs Controls
All nonrheumatic heart disease and hypertension	15.1	9.6	2.1	7.3	4.6
Ischemic heart disease	13.0	4.1	2.0	6.4	2.0
Malignant hypertension	0.0	2.5	0.0	—	—
All cerebrovascular disease	10.1	18.2	5.0	2.0	3.6
Subarachnoid hemorrhage	7.3	10.2	2.3	3.2	4.5
Cerebral thrombosis, hemorrhage, and embolism	2.7	8.1	2.7	1.0	3.0
Pulmonary embolism and thrombophlebitis	2.8	2.2	0.0	—	—
Other vascular diseases	0.8	0.9	0.0	—	—
All circulatory diseases	28.6	30.9	7.2	4.0	4.3

*Mortality rate per 100,000 women-years.

Table 16–7. Oral Contraceptives by Potency and Type of Progestin

Drug	Progestin* (mg)	Estrogen (mg)	Type of Estrogen†
Low Dose Preparations			
Norethindrone (weak)			
Nor-Q.D (Syntex)	7.4	0	
Micronor (Ortho)	7.4	0	
Ovcon-35 (Mead Johnson)	8.4	0.74	EE
Brevicon (Syntex)	10.5	0.74	EE
Modicon (Ortho)	10.5	0.74	EE
Tri-Norinyl (Syntex)	15.0	0.74	EE
Ortho-Novum 7/7/7 (Ortho)	15.8	0.74	EE
Ortho-Novum 10/11 (Ortho)	16.0	0.74	EE
Norinyl 1 + 35 (Syntex)	21.0	0.74	EE
Ortho-Novum 1/35 (Ortho)	21.0	0.74	EE
Norethindrone acetate (weak)			
Loestrin 1/20 (Parke-Davis)	21.0	0.42	EE
Loestrin 1.5/30 (Parke-Davis)	31.0	0.63	EE
Levonorgestrel (moderate)			
Triphasil-21 (Wyeth), Tri-Levlen (Berlex)	1.9	0.68	EE
Nordette-21 (Wyeth), Levlen (Berlex)	3.2	0.63	EE
Norgestrel (moderate)			
Ovrette (Wyeth)	1.6	0	
Lo/Ovral (Wyeth)	6.3	0.63	EE
Ethynodiol diacetate (potent)			
Demulen 1/35 (Searle)	21	0.74	
Moderate Dose Preparations			
Norethindrone (weak)			
Ovcon-50 (Mead-Johnson)	21.0	1.1	EE
Ortho-Novum 1/50 (Ortho)	21.0	1.1	ME
Norinyl 1 + 50 (Syntex)	21.0	1.1	ME
Norethindrone acetate (weak)			
Norlestrin 1/50 (Parke-Davis)	21.0	1.1	EE
Ethynodiol diacetate (potent)			
Demulen 1/50 (Searle)	21.0	1.1	EE
High Dose Preparations			
Norethindrone (weak)			
Ortho-Novum 1/80 (Ortho)	21.0	1.7	ME
Norinyl 1 + 80 (Syntex)	21.0	1.7	ME
Ortho-Novum 2 (Ortho)	42.0	2.1	ME
Norinyl 2 (Syntex)	42.0	2.1	ME
Norethindrone acetate (weak)			
Norlestrin 2.5/50 (Parke-Davis)	52.5	1.1	EE
Norgestrel (moderate)			
Ovral (Wyeth)	10.5	1.1	EE
Norethynodrel (moderate)			
Enovid-E (Searle)	52.5	2.1	ME
Enovid 5 (Searle)	105.0	2.1	ME
Ethynodiol diacetate (potent)			
Ovulen (Searle)	21.0	2.1	ME

*The six different synthetic progestins shown are not necessarily equivalent in potency or their milligram-for-milligram effect on serum lipids and carbohydrates.
†The two different estrogens shown are approximately equivalent in potency and metabolic effects. EE, ethinyl estradiol; ME, mestranol.

Table 16–8. Pertinent Clinical Information Before Oral Contraceptive Therapy

History	Physical Examination
Current Medical Illnesses	Blood pressure
Hypertension	Skin: stigmata of hyperandrogenism (acne,
Hyperlipidemia	hirsutism), hyperlipidemia
Congestive heart failure	Breast
Diabetes mellitus	Abdomen: liver size and texture
Migraine headaches	Pelvic with Pap smear
Blood dyscrasias	Cardiovascular: signs of congestive heart failure
Primary or secondary amenorrhea	
Oligomenorrhea	**Laboratory Analyses**
Cholelithiasis	
Acute hepatitis or chronic liver disease	Lipid profile if age over 35 or family history of
Epilepsy	hyperlipidemia or premature atherosclerosis
Breast cancer	Liver profile if past history of liver disease
	Fasting glucose test if history of gestational diabetes
Past history of	mellitus or family history of type II diabetes
Deep venous thrombosis	mellitus
Cerebrovascular disease	
Myocardial infarction	
Hepatitis or other liver disease	
Primary or secondary amenorrhea	
Gestational diabetes mellitus	
Pruritus or jaundice with pregnancy	
Pre-eclampsia	
Breast cancer	
Habits	
Tobacco use	
Family history	
Type II diabetes mellitus	
Hypertension	
Premature myocardial infarction (< age 55 in males,	
< age 60 in females)	

tially serious complication of oral contraceptives. Two histopathologic forms, focal nodular hyperplasia and adenomas, develop in 5 to 20 of 1 million users. Adenomas are the greater clinical concern because of the risk of spontaneous rupture and massive hemorrhage. The risk of adenoma formation increases with higher oral contraceptive doses and after 5 years of combination agent use. Adenomas can be clinically suspected if there are symptoms of right upper quadrant pain and clinical evidence of hepatomegaly.

Hyperlipidemia. Oral contraceptives generally raise triglyceride levels by 25 to 50% and total cholesterol levels by 5 to 7%. The triglyceride elevation is estrogen-dependent and usually inconsequential. However, rare patients with genetic hypertriglyceridemia may develop severe triglyceride elevations and significant complications such as pancreatitis. Estrogens and progestins exert different effects on cholesterol metabolism. In general, estrogens raise very low density lipoprotein (VLDL) and high density lipoprotein (HDL) cholesterol and lower low density lipoprotein (LDL) cholesterol. Progestins tend to antago-

nize the effects of estrogen; progestins with a low antiestrogen effect (norethynodrel) are associated with higher HDL levels than progestins with high antiestrogen effects (norgestrel). Data indicate that certain oral contraceptives (low estrogen, high progestin formulations like Ovral) may be potentially atherogenic by lowering HDL cholesterol and raising LDL cholesterol. There is no evidence, however, that long-term use of oral contraceptives accelerates the rate of atherosclerosis in patients without other risk factors.

Carbohydrate Metabolism. Oral contraceptives cause insulin resistance, hyperinsulinism, and impaired glucose tolerance. These effects may be clinically significant in patients who are susceptible to diabetes mellitus (gestational diabetes or positive family history) or those with established diabetes mellitus.

Thyroid Function. Oral contraceptives stimulate the hepatic production of TBG and raise the total thyroxine level. Despite the resulting hyperthyroxinemia, a patient's clinical thyroid status is unchanged because the free thyroxine level is unaffected.

Hypertension. Users of combination oral

Table 16–9. Absolute (A) and Relative (R) Contraindications to Oral Contraceptive Use

Cardiovascular System
A—Thrombophlebitis
A—Deep venous thrombosis
A—Pulmonary embolism
A—Transient ischemic attacks or cerebrovascular accident
A—Angina or myocardial infarction
Liver
A—Acute or chronic hepatitis
A—Cirrhosis
A—Jaundice of pregnancy
A—Hepatic prophyria
Metabolic Disorders
R—Diabetes mellitus
R—Predisposition to diabetes mellitus
   Family history
   Family history and obesity
   History of large babies (> 9 lb)
A—Hypertension
A—Hyperlipidemia
Reproductive Tract
A—Pregnancy
R—Lactation
A—Primary amenorrhea
R—Secondary amenorrhea
R—Chronic, unpredictable breakthrough bleeding when taking oral contraceptives
A—Chronic cystic mastitis in a smoker or heavy caffeine user
A—Undiagnosed genital bleeding
Miscellaneous Concurrent Diseases
R—Epilepsy
R—Migraine headaches
A—Acute intermittent porphyria
A—Blood dyscrasias (leukemia, sickle cell anemia, and polycythemia are associated with diffuse intravascular coagulation)
R—Uterine fibroid tumors
R—Benign breast tumors
R—Varicose veins (severe)
R—Cholelithiasis (known) or chronic biliary symptoms
A—Breast cancer
Associated Side Effects and Symptoms
R—Chronic weight gain
R—Chronic edema, unknown etiology
R—Chronic gastrointestinal symptoms (nausea, dyspepsia, vomiting)
R—Chronic unmanageable leg cramps
R—Recurrent vaginal (*Candida*) infections

contraceptives develop elevations in both systolic and diastolic blood pressures. In a study by Weir and colleagues, the average systolic and diastolic increases were 13.5 and 6.2 mmHg, respectively. A large prospective study at Kaiser Permanente demonstrated a mean systolic rise of 4 to 6 mmHg and a mean diastolic rise of 1 to 2 mmHg. Women using oral contraceptives are six times more likely to develop hypertension than are age-matched nonusers; hypertension appears in 5% of those taking oral contraceptives for 5 years. Risk factors for contraceptive-induced hypertension

are a family history of hypertension, age above 35, obesity, and smoking. The blood pressure generally increases within the first 3 months of use, follows a mild course, and in over one half of these women, returns to normal when oral contraceptives are stopped. Only rarely does malignant hypertension supervene. The proposed mechanism of hypertension is estrogen-augmented production of angiotensin II, which results in vasoconstriction and sodium retention, and the mineralocorticoid effects of synthetic progestins.

Vitamin and Mineral Metabolism. Studies demonstrate that oral contraceptives decrease serum levels of the B complex vitamins and vitamin C. There is little evidence, however, that clinical manifestations of vitamin deficiency accompany these lowered blood levels, and vitamin supplementation, although theoretically justified, is usually not necessary. The serum levels of several minerals, including copper, iodine, and iron, are increased but not to clinically significant values.

Thromboembolism. Combination oral contraceptives can cause hypercoagulability and predispose users to venous thromboembolism. In a prospective study, The Royal College of General Practice (U.K.) correlated the incidence of deep venous thrombosis to the dose of synthetic estrogen. Use of a low dose (35 μg of ethinyl estradiol) pill is not associated with increased risk. The incidence for the 50 and 100 μg estrogen pill was 81 and 111 cases of thrombosis per 100,000 users, respectively. The overall risk in oral contraceptive users was 5.6 times greater than that in nonusers. The mechanism of hypercoagulability is attributed mainly to the effect of estrogens on increasing the levels and activity of vitamin K–dependent coagulation factors, lowering the levels of antithrombin III (a natural anticoagulant), accelerating platelet aggregation time, and raising fibrinogen levels. Certain progestins interact with estrogens to lower antithrombin III levels.

Cardiovascular and Cerebrovascular Diseases. Combination oral contraceptive use confers an increased risk of cerebrovascular disease correlated with the estrogen dosage and the presence of underlying vascular disease. According to British data, the relative risk of developing a cerebrovascular accident is fourfold higher. However, the actual incidence remains quite low, about $\frac{1}{20,000}$ to $\frac{1}{30,000}$ users per year.

The risk of myocardial infarction in oral contraceptive users increases with age, tobacco use, hypertension, and hypercholesterolemia.

Table 16–10. Guidelines to Selection of Combination Oral Contraceptives

Estrogenic Combination	Intermediate	Androgenic Combination
Low Dose (First Choice)		
A. Demulen 1/35	B. Modicon 0.5/35, Ortho-Novum 1/35	C. Lo/Ovral, Levlen, Triphasil, Tri-Levlen
Intermediate Dose (Alternate Choice)		
D. Demulen 1/50	E. Ortho-Novum 1/50, Ortho-Novum 10/11, Ortho-Novum 7/7/7	F. Ovral
High Dose (Final Choice)		
G. Ovulen	H. Ortho-Novum 1/80, Ortho-Novum 2 mg	I. Ovral
J. Provera 10 mg (days 15–25) with barrier contraception		

	Puberty and Adolescence (Age 11–18)	
A,B,C,	1. Contraception: mature secondary sex characteristics	
A,B,C	2. Contraception: regular menstrual periods	
D,G	3. ± Hyperandrogenism: acne, hirsutism	
D,E,F,G	4. ± Dysmenorrhea: cramps with menstrual periods	
J	5. Amenorrhea	
J	6. Infrequent menstrual periods (2–8/year)	
D,G	7. Infrequent menstrual periods (2–8/year) with evidence of transient or early hyperandrogenism, premenstrual acne, acne, or hirsutism*	
D,E,F,G	8. Irregular menstrual periods†	

	Reproductive Years (Age 15–40) and Pregnancy Spacing	
A,B,C	1. Contraception: regular menstrual periods	
D,G	2. Contraception: hyperandrogenism (acne, hirsutism)‡	
D,E,F,G	3. Contraception: dysmenorrhea (cramps with menstrual period)§	
C,D,E,F,G	4. Contraception: with or without irregular menstrual periods	
D,E	5. Contraception: with or without infrequent menstrual periods (3–6/year)‖	
A,B,C	6. Contraception: with cessation of menstrual periods	
D,E,F,G	7. Alternate choice for breakthrough bleeding	
A,B,C	8. Alternate choice for weight gain, nausea, headache, fatigue, lassitude	
A,B,C	9. Alternate choice for recurrent vaginitis	
A,B,C	10. After 40 years, medical indications only	
A,B	11. Hyperlipidemia, coronary disease, atherosclerosis: with discretion‡	

*An option is C or F days 15–25 of treatment cycle.
†An option is C, D, E, F, G days 15–25 of treatment cycle.
‡An option is days 15–25 of treatment cycle, with barrier contraception.
§With antiprostaglandins: (1) ibuprofen (Motrin), (2) mefenamic acid (Ponstel).
‖Administer days 5–25 or 15–25, the latter with barrier contraception.

The overall relative risk is two- to six-fold greater than among non–pill users (Table 16–6) and is most strongly related to age and smoking. The amount of smoking is important; the relative risk increases from 3.4 in women who smoke 1 to 24 cigarettes per day to 7.8 in those who smoke more than 25 cigarettes per day. In general, oral contraceptives are considered to be safe in women: (1) under age 45 who are nonsmokers, normotensive, and normolipidemic; and (2) under age 35 who smoke but do not have hypertension or lipid abnormalities. These agents should be used cautiously in any patient with either illnesses predisposing to vascular disease or established atherosclerosis.

Treatment Guidelines

Selection of oral contraceptives requires pertinent clinical information and knowledge of the available drugs (Table 16–7). Pertinent aspects of the clinical evaluation are noted in Table 16–8. Table 16–9 lists those conditions in which oral contraceptives are either relatively or absolutely contraindicated. Another temporary method (diaphragm, condom) or permanent method (vasectomy, tubal ligation) of contraception may be preferred in these cases.

Oral Contraception Selection, Patient Education, and Follow-up

It is important to remember that women using oral contraception do not receive this medication because they are ill but rather for purposes of family planning. Therefore, the medication should fulfill the following criteria: (1) not initiate any medical problems; (2) not aggravate any pre-existing medical problems; (3) successfully eliminate unwanted pregnancies; and (4) not be associated with any danger to an inadvertent pregnancy or interfere with future pregnancies. Table 16–10 provides guidelines to combination oral contraceptive selection. It is preferable to begin with a low dose preparation (i.e., 35 μg of ethinyl estradiol). A change to an intermediate dose or eventually a high dose is necessary if breakthrough bleeding occurs. The adolescent desiring oral contraceptives or the patient who is between pregnancies requires special attention (Table 16–10). Progestin-only tablets have a higher failure rate and cause a greater frequency of irregular bleeding. They should be considered for use only by women who are breast-feeding or who have specific contraindications to estrogens (such as a history of thrombosis).

Recommendations for patient education include the following:
1. Use barrier contraception during the first 2 months of oral contraceptive use.
2. Report the following symptoms to your physician:
   a. Headaches
   b. Chest pain
   c. Lower extremity swelling or pain
   d. Right upper quadrant pain
   e. Midepigastric pain
   f. Galactorrhea
   g. Generalized pruritus
   h. Blurred vision
   i. Neurologic deficits
3. Avoid concomitant tobacco use, which increases the risks of complications from oral contraceptives.
4. Use barrier contraception, in addition to oral contraceptives, when taking antibiotics or barbiturates or if diarrhea occurs.
5. Examine breasts monthly.
6. Take the oral contraceptive daily.

Clinical follow-up visits should be scheduled at 3 months and 1 year after the patient starts taking oral contraceptives.

Three months after oral contraceptives are begun:

- Obtain a nondirected history.
- Ask specific questions about symptoms related to deep venous thrombosis, myocardial infarction, or cerebrovascular disease.
- Clinical examination: measure blood pressure.
- Laboratory analyses: obtain a lipid profile if: age > 35, family history of either hyperlipidemia or premature atherosclerosis; fasting glucose level if: history of gestational diabetes or family history of type II diabetes mellitus.

One year after oral contraceptives are begun:

- Use same measures as for 3-month examination.
- Perform breast examination.

Bibliography

D'Arcy PF. Drug interactions with oral contraceptives. Drug Intell Clin Pharm 20:353–362, 1986.
Specific potential problems and oral contraceptives.

Deslypere JP, Thiery M, Vermeulen A. Effect of long term hormonal contraception on plasma lipids. Contraception 31(6):633–642, 1985.
Specific potential problems and oral contraceptives.

Dickey RP. Managing contraceptive pill patients, in Oral Contraception Handbook, ed 5. Durant, OK, Creative Informatics (PO Box 1607), 1987.
General review of oral contraceptives.

Diczfalusy E. New developments in oral, injectable and implantable contraceptives, vaginal rings and intrauterine devices. Contraception 33(1):7–22, 1986.
Alternatives to oral contraceptives.

Fuller JH, Shepley MV, Rose G, et al. Coronary heart disease risk and impaired glucose tolerance. The Whitehall study. Lancet 1:33–37, 1980.
Specific potential problems and oral contraceptives.

Mishell DR Jr. Contraceptive use and effectiveness, in Mishell DR Jr, Davajan J (eds). Infertility, Contraception and Reproductive Endocrinology, 2. Oradell, NJ, Medical Economics Books, 1986, pp 583–622.
General review of oral contraceptives.

Mishell DR Jr. Oral steroid contraceptives, in Ayless TM, Brain MC, Cherniack RM (eds). Current Therapy in Internal Medicine-2. Toronto, BC Decker, 1987, pp 529–533.
General review of oral contraceptives.

Shearman RP. Oral contraceptive agents. Med J Aust 144:201–205, 1986.
General review of oral contraceptives.

U.S. Food and Drug Administration. Oral contraceptives and cancer. FDA Drug Bull 141:2–3, 1984.
Specific potential problems and oral contraceptives.

Vorys N, Rayburn WF. Oral contraceptives, in Rayburn W, Zuspan F (eds). Drug Therapy in Obstetrics and Gynecology. Norwalk, CT, Appleton-Century-Crofts, 1986, pp 197–224.
General review of oral contraceptives.

17

Unintentional Weight Loss

KEITH I. MARTON, M.D.

Weight loss, which may be seen in between 3 and 8% of both inpatients and outpatients, is like headache, dizziness, and fever. It is a symptom that requires a careful and thoughtful approach; it may be the only symptom the patient has or it may be accompanied by multiple findings; it may be a minor problem or it may be associated with a fatal illness. Like most other problems encountered in ambulatory care, its accurate evaluation depends primarily on a careful history and physical examination. The laboratory plays a secondary role. In fact, in most situations the cause of involuntary weight loss should be readily apparent to the physician after the initial visit. The less apparent the cause of the problem, the less likely there is a serious physical illness. Moreover, many patients with weight loss have a chief complaint other than weight loss that takes precedence in the evaluation. When the symptom of concern is weight loss, there are three phases in the evaluation: (1) establishment of the validity of the symptom; (2) initial evaluation: physical versus nonphysical causes; and (3) focused evaluation for specific causes.

Phase 1: Establishment of the Validity of the Symptom

Before one looks for the cause of weight loss, its presence should be established because as many as half of the patients who claim to have lost weight actually have not. Proof of weight loss may come in the form of medical records or a convincing story such as a change of clothing size or confirmation of weight loss by a family member. Absence of clinical weight loss or exaggeration of the amount of weight lost is a useful diagnostic sign: it is a strong predictor of the absence of organic illness. Underestimation of the amount of weight lost occurs more often in patients with cancer.

Furthermore, the degree of weight loss also has diagnostic meaning. Nearly all patients with weight loss resulting from organic illness lose at least 2.5 kg of body weight (sensitivity = 0.96). Nearly all patients with a weight loss of more than 15 kg have a serious illness (predictive value approaches 1.0).

If the patient does not have a documented weight loss and does not have a convincing story for weight loss, the clinician must decide either to evaluate other symptoms (as is often the case) or to observe the patient for a period of time.

Phase 2: Physical Versus Nonphysical Causes of Weight Loss

Because there are so many potential causes of weight loss, the initial evaluation serves as a form of triage that allows subsequent evaluations to be more focused. The main issue to be resolved by this phase is whether the weight loss is due to an organic (i.e., physical) illness or a nonphysical cause. Because the two categories have such different evaluations and treatments, this distinction is crucial. This formulation is also helpful for avoiding the common misconception that weight loss is often due to occult diseases. Weight loss is usually a late complication of physical illness and its cause is usually readily apparent. In fact, a negative initial evaluation for physical illness rarely signals the need for further testing for organic disease. Instead it indicates the need to focus on nonphysical illness.

Although a complete history and physical examination should be performed for any patient complaining of weight loss, several questions should figure prominently in the history. These questions were identified via multivariate analysis of a large number of questions asked of 91 patients with physical and non-physical causes of weight loss (Fig. 17–1). Patients with a history of heavy smoking; a decrease in functional status because of fatigue, nausea, or vomiting; a cough that recently changed; or an increase in appetite are more likely to have a physical cause of weight loss. In addition, abnormalities noted during the physical examination may point to a phys-ical cause of weight loss. Patients who answer no to the above questions and who have a completely normal physical examination are unlikely to have a significant physical illness. For such patients, observation coupled with a more complete discussion of psychosocial issues may be required.

If after the history and physical examination the clinician is still uncertain or abnormalities

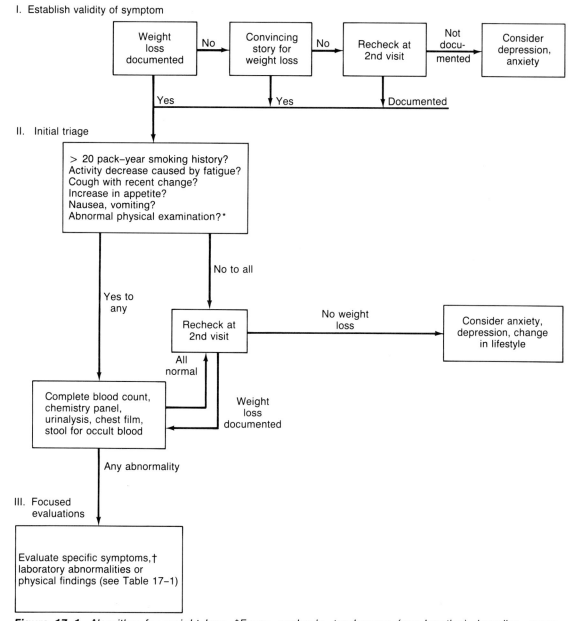

Figure 17–1. Algorithm for weight loss. *Fever, cachexia, tenderness (any location), jaundice, mass, hepatomegaly, adenopathy, thyroid nodule, thyromegaly, neurologic abnormality, evidence of congestive heart failure or chronic obstructive pulmonary disease. †Change in bowel habits, dysphagia, localized pain, cough, dyspnea, melena, hemoptysis, polyuria, polyphagia.

have been discovered, a screening laboratory evaluation may be obtained. This should include a complete blood count, urinalysis, chemistry panel (including liver function tests, glucose concentration, electrolytes, renal function tests, and serum protein analysis), and a chest x-ray. Patients whose laboratory evaluations are normal almost never have a physical cause of weight loss. Note that a sedimentation rate is not included in this list; its nonspecificity makes it much less helpful than the other tests. Thyroid function tests (e.g., thyroxine and free thyroxine index) may be helpful in elderly patients, who are more likely to have a paucity of symptoms when they develop thyrotoxicosis.

Thus, patients without a suggestive history and with normal results of a physical examination (and, if the clinician wishes to obtain it, a normal laboratory evaluation) may be reassured about the absence of physical disease. Equally important is an attempt to address issues that might have prompted the visit to the physician in the first place. Depression, anxiety, and lifestyle changes (particularly those resulting in alterations in caloric intake or requirement) are important nonphysical causes of weight loss. Occasionally, when the picture is still unclear, it may be necessary to have patients record their eating activities for several days to ascertain more clearly the actual caloric intake.

Phase 3: Specific Causes of Weight Loss

After the initial evaluation, one can approach the patient either by considering potential mechanisms for weight loss or by searching for specific causes of weight loss. Sometimes a combination of the two must be used. Nearly all of the known causes of weight loss can be classified according to the mechanism by which they cause weight loss. There are only two basic mechanisms: inadequate caloric intake or excessive caloric expenditure. The latter includes increased use of calories (e.g., thyrotoxicosis) as well as increased loss of calories (e.g., diarrhea). For some conditions, both mechanisms are involved; in some situations, such as cardiac cachexia and the weight loss associated with some malignancies, the mechanism is unknown.

As noted earlier, the initial evaluation usually provides important hints about the cause of the patient's weight loss: specific symptoms or findings should be actively pursued, usually by imaging procedures or biochemical or histologic tests. Thus, a patient with weight loss and jaundice usually requires imaging of the liver and biliary tract, whereas the patient with weight loss, anemia, and occult blood in the stool should have the gastrointestinal tract visualized. In some situations, conditions producing the weight loss may interfere with the accuracy of the history, such as with alcoholism, drug abuse, anorexia nervosa, and depression. In other cases, the illness may be noted in the absence of specific findings: lymphoma, pancreatic cancer, Addison's disease, panhypopituitarism, and lung cancer can be such conditions. It should be extremely rare for the clinician to go on a "hunting expedition" for disease (e.g., performing abdominal computerized tomography or intestinal radiography in the absence of any indicators). A more appropriate approach is the test of time—observation of the patient during several visits—which will allow the cause of weight loss to become apparent. Although this last approach may cause some discomfort because of concern about a delay in diagnosis, most patients with physical causes of weight loss are diagnosed rapidly. Moreover, nearly all causes of weight loss become apparent within several months; such a delay should not actually affect outcome. In our prospective study of 91 patients, only one had a truly occult cause of weight loss. In all cases, the cause of weight loss was apparent within 6 months of initial presentation.

Among the physical causes of weight loss, malignancy—especially lung, gastrointestinal, and lymphoma—is the most common and may account for 20 to 35% of causes of weight loss. Among the other causes (Table 17–1), gastrointestinal tract disease is the next most common disorder and accounts for approximately 15% of these patients.

The long-term outcome in patients with weight loss clearly depends on the cause of the symptoms. Patients with cancer are most likely to succumb (up to 50% may be dead within a year), whereas patients with no discernible cause of weight loss are most likely to survive.

In general, physical causes of weight loss are more common than nonphysical causes when significant (greater than 5 kg) weight loss is present. On the other hand, fruitless searches for illness when a careful but simple evaluation can reduce uncertainty are costly and harmful. As such, weight loss is a challenge to the clinician's diagnostic skill.

Table 17–1. Causes of Weight Loss

Nonphysical Causes	Physical Causes
Depression	Alcoholism/drug abuse
Anxiety	Poor dentures, painful oral lesions
Eating disorders	Medications (e.g., those producing intestinal irritations)
Change in lifestyle (diet, activity)	Intestinal malabsorption
	Neurologic diseases that interfere with eating
	Hyperthyroidism
	Diabetes
	Cancer (especially lung, stomach, pancreas, lymphoma)
	Leukemia
	Acquired immunodeficiency syndrome
	Tuberculosis or other chronic infections
	Parasitic infestations
	Liver disease
	Renal disease
	Addison's disease
	Panhypopituitarism
	Pernicious anemia
	Severe heart failure
	Severe pulmonary insufficiency

References

Karsh HB. Unexplained weight loss, in Friedman HH (ed). Problem-Oriented Medical Diagnosis. Boston, Little, Brown & Co., 1977, pp 13–15.
A brief outline of a more traditional approach to weight loss.

Marton KI, Sox HC, Krupp JR. Involuntary weight loss: diagnostic and prognostic significance. Ann Intern Med 95:568–574, 1981.
A prospective study of nearly 100 patients with weight loss. Discusses a simplified approach to diagnosis.

Pittman JG, Cohen P. The pathogenesis of cardiac cachexia. N Engl J Med 271:403–409, 453–460, 1964.
Discussion of weight loss in cardiac disease.

Rabinowitz M, Pitlik SD, Leiter M, et al. Unintentional weight loss. A retrospective analysis of 154 cases. Arch Intern Med 146:156–187, 1986.
Findings of Marton's study are confirmed with inpatients.

Ramboer C, Varhomme M, Verwere L. Patient's perception of involuntary weight loss: implications of underestimation and overestimation. Br Med J 291:1091, 1985.
Indicates that patients tend to misestimate the degree of weight loss.

Theologides A. Weight loss in cancer patients. Cancer 27:205–208, 1977.
Discussion of mechanisms of weight loss in cancer.

Winfield PA. Weight loss and the belt. Ann Intern Med 79:910, 1973.
A useful hint for establishing the validity of a complaint of weight loss.

18

Withdrawal of Corticosteroid Therapy

RICHARD L. BYYNY, M.D.
STEVEN S. LEVINE, M.D.

Glucocorticoids, such as hydrocortisone, cortisone, prednisone, prednisolone, and dexamethasone are prescribed as physiologic replacement for adrenal insufficiency or as pharmacologic treatment for a wide variety of conditions, including asthma, sarcoidosis, nephrotic syndrome, inflammatory bowel disease, collagen-vascular disorders, malignancies, immune system–mediated blood dyscrasias, dermatitis, and hypersensitivity reactions.[1]

Risks of Glucocorticoid Therapy

When glucocorticoids are prescribed as a physiologic replacement, side effects are not a significant concern. Pharmacologic treatment employs supraphysiologic doses of glucocorticoids to suppress inflammatory or immune responses or to stabilize membranes. Except for replacement therapy, steroids rarely treat the cause of disease. Instead they suppress the detrimental immune or inflammatory response to the disease-producing stimulus. This often results in chronic use of glucocorticoids. They are frequently of great benefit, but they also often cause the well-known Cushing's syndrome characterized by obesity, hypertension, diabetes mellitus, fragile skin, osteoporosis, nephrolithiasis, cataracts, ecchymoses, phlebitis, phlethora, activation of infection, increased susceptibility to infection, immune suppression, and other complications. Before the advent of therapy for endogenous Cushing's syndrome, the 5-year mortality from untreated hypercortisolism was 50%, with most deaths resulting from vascular disease or infection.[2] The other major side effect of prolonged

glucocorticoid use is hypothalamic-pituitary-adrenal (HPA) suppression. Cortisol secretion is regulated by the anterior pituitary hormone adrenocorticotropin (ACTH), which is controlled by the hypothalamic corticotropin-releasing factor (CRF) and the level of cortisol that modulates the response to CRF. Under normal circumstances, the control of ACTH and cortisol is characterized by the following: circadian rhythm; cortisol release in response to stress; and a negative feedback mechanism whereby an increase in circulating glucocorticoid inhibits CRF and ACTH secretion and limits adrenal glucocorticoid production.[3] The feedback mechanism explains the HPA suppression and adrenal atrophy with subsequent lack of response to usual provocative stimuli when supraphysiologic glucocorticoid is administered.[4, 5] As long as steroid is administered in doses appropriate for the condition of the patient, the patient remains stable. However, if the steroid use is stopped abruptly or if the patient becomes ill or experiences increased stress, the demand for the required cortisol cannot be met by the atrophic adrenal glands.

Minimization of Side Effects

To minimize the risks of glucocorticoid therapy, the clinician must carefully weigh the continued benefit from glucocorticoids with the risks of serious side effects that cause iatrogenic morbidity and mortality. Physicians frequently see patients with serious morbidity who began steroid therapy for a dubious indication such as chronic obstructive pulmonary disease and who demonstrated no subjective

Table 18–1. Approach for Initiation of Glucocorticoid Therapy

1. Establish a high probability of the diagnosis.
2. Consider the prognosis and determine the severity of the disease.
3. Weigh the risks and benefits of glucocorticoids.
4. Decide how to assess improvement.
5. Collect baseline data.
6. Determine if local steroid therapy can be used.
7. Decide which glucocorticoid preparation to use.
8. Choose the lowest effective initial dosage.
9. Evaluate the patient for alternate-day steroids.
10. Estimate the duration of glucocorticoid therapy.
11. Individualize management strategies for each patient after judging susceptibility to glucocorticoids.

Adapted from Axelrod L. Medicine 55:39–65, 1976, and Thorn GW. N Engl J Med 274:775–781, 1976, with permission.

or objective improvement. In fact, some patients have developed an infection or vertebral compression fracture due to osteoporosis, which makes the lung disease worse than when they were untreated. To avoid this unfortunate sequence of events, it is imperative that the clinician carefully plan the therapeutic use of glucocorticoids in each patient. Explicit measurable end points of therapy must be chosen and evaluated regularly. There must be a clear definition of success or failure and the time allowable to reach success. The probability of success should be stated a priori. Then decision points must be chosen to continue or terminate glucocorticoid treatment.

One can use the approach in Table 18–1 to initiate glucocorticoid therapy. Because of the serious side effects of glucocorticoid treatment, the physician should discuss the goals of treatment and side effects with the patient, reach a consensus, make a contract, and then implement therapy.

When prescribing systemic steroids, one should usually choose the shortest-acting steroid at the lowest effective dose and least frequent regimen compatible with therapeutic success to minimize side effects. Some steroids may be administered topically or locally, e.g., by inhalation or by local injection, which may minimize systemic side effects and pituitary-adrenal suppression. One example of this type of steroid is beclamethasone, which is effective locally when inhaled but whose absorption via the lung is minimal. Also, swallowed beclamethasone is rapidly metabolized during the first pass through the liver. However, as with most steroids, very high doses may still cause systemic effects and demonstrable reduction in HPA responsiveness. It is unclear if the latter effect is clinically important.

Alternate-Day Therapy

An alternate-day regimen of prednisone, if effective in treating the disease process, will dramatically decrease side effects; modest doses do not result in significant pituitary-adrenal suppression. Alternate-day use of long-acting steroids, e.g., dexamethasone, does not decrease side effects sufficiently. Even if the disease being treated initially requires a daily dose, the response can often be maintained with alternate-day steroids. Some basic principles of alternate-day steroid use are given in Table 18–2.

The clinician may want to switch a patient from daily to alternate-day steroid therapy. Table 18–3 illustrates a sample schedule for conversion from 50 mg of prednisone daily to alternate-day dosing.

Prevention of Side Effects of Steroid Therapy

The clinician should always assess the use of ancillary measures to prevent complications caused by steroids. For example, most postmenopausal women should be treated with estrogen replacement therapy in an attempt to prevent osteoporosis. The roles of supplemen-

Table 18–2. Basic Principles of Alternate-Day Steroid Therapy

1. Do not use for the patient with Addison's disease.
2. For some disorders, alternate-day steroid therapy is initially prescribed, but most often it is used to maintain a response achieved with daily dosing.
3. The switch from daily dosing should begin as soon as possible to avoid undue HPA suppression. Patients taking daily steroids for months before the transition may have a difficult time. For these patients, the clinician may have to use more than twice the previous daily dose on the "on" day to control the disease or prevent withdrawal symptoms. The conversion may extend to months, not weeks, as the adrenal gland recovers on the "off" day.
4. Use once-daily dose, not divided doses, because divided daily doses cancel the benefits.
5. The steroid should be given early each day to preserve the diurnal rhythm.
6. Initially, low doses of steroids can be used the morning of the off day to control symptoms, but the goal should be to eliminate glucocorticoids entirely on the off day. Nonsteroidal anti-inflammatory agents or intensified conventional therapy should be given to control minor disease flare-ups.
7. An intermediate-acting steroid, prednisone, should be used. The biologic half-life of dexamethasone is too long.

Reprinted with permission from The New England Journal of Medicine, 269:591–596, 1963.

Table 18–3. Conversion from Once-Daily Prednisone to Alternate-Day Prednisone

Day	Prednisone (mg)	Day	Prednisone (mg)
1	60	8	10
2	40	9	95
3	70	10	5
4	30	11	100
5	80	12	0
6	20	13	95
7	90	14	0
		15	Gradual reduction

From Swartz S, Dluhy RG. Drugs 16:238–255, 1978, with permission.

tal calcium and vitamin D are controversial. In hypertensive patients or patients with fluid retention, one can choose a steroid free of salt-retaining potential, e.g., dexamethasone. Often a distal tubular diuretic minimizes sodium retention. Older myopic patients and diabetics are more susceptible to glaucoma and should have intraocular pressures measured periodically.

The risk of reactivation of tuberculosis should be assessed and if necessary isoniazid should be prescribed. Although the association between glucocorticoids and peptic ulcer disease is still controversial, some high risk patients may benefit from simultaneous use of antacids, histamine-2 receptor blockers, or local agents such as sucralfate.

Glucocorticoids can exacerbate or induce a wide variety of psychologic effects. They range from irritability or poor judgment and euphoria to serious sleep disturbance, depression, and psychosis. The premorbid personality of the patient frequently predicts the psychologic response. For example, a patient with a prior episode of depression is more likely to become depressed while taking the drug. Such responses should be anticipated and preventive measures should be considered.

Some patients become psychologically and physiologically addicted to steroids. They may abuse the drugs or have serious withdrawal syndromes when the drug dosage is reduced or the drug is withdrawn. The clinician should deal with these addicted patients in a fashion similar to that used for patients addicted to other medications. Addiction makes logical management more difficult and clinical assessment of the response and side effects extremely difficult.

Tapering of Glucocorticoid Treatment

During treatment of any systemic disease with glucocorticoids, the initial reduction from pharmacologic to physiologic doses is determined largely by the likelihood of an exacerbation of the underlying disease.[9] The rapidity of reduction should usually be determined by an empiric reduction in frequency and/or dosage of the steroid with careful monitoring of the disease being treated.

HPA Suppression

Next in importance in withdrawing steroids is the degree of treatment-induced HPA suppression. The likelihood of this suppression is dependent on the following: the type of glucocorticoid[10]; dose; duration of action[11]; frequency and route of administration[12–14]; and duration of treatment. Glucocorticoid preparations can be grouped on the basis of three characteristics: anti-inflammatory potency, mineralocorticoid and salt-retaining effect, and biologic half-life. All of the drugs are compared with cortisol as the reference. Steroid chemists have been able to modify glucocorticoids to omit the salt retention potential, but they have been unable to uncouple the anti-inflammatory effects from the typical steroid side effects or HPA suppression. Greater potency and duration of anti-inflammatory effect increase the risk of HPA suppression.

Table 18–4 summarizes some of the characteristics of corticosteroid preparations including half-life, anti-inflammatory potency, and mineralocorticoid activity. Hydrocortisone is usually the drug of choice for glucocorticoid replacement therapy and management of stress related to primary or secondary adrenal insufficiency. Prednisone is usually the glucocorticoid of choice for systemic anti-inflammatory and immunosuppressive therapy. Dexamethasone is the drug of choice for cerebral edema and some endocrine diagnostic testing and may be preferred for patients with hypertension, congestive heart failure, and other salt-retaining conditions, but it is the most expensive.

The following is a summary of clinically helpful generalities about the risk of HPA suppression. Lower doses of glucocorticoid, e.g., less than 40 mg of prednisone once each morning for fewer than 5 to 7 days, do not usually result in clinically significant pituitary-adrenal suppression.[16] Statistically significant HPA suppression is demonstrable when prednisone, 25 mg twice daily, is administered for 5 days. However, the clinical importance of this HPA suppression has not been demonstrated.[17] Therefore, short courses of high

Table 18–4. Characteristics of Corticosteroid Preparations

Drug	Half-life	Relative Anti-inflammatory Potency	Relative Mineralo-corticoid Potency
Cortisone acetate	Short	1.0	1.0
Hydrocortisone	Short	0.8	0.8
Prednisone, prednisolone	Intermediate	4.0	0.8
Dexamethasone,* betamethasone	Long	25.0	0

*Certain data on dexamethasone indicate that it may be 52 times more potent than hydrocortisone 8 h after administration and 154 times more potent at 14 h.[15]

doses or long courses of lower doses of glucocorticoid may produce clinically significant HPA suppression. Alternate-day therapy with less than 40 mg of prednisone per day is not associated with clinically important HPA suppression.[12] Steroid doses administered at night suppress the HPA axis much more than those administered in the morning.[18]

The problem with predicting HPA suppression relates to the tremendous variability from patient to patient despite the above principles. We have assumed that HPA suppression may occur within 1 to 2 weeks with a daily regimen of 15 to 20 mg of prednisone each day or its equivalent. HPA suppression has enormous clinical importance because sudden steroid withdrawal or increased steroid demand with stress can cause morbidity or death from adrenal insufficiency.[19-23] Most of the time, acute adrenal crisis does not occur with steroid withdrawal. However, chronic adrenal insufficiency is often symptomatic, with fatigue, lassitude, weakness, loss of appetite, weight loss, arthralgias, nausea, hypotension, orthostasis, fainting, dyspnea, or hypoglycemia. Even mild illness will be exaggerated in severity, and there may be a symptomatic flare-up of the underlying disease. Because of the psychologic and physiologic dependence, the patient may crave or demand higher doses of steroid.[19-23]

Unfortunately the diminished release of ACTH cannot be restored to normal by repetitive administration of exogenous ACTH. However, cortisol secretion can be restored to normal with repetitive ACTH injection, but it falls rapidly to suppressed levels when the ACTH is stopped.[24] There is insufficient evidence that corticotropin-releasing hormone can hasten the recovery of the HPA axis. Recovery of the HPA axis is highly variable, but it may take 9 months for return of the HPA function to normal when steroids are withdrawn completely.[25] Table 18–5 illustrates the typical recovery sequence of prolonged HPA suppression.

Glucocorticoid Withdrawal

Christy has recommended that physicians consider the following when anticipating steroid withdrawal: define successful withdrawal; carefully assess the status of the disease being treated by the steroids and be sure why steroids were used initially and why they are being stopped; review the current steroid treatment; anticipate, identify, and deal with manifestations of steroid withdrawal; and assess the patient's personality and dependence on or beliefs about steroid therapy.[26]

Success would be the gradual reduction and elimination of exogenous steroids without exacerbation of the underlying disease and with no manifestation of adrenal insufficiency. This may be possible when patients have been given low doses for a short time or with routes or frequency of administration that cause less HPA suppression. Withdrawal of glucocorticoids needs to be carefully planned after reviewing the above considerations.

Because there is no single simple, inexpensive, convenient, safe way to rapidly assess the degree of HPA suppression, the approach to steroid withdrawal is usually empiric. Simply stated, the dose of prednisone is slowly reduced by an arbitrary amount, usually 2.5 to 5.0 mg, every few days. If the underlying disease flares up, the dose is increased and tapering is done more slowly. The dose should be reduced to physiologic levels, e.g., about 20 mg of hydrocortisone, 5 mg of prednisone, and 0.5 mg of dexamethasone. At this point one decides about reducing the exogenous steroid to zero or maintaining basal physiologic replacement. For many patients given long-term steroid therapy who have chronic conditions such as chronic obstructive pulmonary disease or rheumatoid arthritis, further reduction in steroids is associated with unnecessary morbidity and dysfunction. In these patients it is best to act as if the patient had permanent adrenal insufficiency and to maintain chronic steroid therapy with adequate basal glucocor-

Table 18–5. Typical Recovery of Pituitary-Adrenal Axis after Withdrawal of Long-Term Glucocorticoids

Months after Steroid Withdrawal	Plasma Cortisol Values	Plasma ACTH Values	Adrenal Response to ACTH or Stress
1	Low	Low	Low
2–5	Low	High	Low
6–9	Normal	High to normal	Low
9	Normal	Normal	Normal

Adapted from Graber AL, Ney RL, Nicholson WE, et al. Clin Endocrinol Metab 25:11–16, 1965, © by The Endocrine Society, with permission.

ticoid replacement and with supplementation for exacerbation of the illness or for stress.

If one plans to reduce the steroid level to below physiologic levels with the goal of complete withdrawal of steroids, it is usually best to decrease the amount slowly and in increments rather than to cease therapy suddenly. The latter is usually associated with a symptomatic period of steroid deficiency before the adrenals recover, and this symptomatic phase can be very prolonged.

One approach is to switch the patient to hydrocortisone 20 mg each morning or to prescribe prednisone 5 mg each morning. The dose is reduced in increments of 2.5 mg /week to hydrocortisone 10 mg or prednisone 2.5 mg each morning. HPA recovery may be further delayed but is likely to occur without symptoms of adrenal insufficiency. Some clinicians advocate switching to alternate-day steroids, but this is often associated with symptoms on the off day. However, if there are no symptoms, HPA recovery would probably occur more rapidly. Because both of these regimens maintain homeostasis with physiologic levels of glucocorticoid, steroid side effects do not occur or resolve with time.

Until complete recovery has occurred (discussed later), it is best to assume that the patient needs supplementary glucocorticoid therapy when there is stress, an illness, or surgery.

To use this empiric approach optimally, the clinician needs to understand the steroid withdrawal syndromes described in Table 18–6.[26]

During this period, the patient requires steroid replacement therapy for increased stress, e.g., a withdrawal syndrome, acute illness, trauma, or surgery. However, the dose of the steroid supplement has become somewhat controversial. There is a poor correlation between biochemical assessment of HPA function and the clinical response to stress in surgery.[27–29] Kehlet and Binder reported on 203 glucocorticoid-treated patients who underwent surgery without supplemental glucocorticoids. Although some patients had complications, these could be attributed to other causes or were not associated directly with tests demonstrating HPA suppression. In fact, rarely has postoperative collapse been reported in patients receiving glucocorticoids preoperatively.[26] Therefore, the theoretical risk of these complications is much greater than the practical risk if the patient is receiving physiologic replacement therapy before surgery or has recovered.

The fact remains that the standard practice is to administer glucocorticoids for stress and illnesses in patients suspected of having HPA suppression. We assume that any patient given other than alternate-day steroids in the last year or patients with the clinical appearance of hypercortisolism have HPA suppression and require glucocorticoid supplementation. Thus, clinicians always add to the historical questions asked, "Have you taken cortisone, prednisone, or other steroid hormones for any condition during the last year?" Therapy is then designed to mimic the physiologic adrenal response to maximum stress in which the adrenals secrete 200 to 300 mg of hydrocortisone in 24 hours.[1] For minor febrile illness, psychologic stress (i.e., sudden loss of a family member or devastating financial loss), or the equivalent, the usual replacement dose is administered twice a day for several days and then reduced to basal levels or eliminated. Higher doses may be needed for more prolonged or severe illness, e.g., influenza, urinary tract infections, or gastroenteritis.

For elective procedures, e.g., lumbar puncture, dental extractions, or endoscopy, one administers 100 mg of hydrocortisone hemisuccinate intravenously with the preprocedure medication or instructs the patient to take 100 mg of hydrocortisone orally on the morning of the procedure. An extra 20 mg of hydrocortisone is then taken orally that evening, and the usual dose is resumed the next day.

For elective minor surgery, major surgery, or major medical illness trauma, one administers 100 mg of hydrocortisone hemisuccinate intravenously or intramuscularly every 6 hours

Table 18–6. Steroid Withdrawal Syndromes

Type	Characteristics
I	The patient has symptomatic and biochemical evidence of HPA insufficiency. The symptoms respond to physiologic replacement doses of glucocorticoids, and there is no evidence of recurrent disease. This patient should continue receiving physiologic replacement doses of hydrocortisone, should receive supplementation for stress, and should be evaluated at 4-wk intervals.
II	In this syndrome, the patient has a flare-up of the basic disease but a normally functioning HPA system. The flare-up should be treated.
III	The patient is symptomatic but exhibits normal HPA responsiveness with no signs of recurrent disease. Symptoms are relieved only by greater than physiologic doses of hydrocortisone or its equivalent. The symptoms and signs a patient experiences may lead to self-medication or to a boost of the dosage beyond levels required for control of the disease. The clinician should continue to taper the glucocorticoids, explaining the rationale while continually reassuring the patient. It may be difficult to withdraw drugs from these patients, and subspecialty or psychiatric consultations may help.
IV	These patients have no symptoms of HPA insufficiency or of recurrent disease but have documented HPA insufficiency. They should receive supplemented therapy for stress and be tested as outlined.

Adapted from Dixon R, Christy N. Am J Med 68:224–230, 1980, with permission.

for four doses, the first doses being given with premedication. The dose is then tapered by 50% each day until the patient is on a total of 50 mg/day in divided doses. At this point, 20 mg of hydrocortisone orally twice daily is used until the patient is fully recovered, and then the maintenance dose is resumed. The dose is increased if the patient develops complications, has a prolonged postoperative or hospital course, or exhibits hypoadrenalism.

The patient may present with acute adrenal insufficiency. The manifestations of secondary adrenal insuffiiency differ from those of Addison's disease in that there is no mineralocorticoid insufficiency. Volume deficiency and hyperkalemia are not usually a problem; however, nausea, vomiting, hypotension, and an exaggerated febrile response to illness are present. The patient should be empirically treated with fluids and 100 mg of hydrocortisone intravenously every 6 to 8 hours. After resolution of the syndrome, the hydrocortisone dose can be reduced to replacement levels.

Recovery of HPA Function

One of the problems associated with glucocorticoid withdrawal is the difficulty in determining when the patient has satisfactorily recovered from steroid suppression of the HPA axis. This is often done empirically by withdrawing steroids and observing no manifestation of adrenal insufficiency over time. This may be acceptable because with medical attention, few patients die from this process. The adrenal insuficiency, if it occurs, is usually gradual in onset and the patient usually seeks medical attention for the stressor.

Some patients and physicians want to know when there has been recovery of the HPA axis. Basal recovery can be simply assessed by withholding the morning hydrocortisone dose and obtaining a plasma cortisol level at 7 to 9 a.m. Although the lower limit of normal for the plasma cortisol level is about 7 μg/dl, the normal range goes to 25 μg/dl.

What is a satisfactory plasma cortisol level for your patient? Probably any value above 7 μg/dl in an asymptomatic person is satisfactory, and values from 7 to 14 μg/dl in a patient with fatigue, lassitude, weakness, loss of appetite, weight loss, and low blood pressure are too low. We often arbitrarily assume basal secretion has recovered if the plasma cortisol level is higher than 10 μg/dl. If it is less than 10 μg/dl or if the patient is symptomatic, we continue basal hydrocortisone replacement and repeat the test in 4 weeks. If the plasma cortisol value is higher than 10 μg/dl, we stop basal supplementation and continue to supplement for stress.

At this point, one still does not know if the HPA response to stress will be adequate. If patients have not received steroids except as supplementation for 9 to 12 months, one can presume that they have recovered. One can decide to supplement for stress for 1 year and then assume recovery. This is least expensive. Earlier in the recovery period, one must test the HPA axis to establish recovery if one wants to be certain.

TESTS FOR HPA RECOVERY

The method of testing the HPA axis is somewhat controversial. If a patient presents with a serious stress, one could obtain a plasma cortisol value, then supplement with hydrocortisone, and await the result. If the plasma cortisol level is higher than 20 to 25 μg/dl, the patient has probably recovered; if less than 20 μg/dl the patient should continue to receive supplemental hydrocortisone.

Tests for the HPA axis include use of corticotropin-releasing hormone; insulin hypoglycemia; metyrapone; vasopressin; and ACTH. The corticotropin-releasing hormone test has great variability at any time after administration. Therefore, multiple samples are required, and there is no established response dividing HPA-suppressed from normal subjects. Insulin hypoglycemia is probably the gold standard test because it mimics acute stress. However, it is expensive, requires time and multiple blood samples, and is perceived as potentially hazardous.

Metyrapone tests feedback responsiveness and not stress, and discrepancies between metyrapone and insulin hypoglycemia tests have been shown. The drug must be absorbed to be effective. Drug interactions cause an increased rate of catabolism of metyrapone, which can result in low plasma metyrapone levels and a subnormal response.

The 30-minute ACTH stimulation test is controversial but most practical. It is convenient, simple, and relatively inexpensive. It involves obtaining a baseline plasma cortisol value, administering synthetic ACTH (cosyntropin) at 250 μg intravenously, and repeating the plasma cortisol test after 30 minutes. An increment greater than 6 μg/dl and to more than 20 μg/dl is normal.[30] A highly significant correlation has been reported between the preoperative adrenocortical response to ACTH and the HPA response to surgery.[31] A normal response was never followed by a greatly impaired response to surgery. The authors concluded that the ACTH test is reliable in predicting the response to major stress in glucocorticoid-treated patients undergoing surgery without supplementary glucocorticoid administration. Those with an adequate response usually do well during surgery. A large number of patients with minimal adrenocortical function had no signs of adrenocortical insufficiency related to surgery.[29] When the ACTH test is normal, one can consider recovery to be complete. However, if such a patient has manifestations of chronic or acute adrenocortical insufficiency, good clinical judgment indicates the need for temporary glucocorticoid replacement therapy.

Recovery of HPA function may be brief or prolonged. In some cases it is best to continue physiologic replacement chronically and not attempt recovery. However, in most cases, function returns to normal with sufficient time.

References

1. Liddle GW. The adrenal cortex, in Williams RH (ed). Textbook of Endocrinology, ed 5. Philadelphia, WB Saunders, 1974, pp 233–283.
2. Plotz CM, Knowlton AI, Ragan C. The natural history of Cushing's syndrome. Am J Med 13:597–614, 1952.
3. Steroid therapy and the adrenals. Lancet 2:537–538, 1975 (editorial).
4. Fraser CG, Preuss FS, Bigford WD. Adrenal atrophy and irreversible shock associated with cortisone therapy. JAMA 149:1542–1543, 1952.
5. Slaney G, Brooke BN. Postoperative collapse due to adrenal insufficiency following cortisone therapy. Lancet 1:1167–1170, 1957.
6. Axelrod L. Glucocorticoid therapy. Medicine 55:39–65, 1976.
7. Thorn GW. Clinical considerations in the use of corticosteroids. N Engl J Med 274:775–781, 1976.
8. Swartz S, Dluhy RG. Corticosteroids, clinical pharmacology and therapeutic use. Drugs 16:238–255, 1978.
9. Haynes RC, Larner J. Adrenocorticotropic hormone; adrenocortical steroids and their synthetic analogs; inhibitors of adrenocortical steroid biosynthesis, in Goodman LS, Gilman A (eds). The Pharmacological Basis of Therapeutics, ed 5. New York, Macmillan, 1975, pp 1472–1506.
10. Christy NP, Wallace EZ, Jailer JW. Comparative effects of prednisone and of cortisone in suppressing the response of the adrenal cortex to exogenous adrenocorticotropin. J Clin Endocrinol Metab 16:1059–1074, 1956.
11. Treadwell BLJ, Savage O, Sever ED, et al. Pituitary-adrenal function during corticosteroid therapy. Lancet 1:355–358, 1963.
12. Ackerman GL, Nolan CM. Adrenocortical responsiveness after alternate-day corticosteroid therapy. N Engl J Med 278:405–409, 1968.
13. Nichols T, Nugent CA, Tyler FH. Diurnal variation of suppression of adrenal function by glucocorticoids. J Clin Endocrinol Metab 25:343–349, 1965.
14. Maberly DJ, Gibson GJ, Butler AG. Recovery of adrenal function after substitution of beclomethasone dipropionate for oral corticosteroids. Br Med J 1:778–782, 1973.
15. Meikle A, Tyler FH. Potency and duration of action of glucocorticoids. Effects of hydrocortisone, prednisone and dexamethasone on human pituitary-adrenal function. Am J Med 63:200–207, 1977.
16. Livanou T, Ferriman D, James VHT. Recovery of hypothalamopituitary-adrenal function after corticosteroid therapy. Lancet 2:856–859, 1967.
17. Streck WF, Lockwood DH. Pituitary-adrenal recovery following short-term corticosteroid therapy. Lancet 1:630–633, 1979.
18. Nichols T, Nugent CA, Tyler FH. Diurnal variation in suppression of adrenal function by glucocorticoids. J Clin Endocrinol Metab 25:343–349, 1965.
19. Fraser CG, Preuss FS, Bigford WD. Adrenal atrophy

and irreversible shock associated with cortisone therapy. JAMA 149:1542–1543, 1952.

20. Slaney G, Brooke BN. Postoperative collapse due to adrenal insufficiency following cortisone therapy. Lancet 1:1167–1170, 1957.

21. Sampson PA, Brooke BN, Winstone NE. Biochemical confirmation of collapse due to adrenal failure. Lancet 1:1377, 1961.

22. Sampson PA, Winstone NE, Brooke BN. Adrenal function in surgical patients after steroid therapy. Lancet 2:322–325, 1962.

23. Jasani MK, Freeman PA, Boyle JA, et al. Studies of the rise in plasma 11-hydroxycorticosteroids (11-OCHS) in corticosteroid-treated patients with rheumatoid arthritis during surgery. Q J Med 37:407–421, 1968.

24. Fleischer N, Abe K, Liddle GW, et al. ACTH antibodies in patients receiving depot porcine ACTH to hasten recovery from pituitary-adrenal suppression. J Clin Invest 46:196–204, 1967.

25. Graber AL, Ney RL, Nicholson WE, et al. Natural history of pituitary-adrenal recovery following long-term suppression with corticosteroids. J Clin Endocrinol Metab 25:11–16, 1965.

26. Dixon R, Christy N. On the various forms of corticosteroid withdrawal syndrome. Am J Med 68:224–230, 1980.

27. Danowski T, Bonessi J, Sabeh G, et al. Probabilities of pituitary-adrenal responsiveness after steroid therapy. Ann Intern Med 61:11–26, 1964.

28. Plumpton L, Besser GM, Cole PV. Corticosteroid treatment and surgery. Anaesthesia 24:3–18, 1969.

29. Kehlet H, Binder C. Adrenal-cortical function and clinical course during and after surgery in unsupplemented glucocorticoid-treated patients. Br J Anaesth 45:1043–1048, 1973.

30. Wood JB, James VHT, Franckland AW, et al. A rapid test of adrenocortical function. Lancet 1:243–245, 1965.

31. Kehlet H, Binder C. Value of an ACTH test in assessing hypothalamic-pituitary-adrenocortical function in glucocorticoid-treated patients. Br Med J 2:147–149, 1973.

32. Harter J, Reddy W, Thorn G. Studies on an intermittent corticosteroid dosing regimen. N Engl J Med 269:591–596, 1963.

Bibliography

Axelrod L. Glucocorticoid therapy. Medicine 55:39–65, 1976.

This classic, extensively referenced review discusses the advantages of morning, single-dose therapy or alternate-day therapy, and the recovery of the HPA axis.

Byyny R. Withdrawal from glucocorticoid therapy. N Engl J Med 295:30–32, 1976.

This concise review includes a protocol for monitoring corticosteroid withdrawal and assessing the recovery of the HPA axis.

Christy N. Corticosteroid withdrawal, in Bayless T, Brain M, Cherniack R (eds). Current Therapy in Internal Medicine 2. Toronto, BC Decker, 1987, pp 597–605.

This is a thorough review discussing the principles of and approach to corticosteroid withdrawal.

Dixon R, Christy N. On the various forms of corticosteroid withdrawal syndrome. Am J Med 68:224–230, 1980.

There are four subgroups of corticosteroid withdrawal syndrome: (1) both symptomatic and biologic evidence of HPA suppression; (2) recrudescence of the disease for which the drug was originally prescribed; (3) either physical or psychologic dependence on corticosteroids with normal HPA function; and (4) biologic evidence of HPA suppression without either disease recrudescence or symptoms of withdrawal. The rapid ACTH test is a clinically useful way to assess HPA function.

Meikle AW, Tyler F. Potency and duration of action of glucocorticoids. Am J Med 63:200–207, 1977.

The two most important factors determining the relative potency of orally administered glucocorticoids are their intrinsic potency and their relative rate of disappearance from plasma. The relative potency of dexamethasone may be generally underestimated; in this study, dexamethasone was 52 times more potent than hydrocortisone at 8 hours after administration, and 154 times greater at 14 hours. Usual estimates give dexamethasone a potency of 30 compared with 1 for hydrocortisone.

PART FOUR

Gastroenterology

19

Management of Common Anorectal Disorders by the Internist

DAVID A. LIEBERMAN, M.D.

Modern textbooks of medicine and surgery devote little or no attention to common anorectal problems. In ancient times, anal function was recognized for what it is—crucial to our well-being. Proctologists were among the most prominent physicians of the middle ages and anorectal disease has had some influence on modern history. Anorectal disorders are frequently encountered in general practice but are poorly understood, which may explain the lack of emphasis in modern medical training. There is also a certain degree of avoidance behavior practiced by both physicians and patients with regard to anorectal disease. Patient embarrassment about anorectal complaints is exacerbated by fears of what the physician may do (e.g., a sigmoid examination) or find (e.g., cancer). Physicians may omit questions about anorectal problems from the review of systems and avoid rectal or sigmoid examinations. The ubiquity of anorectal complaints does not diminish their importance or the need for a complete evaluation.

In this review I will focus on anorectal disease seen by the internist and will discuss the approach to rectal pain, bleeding, itching, and incontinence.

Anorectal Pain and Bleeding

The differential diagnosis of anorectal pain includes a wide spectrum of benign and malignant diseases (Table 19–1). The history may help distinguish between rectal and anal causes of pain (Table 19–2). Pain patterns differ because the rectal mucosa is not supplied by

Table 19–1. *Causes of Anorectal Pain*

Location	Cause
Rectum	Malignancy
	Proctitis
	Ulcer
Anus	Malignancy
	Hemorrhoids
	Fissure in ano
	Anorectal abscess
	Anal fistula
Other	Proctalgia fugax
	Coccygodynia

cerebrospinal peripheral nerves and is insensitive to direct painful stimuli. In contrast, the anoderm is composed of a thin layer of squamous epithelium and is supplied by one of the most elaborate networks of sensory nerve endings in the body. This sensitive anal mucosa distinguishes gas, liquid, and solid material and provides the sensory input to enable a person to determine the urgency of reaching a toilet. Pain caused by rectal pathology is often exacerbated by rectal distention before bowel movements and is partially or completely re-

Table 19–2. *Symptoms of Anorectal Pain*

Location	Symptom
Rectum	Increased pain by rectal distention
	Relief of pain with passage of flatus or stool
	Tenesmus
	Sensation of incomplete evacuation
Anus	Increased pain by passage of stool or straining
	Throbbing pain with sitting or activity
	Protrusion of mass with bowel movement

lieved by passing flatus or stool. Tenesmus (urge to defecate) may occur with edema of the rectal mucosa, and a sensation of incomplete evacuation may occur with edematous proctitis or rectal masses. Pain caused by anal disease may be exacerbated by the passage of hard scybalous stools or with straining. Pain may be so severe that patients defer defecation for fear of pain. Throbbing or persistent anal pain suggests inflammation and edema, which may be associated with an abscess or chronic anal fissure. When edema or inflammation affects both the rectum and anus, these distinctions may be vague.

The possibility of rectal cancer should be considered in most if not all patients with anorectal pain and bleeding. A sensation of rectal fullness, tenesmus, or change in stool caliber should heighten suspicion of malignancy. Unfortunately there is no single discriminating feature of the clinical picture of rectal cancer. Therefore, the evaluation of anorectal pain should rule out the possibility of malignancy (Fig. 19–1). A complete history should elicit symptoms of inflammatory bowel disease, travel, anorectal trauma, rectal intercourse, weight loss, change in bowel habits, or family history of colorectal malignancy. The presence or absence of gross bleeding or a hemoccult-positive stool should be determined. A visual examination of the anus (with cheeks maximally spread) and digital examination of the anal canal and rectum should be performed. Anoscopy is a simple bedside procedure in which anal mucosa is viewed as it protrudes through a slit in the anoscope. This may provide a somewhat better examination than can be achieved with flexible sigmoidoscopy, although no comparison study has been performed. The finding of hemorrhoids should not preclude further evaluation unless an obvious thrombosed external hemorrhoid is present. Examination of the rectal mucosa should be performed for most if not all patients with persistent anorectal pain. Flexible sigmoidoscopy currently offers the simplest and most comfortable way to accomplish this, although a rigid proctoscope can also be used. We try to improve the yield of flexible sigmoidoscopy by attempting to retroflex the sigmoidoscope in the rectum to better visualize the anorectal junction and to identify internal hemorrhoids. At this point in the evaluation, further diagnostic studies or treatment depends on the findings. It is beyond the scope of this chapter to discuss malignancy in detail, but the possibility of malignancy should be considered in *every* patient with anorectal complaints.

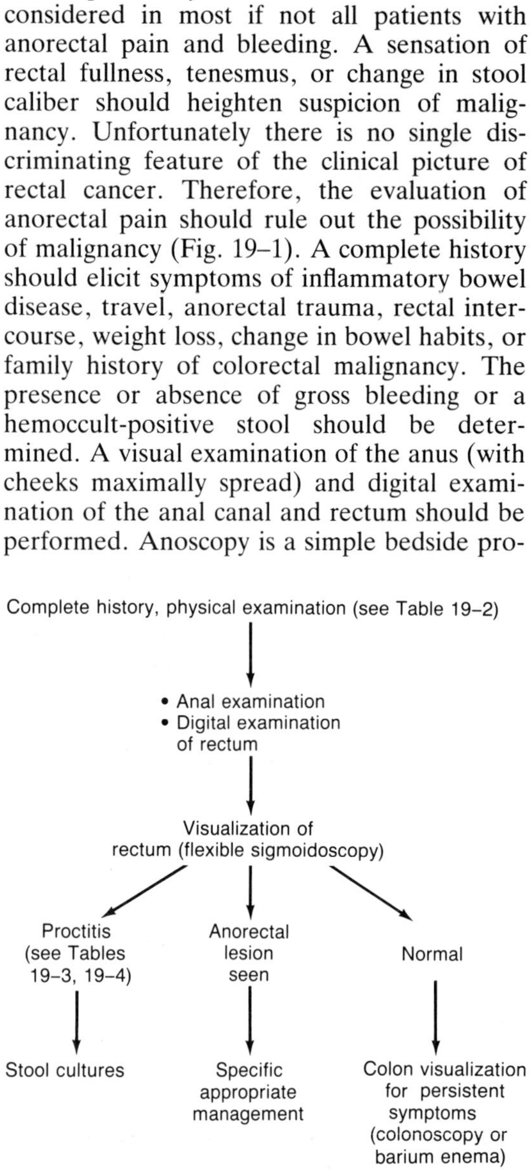

Proctitis

Inflammation of the rectum may be due to infection, radiation, trauma, or nonspecific causes. Symptoms include crampy rectal discomfort exacerbated by rectal distention resulting from stretching of inflamed tissues. Patients may note rectal urgency, tenesmus, and hematochezia. A sensation of rectal fullness and incomplete evacuation is not unusual. Stools may be watery, loose, or of normal consistency depending on the amount of colon involved. A sigmoidoscopic examination may reveal rectal edema, granularity, friability, or ulceration. The differential diagnosis of proctitis is lengthy (Table 19–3) and ever-growing as new pathology is discovered. Chemically induced colitis (caused by soapsuds or hydrogen peroxide enemas) and radiation colitis (caused by prior pelvic irradiation) should be considered in patients at risk. Sexually transmitted proctitis is a common problem in homosexual men who may harbor a baffling array of microorganisms (see Chapter 37). Travel outside the United States should raise the possibility of infection with amebae, shigella, or salmonella organisms. Recent antibiotic therapy raises the specter of pseudomembranous colitis caused by *Clostridium difficile*. Symptoms caused by *Campylobacter* species and hemorrhagic colitis caused by *Escherichia*

Figure 19–1. Evaluation of anorectal pain and bleeding.

Complete history, physical examination (see Table 19–2)

• Anal examination
• Digital examination of rectum

Visualization of rectum (flexible sigmoidoscopy)

Proctitis (see Tables 19–3, 19–4) → Stool cultures

Anorectal lesion seen → Specific appropriate management

Normal → Colon visualization for persistent symptoms (colonoscopy or barium enema)

Table 19–3. Differential Diagnosis of Proctitis

Inflammatory bowel disease
  Ulcerative colitis
  Crohn's disease
Infection
  Shigella
  Salmonella
  Campylobacter jejuni
  Clostridium difficile
  E. coli species
  Sexually transmitted pathogens
    Neisseria gonorrhoeae
    Treponema pallidum
    Chlamydia
    Herpes
    Chlamydia trachomatis
    Amebae
    Cytomegalovirus
Nonspecific proctitis
  Ischemia
  Radiation
  Lipid proctitis
  Collagenous colitis
  Soap colitis
  Hydrogen peroxide colitis
  Trauma

coli 0157:H7 may mimic idiopathic inflammatory bowel disease. The diagnosis of inflammatory bowel disease (ulcerative colitis or Crohn's disease) depends on ruling out known infectious causes of proctitis. Stool samples should be examined for pathogens, particularly in the high risk groups mentioned above. Anorectal swabs should be obtained for patients who had rectal intercourse to examine for evidence of herpes simplex infection, gonorrhea, or syphilis. A rectal biopsy is recommended if no pathogens are found.

Treatment is generally specifically targeted for the disease process. Antibiotic therapy for infectious proctitis is outlined in Table 19–4. The management of ulcerative colitis, Crohn's disease, and radiation proctitis has been reviewed elsewhere. The keys to the management of proctitis are the recognition of rectal pathology (which requires direct visualization) and a thorough search for infectious causes.

The solitary rectal ulcer should be recognized as an entity distinct from proctitis. Patients may have rectal bleeding and anorectal or left iliac fossa pain. There is a very strong association with rectal prolapse. Sigmoidoscopy may reveal one or more isolated ulcers in the rectum, often with associated "lumpy" mucosa, which may represent localized submucosal cysts (colitis cystica profunda). The differential diagnosis of the endoscopic finding includes all of the aforementioned causes of colitis as well as rectal neoplasms, trauma, drug-induced ulcers, and an assortment of miscellaneous causes. Medical treatment with azulfidine, steroids, and antibiotics is usually not successful. Dietary fiber and avoidance of straining may be helpful but in many cases are unsatisfactory. Local surgical excision of the lesions is often associated with recurrence. Surgical correction of rectal prolapse is unproved but may provide better long-term results.

Hemorrhoids

Hemorrhoids are among the most common and the most poorly understood of human afflictions. The only consensus about etiology is that hemorrhoids represent enlarged vascular tissues. The current most widely accepted theory of hemorrhoid formation proposes, that there are anal cushions containing vascular and muscular tissue that slide distally during defecation. This vascular tissue probably includes arteriovenous communications resulting in the bright red blood associated with hemorrhoidal bleeding. Normally, longitudinal smooth muscles help retract these tissues after they protrude. However, the tissues may become congested and trapped (in a distal position) by a tight anal sphincter. In other patients, weakened pelvic musculature may be unable to retract the tissue. Prolonged straining, which stretches pelvic muscles and diminishes muscle

Table 19–4. Specific Treatments for Infectious Proctitis

Disease	Treatment
Neisseria gonorrhoeae	Aqueous procaine penicillin 4.8 million U intramuscularly + probenecid (1.0 g)
Treponema pallidum	Benzathine penicillin 2.4 million U
Chlamydia trachomatis	Tetracycline 2 g/day for 2–3 wk
Amebae	Metronidazole 750 mg t.i.d. for 10 days
Campylobacter species	Erythromycin (for severe disease only) 250–500 mg t.i.d. for 7 days
Clostridium difficile	Vancomycin 125–500 mg q.i.d. for 7–10 days
	Metronidazole 500 mg t.i.d. for 7–10 days
	Bacitracin 20,000 U q.i.d. for 7 days
	Cholestyramine 4 g t.i.d. for 7–10 days (for mild disease only)

tone, may be an important factor in pathogenesis. This theory explains many of the clinical aspects of hemorrhoids and the response to specific therapies. Remissions and exacerbations may be directly related to straining or irritation of the anal sphincter (causing spasm).

Patients usually visit physicians because of persistent perianal discomfort or bleeding. Severe anal pain is seldom due to hemorrhoids alone, unless there is acute thrombosis with edema and secondary anal spasm, or an associated fissure. Fecal and mucus soilage may occur, particularly in the presence of hemorrhoid prolapse, which can also cause pruritus. Blood associated with bleeding from hemorrhoids is usually bright red, and bleeding is occasionally profuse. Hemorrhoids are defined by their anatomic location. External hemorrhoids are distal to the anorectal junction (pectinate line) and covered by the sensitive anoderm. Acute thrombosis seen in young people can be exquisitely painful. Internal hemorrhoids are proximal to the pectinate line covered with rectal mucosa and may prolapse into the anal canal. The degree and severity of prolapse determine the classification of the hemorrhoid: primary lesions are small and nonprolapsing; secondary hemorrhoids prolapse with defecation but reduce spontaneously; third-degree lesions may be reduced manually; and fourth-degree hemorrhoids are not reducible.

No patient should be presumed to have rectal bleeding or pain secondary to hemorrhoids and be dismissed without evaluation. The mere presence of hemorrhoids does not preclude coexistent inflammatory proctitis or malignancy of the anus or rectum. Therefore, visualization of the rectum is necessary in most patients. The decision to pursue a more complete evaluation of the colon in the presence of anorectal bleeding should be individualized. In most cases, if bleeding hemorrhoids are seen at sigmoidoscopy, further diagnostic evaluation is probably not necessary. However, if stool obtained from above the rectum during sigmoidoscopy is hemoccult positive, a barium enema or colonoscopy should be considered even with coexisting hemorrhoids because of the incidence of other lesions in this setting. A recent study from Australia found that the clinical assessment of the source of rectal bleeding was often inaccurate but was improved by sigmoid examination. Nevertheless, there may be a high prevalence (60%) of hemorrhoids concurrent with other colonic lesions. It is also clear that rectal bleeding can originate from malignancies beyond the reach of the flexible sigmoidoscope. Therefore, patients with persistent bleeding or a family history of colon cancer should undergo full colon examinations.

Tedesco and colleagues studied 258 patients over age 40 who had rectal bleeding and negative sigmoidoscopy results. Significant colonoscopic findings were present in 41%, with carcinoma present in 11.2%. These data further reinforce the need to pursue a complete evaluation of rectal bleeding, especially in patients more than 40 years old.

Lack of consensus about the cause of hemorrhoids has led to a confusing array of treatments. That many empiric treatments appear to be successful is a tribute to the variable course of hemorrhoids as well as the salutary effect of visiting a physician. The cornerstone of conservative medical treatment for hemorrhoids is avoidance of straining. All current theories of hemorrhoid formation place some of the blame on straining during defecation. Epidemiologic evidence indicates that hemorrhoids and constipation are common in "low fiber" societies like Great Britain and are rare in rural Africa and communities where people consume high fiber diets and exercise regularly. Such evidence would support the notion that softening stools and avoidance of straining may prevent hemorrhoids. However, the few studies evaluating bulk diet therapy in a scientific manner have shown no benefit. The public is deluged with advertisements for ointments, creams, and suppositories, but no placebo-controlled studies have been performed to evaluate these products. In the existing uncontrolled studies, it is unclear if resolution on treatment reflects the natural history of hemorrhoid inflammation. It certainly seems reasonable that the anti-inflammatory properties of local corticosteroids and the local anesthetic properties of other ingredients and emollients may relieve some hemorrhoid symptoms. Adverse reactions are unusual, but local allergic skin reactions may occur. Sitz baths have long been recommended by proctologists and have uncertain efficacy; possible benefits include nontraumatic cleansing and relaxation of the anal sphincter.

Fortunately the vast majority of patients have improvement in symptoms either because of or in spite of the aforementioned conservative therapies. If bleeding, pain, or prolapse persists, invasive procedures should be considered. Because hemorrhoids probably represent engorged prolapsed vascular tissue, measures to reduce prolapse or decrease engorgement seem more prudent than resection of otherwise normal tissue. Three categories of surgical treatment are prevention of mucosal prolapse, reduction of sphincter tone, and resection of hemorrhoids. Prevention of mucosal prolapse is achieved by inducing a submucosal injury by application of a sclerosant, cryosurgery, rubber band ligation, or laser to a portion of an internal hemorrhoid. The subsequent fibrosis and fixation eliminate the downward movement of the anal cushions during bowel movements. As long as the procedure is performed proximal to the pectinate line, it is not painful. Patients with permanently prolapsed hemorrhoids are not likely to benefit from fixation procedures. When rubber band ligation was compared with the other methods of fixation in several studies, ligation results were the most favorable. Complications include hemorrhage 7 to 14 days after ligation, when necrotic tissue sloughs and separates. Most patients resume their normal activities within days.

The proponents of the theory that a tight anal sphincter is the primary cause of hemorrhoids recommend reduction of sphincter tone by dilation or internal anal sphincterotomy. Young patients seem most likely to benefit and elderly patients seem most likely to suffer complications (fecal incontinence, fissure, hematoma, prolapse) from these procedures. Few direct comparisons with other forms of therapy exist, and even the most enthusiastic advocates of sphincter dilation would limit the procedure to patients with documented elevation of sphincter pressure.

The excision of hemorrhoidal tissue results in excellent relief of symptoms but at a tremendous cost—hospitalization, operating room time, and up to 6 weeks of recovery time. Fecal soilage after resection is not unusual (in 10 to 25%).

The following approach to the management of symptomatic hemorrhoids is recommended. Careful examination of the anorectum is mandatory, and further study of the colon may be indicated for older patients, particularly if there is bleeding. Initial management should include advice regarding stool softeners, exercise (to enhance gut motility), and the avoidance of straining and rectal trauma. The sitz bath is a harmless homeopathic, noninvasive treatment that is often recommended by physicians. Ointments, creams, and suppositories are not always harmless but may indeed provide symptom relief. Adverse effects are unusual, but allergic skin reactions can exacerbate pruritus. Although the benefit of these drugs remains unproved, anecdotal successes and the need to prescribe something have perpetuated their use. More aggressive therapy should be considered only in patients with persistent symptoms. Rubber band ligation is a cost-effective, relatively painless procedure with little morbidity. Acutely thrombosed internal hemorrhoids, severe bleeding, and permanent prolapse are best managed with hemorrhoid resection. Thrombosed external hemorrhoids are distinctive bluish masses distal to the pectinate line and can be treated conservatively with analgesics or warm baths or with a simple elliptical incision under local anesthesia. Skin tags that are cutaneous remnants of formerly active hemorrhoid disease require no treatment.

Anal Fissure

Perhaps the most painful of anorectal diseases is the fissure in ano: a longitudinal ulcer in the anal canal usually located along the posterior wall. This condition may be so painful as to preclude a digital rectal examination without anesthesia. Traditionally, the fissure is thought to be the result of passage of large firm stools through a nonpliable anal canal. Prior injury, trauma, or surgery to the anus may result in scarring that may predispose to fissure formation. If the fixed anoderm does not glide during stool passage, the canal wall may tear. The subsequent submucosal inflammation and edema may stimulate internal sphincter spasm, which can prevent healing and result in a chronic, nonhealing fissure. The patient complains of severe tearing anorectal pain worsened by the passage of stool but often persisting between bowel movements. Many patients defer defecation for fear of pain, which results in worsening constipation. Gentle eversion of the anal mucosa while the patient strains often reveals the fissure. The differential diagnosis includes Crohn's disease and infective ulcers (from gonorrhea, syphillis, or tuberculosis). Any association with hemorrhoids is probably coincidental.

Nonoperative treatment for an acute posterior fissure includes stool softeners, analgesics, and warm baths to break the pain-spasm cycle. Suppositories should be avoided because of the possibility of further injury during insertion. A recent randomized trial compared a warm sitz bath plus ingestion of bran daily with hydrocortisone ointment and lignocaine ointment in 103 patients with new onset posterior anal fissure. Symptomatic relief occurred more rapidly in the sitz bath–bran group. This conservative approach avoids the use of potentially irritating ointments. Anal dilators with anesthetic jelly have been used to stretch the anal sphincter; however, recent controlled studies have failed to demonstrate clinical benefit. Moreover, patients have been reported to misplace dilators in the rectum. Fortunately, most acute fissures heal spontaneously in 1 to 2 weeks.

Chronic fissures may require surgical therapy. Lateral internal anal sphincterotomy is associated with little or no recurrence of fissures and is far superior to forceful dilation of the sphincter. The success of sphincterotomy may indicate that sphincter spasm does indeed play a major role in the chronicity of fissures.

Anorectal Abscess and Fistula

Anorectal abscesses are infections localized to the tissue spaces in and around the anus and occur most commonly in patients with Crohn's disease or during immunodeficient states. Otherwise normal individuals may uncommonly develop an anal abscess, with infection arising from the anal crypt. The symptoms depend on the location and size of the abscess. Throbbing constant pain exacerbated by sitting or walking is typical, but some patients may have a chief complaint of lower abdominal discomfort. Examination may reveal an indurated, tender erythematous mass if the lesion is superficial, or digital detection of fullness and tenderness if the lesion is deep. Patients should be examined closely for the presence of a fistula or clinical evidence of Crohn's disease. If an abscess is present, careful incision and drainage should be performed by an experienced surgeon because of the proximity of vital sphincters and difficulties with wound healing in this area.

Fistulas may be due to trauma, chronic fissure, tuberculosis, Crohn's disease, carcinoma, or radiation therapy. Perianal drainage of pus, blood, mucus, or stool may be evident on examination. Openings in the perianal skin may appear as raised papules.

Although surgical drainage is often necessary, the internist must recognize the abscess and distinguish it from other causes of anorectal pain.

Miscellaneous Causes of Anorectal Pain

LEVATOR SYNDROME

The levator syndrome is characterized by a dull, aching pain high in the rectum. Patients may complain of a sensation that there is a ball in their rectum. Symptoms may worsen during bowel movements when stool presses against the levator muscles. Examination reveals moderate tenderness and spasm of the levator muscles that form the sling that pulls the rectum anteriorly toward the symphysis pubis. Palpation along the lateral walls of the rectum characteristically elicits tenderness. There may be some tenderness with motion of the coccyx. The syndrome is more common in females and is often the result of prolonged sitting. The differential diagnosis includes perineal descent syndrome, prostatitis, and internal procidentia, all of which can give a sensation of a rectal ball but are not associated with levator tenderness during the examination. Coccygodynia refers to tenderness of the coccyx, which may be the result of trauma or prolonged pressure from sitting. Once again, the digital rectal examination usually permits a distinction between coccyx pain and levator tenderness. Sigmoidoscopy should also be performed to rule out rectal neoplasms. Some patients respond to firm massage of this muscle sling from anterior to posterior. Rubbing back and forth against the tender muscle multiple times may alleviate the spasm. Sitz baths and muscle relaxants have also been used with some success. Electrogalvanic stimulation with a low frequency oscillating current has also been employed to break the spastic cycle. In many cases, however, reassurance that this is a benign process and avoidance of prolonged sitting are sufficient.

PROCTALGIA FUGAX

Proctalgia fugax is a sudden, severe episode of rectal pain that may last seconds to minutes. This may be a fleeting variant of the levator syndrome. It occurs in 14% of apparently healthy adults and has been linked to the ubiquitous irritable bowel syndrome. Half of patients complaining of proctalgia have other functional gastrointestinal symptoms. The cause is unknown, but some authorities propose that spasm of the levator muscles is the cause of pain, whereas others suggest that pain is a result of contractions of the sigmoid colon.

The condition is most common in compulsive young men. No precipating events have been identified. Diagnosis is based on the exclusion of other pathologic conditions plus a consistent history. Although many treatments have been used, none have been of proven benefit. Reassurance may be salutary for some patients, and mild analgesics may be necessary in a minority of patients.

Pruritus Ani

Itching of the perianal skin is common and is often due to too much or too little hygiene (Table 19–5). Overzealous cleansing with tissue paper, soaps, and creams can produce mucosal irritation or sensitivity reactions to perfumes and chemicals in these substances. For some patients, gentle anal cleansing with water or witch hazel and avoidance of irritants may be therapeutic. Inadequate hygiene and perianal soilage may produce pruritus in some individuals. Mucus seepage associated with hemorrhoids, tumors, fissures, fistulas, condylomas, or sphincter dysfunction may be irritating to perianal skin. Careful but not too vigorous anal cleansing is recommended. Some individuals note perianal irritation in association with diarrhea. The alkaline pH of diarrheal stool may induce an anal cryptitis. Based on this theory, acidification of stools with *Lactobacillus acidophilus* or malt soup and avoidance of alkaline ointments and creams have been advocated, although the efficacy of this approach remains uncertain. Finally, a variety of infections can produce pruritus, including fungal infections, condyloma acuminata, and parasites. Primary dermatologic disorders like psoriasis, eczema, lichen planus, and seborrheic dermatitis are often apparent on examination and are not limited to the perianal skin.

Table 19–5. *Causes of Pruritus Ani*

Inadequate hygiene or mucus seepage caused by
    Inappropriate sphincter relaxation or incontinence
    Rectal or hemorrhoidal prolapse
    Anal polyps or condylomata
    Anal fistulas
Overzealous hygiene
Diarrhea
Infections (parasitic, fungal, viral, bacterial)
Primary dermatologic disorders (psoriasis, atopic
    eczema, lichen planus, seborrheic dermatitis)
Inflammatory bowel disease
Anorectal neoplasm

Adapted, with permission, from Lieberman DA. Common anorectal disorders. Ann Intern Med 1984; 101:837–846.

A careful history and examination often reveal a cause for pruritus ani. If a diffuse perianal skin rash is present, dermatologic causes and fungal infection should be considered. Tissue scraping for fungi may be helpful. Locally applied creams or ointments should be discontinued. Nontraumatic gentle hygiene may relieve symptoms for most patients. If mucus seepage appears to be an underlying problem, a careful anorectal examination should be completed to rule out malignancy.

Fecal Incontinence

Fecal incontinence exacts a terrible psychological toll and severely impairs activity and socialization in the elderly. It is estimated that 16 to 60% of the institutionalized elderly have some degree of fecal incontinence. The preservation of continence is complex and its failure is multifactoral in most cases. Defecation is part reflex, part voluntary. After rectal distention with feces, there is reflex relaxation of the internal anal sphincter, which is under autonomic control. This relaxation permits contact of feces with the sensitive anoderm of the upper anal canal, which can be sensed at a conscious level. Contraction of the voluntary external anal sphincter prevents stool spillage. It is now clear that some individuals have diminished myoelectric activity of the external sphincter resembling denervation and resulting in histologic loss of muscle fibers. Denervation may be due to entrapment or stretching of nerves caused by straining or pelvic descent. A vicious cycle of pelvic floor weakness and further straining can lead to diminished external sphincter activity. Anal sensation is impaired in some patients who fail to recognize the movement of stool into the anal canal. Internal anal sphincter dysfunction resulting from autonomic neuropathy, diabetes mellitus, spinal cord lesions, or prior anal surgery may impair continence mechanisms. Diarrhea may overwhelm otherwise normal sphincter mechanisms but can be quite problematic in elderly patients with marginal neuromuscular function. Finally, impaction or obstruction can result in overflow incontinence.

The evaluation of the incontinent patient may involve a coordinated effort of geriatricians, endocrinologists, neurologists, and gastroenterologists. The relationship of sphincter tone on digital examination and recorded pressure measurements is not good, but the inability of a patient to voluntarily squeeze the external sphincter suggests dysfunction. An aggressive search for treatable problems is warranted. The effect of drugs on mentation should be carefully examined, and unnecessary drugs should be discontinued. If drugs have depressed the level of consciousness, the patient may not be aware of anal sensations. When constipation and impaction are present, the fecal mass should be removed and bowel habits assessed. If diarrhea is a contributing factor, the underlying cause of the diarrhea should be treated if possible. Nonspecific diarrhea (which may occur in diabetes mellitus) can be treated with antidiarrheal drugs and sphincter exercises. Neurogenic incontinence with impaired sphincter function can sometimes be treated by taking advantage of an intact gastrocolic reflex with a visit to the commode immediately after a meal. For some patients, a regular program of enemas can achieve bowel cleansing and avert incontinent episodes.

Simple exercises consisting of repetitive (10 to 20) contraction-relaxation cycles of the external sphincter (Kegel's exercises) may help augment sphincter tone in patients with otherwise intact reflexes. Patients should perform these exercises several times a day. More recently, biofeedback therapy has been applied to the treatment of fecal incontinence. Successful treatment requires a well-motivated subject who has intact anal sensation and an external sphincter capable of responding to rectal distention. A three-balloon system provides simultaneous pressure measurements from the external and internal anal sphincters and proximal rectum. Patients can see a normal external sphincter tracing during rectal sensation and try to reproduce that pattern on the physiologic tracing, which provides the visual feedback. Rectal sensitivity is gradually increased by using decreasing distending volumes. A less cumbersome method was recently described that employs a small anal plug containing two electrodes to record external sphincter contractions. Patients are reinforced by the visual image of their contractions on a computer screen. The biofeedback approach has been successful in more than two thirds of eligible patients. By individualizing therapy, many patients can achieve continence.

Conclusion

Anorectal disorders are ubiquitous and troubling to many patients who nevertheless are reluctant to mention their problems during the routine medical history. Physicians should elicit a complete history and perform a thorough anorectal examination. The diagnosis of rectal malignancy should be considered in all patients with persistent rectal pain and bleeding. Therefore, direct visualization of the rectum is mandatory in most patients with these complaints. The treatment of common disorders like hemorrhoids and pruritus ani remains unscientific. Reassurance and common sense have remarkable salutary effects.

Bibliography

Blaser MJ, Reller LB. *Campylobacter* enteritis. N Engl J Med 305:1444–1452, 1981.
   This review discusses epidemiology, diagnosis, and therapy and emphasizes that C. jejuni infection may mimic other forms of colitis.

Buser WD, Miner PB. Delayed rectal sensation with fecal incontinence. Successful treatment using anorectal manometry. Gastroenterology 91:1186–1191, 1986.
   Manometric techniques were applied to improve recognition of rectal distention in patients with incontinence. Clearly, continence depends not only on sphincter function but also on recognition of rectal distention.

Ford MJ, Anderson JR, Gilmour HM, et al. Clinical spectrum of "solitary ulcer" of the rectum. Gastroenterology 84:1533–1540, 1983.
   The clinical presentation, etiology, and treatment of 40 patients with rectal ulcers are described. The authors suggest that rectal prolapse is commonly associated with rectal ulcers.

Gebhard RL, Gerding DN, Olson MM, et al. Clinical and endoscopic findings in patients early in the course of *Clostridium difficile*–associated pseudomembranous colitis. Am J Med 78:45–48, 1985.
   This is a good review of the early clinical features of this disease in 39 patients.

Goulston KJ, Cook I, Dent OF, et al. How important is rectal bleeding in the diagnosis of bowel cancer and polyps. Lancet 2:261–265, 1986.
   In a population of patients with rectal bleeding, the source of bleeding was confirmed by colonoscopy. The clinical prediction of the source of bleeding was often inaccurate, which emphasizes the need for a thorough evaluation for persistent rectal bleeding.

Jensen SL. Treatment of first episodes of acute anal fissure: prospective randomized study of lignocaine ointment versus hydrocortisone ointment or warm sitz baths plus bran. Br Med J 292:1167–1169, 1986.

Levine DS. "Solitary" rectal ulcer syndrome. Gastroenterology 92:243–253, 1987.
   The relationship among rectal prolapse, colitis cystica profunda, and rectal ulcers is explored.

Lieberman DA. Common anorectal disorders. Ann Intern Med 101:837–846, 1984.
   This comprehensive review of recent literature discusses current concepts in the pathogenesis and treatment of hemorrhoids, anal fissure, pruritus ani, and fecal incontinence.

MacLeod JH. Management of anal incontinence by biofeedback. Gastroenterology 93:291–294, 1987.
   Two techniques for biofeedback for anal incontinence

are discussed that achieve successful control in two thirds of properly selected patients.

Pai C, Gordon R, Sims H, et al. Sporadic cases of hemorrhagic colitis associated with *Escherichia coli* 0157:H7. Ann Intern Med 101:738–742, 1984.
This newly recognized pathogen must be added to the list of infections that mimic inflammatory bowel disease. Specific cultures are available.

Quinn TC, Stamm WE, Goodell SE, et al. The polymicrobial origin of intestinal infections in homosexual men. N Engl J Med 309:576–582, 1985.
The spectrum of enteric pathogens identified in 119 homosexual men is described, and an algorithm for diagnosis and management is presented.

Salvati EP. The levator syndrome and its variant. Gastroenterol Clin North Am 16:71–78, 1987.

Schuster MM. The riddle of the sphincters. Gastroenterology 69:249–262, 1975.
This article is an excellent review of anorectal physiology.

Tedesco FJ, Wayne JD, Raskin JB, et al. Colonoscopic evaluation of rectal bleeding: a study of 304 patients. Ann Intern Med 89:907–909, 1978.
This landmark study presents the results of complete colonoscopy in patients with rectal bleeding. The incidence of significant lesions was 41%, and 11.2% had cancer. The predictive value of rectal bleeding was high and justifies evaluation.

Thompson WG. Proctalgia fugax. Dig Dis Sci 26:1121–1124, 1981.

Thomson WHF. The nature of haemorrhoids. Br J Surg 62:542–552, 1975.
A theory of hemorrhoids formation is presented based on autopsy findings. The sliding anal cushion concept is now widely accepted and explains much of the natural history of hemorrhoids.

Wald A. Biofeedback therapy for fecal incontinence. Ann Intern Med 95:146–149, 1981.
Two techniques for biofeedback for anal incontinence are discussed that achieve successful control in two thirds of properly selected patients.

20

Diagnosis and Management of Dyspepsia

FERMIN MEARIN, M.D.
JUAN-RAMON MALAGELADA, M.D.

What is Dyspepsia?

Dyspepsia comes from the Greek words *dus* (bad) and *pepto* (digestion). It is a variably defined clinical syndrome of episodic or persistent epigastric discomfort, often related to feeding and sometimes associated with early satiety, belching, bloating, nausea, and vomiting. Dyspepsia is extremely common, with a point prevalence of nearly 30% in the general population, and is the reason for 1 to 3% of visits to primary care practitioners. Hundreds of millions of dollars are spent annually on antacids and histamine-2 (H_2) receptor antagonists to treat dyspepsia. After the common cold, it is the second most frequent cause for time lost from work.

Dyspepsia has many causes (Table 20–1). Etiologies not involving the upper gastrointestinal tract can generally be diagnosed or strongly suspected on clinical grounds. However, it is not easy to differentiate clinically among the various upper gastrointestinal causes of dyspepsia, and endoscopy and other more sophisticated studies are required for precise diagnosis. Endoscopic studies of dyspeptic patients who consult physicians have revealed duodenal ulcer in 12 to 22% of patients, gastric ulcer in 2 to 14%, gastric cancer in ≤ 1%, and gastritis and/or duodenitis in 5 to 40%. However, the relationship between endoscopically documented gastritis or duodenitis and dyspepsia remains uncertain.

In 15 to 30% of patients with dyspepsia, no underlying cause is found after clinical, analytic, radiologic, and endoscopic examinations, and the symptoms are assumed to be due to a "functional" disorder of the upper gut. Several terms are used to describe it: essential dyspepsia, nonulcer dyspepsia, epigastric distress syndrome, or Moynihen's disease. We prefer to use the term functional dyspepsia because it excludes peptic ulcer disease and other lesions and indicates the supposed functional cause of the syndrome. Thus, functional dyspepsia is defined as dyspepsia that is not attributable to structural, drug-induced, alcohol-induced, or metabolic diseases but is related to disorders of upper gut function or to the patient's abnormal perception of normal physiology.

The physician caring for dyspeptic patients faces two major dilemmas. First, should all

Table 20–1. *Causes of Dyspepsia*

Upper gastrointestinal tract
  Peptic ulcer disease
  Gastroesophageal reflux
  Gastric cancer
  Disorders of gastrointestinal motility
  Gastritis and/or duodenitis (?)
Hepatobiliary tract
  Cholelithiasis
  Hepatic congestion
Chronic pancreatitis
Small and large bowel
  Irritable bowel syndrome
  Idiopathic intestinal pseudo-obstruction
  Intestinal angina
Metabolic disorders
  Diabetes mellitus
  Adrenal insufficiency
  Uremia
  Electrolyte disorders
Medications
  Nonsteroidal anti-inflammatory agents
  Others
Alcohol
Functional dyspepsia

patients with dyspepsia undergo detailed evaluation, including endoscopy, to make a precise diagnosis and particularly to exclude serious organic disorders such as peptic ulcer disease and gastric cancer? The high prevalence of dyspepsia and the considerable expense of the diagnostic techniques in this era of cost containment mandate the use of an effective diagnostic strategy. Second, how should the large group of patients with functional dyspepsia be managed? We discuss the clinical approach to these two questions in the remainder of this chapter.

Diagnosis of Dyspepsia

The diagnostic evaluation should always begin with a detailed history and physical examination. The time of onset and duration of symptoms, the location, radiation, and character of the abdominal discomfort, and the presence or absence of other associated symptoms should all be determined. The symptoms of gastroesophageal reflux, cholelithiasis, and the irritable bowel syndrome (see Chap. 22) can most often be distinguished from the other causes of dyspepsia. However, the symptoms associated with the various upper gastrointestinal etiologies of dyspepsia, including functional dyspepsia, overlap to such an extent that these conditions cannot be distinguished on clinical grounds. Still, useful information can be obtained from the history and physical examination to help guide subsequent diagnostic efforts. Dyspeptic patients with significant weight loss (more than 5 lb), protracted vomiting suggestive of upper gastrointestinal obstruction, lymphadenopathy, abdominal masses, or positive fecal occult blood tests are more likely to have significant organic lesions than patients with uncomplicated dyspepsia. Alcohol and a number of medications, including nonsteroidal anti-inflammatory agents, may either cause or exacerbate dyspepsia. Cigarette smoking may exacerbate peptic ulcer disease. When compared with age- and sex-matched controls, patients with functional dyspepsia have a several-fold increase in the frequency of headache, dizziness, chest discomfort, palpitations, and sweating. They are frequently anxious and occasionally depressed, but no more so than dyspeptic patients with ulcers.

After this initial evaluation, the physician must decide whether to visualize the patient's upper gastrointestinal tract with either endoscopy or an upper gastrointestinal barium series. Patients with symptoms or signs of gastrointestinal bleeding or obstruction or of systemic illness (e.g., weight loss or fever) certainly require an early diagnostic evaluation. However, the necessity of obtaining a precise diagnosis on initial presentation in other dyspeptic patients is controversial. Several investigators recommend an initial empiric course of therapy for 6 to 8 weeks with H_2 receptor antagonists in patients with uncomplicated dyspepsia. They reserve further diagnostic evaluation for patients who fail to improve after the first 10 days of treatment or for patients whose dyspepsia does not completely resolve or recurs after a 6- to 8-week course of therapy. However, given the high cost of H_2 antagonists and because most dyspeptic patients eventually require endoscopic examination, the cost/benefit relationship of this approach is doubtful. Moreover, a positive diagnosis helps both the practitioner and the patient to pursue a more rational course of treatment.

Esophagogastroduodenoscopy is superior to an upper gastrointestinal barium series for the diagnosis of upper gut pathology. The double-contrast barium study has a higher false-negative rate (10 to 15%) and false-positive rate (10%) than endoscopy and does not allow for biopsy of suspicious lesions. Gastric and duodenal biopsies should probably be obtained at the time of endoscopy, because histologic gastroduodenitis may be present despite the absence of visible abnormalities. A biliary tract ultrasound examination should be performed only if cholelithiasis is suspected after the history and physical examination. The presence of stones does not imply that dyspepsia originates in the biliary tract. Moreover, prospective studies have demonstrated that patients with functional dyspepsia have a prevalence of cholelithiasis no higher than that for the general population. Tests of gastric acid secretion are generally not helpful for dyspeptic patients. In some cases, esophageal manometry, use of a pH meter, and acid perfusion tests are useful for detecting esophageal disease and gastroesophageal reflux. In some patients with severe functional dyspepsia, special procedures to investigate gastrointestinal motility may be helpful. The most important of these procedures are gastrointestinal manometry, radioisotopic measurement of gastric emptying, and electrogastrography. These investigations may facilitate more rational treatment for some patients.

Management of Dyspepsia

When endoscopy or other diagnostic studies have revealed an organic etiology for dyspepsia, specific treatment may be initiated. However, in most studies, 15 to 30% of patients have persistent or recurrent dyspepsia with no visible lesions seen by endoscopy. How should this large group of patients with functional dyspepsia be managed?

Functional Dyspepsia: Clinical Presentation

Functional dyspepsia requiring medical attention is more frequent in women than men, with a ratio of about 1.5:1. Most patients are first seen between the third and fifth decades of life. The onset of symptoms may be insidious or abrupt and in some cases is preceded by an influenza-like syndrome. The predominant symptom is epigastric pain, usually without radiation and frequently aggravated by food intake; a variety of foods are reported to cause or aggravate the pain. Up to 20% of patients report nocturnal pain and relief of pain by food intake, a combination of symptoms generally believed to suggest peptic ulcer disease. About one half of functionally dyspeptic patients report associated symptoms of nausea, feelings of fullness, heartburn, and belching (Table 20–2). Symptoms of the irritable bowel syndrome (looser or more frequent bowel movements with the onset of abdominal pain, relief of pain with the passage of stool, abdominal distention, and a sensation of incomplete evacuation) may occur in some patients with functional dyspepsia. Compared with age- and sex-matched controls, these patients appear to have a propensity for multiple somatic complaints including headaches, dizziness, chest pain, palpitations, and sweating (Table 20–3). It is controversial whether anxiety and depression are more common in these patients than in patients with peptic ulcer disease or in control subjects in the community. The majority of patients have weekly or more frequent symptoms, which may persist from hours to weeks. The clinical course of functional dyspepsia is variable with periods of relapse and recovery.

Functional Dyspepsia: Pathophysiology

The pathophysiology of functional dyspepsia is unknown. It is presumed to be a heterogeneous syndrome with several mechanisms producing a similar clinical picture (Fig. 20–1).

Gastric or Duodenal Nonulcerated Mucosal Lesions (Gastroduodenitis). The relationship of gastroduodenitis to dyspepsia is uncertain. In some studies gastroduodenitis has been as frequent in asymptomatic control subjects as in dyspeptic patients. Recent investigations suggest the possible existence of different subsets of gastroduodenitis patients. Gastroduodenitis appears to be the cause of functional dyspepsia in patients with endoscopic evidence of nonulcerated mucosal lesions associated with neutrophilic infiltration in biopsy specimens. The dyspepsia in these patients is similar to that of classic peptic ulcer disease with preprandial onset, periodicity, and relief by antacids; this subgroup may constitute one end of the spectrum of peptic ulcer disease. Other patients with gastroduodenitis and dyspepsia may have an unrelated disorder because they respond poorly to antiulcer therapy.

Infection. *Campylobacter pyloridis* has been proposed as a cause of functional dyspepsia. Ingestion of *Campylobacter* induces dyspepsia and gastritis, and the organism is found in the gastric mucosa of 60% of dyspeptic patients. However, this postulated relationship is weakened by the inconsistent association of *Campylobacter* with both inflammation and symptoms in many patients.

Upper Gut Motor Abnormalities. A motility disorder has been suspected to cause functional dyspepsia. Some manifestations of dyspepsia, such as vomiting and regurgitation, suggest abnormal motility of the upper gut. Manomet-

Table 20–2. *Gastrointestinal Symptoms in Patients with Functional Dyspepsia*

Symptom	Percentage of Patients Reporting Symptoms
Epigastric pain	100
Nausea	66
Feeling of fullness	57
Acid regurgitations	50
Eructations	46
Borborygmus	44
Heartburn	39
Early satiety	31
Diarrhea	23
Vomiting	21
Obstipation	17
Water brash	13
Dysphagia	10

Adapted from J Clin Gastroenterol. The epigastric distress syndrome. Nyren O, Adami HO, Gustavsson S, et al., vol 9, 1987, pp 303–309, with permission.

Table 20–3. Associated Symptoms in Patients with Functional Dyspepsia Compared
with Age- and Sex-Matched Healthy Control Subject

Symptom	Percentage of Patients Reporting Symptoms	Percentage of Controls Reporting Symptoms
Headache	47	19
Dizziness	36	7
Chest discomfort	23	2
Palpitations	21	2
Sweating	17	5
Smothering sensation	14	1

Adapted from J Clin Gastroenterol. The epigastric distress syndrome. Nyren O, Adami HO, Gustavsson S, et al., vol 9, 1987, pp 303–309, with permission.

ric abnormalities of the stomach and small bowel have been demonstrated in about one half of patients with functional dyspepsia. The most common manometric finding is antral hypomotility. Such hypomotility is most evident after ingestion of a solid meal (Fig. 20–2). In such patients, the frequency and amplitude of the gastric waves are decreased. Small bowel abnormalities include unpropagated bursts of phasic and tonic contractile activity, defective propagation of interdigestive motor complexes in the intestine, and abnor-

mal patterns suggesting disorganized motor activity. Thus, not only gastric but also small bowel dysmotility may be responsible for functional dyspepsia.

As a result of abnormal upper gut motility, gastric emptying is impaired and both esophagogastric and duodenogastric reflux may increase. Slow gastric emptying, mainly of solids, has been demonstrated in dyspeptic patients (Fig. 20–3). Moreover, decreased gastric emptying might predispose to gastroesophageal reflux. Duodenogastric reflux has also been

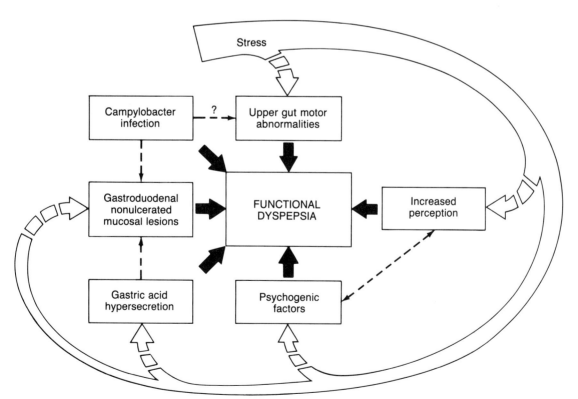

Figure 20–1. Possible underlying mechanisms in functional dyspepsia.

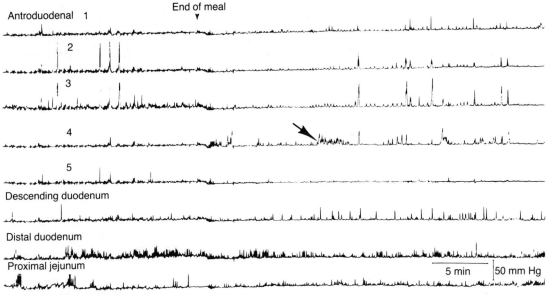

Figure 20–2. *Antral hypomotility in a patient with functional dyspepsia. Postcibal tracing shows a paucity of antral phasic pressure waves. The arrow indicates the pylorus.*

regarded as a determinant of dyspeptic symptoms.

Secretory or Motor Abnormalities Related to Stress. It is well-known that some emotions can modify secretion and motility of the upper gut. In healthy volunteers, cold pain, as an experimental stressor, produced a biphasic alteration in gastric secretion, with an initial reduction in secretion occurring during the application of the stress followed by an in-

crease in secretion after cessation. Such studies have not yet been performed with functional dyspeptic patients.

Acute stress in normal volunteers inhibits postcibal antral contractile activity and retards gastric emptying. Gastric motility responses to experimentally induced stress in patients with functional dyspepsia differ according to the basal motor activity: in the subgroup of patients with postprandial antral hypomotility,

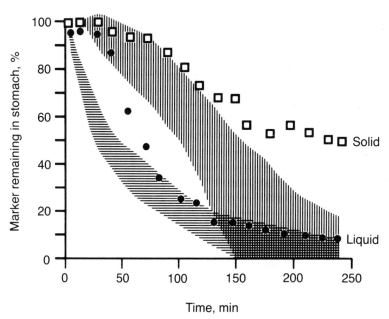

Figure 20–3. *Gastric emptying of a mixed radiolabeled meal in a patient with functional dyspepsia: gastric emptying of the solid phase is delayed, whereas emptying of the liquid phase is normal.*

gastric motility is not further suppressed by somatic stressful stimulation. These patients are probably afflicted by a primary gastric motor disorder. In contrast, in the dyspeptic patients with normal postcibal antral motility, gastric motor activity is normally suppressed by stress. It is unlikely that a motility disturbance is the cause of the symptoms in these patients; an increased perception or awareness of normal gut functions is a possibility.

Psychogenic Factors. In some patients, dyspeptic symptoms probably have a psychogenic basis. Conversion reaction is suspected in some cases, and in others, the profusion of somatic complaints implies that illness behavior has been learned.

Functional Dyspepsia: Therapy

Progress in the therapy of functional dyspepsia has been hampered by its largely unknown and probably heterogeneous pathophysiology. Current modes of treatment are therefore empiric, and it appears unlikely that a single form of treatment benefits all patients.

Several types of nonpharmacologic therapy are frequently prescribed for patients with functional dyspepsia. Simple dietary changes (e.g., small, frequent, low fat meals) and elimination of smoking, alcohol, nonsteroidal anti-inflammatory medications, or other drugs likely to cause or exacerbate dyspepsia may ameliorate symptoms in some patients. However, the efficacy of these recommendations has not been documented in clinical trials.

A number of drugs have been used to treat functional dyspepsia. However, their efficacy is uncertain because many of the published studies are complicated by inadequate definitions of functional dyspepsia and/or variable patient selection criteria. The fluctuating clinical course with frequent spontaneous recovery and the high placebo response of functional dyspepsia (25 to 50% of patients improve with placebo in most studies) increase the difficulty of interpreting these studies.

As previously discussed, the role of gastric acid in the pathogenesis of functional dyspepsia is questionable. Most of the controlled, double-blind trials have shown no significant

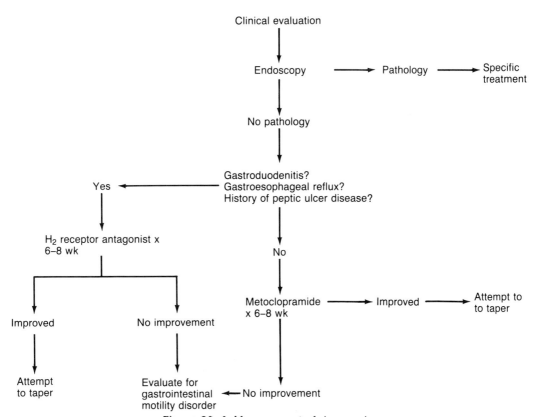

Figure 20–4. *Management of dyspepsia.*

difference among antacids, H_2 antagonists, and placebo. However, these studies do not definitively exclude the benefit of antisecretory or acid-neutralizing drugs for some subgroups of patients. It is possible that H_2 antagonists, antacids, or the protective agent sucralfate may benefit patients with (1) erosive prepyloric changes seen by endoscopy; (2) histologically proven gastroduodenitis with neutrophilic infiltration; (3) associated symptoms of gastroesophageal reflux; or (4) prior history of peptic ulcer disease. The response to 6 to 8 weeks of therapy should be carefully assessed in these patients. The indiscriminate use of antiulcer drugs in all patients with functional dyspepsia is not appropriate.

Consideration of gastrointestinal hypomotility as a possible etiology for functional dyspepsia has led to the use of prokinetic drugs including metoclopramide, domperidone, and cisapride (the latter two drugs are not available in the United States). It has been suggested that dyspeptic patients with delayed gastric emptying are more likely to respond to prokinetic drugs. However, there is not always a strict correlation between improvement in symptoms and enhancement of gastric motility.

Bismuth compounds (which may eliminate *Campylobacter* from the gastric mucosa) cannot be recommended for routine use at this time.

On the assumption that psychogenic or stress-induced gastric secretory and motor disturbances are pathogenically important in dyspepsia, treatment sometimes involves psychotherapy, behavioral modification, or psychoactive drugs. The efficacy of these therapies has not been proved.

In rare cases, surgical treatments, such as vagotomy, antrectomy, or bypass procedures, have been carried out, but there is little rationale for their use and they are as a rule ineffective.

Figure 20–4 summarizes the therapeutic approach to patients with functional dyspepsia. Patients with gastroduodenitis demonstrated by endoscopy or biopsy, with symptomatic gastroesophageal reflux, or with a past history of peptic ulcer disease should be treated with a 6- to 8-week course of H_2 receptor antagonists. Patients with mild to moderate dyspepsia but without abnormalities may be treated with a 6- to 8-week course of therapy with metoclopramide, 10 to 20 mg orally, 30 minutes before each meal and at bedtime. Patients who fail to respond to these two regimens and who have severe dyspepsia should be referred to a gastroenterologist for more detailed evaluation. Patients with apparent psychologic abnormalities may be referred for psychiatric consultation. As with other functional disorders of the gastrointestinal tract, a close relationship between patient and physician with frequent, regularly scheduled follow-up visits is essential (see Chap. 22).

Bibliography

American College of Physicians. Endoscopy in the evaluation of dyspepsia. Ann Intern Med 102:226–229, 1985.
  Recommendations are given for clinical management and diagnostic approach in dyspeptic patients.
Camilleri M, Brown ML, Malagelada JR. Relationship between impaired gastric emptying and abnormal gastrointestinal motility. Gastroenterology 91:94–99, 1986.
  Gastric stasis in gut dysmotilities occurs because of impaired antral peristalsis resulting from antral hypomotility or increased resistance to flow into the small intestine caused by intestinal dysmotility.
Camilleri M, Malagelada JR, Kao PC, et al. Gastric and autonomic responses to stress in functional dyspepsia. Dig Dis Sci 31:1169–1177, 1986.
  There are two subtypes of antral motility in functional dyspepsia: (1) antral hypomotility under basal conditions and (2) normal basal antral motility and autonomic and gastric motor responses to stress.
Camilleri M, Thompson DG, Malagelada JR. Functional dyspepsia: symptoms and underlying mechanism. J Clin Gastroenterology 8:424–429, 1986.
  The physiopathology of functional dyspepsia is reviewed with special interest in manometric, gastric emptying and electrogastrographic studies.
Malagelada JR, Camilleri M, Stanghellini V. Manometric Diagnosis of Gastrointestinal Motility Disorders. New York, Thieme Medical Publishers, 1986.
  This book provides an overview of the physiology of gastric and intestinal motility; multiple examples and figures are shown.
Malagelada JR, Stanghellini V. Manometric evaluation of functional upper gut symptoms. Gastroenterology 88:1223–1231, 1985.
  In patients with functional-type symptoms, gastrointestinal manometry is a useful technique to discover the underlying gut motor disturbance that is present in a relatively high proportion of these patients.
Nyren O, Adami HO, Gustavsson S, et al. The epigastric distress syndrome. J Clin Gastroenterol 9:303–309, 1987.
  A review and personal experience are provided about the clinical aspects of functional dyspepsia. Epigastric distress syndrome is proposed as a new term to describe dyspepsia of unknown origin.
Rees WDW, Miller LJ, Malagelada JR. Dyspepsia, antral motor dysfunction, and gastric stasis of solids. Gastroenterology 78:360–365, 1980.
  Extensive gastric manometric and emptying studies were performed with a patient having postprandial dyspeptic symptoms.
Stanghellini V, Malagelada JR, Zinsmeister AR, et al. Stress-induced gastroduodenal motor disturbances in humans: possible humoral mechanism. Gastroenterology 85:83–91, 1983.

Centrally acting external stimuli may severely disrupt antral feeding activity.

Talley NJ, Phillips SF. Non-ulcer dyspepsia: potential causes and pathophysiology. Ann Intern Med 108:865–879, 1988

This is a current, thorough review with an extensive list of references.

Talley NJ, Fung LH, Gilligan IJ, et al. Association of anxiety, neuroticism, and depression with dyspepsia of unknown cause. Gastroenterology 90:886–892, 1986.

Patients with dyspepsia of unknown cause are more likely to be neurotic, anxious, and depressed than dyspepsia-free control subjects.

Talley NJ, McNeil D, Piper DW. Discriminant value of dyspeptic symptoms: a study of the clinical presentation of 221 patients with dyspepsia of unknown cause, peptic ulceration and cholelithiasis. Gut 28:40–46, 1987.

Clinical assessment may be of value in the differential diagnosis of dyspepsia of unknown cause.

Talley NJ, Piper DW. Major life event stress and dyspepsia of unknown cause: a case control study. Gut 27:127–134, 1986.

Life stress events are not more frequent or significantly different in type in patients with dyspepsia of unknown cause than in community control subjects.

Working party. Management of dyspepsia: report of a working party. Lancet 1:576–579, 1988.

A practical approach to the management of dyspepsia is proposed by an international panel of 10 gastroenterologists. It is current and well referenced.

21

Evaluation and Management of Acute Diarrhea

SUSAN W. TOLLE, M.D.
DIANE L. ELLIOT, M.D.

Diarrheal illnesses may be classified as either acute or chronic, with the latter lasting more than 3 weeks. This differentiation is useful, because acute diarrheas are usually infectious, and most will resolve in time without specific therapy. At their onset, the symptoms of chronic diarrhea may resemble acute illness; however, as the evaluation involves excluding the acute etiologies, the initial diagnostic approach is the same as that used for acute diarrhea. This review will focus on the clinical features, diagnostic approach, and management of acute diarrhea.

Clinical Manifestations

Acute diarrheal illnesses can be grouped into noninflammatory and inflammatory, each having different clinical manifestations. The features of a noninflammatory diarrhea are large volumes of watery stool, often associated with cramping, bloating, and periumbilical pain. Constitutional symptoms are minimal or absent. This is in contrast to inflammatory diarrhea, caused by organisms that tend to invade the mucosa. Inflammatory diarrhea is commonly accompanied by fever and other constitutional symptoms, lower abdominal pain, and tenesmus. Inflammatory diarrheas can progress to dysentery with small stool volumes containing gross blood and mucus. When a patient has features of both inflammatory and noninflammatory diarrhea (i.e., watery diarrhea with systemic symptoms), he or she should be approached as having an inflammatory diarrhea. Table 21–1 summarizes the important features of both noninflammatory and inflammatory diarrheas.

Viral agents are the most common cause of noninflammatory diarrheal disease in the United States. In children, rotavirus infections predominate and cause diarrhea of 5 to 8 days' duration. Adult illness is usually due to Norwalk or other viral infections, and the diarrhea is self-limited, lasting 24 to 48 hours. Other causes of noninflammatory diarrhea include enterotoxigenic *Escherichia coli*, *Vibrio cholerae*, *Giardia lamblia*, and *Cryptosporidium*. In addition, the preformed bacterial toxins associated with food poisoning have a similar clinical picture. Because the mucosa is not invaded, systemic symptoms, hematochezia, and the presence of fecal leukocytes are rare.

Diarrhea among travelers is commonly noninflammatory. Among those going to Mexico, enterotoxigenic *E. coli* is the most frequent pathogen. A recent travel history should also lead to consideration of *G. lamblia* and, when symptoms are severe, *V. cholerae*. Most cases of cholera are acquired in developing nations. However, *V. cholerae* is endemic in the bayous of Louisiana, and sporadic cases continue to be reported from these areas. When a traveler has watery diarrhea that persists for more than a week, *Giardia* should be considered. Although international and wilderness travel increases the risk of giardiasis, the illness is frequently seen throughout the United States. Suggestive symptoms include bloating, cramping, and periumbilical pain associated with prolonged foul-smelling watery stools, which develop 2 weeks after exposure.

Potential causes of inflammatory diarrhea are *Shigella*, *Campylobacter jejuni*, *Yersinia enterocolitica*, invasive *E. coli*, *Salmonella*, and *Entamoeba histolytica*. *Shigella* is a highly infectious organism, and a small inoculum can spread the organism. *Shigella* has traditionally

Table 21–1. Clinical Features of Diarrhea

Parameter	Noninflammatory	Inflammatory
Mechanism	Enterotoxin (or reduced absorption)	Mucosal invasion
Relative incidence in ambulatory setting	95%	5%
Systemic symptoms	Absent	Often present
Location	Small bowel	Colon
Character of diarrhea	Large volume, watery	Small volume, may be bloody or mucoid
Fecal leukocytes	Absent	Present

been considered the most common cause of illness in patients with blood-streaked diarrhea. However, in recent years, *Campylobacter* has been identified with greater frequency than *Shigella,* particularly in the western United States.

Shigellosis is often a biphasic illness. Patients initially have large volumes of watery stool suggesting a noninflammatory diarrhea. However, concurrent malaise and fever should suggest an invasive organism even before other symptoms of mucosal invasion develop. By the second day of illness, the patient's symptoms are usually fever and lower abdominal pain, and the stools have changed to small volumes and are often streaked with blood and mucus.

Transmission patterns for *Campylobacter* are not well understood, and person-to-person transmission has not been documented. Most cases are sporadic, and contact with infected pets has at times been temporally associated. *Campylobacter* is a relatively common cause of diarrhea in travelers, especially summertime campers and hikers. Diarrheal illness after the ingestion of raw milk contaminated with *Campylobacter* has also been confirmed in several outbreaks. The usual incubation period is 2 to 7 days, and the patient's symptoms are abdominal pain, vomiting, malaise, fever, and often grossly bloody diarrhea.

Y. enterocolitica also has a clinical spectrum that can include bloody diarrhea. Symptoms range from dysentery to profuse watery diarrhea with an incubation period of 4 to 10 days. The modes of transmission to humans have not been clearly defined but include ingestion of contaminated raw milk. *Y. enterocolitica* is found mainly in northern countries such as Canada and Finland. Laboratory identification of this organism is difficult, requiring special culture techniques with enrichment at low temperatures.

Food poisoning can cause a noninflammatory diarrhea when preformed bacterial toxins are ingested. Food-borne illnesses can also follow the ingestion of invasive pathogens. When outbreaks of diarrhea are suspected to have been food-borne, the Public Health Department should be notified. The etiologic agent may be suggested by the clinical setting (Table 21–2). Symptoms that begin within 8 hours of the meal suggest staphylococcal toxin. This toxin may contaminate meats, poultry, salads, or cream-filled pastries. Nausea and vomiting begin abruptly, and shortly after the patient usually develops abdominal cramping and diarrhea. The onset of symptoms is more gradual when disease is caused by *Clostridium perfringens*. Patients tend to have abdominal cramping and watery diarrhea appearing 8 to 14 hours after the ingestion of contaminated meats. Symptoms last for about 24 hours, and vomiting is not a prominent feature.

Food poisoning can also be associated with marine organisms. When outbreaks of watery diarrhea occur 4 to 96 hours after the ingestion

Table 21–2. Features of Food Poisoning–Induced Diarrheas

Type of Diarrhea and Causative Organism	Sources	Incubation Time
Predominately Noninflammatory		
Staphylococcus aureus	Meats, poultry, salads, cream-filled pastries	1–8 h
Clostridium perfringens	Meats	8–14 h
Bacillus cereus	Rice	1–6 h
Predominately Inflammatory		
Nontyphoidal *Salmonella*	Raw milk, eggs, poultry	6–24 h
Campylobacter jejuni	Raw milk, contaminated water	2–7 days
Yersinia enterocolitica	Raw milk, meats	4–10 days
Vibrio parahaemolyticus	Poorly cooked seafood or shellfish	4–96 h
Shigella	Contaminated water, mixed salads	12–72 h

of contaminated seafood or shellfish, *Vibrio parahaemolyticus* should be considered. If the diarrhea is severe and the shellfish may have been from Louisiana, the patient should be treated for cholera pending further investigation.

Inflammatory diarrhea may also be acquired through the ingestion of contaminated food and water. Nontyphoidal *Salmonella* is the most common infectious agent linked to cases of food-borne diarrhea. The clinical picture with *Salmonella* infection may have features of both inflammatory and noninflammatory diarrheas. An enterotoxin-induced watery diarrhea usually begins 6 to 24 hours after ingestion. If the infection progresses to mucosal invasion, malaise, fever, and bloody diarrhea can occur. The most frequent types of foods contaminated with *Salmonella* are raw milk, eggs, and poultry. Several other food-borne organisms have the potential to cause inflammatory diarrhea (i.e., *Shigella, C. jejuni, Y. enterocolitica,* and invasive *E. coli*).

In addition to inquiries about travel and recent food ingestion, a detailed medication history should be part of the evaluation. Noninflammatory diarrhea may be caused or worsened by the use of stimulant laxatives or the extensive use of sorbitol, which is used as an artificial sweetener. Magnesium-containing antacids often cause an osmotic diarrhea. Diarrhea is commonly associated with broad-spectrum antibiotic therapy and with the use of quinidine and colchicine. Drug-induced diarrhea usually follows a noninflammatory course, and symptoms disappear with discontinuation of the medication.

Diarrhea in patients who have recently taken antibiotics deserves special consideration. Most antibiotics have been associated with colitis caused by the overgrowth of *Clostridium difficile*. Nearly half of patients with *C. difficile* have a noninflammatory watery diarrhea, which can develop as long as 6 weeks after antibiotic therapy. In more severe cases, dysentery and high fever occur.

When evaluating diarrheal illnesses, the patient's sexual practices should be considered. Multipartnered homosexual men are at increased risk of infections with *C. jejuni, Shigella, G. lamblia, E. histolytica,* and perhaps *Cryptosporidium.* (See Chap. 37 for a discussion of the evaluation of diarrhea and proctitis in this population.)

The epidemiologic importance of day-care centers in the spread of diarrheal pathogens has recently been confirmed. Outbreaks of diarrhea in day-care centers most frequently have been associated with the spread of *Shigella* and *Giardia.* However, *C. difficile, Campylobacter, Cryptosporidium,* and rotavirus have all been linked to this setting. The secondary infection rate for members of the families of affected children is 10 to 30%.

Acute diarrhea occasionally occurs as the initial manifestation of ulcerative colitis. Negative results of cultures and following the patient's clinical course are required to make this distinction.

Laboratory Evaluation

Patients with clinical features of an inflammatory diarrhea should have a fresh stool specimen examined for fecal leukocytes. This test is performed by placing a thin layer of feces or mucus on a slide and mixing it with one drop of Löeffler's methylene blue. The presence of more than five polymorphonuclear leukocytes per high power field is considered a positive result and suggests colonic mucosal invasion. This finding increases the probability of infection with *Campylobacter, Shigella,* invasive *E. coli,* or an overgrowth of *C. difficile,* or of ulcerative colitis. False-positive results are increased when slides are interpreted by inexperienced personnel. In addition, ameba may be mistaken for leukocytes. Because colonic invasion does not occur in all patients infected with invasive pathogens, false-negative results are common. For example, fecal leukocytes were found in only 69% of *Shigella* infections in one study. Similar results have been reported for *Campylobacter.*

Fecal leukocytes are rarely found in noninflammatory diarrhea caused by viruses, toxins, enterotoxigenic *E. coli,* or *G. lamblia.* When colitis is due to the overgrowth of *C. difficile,* leukocytes are few or absent in mild cases but may be seen in severe cases. Likewise, the findings are variable and depend on the extent and severity of the disease with infections caused by *Salmonella, E. histolytica, Y. enterocolitica,* and *V. parahaemolyticus.*

Microscopic examination of saline wet mount preparations of the stool can be useful in the preliminary diagnosis of *Campylobacter* infection. This organism is motile with polar flagella and makes random darting movements about the slide. The combination of this characteristic motion and fecal leukocytes is presumptive evidence for *Campylobacter* enteritis. A Gram's stain of the stool allows prompt, reliable identification of gram-negative vibrio organisms but has a sensitivity of only 50%.

As most diarrheal illnesses are caused by viruses, stool cultures are useful for a minority of patients. Reserving cultures for specific indications is cost effective. Cultures should be performed when the test for fecal leukocytes is positive or when occult blood is present (Fig. 21–1). Stool cultures are also advisable in evaluating diarrhea in patients who are febrile, require admission to the hospital, work as food handlers, or have diarrhea for longer than 1 week. When a stool culture is indicated, methods should be used to identify *Shigella, Salmonella, Campylobacter,* and *Yersinia.* Because efficacy is questionable, many providers have reserved the *Yersinia* stool culture for patients with persistent diarrhea with a prior negative diagnostic evaluation. A *C. difficile* toxin titer should be obtained for patients with a recent history of antibiotic use. If a culture result is positive, a repeat stool culture is

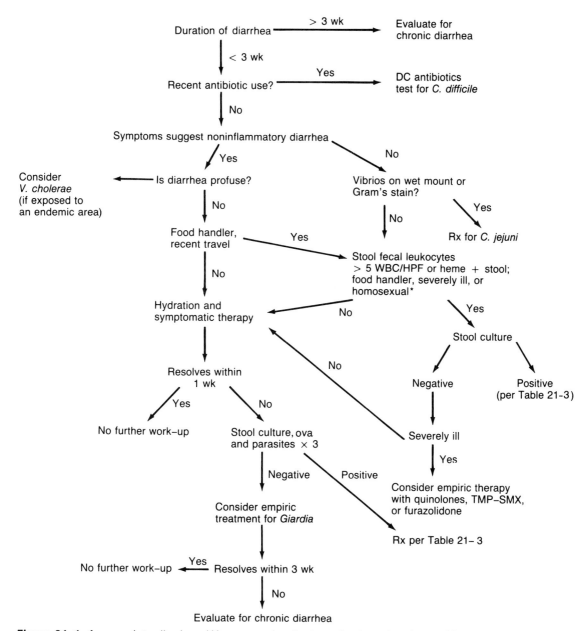

Figure 21–1. Approach to diarrhea. *Homosexual patients and selected patients with recent travel history should also have stool tested for ova and parasites × 3.

needed only for food handlers and those who fail to respond to therapy.

Sigmoidoscopic examination is rarely indicated in the diagnostic evaluation of patients with acute diarrhea. It is useful primarily to establish the diagnosis of amebic and ulcerative colitis. About 10% of those with ulcerative colitis have acute diarrhea as their initial symptom. The diagnosis can be established only in the absence of other pathogens and by following the patient's clinical course over time. Both ulcerative colitis and inflammatory diarrheas reveal a diffusely erythematous and friable mucosa. In amebiasis, proctoscopy allows direct visualization of localized colonic ulcerations and access to mucus for microscopic examination. Specimens should be obtained by suction or scraping, as amebas tend to adhere to cotton swabs. Serologic confirmation with gel diffusion precipitin or indirect hemagglutination tests is positive in 85 to 90% of patients with invasive amebic colitis. Antibiotic-associated colitis may also have a characteristic appearance. However, the ability to evaluate stool for *C. difficile* toxin has reduced the need for sigmoidoscopy to establish this diagnosis.

Parasitic examination is most useful when the patient's travel history, sexual preference, or duration of symptoms increases the probability of amebiasis or giardiasis. The numbers of amebas are decreased for weeks by prior barium examination and for several days by recent enemas, laxatives, and certain antibiotics. Parasites are reliably identified in stool specimens only in the acute phase of giardiasis. As the transit time slows, trophozoites, although still multiplying in the small bowel, are destroyed in the colon, and stool specimens frequently have negative results. A small bowel biopsy or the use of a gelatin capsule on a string may be required to confirm an established infection. We empirically treat patients with suspected giardiasis without confirmation by small bowel biopsy or duodenal aspirate.

Barium enema examination is contraindicated in the evaluation of patients with acute diarrhea. The procedure rarely contributes diagnostic information and carries the risks of megacolon and perforation.

Obtaining electrolyte studies for acute diarrhea is rarely indicated. When oral rehydration has been unsuccessful and the patient requires hospitalization, serum electrolytes should be tested.

Therapy

During management of patients with acute diarrhea, emphasis is on supportive measures. Care consists primarily of rehydration. When the degree of dehydration is mild, it can be corrected with fruit juices or caffeine-free soft drinks. More severe dehydration should be treated with a balanced glucose and electrolyte oral rehydration solution because glucose facilitates absorption in the small bowel. A simple approximation for home use is ½ tsp table salt, ½ tsp baking soda, and 1 cup orange juice plus 4 tbsp sugar dissolved in 1 qt of water. The World Health Organization has found that even severe diarrheas can often be treated with careful oral rehydration. Hospitalization is rarely necessary but is indicated for dehydrated patients who are vomiting and for elderly patients and infants with profuse diarrhea and dehydration.

Caffeine, alcohol, and dairy products should be avoided. Caffeine and alcohol increase intestinal motility, and transient lactose intolerance is common after acute diarrheal illnesses.

Symptomatic therapy is often useful for patients with noninflammatory diarrheas. Bismuth subsalicylate (Pepto-Bismol) has been shown to improve patient comfort by reducing stool volumes and relieving abdominal cramping. To be effective, large volumes of this preparation are required (60 ml every half hour for eight doses).

Recent studies concluded that loperamide is an effective alternative to bismuth subsalicylate for the treatment of nondysenteric travelers' diarrhea. Loperamide decreases stool volumes and relieves cramping. Caution has been advised because of concerns that antiperistaltic agents could exacerbate bacillary dysentery. However, for nonpregnant adults without fever or dysentery, loperamide has proved both safe and effective. Pregnant patients may benefit from kaolin with pectin.

Most acute diarrheal illnesses are noninflammatory and self-limited and respond to volume repletion and symptomatic therapy. Antibiotic therapy is indicated for the treatment of specific pathogens and for selected circumstances (Table 21–3). Antibiotics are indicated for only two of the pathogens associated with noninflammatory diarrhea: *G. lamblia* and *V. cholerae*. In giardiasis, quinacrine rapidly eradicates the pathogen, and metronidazole is also effective. Furazolidone is slightly less effective but is available as a suspension and, because

Table 21–3. Pathogen-Specific Antimicrobial Therapy

Pathogen	Effective Antimicrobial Agents	Regimen*
Giardia lamblia	Metronidazole	Adults: 250 mg t.i.d./10 days
	Quinacrine	Adults: 100 mg t.i.d./7 days
	Furazolidone	Children: 8 mg/kg/day, in 3 doses/7 days
Vibrio cholerae	Tetracycline	Adults: 250 mg q.i.d./5 days
	TMP-SMX	Children: same as for *Shigella*
Shigella	TMP-SMX	Adults: 160 mg trimethoprim and 800 mg sulfamethoxazole every 12 h/5 days
		Children: 50 mg TMP/kg/day in 2 divided doses/5 days
	Ampicillin	Adults: 500 mg q.i.d./5 days
		Children: 100 mg/kg/day in 4 divided doses/ 5 days
Salmonella spp† (compromised patients)	Ampicillin	Adults: 1 g IV every 4 h/14 days
		Children: 100 mg/kg/day IV in 4 divided doses/10 days
	TMP-SMX	Adults and children: doses as for *Shigella* but for 14 days
Campylobacter jejuni	Erythromycin	Adults: 250 mg q.i.d./7 days
		Children: 40 mg/kg/day in divided doses every 6 h
Yersinia enterocolitica‡	TMP-SMX	Adults and children: doses as for *Shigella*
Entamoeba histolytica	Metronidazole	Adults: 750 mg t.i.d./5–10 days plus iodoquinol, 650 mg every 8 h/21 days
		Children: 50 mg/kg/day in 3 doses/10 days
Clostridium difficile	Vancomycin	Adults: 125 mg q.i.d./10 days
		Children: 10 mg/kg/day in 4 divided doses
	Metronidazole	Adults: 500 mg t.i.d./10 days
		Children: 20 mg/kg/day in 3 divided doses/ 10 days

*All drugs are given by mouth unless otherwise stated.
†Antibiotics are not indicated except in special circumstances.
‡Antibiotics are reserved for severe illness.

of better compliance, is often the treatment of choice for giardiasis in children. Cholera, caused by *V. cholerae* 01, with its copious purging ability, is usually susceptible to tetracycline. Tetracycline is superior to other oral antibiotics for this purpose.

Antibiotics may be considered in the management of inflammatory diarrheas caused by bacterial pathogens. We recommend treating *Shigella* infections with trimethoprim-sulfamethoxazole (TMP-SMX), which is effective in diminishing the number of days of diarrhea, fever, and excretion. *Shigella* species are often resistant to tetracycline and ampicillin, and problems of resistance to other drugs are developing.

The effectiveness of antibiotic therapy in the treatment of *C. jejuni* has been questioned. Studies have shown that the duration of excretion of *C. jejuni* was significantly reduced by giving erythromycin, and the incidence of relapses may also be reduced. However, several studies have failed to demonstrate a clinical benefit for patients who had been ill for more than 5 days before receiving antibiotics.

Antibiotic therapy is not indicated for most patients with nontyphoidal *Salmonella* gastroenteritis because it does not diminish the duration or severity of illness, and shedding of *Salmonella* is prolonged in antibiotic-treated patients. However, antibiotics should be given to compromised patients who are at increased risk of developing bacteremia, such as infants; elderly, immunocompromised, and sickle cell patients; and those with prosthetic devices.

Limited information is available on the antibiotic treatment of *Y. enterocolitica*. Only one controlled study has been done, and most patients had been ill more than 5 days before starting antibiotic therapy. Treatment with TMP-SMX did not shorten the duration of illness but did significantly reduce excretion of the pathogen.

Amebic dysentery should be treated with metronidazole, which is effective against trophozoites. If the patient continues to pass amebic cysts after successful treatment of the dysentery, further treatment to eradicate cysts is necessary. This is often done with iodoquinol (650 mg three times a day for 21 days) or diloxanide furoate (available from the Centers for Disease Control).

The growth of *C. difficile* is facilitated by the continued use of the offending antibiotic. The incriminated antibiotic should be withdrawn whenever possible. Successful treatment requires eradication of the *C. difficile* organism, which is most effectively done by giving vancomycin orally. Metronidazole is slightly less effective but substantially less expensive. Relapse rates are fairly high with as many as 20% of patients requiring retreatment with metronidazole or vancomycin.

Bibliography

Gorbach S. Bacterial diarrhoea and its treatment. Lancet 2:1378–1382, 1987.
> *This concise review of bacterial diarrhea utilizes an algorithm for evaluation and management.*

Gorbach SL, Edelman R (eds). Travelers' diarrhea: National Institute of Health Consensus Development Conference, Bethesda, Maryland, January 28–30, 1985. Rev Infect Dis 8(Suppl 2):S109–233, 1986.
> *This excellent, current, comprehensive review of travelers' diarrhea covers all aspects from epidemiology and prevention to drug resistance and treatment.*

Johnson PC, Ericsson CD, DuPont HL, et al. Comparison of loperamide with bismuth subsalicylate for the treatment of acute travelers' diarrhea. JAMA 255:757–760, 1986.
> *The authors conclude that loperamide is a safe and effective alternative to bismuth subsalicylate for travelers with noninflammatory diarrhea.*

Krejs GJ (ed). Diarrhoea. Clin Gastroenterol 15:477–741, 1986.
> *This volume addresses acute and chronic diarrheal diseases. Pathophysiologic mechanisms are addressed in detail.*

Walker-Smith JA (ed). Paediatric Gastroenterology. Clin Gastroenterol 15:21–37, 39–53, 1986.
> *Chapters address bacterial diarrhea and viral diarrhea in the pediatric patient. Pathophysiology and epidemiology are stressed.*

Williams EK, Lohr JA, Guerrant RL. Acute infectious diarrhea. II. Diagnosis, treatment and prevention. Pediatr Infect Dis 5:458–465, 1986.
> *This is a good review of infectious diarrhea in children. A management algorithm is provided.*

Yungbluth PM. Practical approach to the use of the laboratory in infectious enteritis. Pract Gastroenterol 11:35–42, 1987.
> *The cost-effective use of direct examination of stool, bacterial cultures, and parasitic examination is reviewed.*

22

Management of the Irritable Bowel

W. GRANT THOMPSON, M.D., F.A.C.P., F.R.C.P.C.

Functional gastrointestinal disease has been defined by an international working team (see report by Thompson and colleagues) as "a variable combination of chronic or recurrent gastrointestinal symptoms not explained by structural or biochemical abnormalities. This may include syndromes attributed to the esophagus, stomach, biliary tree, small or large intestine or anus." It is sobering that patients with functional gastrointestinal disturbances constitute up to 50% of those referred to gastroenterologists. Even more thought-provoking is the notion that gastrointestinal disturbances occur in up to 30% of apparently healthy people, most of whom do not see a physician let alone get referred to a specialist (Fig. 22–1).

When a patient presents with an organic disease such as peptic ulcer or inflammatory bowel disease, the physician's course of action is usually clear. On the other hand, the correct treatment for functional disease is more obscure. No recognizable or verifiable anatomic, physiologic, or biochemical disturbance is present; no pathognomonic feature can be expected to be found on investigation; and no cure is forthcoming. The outlook in terms of life expectancy or physical disability is good, but the condition tends to persist or recur throughout a lifetime despite a variety of treatments.

The cost of investigation and management of these prevalent and long-lasting disorders can only be imagined. The total health care bill is at least as great as that for inflammatory bowel disease. Because most patients and physicians are concerned about the possible presence of organic disease, many consultations,

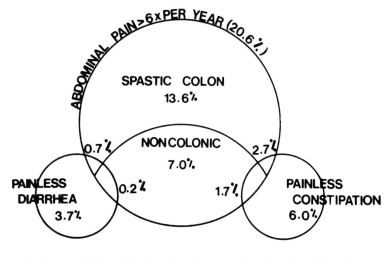

Figure 22–1. *Functional bowel disorder in 91 (30.2%) of 301 apparently healthy individuals. The large circle indicates 65 persons (20.6%) who have abdominal pain more than six times a year. It is divided to show 41 (13.6%) with irritable bowel syndrome and 21 (7%) with noncolonic pain (dyspepsia). The small circles represent 14 patients with diarrhea and 31 with constipation. The overlap of these with the large circle indicates that some patients with diarrhea and constipation also had abdominal pain. Most of the individuals reporting symptoms had not consulted a doctor about them. Reprinted with permission from Functional bowel disorders in apparently healthy people, by Thompson WG, Heaton KW. Gastroenterology, vol 79, 283–288. Copyright 1980 by The American Gastroenterological Association.*

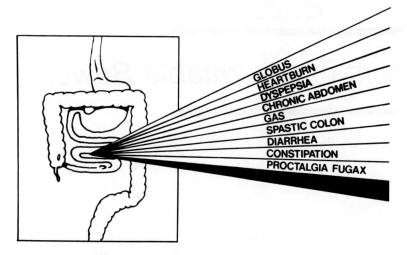

Figure 22–2. Gut dysfunction may occur at all levels, leading to functional symptoms from gullet to anus.

x-rays, and endoscopies are performed. Drugs such as laxatives, tranquilizers, and anticholinergic agents are often expended at great cost and some risk in an effort to quell the symptoms. It is even established that individuals with such functional symptoms are liable to suffer unnecessary surgery. Fielding found that 25 of 50 patients with irritable bowel syndrome (IBS) had more than one operation and 16 had more than two. The corresponding figures are five and zero for age-matched controls. Perhaps the greatest costs are the anguish engendered in these patients and the diversion of health care resources from application to more serious disease.

The following is a strategy of management for these conditions. Because there are many irritable gut syndromes (Fig. 22–2), I have selected the IBS as a prototype. The general approach suggested here may be employed with all types of functional gastrointestinal disease.

Management Strategy

The irritable bowel has been defined (see report by Thompson and colleagues) as "a functional disorder attributed to the intestines: abdominal pain; disturbed defecation (ur-

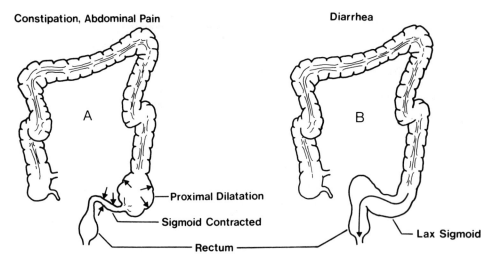

Figure 22–3. Contraction and relaxation of the gut may hold up or release fecal flow, contributing to (A) constipation and abdominal pain and (B) diarrhea. Although this is a useful concept, it cannot be demonstrated in all cases.

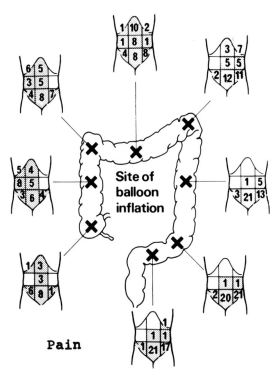

Figure 22–4. *Balloon distention at various gut levels may reproduce abdominal pain. Such trigger points are found in the small bowel as well. From Swarbrick ET, et al. Lancet 2:444–446, 1980, with permission.*

gency, straining, feeling of incomplete evacuation, altered stool form [consistency] and altered bowel frequency/timing); bloatedness (distension)." The many subtypes have been alluded to (Fig. 22–2). Symptoms have been believed to be due to motility disturbance of the gut, but characterization of this disturbance has been elusive (Fig. 22–3). Currently, the disturbance is believed to affect both small and large intestines. Balloon distention studies of the entire gut have suggested that affected individuals may have one or more trigger points from which the abdominal discomfort emanates (Fig. 22–4). It remains uncertain to what extent IBS symptoms are a normal perception of abnormal physiology rather than an abnormal perception of normal physiology.

The cause of the irritable bowel is unknown. The three most important theories are that (1) it is a physiologic disorder awaiting definition, (2) it is a physiologic expression of an emotional or psychiatric disturbance, and (3) the symptoms result from disturbed handling of our Western, fiber-deficient diet. Drugs, attacks of gastroenteritis, and other environmental factors no doubt interact as well.

The approach to a patient with IBS will be discussed in three phases (Table 22–1). Phase I is based on the establishment of a positive diagnosis, reassurance that no serious disease exists, explanation of the possible mechanisms of the syndrome, and establishment of a high bulk diet. Phase II consists of a follow-up visit to ensure compliance and comprehension and to detect previously overlooked organic or inorganic factors. Phase III is the long-term management of the intractable, difficult, or psychologically handicapped patient.

Phase I: The First Clinical Encounter

For reasons that will become apparent, it is important that a *positive diagnosis* be firmly implanted in the physician's and patient's minds on the first clinical visit. The physician must establish credibility with the patient through a careful history and physical examination. There is much evidence that the alert physician may make a diagnosis of the irritable bowel with a high degree of specificity and sensitivity via the patient history. Table 22–2 indicates symptoms found to be more common in IBS than in organic abdominal disease. Figure 22–5 shows how this information may be used. Abdominal pain relieved by defecation, abdominal distention, and looser and more frequent stools with pain onset are individually suggestive of IBS rather than peptic ulcer or inflammatory bowel disease. The more symptoms that are present, the more likely the

Table 22–1. *Management Strategy for the Irritable Bowel*

Phase	Steps in Approach
I	A positive diagnosis
	Establish patient's expectations and reason for consultation
	Reassurance about absence of cancer, benign prognosis
	Explanation of how symptoms are generated
	Initiate bran or other fiber therapy
	Schedule follow-up visit
II	Follow-up visit
	Ensure comprehension
	Encourage compliance
	Develop new strategy for unimproved patient
	Consider alternate diagnoses but resist unindicated tests
	Select drugs suitable for certain syndromes
III	Special strategies for the patient with intractable disease
	Obtain opinion of esteemed colleague in another medical center
	Provide emotional support and continued access to good health care

Table 22–2. *Symptoms More Likely to be Found in IBS Than in Organic Abdominal Disease*

Symptom	Incidence		Significance, P
	Organic Disease	IBS	
Pain eased after bowel movement*	9/30	25/31	<0.01
Looser stools at onset of pain	8/30	25/31	<0.001
More frequent bowel movements at onset of pain	9/30	23/31	<0.01
Abdominal distension	7/33	17/32	<0.01
Mucus per rectum	7/33	15/32	0.05<P<0.1
Feeling of incomplete emptying	11/33	19/32	0.05<P<0.1
	(n = 299)	(n = 108)	
A. Abdominal pain†	55%	96%	0.61
B. Flatulence	50%	85%	<0.4
C. Irregularity	42%	85%	<0.025
A + B + C	10%	70%	<0.0005
Symptoms more than 2 yr	39%	70%	<0.0005
Diarrhea *and* constipation	30%	65%	<0.0005
Pellety stools or mucus	38%	76%	<0.0005

*Manning ARP, Thompson WG, Heaton KW, et al. Bri Med J 2:653–654, 1978 (upper part of table).
†Lower part of table reprinted with permission from A diagnostic score for the irritable bowel syndrome, by Kruis W, Thieme C, Weinzierl M, et al. Gastroenterology, vol 87, pp 1–7. Copyright 1984 by The American Gastroenterological Association.

diagnosis is IBS. Obviously, symptoms such as weight loss, anemia, blood in the stool, and fever cannot be explained by the IBS and require further investigation. A physical examination helps exclude organic disease. Other than the presence of multiple abdominal scars resulting from negative exploratory surgery, there are few agreed upon signs of the irritable bowel. No doubt this process has a therapeutic effect in itself.

Sigmoidoscopy also has an important symbolic or placebo effect on the patient. There are diagnostic benefits, to be sure. Local diseases such as colitis or fissures may be found. Some physicians believe that a finding of scybalous stool, sigmoid spasm, or melanosis coli assists in the diagnosis of functional disease. However, the most important benefit of sigmoidoscopy may be the increased credibility that it imparts to the physician. In patients with noncardiac chest pain, the use of electrocardiography and tests for transaminase levels reassures the patient, lessens symptoms, and returns him or her to work more quickly. The

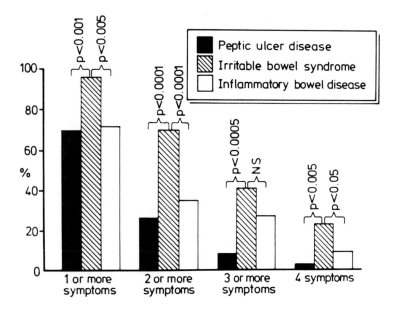

Figure 22–5. *Cumulative symptoms (pain relief with defecation, looser and more frequent bowel movements with pain onset, abdominal distention) in IBS, inflammatory bowel disease, and peptic ulcer. Shown are the percentages of patients with one or more, two or more, three or more, and four of these symptoms. From Thompson WG. Gut 25:1089–1092, 1984, with permission.*

irritable bowel patient may see sigmoidoscopy in a similar light.

A white blood count, hemoglobin, and erythrocyte sedimentation rate are useful screening tests because abnormalities here cannot be explained by functional disease. In the diarrhea-dominant IBS, it may be prudent to measure daily stool weight and analyze the stool for parasites or laxatives; stool weight higher than 500 g/day suggests small bowel disease. The symptoms of the irritable bowel are not those of colon cancer. Nonetheless, colon cancer is a common and much feared disease that one cannot afford to overlook even if it is only incidentally present. Therefore, patients over age 40 should have a barium contrast study of the lower bowel. Once a positive diagnosis of the IBS has been established, the physician is in a position to reassure the patient. This positive approach to diagnosis has recently been endorsed by a working team at the Thirteenth International Congress of Gastroenterology in Rome (see report by Thompson and colleagues).

It has already been stated that up to one third of individuals suffer irritable bowel symptoms but most of them do not go to a physician. Psychosocial or cultural factors may influence this decision. In clinics in the West, 80% of IBS patients are women; on the Indian subcontinent, the opposite is the case. It is therefore important to establish why the patient has chosen this occasion to visit a doctor and what are his or her expectations of the visit. The severity of symptoms is unlikely to be the only reason for consultation. Fear of cancer, recent death in the family from bowel disease, and pressures at home or work may point to the single most important service the physician can render to the IBS patient: reassurance.

Of course, drugs may have an effect on the gut. Dietary factors such as excessive use of coffee, alcohol, and diet drinks should be noted. Lactose intolerance may be encountered in individuals not descended from Northern Europeans. An irritable bowel might be triggered by an attack of acute gastroenteritis. Individuals with this phenomenon are said to have a better prognosis, particularly when they are reassured that the organism that originally caused their diarrhea has long since departed.

In addition to reassurance, an explanation of how the patient's symptoms come about may be useful. Most patients do not know that the large and small intestines constitute up to 20 feet of bowel all curled up in their abdomen. The discomfort and bloating may be confined to the upper abdomen, and patients need to know that there is bowel, as well as stomach, in that area. An explanation, perhaps with the aid of diagrams, is very important. A description of pain emanating from stretching or spasm of the bowel in the area of the gut, or of disordered peristaltic and segmenting movements of the gut causing altered bowel habits may help the patient understand the complexities of the symptoms. This sort of supportive psychotherapy has been long believed to be important in the management of many medical disorders. Such a notion is difficult to prove in the case of the irritable bowel, but Swedish physicians (see Svedlund and colleagues) did show that those individuals treated with eight sessions of "supportive psychotherapy which could be performed in any physician's office" had less abdominal pain and psychological disability at 3 months than those patients not receiving such therapy. This improvement was even more marked 1 year later.

It must also be established that the patient has no serious mental disturbance. Those individuals who see a physician and are referred to specialists are a particularly disturbed subgroup of irritable bowel patients and include some with psychoses, depression, or serious anxieties. I will not discuss their management here. It is important to stress, however, that the IBS patient owes at least some of his or her discomfort to his or her psychosocial environment. Many studies point out that anxiety and depression are common. A threatening life event is more likely to precede the IBS patient's visit to the doctor than that of a patient with organic disease. Among patients undergoing appendectomy, those whose appendix was normal at surgery reported more prior personal difficulties and were more troubled with gut complaints 1 year later than those whose appendix was diseased. The mind and the gut share more than nerves and hormones.

One should also establish the type of irritable bowel from which the patient is suffering (Fig. 22–2). It is unlikely that the spastic type of irritable bowel with dominant abdominal pain, constipation, hard scybalous stools, and the occasional bout of diarrhea has the same pathogenesis as painless diarrhea. Chronic abdominal pain without altered bowel habits, predominant gaseousness, atonic constipation, or other variants may require different therapeutic approaches. These considerations become important if the patient does not respond to initial measures.

In the United States, Canada, and Great

Britain, most physicians employ bran or other commercial bulking agents as a method of increasing dietary fiber. Although the half dozen controlled trials do not strongly support the use of bran, they do show some improvement of constipation and perhaps abdominal pain. The widespread use of this harmless substance attests to most physicians' belief in its usefulness. Unlike pharmacotherapeutic agents, bran has a plausible thesis behind its use based on the epidemiologic studies of Burkett. Bran is unlikely to do harm, although some patients have increased bloating or diarrhea. Irritable bowel symptoms often accompany uncomplicated diverticular disease, and bran is useful for these patients as well.

There are many methods of increasing bulk in the diet. I suggest 1 tablespoon of bran three times a day and ask the patient to increase or decrease this amount according to benefit. I stress to the patient that this is a long-term commitment and that he or she should judge benefit over weeks on the basis of changes in stool consistency and frequency. Patients who tend to pass hard, difficult stools with much straining benefit from the softer, bulkier, more easily passed stools induced by bran. Once the benefits of bran are clear to the patient, it may be integrated into the diet. Fiber substitutes such as bran cookies or psyllium (Metamucil) may be useful for individuals who are unwilling or unable to take bran or who seek a more 'medical" cure for their condition.

In general, drugs should not be used in the treatment of this lifelong, benign condition. Many drugs have been tried and few have shown any benefit. Any assessment of the efficacy of drugs in the irritable bowel must take into account the placebo response, which ranges from 30 to 70%. It is difficult for a pharmacologic agent to improve on that.

Some physicians may choose to use drugs for their placebo effect. This may be justified if there is no risk involved and the cost is moderate. It could be argued, however, that the effect of placebos is transient and that if used at all they should be pharmacologically inert. Certainly, much of the benefit that occurs with the administration of bran or psyllium is a placebo result.

The most important factor in the management of functional disorders is the successful physician-patient encounter. According to Brodie, "a clinical approach that makes the illness experience more understandable to the patient, that instills a sense of care and social support, and that increases a feeling of mastery and control over the course of the illness will be most likely to create a positive placebo response and to improve symptoms." A good physician-patient interaction is not a deception and is indispensable in the management of the irritable bowel. A patient can be helped to understand how the gut works and how it may generate symptoms. With this approach, the patient may be expected to deal more rationally with his or her symptoms and not to "shop for doctors" or turn to charlatans in seeking a cure for a benign but seldom completely curable illness. Under ordinary circumstances, no drug is needed. Careful consideration of the patient's complaint, bran, and reassurance benefit many patients.

It is important to arrange a follow-up visit 6 or 8 weeks after the initial one to ensure compliance and comprehension. Many patients do not understand what they have been told, no matter how skillfully the physician explains. Others may not comply fully with therapy. If the patient has not improved, one may need new tactics. In any event, one must continue to take the patient's symptoms seriously.

Phase II: The Follow-up Visit

A patient who is improved at the follow-up visit may need no further medical care. He or she should, however, have some access to health care should the symptoms return or alter.

The unimproved patient, on the other hand, may require consideration of diagnostic alternatives. An open mind about the irritable bowel sufferer is imperative because he or she is not immune to organic disease even though the original diagnosis may be correct. Thus, a review of the essential features of the history should be carried out. If no new information surfaces, one should resist the temptation to embark on further investigative procedures that may serve only to undermine the patient's confidence in the diagnosis. Patients complaining of altered bowel habits, abdominal pain, and gaseousness need not have procedures such as endoscopy, computerized tomography, ultrasound, or endoscopic retrograde cholangiography.

One might consider the use of drugs for certain specific indications (Table 22–3). For example, in patients with the diarrhea-dominant IBS, loperamide may be effective. Often those with diarrhea suffer incontinence, and

Table 22–3. Drugs Useful for IBS Patients in Certain Situations

Type of IBS	Drug
Diarrhea-dominant IBS	Loperamide, 2–4 mg, PO, t.i.d. maximum
	Cholestyramine, 4 g, PO, t.i.d. maximum
Pain-dominant IBS	Postprandial abdominal pain: dicyclomine, 10–20 mg, PO, before meals
	Chronic pain syndrome: Amitriptyline: individualize dose
	Peppermint oil: placebo
Constipation	Bran, 1 tbsp, PO, t.i.d., and adjust
	Psyllium, 1 tsp, PO, t.i.d., and adjust
Gas	Simethicone, 1 or 2 tablets, PO, t.i.d.

the resulting embarrassment may be the most significant disability. Loperamide appears to increase sphincter tone and, because it does not pass the blood-brain barrier, it is the safest of the opioid antidiarrheal drugs. It might be used selectively by the patient who anticipates a diarrheal attack at the time of an important engagement. The patient who has predictable postprandial abdominal pain may benefit from an anticholinergic administered before meals. The object would be to ensure a maximal anticholinergic blockade when the symptom is expected and minimal side effects. Also, cholestyramine may sometimes be beneficial for the diarrhea-dominant patient. It is probable that the mechanism here is a failure of the ileum to reabsorb endogenous bile salts efficiently. Cholestyramine binds the bile salts in the gut before they can exert their diarrheagenic effect.

Some patients appear to be obsessed with abdominal pain or other severe symptoms. Amitriptyline may provide a dramatic remission even if one cannot determine with certitude that the patient is depressed. The beneficial effect of amitriptyline is not understood, nor is it predictable.

In Great Britain, there has been some excitement about the effect of peppermint oil, a smooth muscle relaxant, on the irritable bowel. However, controlled studies show conflicting results. Peppermint oil appears to be harmless enough, although one should recall that it relaxes the lower esophageal sphincter and may cause heartburn.

Tranquilizing drugs such as the benzodiazepines should be reserved for the obviously anxious patient. There is little evidence to support them as a primary treatment for the irritable bowel. It is worth emphasizing that the IBS affects patients for long periods of their lives and that no drug, especially a tranquilizer, should be considered to be a long-term solution.

Of those patients who are unimproved on the follow-up visit, many are unlikely to achieve satisfaction. Much patience is required for encouragement, discussion, and reassurance because the patient's need for these is great. Certainly, access to continuing medical care is important lest such patients fall into the hands of unscrupulous profiteers.

Phase III: The Unsatisfied Patient

Most physicians see unsatisfied IBS patients in their practice. Such individuals challenge one's skill in dealing with anxiety, depression, and often hostility. Should the physician-patient relationship deteriorate, one may wish to consider certain referral options. If the patient is obviously disturbed, psychiatric consultation may be useful. There are anecdotal reports of success with biofeedback, but such facilities are available in few centers. Hypnosis has been tried in resistant cases, but controlled trials of this method are difficult to perform. It is essential that the physician retain overall control of the patient's care, particularly because the above-mentioned treatments may have no lasting benefit.

Since its recognition, the IBS has been thought to be due to some factor in the diet. Most reports are anecdotal. In diarrhea-dominant IBS patients in Cambridge, an elimination diet was effective in identifying sensitivity (not an allergy) to wheat, milk, poultry, or other foods. Although the Cambridge group reported excellent results when these items were removed from the diet, their data were not confirmed elsewhere.

The patient with intractable disease may lose confidence in the physician. In this event it may be useful to refer him or her to a colleague. It is important for the physician to take the initiative here rather than let the patient seek help on his or her own. The consultant, preferably in another medical center, should reinforce the diagnosis and endorse the plan of management. This may make subsequent care by the primary physician easier.

Prognosis

The irritable bowel is a benign condition and the prognosis in terms of life expectancy is

Table 22–4. Prognosis in the IBS

Author*	Number of Patients	Years of Follow-up	% Symptomatic	Comment
Chaudhary 1962	126	1–10	63	
Waller 1969	50	1	88	
Holmes 1982	77	6	57	Diagnosis changed in 4
Harvey 1987	97	5–8	74	No change in diagnosis (26% severe)

*Chaudhary NA, Truelove SC. The irritable colon syndrome. Q J Med 31:307–322, 1962. Waller SL, Misiewicz JJ. Prognosis in the irritable bowel syndrome: a prospective study. Lancet 2:753–756, 1969. Holmes IM, Salter RH. Irritable bowel syndrome—a safe diagnosis. Br Med J 285:1533–1534, 1982. Harvey RF, Mauad AC, Brown AM. Prognosis in the irritable bowel syndrome: a 5 year prospective study. Lancet 1:963–965, 1987.

excellent. In terms of continued symptoms, the outlook is not as good. Several European studies indicate that more than 50% of individuals with the irritable bowel retain their symptoms 1 to 10 years later (Table 22–4). It would appear that children with recurrent abdominal pain are likely to have the IBS as adults. It is reassuring to note, however, that several of these follow-up studies indicate that there is seldom a need to change the original diagnosis. The results of these studies suggest that not only is the irritable bowel a chronic condition affecting people over long periods of their lives, but also that it is a stable diagnosis infrequently requiring change.

Conclusion

Irritable bowel symptoms occur in almost one third of the population. Most of these patients do not see a physician, but those who do constitute up to 50% of gastroenterology referrals in Western countries. The reason why the person with IBS sees a physician and thereby becomes a patient may be the most important factor in the history. By establishing rapport with the patient, making a positive diagnosis of the irritable bowel, and showing concern for the patient's psychosocial state, the physician may do much to reassure the patient. Bran is very useful in the treatment of constipation and perhaps through a placebo effect can lead to a remission in most patients. Nonetheless, the irritable bowel is often a lifelong disorder, and a follow-up visit and easy access to the physician are important if the patient is not to be overinvestigated and maltreated. In most instances, drugs should be avoided. The unsatisfied patient requires much of the physician's time. He or she may benefit from a judicious referral, but the physician should retain control of overall care because such patients are liable to undergo unnecessary surgery and to suffer inappropriate ministrations of unscrupulous practitioners of alternative medicine.

Bibliography

Brodie H. The lie that heals: the ethics of giving placebos. Ann Intern Med 97:112–118, 1982.
This is a thoughtful discussion of the ethics and efficacy of placebos.
Drossman DA, Sandler RS, McKee DC, et al. Bowel dysfunction among subjects not seeking health care. Gastroenterology 83:529–534, 1982.
This article indicates that most IBS sufferers do not seek medical advice and raises the question "Why?"
Heaton KW. Role of dietary fibre in irritable bowel syndrome, in Read NW (ed). Irritable Bowel Syndrome. London, Grune & Stratton, 1985, pp 203–222.
Heaton reviews the evidence that bran is useful in IBS.
Kingham JGC, Dawson AM. Origin of chronic right upper-quadrant pain. Gut 26:783–788, 1985.
IBS symptoms originate at any level of the gut and may be felt in any quadrant of the abdomen.
Klein KB. Controlled treatment trials in the irritable bowel syndrome: a critique. Gastroenterology 95:232–241, 1988.
Manning AP, Thompson WG, Heaton KW, et al. Towards a more positive diagnosis of the irritable bowel. Br Med J 2:653–654, 1978.
Certain symptoms serve to distinguish IBS from organic bowel disease.
Svedlund J, Sjödin I, Ottosson JO, et al. Controlled study of psychotherapy in the irritable bowel syndrome. Lancet 2:589–592, 1983.
This is, perhaps, proof that supportive psychotherapy by physicians is effective.
Swarbrick ET, Hagarty JE, Bat L, et al. Site of pain from the irritable bowel. Lancet 2:443–446, 1980.
IBS symptoms originate at any level of the gut and may be felt in any quadrant of the abdomen.
Thompson WG. The irritable bowel. Gut 25:305–320, 1984.
This article summarizes current concepts of etiology and pathogenesis.
Thompson WG. Gastrointestinal symptoms in the irritable bowel compared with peptic ulcer and inflammatory bowel disease. Gut 25:1089–1092, 1984.
Certain symptoms serve to distinguish IBS from organic bowel disease.
Thompson WG. A strategy for management of the irritable bowel. Am J Gastroenterol 81:95–100, 1986.

This article evaluates putative treatment methods, with references.

Thompson WG. Irritable bowel syndrome: prevalence, prognosis and consequences. Can Med Assoc J 134:111–112, 1986.

The worldwide occurrence of the IBS and its costs are reviewed.

Thompson WG, Dotevall G, Drossman DA, et al. Working team report: irritable bowel syndrome: guidelines for the diagnosis. Thirteenth International Congress of Gastroenterology, Rome, Italy, September 6, 1988. Gastroenterol Int. In press.

Thompson WG, Keaton KW. Functional bowel disorders in apparently healthy people. Gastroenterology 79:283–288, 1980.

Most IBS sufferers do not seek medical advice and raise the question "Why?"

Whitehead WE, Winget C, Fedaravicious AS, et al. Learned illness behaviour in patients with irritable bowel syndrome and peptic ulcer. Dig Dis Sci 27:202–208, 1982.

This paper discusses the notion that IBS symptoms are learned during childhood.

PART FIVE

Genitourinary System

23

Evaluation of Proteinuria and Hematuria

J. GARY ABUELO, M.D.

Introduction

Proteinuria and hematuria are common abnormalities found in the laboratory. When discovered during the investigation of an illness, they may indicate that the illness involves the kidneys. When found during a routine urinalysis, they may be the first sign of a serious problem such as chronic glomerulonephritis (GN) or a malignancy of the urinary tract. Consequently, the physician must always evaluate the urinary abnormality, even though sometimes it may require the use of costly, painful, or potentially dangerous procedures such as arteriography, retrograde pyelography, or a renal biopsy in well-appearing individuals.

Fortunately, proteinuria and hematuria often are caused by benign and transient conditions such as strenuous exercise or urinary drainage with a Foley catheter. In such cases, the diagnosis may be confirmed by simple observation and extensive testing may be avoided. To guide the physician in the investigation of urinary abnormalities, I will discuss the causes and diagnosis of proteinuria and hematuria. Emphasis will be placed on the early recognition of benign conditions and the tailoring of the evaluation to the specific characteristics of the case.

Proteinuria

Definitions

Normal urine contains many proteins in small amounts, such as transferrin, immunoglobulins, enzymes, and hormones, including insulin. These proteins either are produced within the kidney or genitourinary tract or are filtered from the plasma by the glomeruli. Tamm-Horsfall protein, a glycoprotein of unknown function made in the renal tubule, comprises almost half the urinary protein (~50 mg/day). Albumin is the other major protein in the urine. Because a large amount of albumin circulates through the glomerular capillaries, some 5 to 25 mg/day appears in the urine, despite limited filtration by the glomeruli and up to 90% reabsorption by the tubules.

Proteinuria is urine protein excretion in greater than normal amounts. It is usually defined in terms of protein lost per day. The upper limit of normal is 150 mg/day for adults and 300 mg/day for children, adolescents, and pregnant women.

Nephrotic syndrome is the edematous state produced by hypoalbuminemia that results from heavy loss of albumin in the urine. Nephrotic syndrome may also lead to hyperlipidemia, susceptibility to bacterial infection, and thromboembolic complications. It is always caused by a glomerular disease. The serum albumin concentration is 3 g/dl or less, and the urine protein level is 3 g/day or more in adults and 50 mg/kg per day or more in children.

Nephrotic range proteinuria is urine protein excretion in the range expected in patients with nephrotic syndrome (given above) regardless of the serum albumin level or presence of edema. Like nephrotic syndrome, it indicates a glomerular disease. Edema may not occur either because the liver increases albumin production enough to maintain the serum albumin level higher than 3 g/dl or because factors prevent fluid accumulation, such as use of diuretics or a low salt diet prescribed for hypertension.

Benign proteinuria refers to transient or intermittent proteinuria produced by a variety of conditions (Table 23–1), in which renal involvement is benign or potentially reversible. There are none of the usual signs of kidney disease; blood urea nitrogen (BUN) and serum creatinine (Scr) levels, intravenous pyelography results, and urine sediment tests are normal.

Etiology

The causes of proteinuria are given in Table 23–1. Which of these conditions is most common depends on the setting in which the proteinuria is discovered. In apparently well children, adolescents, and young adults, the incidence of a positive urine test for protein may be 1% or more, but about 90% of these patients have benign proteinuria, either the idiopathic transient or the orthostatic type. Similarly, about 10% of adults admitted to a hospital through an emergency room have proteinuria, but this is almost always a benign functional type. Patients with nephrotic syndrome generally have a primary glomerulopathy like membranous GN or have one of three secondary glomerular diseases: diabetic nephropathy, lupus nephritis, or renal amyloidosis.

Pathogenesis

False proteinuria may be produced in dehydrated individuals whose urine volume is so reduced that normal amounts of protein are concentrated enough to give a positive qualitative (screening) test for proteinuria. Gross hematuria may mimic renal protein loss because of the serum protein in the admixed blood and also possibly because of hemoglobin released from the red cells. False-positive tests for protein may also be produced in a few other situations (Table 23–1).

Overload proteinuria is due to the overproduction of a low molecular weight protein, such as immunoglobulin light chains (Bence Jones protein) in multiple myeloma. The high plasma concentration of these protein molecules together with their small size causes them

Table 23–1. Causes of Proteinuria

Type of Proteinuria	Cause

False	Dipstick method
	    Highly concentrated urine
	    Gross hematuria
	    Highly alkaline urine, pH > 8 (e.g., urinary infection with urea-splitting bacteria)
	    Phenazopyridine (e.g., Pyridium)
	    Antiseptic contamination (chlorhexidine or benzalkonium)
	Protein precipitation methods (qualitative or 24-h urine tests)
	    Highly concentrated urine
	    Gross hematuria
	    Radiographic contrast media
	    Drugs: tolbutamide (e.g., Orinase), sulfonamides, tolmetin (Tolectin), high levels of penicillin or cephalosporin analogues

Overload	Immunoglobulin light chains: monoclonal gammopathies (e.g., multiple myeloma) Lysozyme: myelomonocytic leukemia Myoglobin: traumatic and nontraumatic rhabdomyolysis Hemoglobin: massive hemolysis
Glomerular	Primary glomerulopathies (e.g., lipoid nephrosis) Secondary glomerulopathies (e.g., diabetic nephropathy)
Tubular	Tubular disease (e.g., Fanconi's syndrome, cisplatin or gentamicin toxicity) Interstitial disease (e.g., pyelonephritis, acute interstitial nephritis)

Benign	Idiopathic transient proteinuria
	Functional proteinuria
	    Fever
	    Congestive heart failure
	    Exercise
	    Essential hypertension
	    Emotional stress
	    Burns
	    Acute pancreatitis
	Orthostatic (postural) proteinuria

to filter through the glomeruli in abnormally large amounts, so that tubular reabsorption, which is usually complete, is overwhelmed and the protein appears in the urine.

Glomerular proteinuria occurs when the glomerular capillary wall loses its capacity to act as a filtration barrier and leaks plasma proteins, especially albumin, into the urinary space. The degree of proteinuria may range from minimal to nephrotic. This type of proteinuria is seen with idiopathic primary glomerulopathies and glomerular lesions secondary to multisystem disease. The exact mechanism for the abnormally increased glomerular permeability for proteins is not understood.

Tubular proteinuria is due to low molecular weight proteins (molecular weight 10,000 to 70,000) that are normally filtered by the glomeruli and reabsorbed by the tubules. Incomplete reabsorption by poorly functioning tubules allows these proteins to escape into the urine. The underlying cause may be a variety of tubular and interstitial diseases.

Benign proteinuria includes functional and orthostatic types. The proteinuria in these conditions occurs because of either tubular or glomerular dysfunction, but the exact mechanism is unclear.

Clinical Picture

Severe proteinuria may cause the nephrotic syndrome, but in most cases proteinuria does not produce edema or other symptoms. On the other hand, the patient may have signs of renal disease such as hypertension or uremia or manifestations of whatever systemic disease that is causing the proteinuria.

Diagnostic Process

THE QUALITATIVE PROTEIN TEST

Proteinuria is almost always first detected with a qualitative protein test (Fig. 23–1) carried out as part of the urinalysis. Qualitative tests rather than 24-hour urine tests are used for proteinuria screening because of the collection errors and inconvenience entailed in obtaining a 24-hour urinalysis. The qualitative assay used in most laboratories is the dipstick method, in which a chemically impregnated paper strip changes color in the presence of protein. It detects trace proteinuria with urine

protein concentrations between 10 and 20 mg/dl and gives a clear 1+ (30 mg/dl) or greater positive result in most patients with proteinuria. A result of 3+ (300 mg/dl) or greater usually corresponds to nephrotic-range proteinuria.

If a patient with proteinuria has a high urine volume output, the urine protein concentration may be diluted to below the level of detectibility of the qualitative test. Because high urine volume produces low specific gravity (SG) of the urine, a general rule is that the qualitative test may give a false-negative result and is therefore not reliable if the SG is less than 1.015. Conversely, low urine volume produces a concentrated urine (SG ~1.030) and may cause a false-positive protein test. A rule of thumb that may be used to correct for high (> 1.025) or low (< 1.015) SG is that the upper limit of normal of urine protein concentration is the last two digits in the urine SG (e.g., 5 mg/dl for SG = 1.005; 29 mg/dl for SG = 1.029).

After finding a positive qualitative test for protein, the physician should perform two or more repeat tests during the next several days to determine if the proteinuria is transient, intermittent, or constant.

TRANSIENT PATTERN OF PROTEIN EXCRETION

Proteinuria without hematuria is detected in about 5% of apparently healthy children and young adults during routine urinalysis for athletic teams, school admission, induction into the armed forces, new employment, or life insurance. Most of these individuals have an idiopathic transient proteinuria, and repeated urine protein tests are negative. Transient proteinuria may also be produced by fever, strenuous exercise, seizures, heart failure, and hypertension. This functional proteinuria may disappear within a day or so if the precipitating event is resolved. These two transient forms of benign proteinuria are not associated with adverse long-term renal effects, and no further studies or follow-up investigation is necessary.

INTERMITTENT AND CONSTANT PATTERNS OF PROTEIN EXCRETION (Fig. 23–2)

Patients whose proteinuria is not transient should undergo a complete history and physical examination aimed especially at identifying multisystem conditions, renal signs and symptoms, and previously unrecognized functional

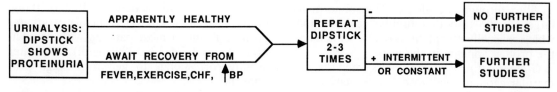

Figure 23–1. *Diagrammatic representation of the initial evaluation of proteinuria.* CHF, *congestive heart failure;* BP, *blood pressure.*

proteinuria. The physician should ask about diabetes mellitus, arthralgia, myalgia, rash, weight loss, fever, gross hematuria, edema, hypertension, urinary tract infections, urinary symptoms, family history of kidney disease, and strenuous exercise. Bone pain or unexplained anemia in a patient older than 40 or 50 years of age raises the question of multiple myeloma. Old medical records need to be examined for previous urinalyses, Scr, and BUN test results, and renal imaging. In reviewing the patient's medications, physicians should be aware that phenazopyridine and other agents may cause false proteinuria (Table 23–1); nonsteroidal anti-inflammatory drugs, particularly fenoprofen, can cause lipoid

nephrosis; many drugs, particularly penicillin and cephalosporin analogues, may trigger allergic interstitial nephritis; and gold, penicillamine, captopril, and trimethadione can cause membranous GN. The physical examination detects fever, congestive heart failure, rash, edema, and hypertension. Further investigation of clues found during the history and physical examination often leads to a diagnosis.

Laboratory Tests. Laboratory studies should include a complete urinalysis, BUN or Scr, and a 24-hour urine test for protein and creatinine to verify and quantitate the degree of protein excretion. Individuals over 40 years of age need to be tested for occult diabetes mel-

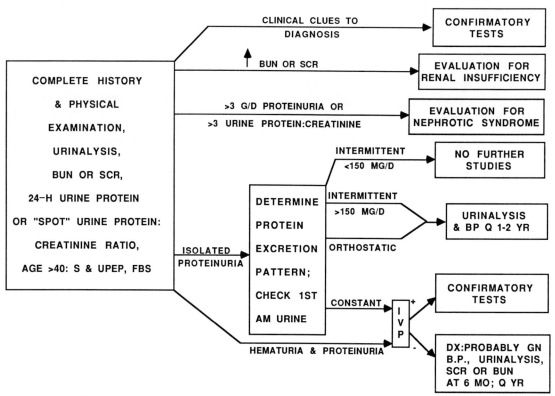

Figure 23–2. *Diagrammatic representation of further steps in the evaluation of proteinuria.* FBS, *fasting blood glucose;* GN, *glomerulonephritis;* IVP, *intravenous pyelogram,* S & UPEP, *serum and urine protein electrophoresis.*

litus and monoclonal gammopathy via a fasting blood glucose analysis and serum and urine protein electrophoresis.

The 24-hour urine test for creatinine is checked to see that the urine specimen was neither an under- nor an over-collection. The amount of creatinine excreted in the urine each day depends on the patient's muscle mass and is constant and predictable. About 1500 mg/day is excreted by an average-sized ($\sim$ 150 lb) young or middle-aged man, and more than 2000 mg/day is excreted by a large muscular man. Young and middle-aged women excrete between 800 and 1400 mg depending on size. Creatinine excretion decreases with age and may be as low as 500 to 700 mg in small elderly individuals. With these figures as guidelines, one can confirm that a proper urine collection was obtained. A formula for predicting creatinine excretion may also be used:

$$\text{Creatinine excreted/day (mg)}$$
$$= \frac{(140 - \text{age}) \times \text{weight} \times 0.85}{5}$$

Where age is given in years, weight is given in kilograms, and 0.85 is used if the patient is female.

Some physicians now use the ratio of protein to creatinine in a single voided urine sample instead of the 24-hour urinary protein test to verify and quantitate proteinuria. The ratio is calculated by dividing protein concentration (mg/dl) by creatinine concentration (mg/dl). The upper limit of normal is 0.2 and the nephrotic range is higher than 3.0. The urine sample may be obtained at any time of day, but the most accurate sample is collected after the first voided morning urine but before noon.

If the quantitation shows nephrotic-range proteinuria when the dipstick test result is only 1 to 2 +, one should consider the possibility of multiple myeloma. The explanation is that the dipstick test is not very sensitive to immunoglobulin light chains, which can be excreted in massive amounts by myeloma patients.

Red blood cells (RBCs) and RBC casts in the urine are evidence of GN. This may be a complication of a multisystem disease like bacterial endocarditis, in which case an investigation of the extrarenal manifestations may lead to a diagnosis without the need for a renal biopsy. More often the GN is a primary renal disease such as immunoglobulin (Ig)A nephropathy. One would need a tissue sample to diagnose the type of GN. However, in the absence of nephrotic-range proteinuria or renal insufficiency, renal biopsies are usually not considered because there is no established treatment for these diseases. Instead, intravenous pyelography should be done to exclude renal cell carcinoma, cystic disease, renal tuberculosis, papillary necrosis, and obstructive or reflux nephropathy. If this pyelogram is normal, the blood pressure, urinalysis, and serum creatinine level should be checked after 6 months and then yearly. The GNs that produce proteinuria and hematuria may resolve, but they also have the potential to produce hypertension, nephrotic syndrome, or chronic renal failure. If hypertension is detected during these follow-up evaluations, it should be treated with the usual medications.

Patients who present with or develop nephrotic-range proteinuria or azotemia should be evaluated according to guidelines given in standard texts. Consultation with a nephrologist is usually advisable in these cases because there may be a need for a renal biopsy, immunosuppressive therapy, or dialysis.

Additional tests should be ordered in certain cases. Patients with arthralgias, rash, or other findings suggestive of systemic lupus erythematosus require an antinuclear antibody test. In patients with a history suggestive of impetigo or streptococcal pharyngitis, serum should be analyzed for antistreptococcal enzyme titers and complement (C3 and C4), and throat or skin cultures should be taken. Complement studies are also helpful for any individual with hematuria and proteinuria because hypocomplementemia occurs with several GNs that produce a nephritic syndrome. The nephritic syndrome is proteinuria and hematuria with or without azotemia and fluid retention.

At this point, the physician may still have an undiagnosed patient with isolated proteinuria, i.e., proteinuria in the face of a normal history, physical examination, urinary sediment test, and other laboratory tests. The management of these patients depends on the pattern of protein excretion. On repeating the qualitative urine protein test, four patterns may be found:

1. The proteinuria may be *transient*. This benign pattern is either idiopathic or functional, as discussed earlier (Fig. 23–1).

2a. Proteinuria may be *intermittent*, i.e., about half the tests are positive, with less than 150 mg protein excreted/day.

Situations 1 and 2a are benign and no further evaluation or follow-up tests are needed.

2b. An *intermittent* pattern may also be associated with more than 150 mg protein excreted/day.

3. The proteinuria may be *orthostatic*, in which urine formed during recumbency (e.g., the first voided urine in the morning) is negative for proteinuria, but urine formed after standing or walking is positive. To identify such a pattern, patients with apparently constant proteinuria should have a first-morning urine sample tested.

Patients with either of these two excretion patterns (2b and 3) are at slight risk, if any, for chronic renal disease and usually become free of proteinuria. They should be seen every year or two for a urinalysis and blood pressure determination until the proteinuria disappears. If the proteinuria becomes constant or does not disappear, the BUN or Scr should also be evaluated at the periodic visits.

4. The proteinuria may be *constant*. This proteinuria is usually associated with mild glomerular abnormalities. Most patients have a benign course and often experience a remission. A more severe glomerular lesion is found in some cases and is probably responsible for the facts that hypertension often develops and perhaps 20% of patients develop renal insufficiency. Renal biopsies are not recommended because proven treatment for these lesions is not available. Patients with constant proteinuria should have intravenous pyelography or a renal ultrasound test to identify the rare cysts, tumors, and other structural abnormalities mentioned earlier. If these results are negative, the patient should have blood pressure, urinalysis, and BUN or Scr checked after 6 months and then yearly. If hypertension is noted, it should be treated with the usual antihypertensive drugs. If azotemia or nephrotic-range proteinuria develops, it should be evaluated by standard methods, and nephrologic consultation is advisable.

Hematuria

Definition

Normal urine contains a variable number of RBCs; their pathway from the blood stream to the urine is unknown. Hematuria is defined as five or more RBCs per high power field on microscopic examination of the urinary sediment. A false-positive dipstick test for blood may be produced by free hemoglobin or myoglobin, so that true hematuria must be confirmed by microscopic examination.

Etiology

Hematuria may be produced anywhere along the urinary tract and has numerous possible causes (Table 23–2). In children and

Table 23–2. Causes of Hematuria

Type of Hematuria	Cause
False	Vaginal bleeding
	Factitious
	Pigmenturia
	Endogenous
	Porphyrin
	Hemoglobin
	Myoglobin
	Exogenous
	Drugs (see Table 23–3)
	Food (beets, blackberries, rhubarb)
Hematologic	Hemorrhagic disorders (including anticoagulation)
	Sickle cell hemoglobinopathies (sickle cell anemia and trait and other forms)
Renal (glomerular)	Primary glomerulopathies (e.g., IgA nephropathy)
	Secondary glomerulopathy (e.g., lupus nephritis)
Renal (nonglomerular)	Infections
	Pyelonephritis
	Tuberculosis
	Leptospirosis
	Viral nephritis
	Malformations
	Cystic
	Vascular
	Neoplasms
	Ischemia
	Embolism
	Cortical or papillary necrosis
	Arterial or venous thrombosis
	Trauma
	Hypersensitivity
	Vasculitis
	Allergic nephritis
Postrenal	Mechanical damage
	Stones
	Obstruction
	Vesicoureteral reflux
	Foreign bodies
	Foley catheter
	Inflammation
	Periureteritis due to an extraureteral process
	Prostatitis
	Epididymitis
	Urethritis
	Cystitis (bacterial, schistosomal, viral, drug-induced, radiation, idiopathic)
	Neoplasms
	Endometriosis
	Benign prostatic hypertrophy
	Strenuous exercise

adolescents, a mild proliferative GN like IgA nephropathy causes about half the cases. This type of GN often produces no hypertension, fluid overload, azotemia, proteinuria, or RBC casts and is easily missed. The second most common cause of hematuria in children is urinary tract infection. In adults, the most common etiologies (and approximate prevalences) are neoplasms (15%), bacterial infections of the urine (15%), urolithiasis (20%), mild proliferative forms of GN (20%), and benign prostatic hypertrophy (20%).

Pathogenesis

False hematuria may be caused by the admixing of extraneous blood in the urine because of vaginal bleeding or the deceptive act of a patient. Blood-tinged urine may be mimicked by a variety of red or brown pigments in the urine (Table 23–2). Some pigments derive from ingested food and drugs; others, like hemoglobin or myoglobin, also give a positive dipstick test for blood.

Hematologic hematuria may be one of two types. The urinary bleeding observed with *sickle cell hemoglobinopathies* probably takes place from dilated capillaries or small infarcts in the medulla of the kidney. Anticoagulants are the most common cause of bleeding related to a *hemorrhagic disorder*. One must fully evaluate these patients, even those who receive excessive amounts of anticoagulants, because an occult urologic malignancy or other lesion that is bleeding as a result of the defective coagulation is often the actual source of hematuria.

Glomerular hematuria may occur when RBCs leak or squeeze through defects or weak points in the glomerular capillary wall. This mechanism is conjectural because it has only rarely been observed during electron microscopy of renal biopsies. The urinary RBCs of patients with GN often appear under the microscope to be fragmented, collapsed, and devoid of hemoglobin. It may be that the RBCs are fragmented by squeezing through the glomerular capillary wall and that they then lose their hemoglobin in the extremely dilute segments of the renal tubule because of osmotic shock. The finding of such dysmorphic or "glomerular" RBCs in exercise-related hematuria is evidence that the glomerular capillaries are the source of hematuria in this condition. The use of urine RBC morphology in the diagnosis of glomerular hematuria is not widely employed because the reliability of the test is not established and it is not performed in most laboratories.

Clinical Picture

Hematuria is usually microscopic and asymptomatic. It may have been present for years and is discovered by chance when a urinalysis is ordered during a routine checkup. On the other hand, macroscopic (or gross) hematuria is a frightening experience and usually brings the patient promptly to medical attention. If the bleeding source is in the bladder, prostate, or urethra, the patient may have gross hematuria only at the beginning or end of micturition. In addition to the hematuria, the underlying disease may produce a variety of signs and symptoms, which will be discussed later.

Diagnostic Process

THE URINALYSIS

The investigation for hematuria begins by confirming its presence by finding five or more RBCs per high power field during a complete urinalysis (Fig. 23–3). Pigmenturia produces bloody colored urine or a positive dipstick test for blood, but no RBCs on microscopic examination. The urinalysis is of additional value in that it shows more than two white blood cells per high power field and more than one bacterium per high power field in most patients with hematuria related to urinary tract infection; a 3 to 4+ (300 to 1000 mg/dl) result for the qualitative protein test in subjects with the nephrotic syndrome; and red cell casts or a qualitative protein result of 1 to 2+ (30 to 100 mg/dl) in patients with renal hematuria, especially if it is due to GN.

Microscopic hematuria is often transient, and one should look for RBCs in urinalyses repeated two or three times during several weeks to see the pattern of blood loss. Patients with constant or intermittent microscopic hematuria require further evaluation, as do all patients with gross hematuria. Because of the increasing incidence of malignancy with age, the physician may also wish to study individuals over 40 years of age having a single urinalysis showing microscopic hematuria, particularly if subsequent "negative" urinalyses reveal one to four RBCs per high power field. The

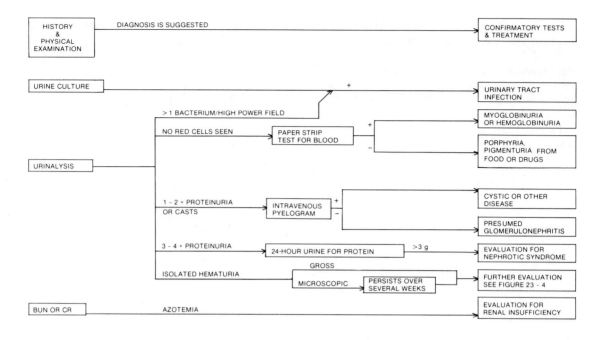

Figure 23–3. *Diagrammatic representation of initial evaluation of hematuria. From Abuelo JG. Urology 21:215–225, 1983, with permission.*

evaluation for hematuria begins with a thorough history and physical examination, BUN or Scr analysis, and a urine culture.

THE HISTORY

Patients with gross hematuria should be asked if they have bloody urine only at the beginning or end of micturition, which would indicate a lower urinary tract source. A lower tract lesion is also suggested by the presence of bright red urine in contrast to the brown or reddish-brown urine that is typical of GN. Moreover, clots in the urine imply a postglomerular source. Patients should also be asked if they have had symptoms of a urinary or upper respiratory tract infection. (Gross hematuria or microhematuria is seen with cystitis and pyelonephritis and with some forms of GN 1 day to 3 weeks after a streptococcal pharyngitis or common cold.) A history of living or traveling abroad raises the possibility of hematuria related to schistosomiasis or tuberculosis. Microscopic or even gross hematuria may occur after strenuous physical activity or after trauma to the urethra, pelvis, flank, or abdomen, so that one must inquire about these causative events. On rare occasion, drugs can induce hematuria by several mechanisms (Table 23–

3). Therefore, a list of medications taken by the patient should be obtained. The physician ought to ask about flank pain, which can accompany urinary obstruction, renal tumors, or acute exacerbations of GN. Renal colic is usually due to a stone that moves through a ureter but may be produced by the passage of a sloughed necrotic papilla or blood clots. The physician must be alert to excessive bruising or bleeding or to symptoms of multisystem disease like fever, arthralgias, or rash. If the history is bizarre or puzzling, factitious hematuria might be considered. The family history may reveal urolithiasis (e.g., cystinuria) or renal disease (Alport's syndrome, benign familial hematuria, or polycystic kidney disease). Finally, previous urinalyses, radiologic studies, and urologic or renal evaluations should be reviewed.

PHYSICAL EXAMINATION

Important physical signs to look for include manifestations of acute GN (hypertension and volume overload); abdominal, pelvic, or prostatic tenderness or masses; and signs of multisystem disease (fever, rashes, arthritis, and so on). Lesions of the urethra may be discovered by palpation of the terminal urethra and inspection of the orifice.

Table 23–3. Drug-Induced Hematuria

Condition	Drug
Allergic interstitial nephritis	Penicillin and cephalosporin analogues, phenindione, phenytoin
Papillary necrosis	Nonsteroidal anti-inflammatory agents
Chemical cystitis	Cyclophosphamide, ifosfamide, mitotane
Malignant neoplasm of the uroepithelium	Cyclophosphamide
Spontaneous bleeding or induction of bleeding by an occult lesion	Anticoagulants
Endogenous pigmenturia (hemoglobinuria caused by glucose-6-phosphate dehydrogenase deficiency)	Nitrofurantoin, primaquine, quinacrine, sulfonamides, and others
Exogenous pigmenturia	Clofazimine, chloroquine phosphate, chlorzoxazone, daunorubicin hydrochloride, deferoxamine mesylate, doxorubicin hydrochloride, ibuprofen, indandione anticoagulants, laxatives with cascara, phenolphthalein or senna, levodopa, methyldopa, nitrofurantoin, phenazopyridine hydrochloride, phenothiazines, phensuximide, quinine sulfate, rifampin, sulfamethoxazole, sulfasalazine

From Abuelo JG. Arch Intern Med May 1983, vol 143, p 969, Copyright 1983, American Medical Association.

FURTHER INVESTIGATION

The diagnosis is often suggested from the history and physical examination and usually can be confirmed by appropriate tests. Although benign prostatic hypertrophy may be a cause of bleeding, other causes must be excluded. Women with symptomatic cystitis may have colony counts less than 10^5 organisms per ml. A positive urine culture result together with pyuria is an indication for antibiotic therapy, after which one must check for the disappearance of hematuria. If the BUN or Scr concentration is elevated, the azotemia should be investigated. Patients with proteinuria are managed as outlined earlier.

As many as 80% of patients with isolated hematuria are still undiagnosed at this point (Fig. 23–4). They should have intravenous pyelography with nephrotomography, urethroscopy, and cystoscopy. Cystoscopy is preferably carried out during the passage of grossly bloody urine to detect unilateral hematuria. If the intravenous pyelogram does not provide a clear view of the kidneys and collecting system, retrograde pyelography can be performed. After these procedures, the proportion of undiagnosed cases falls to about 20%.

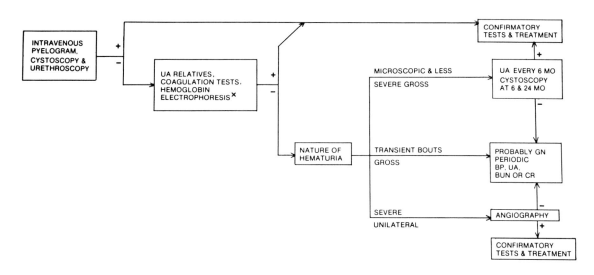

Figure 23–4. Diagrammatic representation of further diagnostic steps in adults with hematuria. UA, urinalysis; URI, upper respiratory infection. From Abuelo JG. Urology 21:215–225, 1983, with permission.

If none of these studies reveals the cause of bleeding, one should look for benign familial hematuria by performing urinalyses in first-degree relatives, evaluate the patient's hemostasis (platelet count, bleeding time, prothrombin time, and partial thromboplastin time), and perform electrophoresis of hemoglobin to exclude sickle cell hemoglobinopathies in individuals of black or Mediterranean ancestry.

Further investigation of individuals still undiagnosed at this point depends on the nature of the hematuria. Some patients have recurrent transient bouts of bilateral gross hematuria triggered in some cases by upper respiratory infections. One can be reasonably certain that they have an IgA or similar nephropathy even without such classic signs of GN as hypertension, azotemia, proteinuria, or RBC casts. These patients may have a remission or may have microhematuria for years or continued bouts of gross hematuria. Chronic renal insufficiency occurs rarely if at all in the absence of proteinuria. One may follow such patients yearly by means of urinalysis and measurement of blood pressure and BUN or Scr levels. Because of the lack of proven therapy for these nephropathies, renal biopsies are not recommended.

Patients with microhematuria probably also have an IgA or similar nephropathy but could have a small radiolucent stone or an occult carcinoma of the bladder. Therefore, urinalyses are done every 6 months for 2 years, and cystoscopy should be repeated at 6 months and 2 years. Thereafter, these patients should have the same yearly follow-up visits as patients with bouts of hematuria triggered by common colds.

Patients with severe, unilateral gross hematuria may also have GN, but one must exclude small renal cell carcinomas or arteriovenous malformations that were not seen on the intravenous pyelogram. Consequently, arteriography and perhaps even dynamic computed tomography of the abdomen should be performed. If no lesion is seen, further investigation should be limited to yearly follow-up visits for the presumed GN.

From time to time the physician may need to evaluate hematuria in an adolescent. The approach outlined earlier should be modified for this age group because of the extreme rarity of bladder malignancy. Thus, cytoscopy is indicated only for patients with severe prolonged gross hematuria which can result from a vascular malformation of a kidney or the bladder. In addition, a 24-hour urine test for creatinine and calcium is necessary to exclude the recently reported association of hematuria with hypercalciuria.

Bibliography

Abuelo JG. Evaluation of hematuria. Urology 21:215–225, 1983.
 A referenced, up-to-date discussion of the etiology and diagnosis of hematuria.
Abuelo JG. Proteinuria: diagnostic principles and procedures. Ann Intern Med 98:186–191, 1983.
 A referenced, up-to-date discussion of the etiology and diagnosis of proteinuria.
Benson GS, Brewer ED. Hematuria: algorithms for diagnosis. II. Hematuria in the adult and hematuria secondary to trauma. JAMA 246:993–995, 1981.
 A good discussion of the evaluation of hematuria secondary to trauma.
Chavers BM, Vernier RL. Proteinuria and enzymuria. Semin Nephrol 6:371–388, 1986.
 A referenced review of the laboratory methods for measurement of urine protein and of the pathophysiology of various types of proteinuria.
Corwin HL, Silverstein MD. The diagnosis of neoplasia in patients with asymptomatic microscopic hematuria: a decision analysis. J Urol 139:1002–1006, 1988.
 The authors use a theoretical argument to advocate the substitution of renal ultrasonography for intravenous pyelography in the evaluation of hematuria because sonography's cost and morbidity are less and its sensitivity and specificity are comparable to those of intravenous pyelography. The discussion is limited to diagnosing neoplasia, and certainly this viewpoint needs verification with a randomized study. In the meantime, the clinician may choose ultrasonography in cases where pregnancy or a previous reaction to contrast media tends to preclude intravenous pyelography.
Dische FE, Weston MJ, Parsons V. Abnormally thin glomerular basement membranes associated with hematuria, proteinuria or renal failure. Am J Nephrol 5:103–109, 1985.
 Reports several patients with hematuria due to thin glomerular basement membranes. This lesion is the hallmark of benign familial hematuria. The lack of familial hematuria in most of these patients may be due to the fact that urinalyses in family members were not performed.
Gilli P, DePaoliVitali E, Tataranni G, Farinelli A. Exercise-induced urinary abnormalities in long-distance runners. Int J Sports Med 5:237–240, 1984.
 A study of urinary abnormalities after long-distance running.
Houser MT, Jahn MF, Kobayashi A, Walburn J. Assessment of urinary protein excretion in the adolescent: effect of body position and exercise. J Pediatr 109:556–561, 1986.
 A study of high school athletes showing greatly increased prevalence of proteinuria after school sports.
Kaysen GA, Myers BD, Couser WG, Rabkin R, Felts JM. Biology of disease: mechanisms and consequences of proteinuria. Lab Invest 54:479–498, 1986.
 Detailed review of pathogenesis of proteinuria and the nephrotic syndrome.
Pettersson E, von Bonsdorff M, Törnroth I, Lindholm H. Nephritis among young Finnish men. Clin Nephrol 22:217–222, 1984.

Renal biopsy results in 174 patients with urinary abnormalities.

Raman GV, Pead L, Lee HA, Maskell R. A blind controlled trial of phase-contrast microscopy by two observers for evaluating the source of haematuria. Nephron 44:304–308, 1986.

A careful evaluation of red cell morphology as an indication of glomerular or nonglomerular hematuria. The test was poorly reproducible from one observer to another and of questionable reliability.

Schuster GA, Lewis GA. Clinical significance of hematuria in patients on anticoagulant therapy. J Urol 137:923–925, 1987.

Seventeen of 29 patients with hematuria while given anticoagulant therapy had significant pathologic findings including four malignancies.

Schwab SJ, Christensen RL, Dougherty K, Klahr S. Quantitation of proteinuria by the use of protein-to-creatinine ratios in single urine samples. Arch Intern Med 147:943–944, 1987.

The latest study showing the reliability of the spot urine protein/creatinine ratio in the quantitation of proteinuria.

Stapleton JB, Roy S, Noe HN, Jerkins G. Hypercalciuria in children with hematuria. N Engl J Med 310:1345–1348, 1987.

Twenty-three of 82 children and adolescents with gross or microscopic hematuria had hypercalciuria. Short-term suppression of the hypercalciuria with low calcium diet or a thiazide diuretic was associated with elimination of hematuria in 20 of 23 cases.

24

Diagnosis and Management of Patients with Urolithiasis

EDWARD T. ZAWADA, JR., M.D.
ANTHONY G. SALEM, M.D.
JAMES R. HORNING, M.D.

Urolithiasis is a common problem in the United States. Up to 5% of females and 12% of males have at least one symptomatic episode with kidney stones during their lifetime, and up to 80% of these patients have a recurrent attack in the succeeding 10 to 20 years. A definite underlying metabolic disturbance can be found in 95% of patients with urolithiasis, and selective therapy reduces stone formation in 88% of patients. Urinary tract stones are small relative to other calculi in the body. As a consequence, the patient frequently passes the stone before seeking medical care and is asymptomatic when seen by his or her physician. The primary care internist must determine when it is cost effective and medically appropriate to perform an extensive metabolic evaluation and to institute therapy. The goal of diagnosis and therapy is to prevent further stone formation, which may result in morbidity, mortality, or economic loss.

Pathophysiology of Urolithiasis

Urolithiasis results from the precipitation of supersaturated crystalloids within the urinary tract. Recurrent stone disease is best understood as a metabolic disturbance leading to the frequent presence of increased amounts of crystalline substances in the urine. Dehydration commonly contributes to the supersaturation phenomenon. Other factors predisposing to urolithiasis are shown in Table 24–1. Note that certain substances in the urine such as citrate, magnesium, and pyrophosphate may actually inhibit stone formation, and reduction in their urinary levels may facilitate stone formation.

The most comprehensive study of the mineral content in urinary tract stones was published by Herring in 1962. Because most of the literature on urolithiasis resides in specialty and subspecialty journals outside of internal medicine, much of the terminology as well as the details of diagnosis and treatment may be unfamiliar to the primary care internist. The mineralogic terms used to define types of renal stones are therefore defined in Table 24–2. Herring demonstrated 29 distinct compounds in urinary calculi along with 85 artifacts. Stones were commonly composed of multiple compounds, but the relative frequency of stones by major component (greater than 50% of the stone) was oxalate, 73%; phosphates, 17%; urates, 7%; cystine, 1%; and miscellaneous/artifact, 2%. Table 24–3 summarizes some of

Table 24–1. *Common Pathogenic Factors for Urolithiasis*

Dehydration
Urine pH
  Acidic urine: increases incidence of uric acid stones
  Alkalines urine: increases incidence of magnesium ammonium phosphate stones
Lithogenic triggers
  Mucoprotein matrix: calcium stones
  Uric acid crystal: calcium stones
  Calcium phosphate: calcium stones
Stone formation inhibitors
  Citrate: calcium stones
  Magnesium: calcium stones
  Pyrophosphate: calcium stones
Anatomic abnormalities
  Spinal cord injury: magnesium ammonium phosphate stones
  Degenerative neurologic disease: magnesium ammonium phosphate stones
  Medullary sponge kidney: calcium stones
  Duplex or horseshoe kidney: calcium stones

Table 24–2. Mineralogic Terms for Urolithiasis

Term	Chemical Composition
Whewellite	Calcium oxalate monohydrate
Weddellite	Calcium oxalate dihydrate
Apatite	Calcium phosphate
Hydroxyapatite	Calcium phosphate
Brushite	Calcium phosphate
Struvite	Magnesium ammonium phosphate hexahydrate
Triple phosphate	Magnesium ammonium phosphate

the clinical characteristics of urolithiasis caused by different stone types.

Calcium Oxalate Stones

Calcium oxalate stones are the most common type and are usually caused by one of three metabolic disorders: idiopathic hypercalciuria, hyperuricosuria, or primary hyperparathyroidism. Idiopathic hypercalciuria is a distinct metabolic entity characterized by hypercalciuria and normocalcemia. It is the most common cause of recurrent stones. The clinical features of this entity include a familial predisposition, an onset of disease between ages 20 and 50, and a higher prevalence in men than in women.

There are two major subtypes of idiopathic hypercalciuria. Renal-leak hypercalciuria is caused by impairment of calcium reabsorption in the proximal renal tubule. The transient decrease in serum calcium stimulates parathyroid hormone (PTH) secretion, which in turn enhances calcium absorption from the gastrointestinal tract. Absorptive hypercalciuria is generally more severe and has a higher frequency of recurrent stone formation. In this subtype, enhanced gastrointestinal tract absorption of calcium causes transient hypercalcemia. The resulting suppression of PTH decreases renal reabsorption of calcium, which causes hypercalciuria.

Uric acid crystals, with or without hyperuricosuria, can serve as a nidus or trigger for calcium crystallization. About 10% of calcium stone formers have hyperuricosuria as the sole metabolic abnormality, and hyperuricosuria is present in up to one third of patients with hypercalciuria and stones. These patients may develop only calcium oxalate stones or both calcium oxalate and uric acid stones. Increased uric acid excretion in these patients may be due primarily to increased dietary intake of purines.

Primary hyperparathyroidism causes hypercalcemia with hypercalciuria. This endocrinopathy is slightly more common in females than in males and has an average age of onset in the 50's. The hypercalcemia is often very mild and may require repeated measurements of the serum calcium level to document it. The ionized serum calcium test is more specific and is the preferred blood measurement for the diagnosis. Because the ionized serum calcium level may be high normal, the best method to separate idiopathic hypercalciuria from hyperparathyroidism is to simultaneously measure ionized serum calcium and PTH levels. In hyperparathyroidism, there is an inappropriately high PTH level for the higher level of ionized serum calcium. In patients with idiopathic hypercalciuria, the PTH may be minimally elevated but only when the ionized serum calcium concentration level is slightly reduced. The most important factor in the development of recurrent stones in these patients is thought to be increased gastrointestinal absorption of dietary calcium from increased 1,25-dihydroxyvitamin D levels.

Other causes of hypercalcemia (e.g., milk-alkali syndrome, vitamin A intoxication, sarcoidosis, and hyperthyroidism) increase renal filtration of calcium and impair renal calcium reabsorption related to suppressed PTH levels. Hypercalcemia from malignancy uncommonly causes urolithiasis because the hypercalciuria is usually brief. The emphasis on calcium supplementation to prevent osteoporosis and as a strategy to treat essential hypertension may result in an increase in stone disease, especially in individuals with occult idiopathic hypercalciuria.

Table 24–3. General Characteristics of Urolithiasis

Stone Composition	Frequency (%)	Age Group	X-Ray Appearance	Major Predisposing Factors
Oxalate	73	Adults/elderly	Opaque	Idiopathic hypercalciuria, hypercalcemia, hyperoxaluria, hyperuricosuria
Phosphate	17	Adults/elderly	Opaque	Hypercalciuria, infection stones
Urate	7	Adults/elderly	Lucent	Gout, hyperuricosuria
Cystine	1	Children	Opaque	Cystinuria
Miscellaneous/artifact	2	Variable	Lucent	See text

A variety of gastrointestinal diseases and hereditary oxaluria cause hyperoxaluria and may occasionally cause calcium oxalate stones. Enteric hyperoxaluria can occur with malabsorption caused by small bowel resection, bacterial overgrowth, jejunoileal bypass for obesity, inflammatory diseases such as Crohn's, or pancreatic or hepatic diseases. Two major factors increase oxalate absorption. First, there is increased colonic permeability to oxalate because of the presence of bile acids and fatty acids in the colon. Second, fatty acids from steatorrhea complex with calcium, thereby decreasing the luminal calcium available to bind oxalate. As a result, the bioavailability of oxalate is increased and a greater amount is absorbed. Primary hyperoxaluria is a disease of childhood and has an autosomal recessive mode of transmission; more than half of patients have urolithiasis by age 4. High doses of vitamin C (4 g/day or more) cause hyperoxaluria, but the clinical significance of this observation is unknown.

Phosphate Stones

The most common metabolic disorder resulting in phosphate stones is idiopathic hypercalciuria in which calcium phosphate is precipitated together with calcium oxalate. Pure calcium phosphate stones suggest deficient urinary acidification with resultant alkaline urine; the most common etiologies are renal tubular acidoses, ingestion of absorbable alkali, and primary hyperparathyroidism. Magnesium ammonium phosphate (MAP or struvite) stones are noted with recurrent urinary tract infections with urea-splitting organisms. These infections increase urinary ammonium and urinary pH and decrease the solubility of magnesium, ammonium, and phosphate. The resulting stones trap bacteria and make eradication of the infection very difficult. The consequence is a vicious cycle that often results in large staghorn calculi that may form a complete mold of the renal collecting system. These patients often develop renal failure because of recurrent obstruction, pyelonephritis, and use of nephrotoxic antibiotics. Underlying anatomic or metabolic abnormalities (usually hypercalciuria) may predispose patients to struvite stone formation. In one study, more than half of patients with struvite stones had such metabolic abnormalities.

Uric Acid Stones

Hyperuricosuria and urine acidity predispose to uric acid stone formation. Of patients with primary gout, 25% have at least one kidney stone, and in approximately 40% of these patients, the stone precedes the articular manifestations of gout. Although most of these gout patients have hyperuricosuria, about 20% do not but instead have a persistently acidic urinary pH of 5.0 or less. Other clinical conditions that cause rapid cell turnover, such as tumor lysis, myeloproliferative disorders, and psoriasis, cause hyperuricosuria. Finally, several enzyme deficiencies such as the homozygous and heterozygous forms of hypoxanthine–guanine phosphoribosyltransferase (HPRT) deficiency result in hyperuricemia and hyperuricosuria. The heterozygous type of HPRT deficiency accounts for a minority of patients with primary gout. The homozygous form of the disease is associated with the Lesch-Nyhan syndrome with mental retardation, self-mutilation, and early death because of renal failure from recurrent stone disease.

Cystine Stones

Cystinuria is a hereditary defect in the gastrointestinal and renal transport of the dibasic amino acids—cystine, ornithine, arginine, and lysine. Patients with cystinuria have increased urinary excretion of cystine, which precipitates in concentrated, acidic urine to form cystine stones. The average age of onset of symptomatic cystine stones is about 20, but a specific diagnosis is usually delayed about 10 years. Even though normal urinary cystine excretion is less than 30 mg/day, cystinuric patients usually do not develop cystine stones until they excrete more than 400 mg/day.

Miscellaneous Stone Types

Other types of stones occur infrequently. Herring found hematin, fibrin, xanthine, indigo, mucin, steatin, cholesterol, bile salts, and sulfonamides in a small percentage of stones. Patients taking excessive doses of triamterene may develop stones composed of both the drug and one of its metabolic products, 6-p-hydroxytriamterene. Urolithiasis is seen in as many as 10% of patients treated with acetazolamide, a carbonic anhydrase inhibitor most commonly used for glaucoma. This agent causes both types 1 and 2 renal tubular acidoses, but its exact role in the pathogenesis of urolithiasis is unclear. High doses of vitamin C may increase endogenous production and excretion of oxalate, but the relationship of this to urolithiasis is uncertain. Nephrocalcinosis is associated with stone formation, particularly in patients with idiopathic hypercalciuria, hyperparathyroidism, renal tubular acidosis, medullary sponge kidney, sarcoidosis, and hypervitaminosis D.

Clinical Presentation of Urolithiasis

The presentation of patients with urolithiasis usually relates to the presence, size, and location of stones. Stones are frequently trapped where the urinary tract changes caliber; the ureteropelvic and ureterovesicle locations are the most common. Stones above the ureteropelvic junction may be asymptomatic but may cause vague flank pain, hematuria, or pyuria. Magnesium ammonium phosphate stones, often in the form of staghorn calculi, are the most common stone type at this site. Mid- or low ureteral sites are the most symptomatic, and stones there can produce excruciating flank pain that radiates into the ipsilateral groin. These stones may progress down the ureter and be passed in the urine or may lodge at the ureterovesicle junction. Calcium oxalate and uric acid stones commonly present in this fashion. Bladder stones are often asymptomatic but may be accompanied by urgency, frequency, and dysuria, suggesting bladder irritation or infection. Uric acid and magnesium ammonium phosphate are the most common components of bladder stones.

Diagnostic Work-up of Patients with Urolithiasis

The diagnostic evaluation of urolithiasis should be performed in the outpatient setting so that patients follow their usual diet and fluid intake. The basic work-up consists of a directed history and physical examination and the selected laboratory and radiologic studies given in Table 24–4. Because patients with a first stone demonstrate metabolic abnormalities similar to those of patients with recurrent stones, all patients should undergo this basic evaluation at the time of their first episode. Whether and how extensively to evaluate patients with a remote history of urolithiasis have not been determined.

Pertinent aspects of the history are noted in Table 24–4. The physical examination is usu-

Table 24–4. Basic Evaluation for Urolithiasis

History
Age of onset
Number and severity of recurrences
Recent immobilization or dehydration
Anatomic abnormalities of genitourinary tract
Prior genitourinary surgery
Medications: calcium-containing antacids; vitamins A, C, and D; triamterene; acetazolamide
Concurrent illnesses: gout, inflammatory bowel disease
Family history: urolithiasis, gout, cystinuria
Diet: 3- to 5-day food diary of calcium, sodium, protein
Physical Examination
Stone Analysis by Crystallography or X-ray Diffraction
Laboratory Studies
Urinalysis, first void in A.M.
Urine culture (if pyuria or bacteriuria present)
Serum uric acid, creatinine, electrolytes: one measurement
Serum calcium and phosphate: two fasting measurements
24-hour urine test for volume, creatinine, uric acid, calcium, sodium
Radiologic Studies
Intravenous pyelogram (or renal ultrasound, if pyelogram is contraindicated)

ally normal. Uncommonly encountered findings that may aid in diagnosis include gouty tophi, band keratopathy (hypercalcemia), and lymphadenopathy and/or splenomegaly (myeloproliferative disease or sarcoidosis).

Laboratory Tests

Stone analysis by optical crystallography or x-ray diffraction, or both, at a reference laboratory may help guide the initial diagnostic work-up. Patients with renal colic should routinely strain their urine through fine mesh gauze in an attempt to recover the stone. If a stone is recovered, further laboratory evaluation should be delayed until the stone analysis is available. Recurrent stones should also be periodically analyzed because stone composition may change with time or therapy.

If a stone is not available for analysis, laboratory testing should include the studies noted in Table 24–4. Urinalysis should be performed on a first-voided a.m. specimen. An early morning urinary pH above 6.0 suggests renal tubular acidosis, whereas a pH less than 5.5 rules out this disorder. The presence of pyuria or bacteriuria is an indication for a urine culture, which if positive suggests the possible presence of struvite stones. Note that 50% of patients with struvite stones have less than 100,000 colonies/ml of urease-producing bacteria, and 20% have fewer than 10,000 colonies/ml. The importance of these low colony counts of urea-splitting organisms must not be overlooked, especially because mixed infections with more than one type of bacteria are common.

Serum uric acid is measured to detect hyperuricemia, which may be seen with gout, whereas serum creatinine and electrolyte analyses assess the presence of renal insufficiency and renal tubular acidosis. Fasting hypercalcemia and hypophosphatemia suggest primary hyperparathyroidism; serum PTH should be measured if they are present.

A careful 24-hour urine collection defines patients with hypercalciuria and hyperuricosuria. The upper limits of normal 24-hour urinary excretion for calcium and uric acid, respectively, are 300 and 800 mg for men and 250 and 750 mg for women. Volume determination helps document fluid intake; urine creatinine tests ensure an adequate collection because males generally excrete 20 mg/kg body weight per day and females excrete 15 mg/kg per day; and the urinary sodium level reflects dietary sodium intake. This latter measurement is important because increased sodium excretion increases calcium excretion. The normal urinary sodium excretion is less than 200 mEq/day.

Additional 24-hour urinary tests may be used selectively. The cyanide nitroprusside test is able to detect 75 mg of cystine and should be used to screen patients with early onset of stone disease (20 years old or younger), multiple stones, or recurrent stones. Urinary oxalate level (elevated if > 45 mg/day) is particularly useful in patients who are young with severe disease, who have recurrent disease and no other identifiable risk factor, or who have gastrointestinal disease. Urinary citrate level (low if < 400 mg/day) is useful during the initial evaluation of patients with systemic acidoses or for patients with diarrhea. During follow-up evaluations, low levels can help guide therapy in patients who are either refractory to conventional treatments or have no obvious metabolic abnormalities. The costs of the diagnostic laboratory evaluation are noted in Table 24–5.

Radiologic Evaluation

Intravenous pyelography (IVP) is the most sensitive radiologic procedure to define urinary

Table 24–5. Cost of Diagnostic Work-up for Urolithiasis

Diagnostic Test	Cost (US $)
Stone analysis	18.00
Urinalysis	7.00
Chemistry panel	16.00
24-hour urine test	
Calcium	16.00
Sodium	9.00
Creatinine	7.00
Uric acid	9.00
Citrate	65.00
Oxalate	34.00
Nitroprusside test	12.00
Intravenous pyelography	82.00
Ultrasonography	130.00

tract anatomy and the presence and location of stones. IVP done emergently may be of poor quality, whereas those done in patients who undergo adequate diet and laxative preparation are usually of high quality. Plain roentgenograms of the abdomen with the patient in the supine position (kidney, ureter, and bladder [KUB]), routinely done before the IVP, can detect radiopaque stones and are useful for following patients with recurrent or retained stones. Because the preparation for IVP may affect serum and urine electrolyte levels, these tests should not be done concurrently with IVP.

Ultrasonography is not as sensitive as carefully performed IVP for detecting urolithiasis. However, this diagnostic modality is useful either when intravenous contrast is absolutely or relatively contraindicated (allergy or renal insufficiency) or when radiation exposure should be limited (pregnancy). Computed tomography is more sensitive than ultrasonography but offers no particular advantage to IVP.

If the initial stone evaluation is negative, the patient should be managed as defined later. If a specific underlying cause is suggested by the initial work-up, further diagnostic studies may be indicated. For example, hypercalciuria may be subclassified into those with renal leak hypercalciuria versus those with absorptive hypercalciuria. Absorptive hypercalciuria can be further subdivided into type I through type III, depending on the underlying pathophysiology. The need to define the subtype of hypercalciuria to recommend specific therapy for each is controversial. We do not recommend that hypercalciuric subtypes be defined routinely. For those who wish to define the subtypes of hypercalciuria, references are provided in the bibliography.*

Therapy

Acute Management of Symptomatic Urolithiasis

Patients with symptoms caused by obstruction at the ureteropelvic junction, uterovesical junction, or elsewhere in the ureter frequently require admission to the hospital for pain control. Intramuscular meperidine or intravenous morphine may be required. Increased fluid intake is designed to accelerate excretion of the stone.

Invasive intervention is required if there is fever, total obstruction, presence of a solitary kidney, or incomplete evacuation of the stone within 24 to 48 hours. Stones impacted in the lower ureter below the pelvic brim on a KUB roentgenogram may be extracted by cystoscopy and retrograde ureteric instrumentation. Stones above the ureteropelvic junction may be approached by either percutaneous or extracorporeal lithotripsy. Lithotripsy is ultrasonographic disintegration of the stone by a probe placed on the calculus or by stereotaxic focusing of ultrasound waves. Stones lodged in the middle or upper parts of the ureters may be removed by either extracorporeal lithotripsy or through a flank incision. Although it would appear that extracorporeal lithotripsy is less invasive than surgery for stone removal, there is a significant incidence of complications such as obstruction, infection, blood loss, and even death. Palliation of upper urinary tract obstruction can be accomplished by retrograde insertion of a double-J stent or by nephrostomy tube placement.

Indications for elective surgery or lithotripsy include episodic pain, recurrent infections, recurrent hematuria, and deterioration of renal function. Elective surgery may also be necessary to correct anatomic defects.

Preventive Management of Urolithiasis

Therapy for urolithiasis is summarized in Tables 24–6 and 24–7. Fluid intake sufficient

---

*An abbreviated outpatient diagnostic work-up for absorptive hypercalciuria (types I and II) and renal leak hypercalciuria can be obtained from Mission Pharmacal Company, Box 1676, San Antonio, Texas 78296, 1–800–292–7364.

Table 24–6. Dietary Restrictions for Patients with Calcium-Containing Stones

600 mg Calcium Diet*	
Foods Highest in Calcium	**Foods Moderately High in Calcium**
Salmon	Baked beans
Sardines	Chard
Cheese	Spinach
Milk	Bologna
Yogurt	Oysters
Rhubarb, cooked	Molasses
Beet greens, cooked	Cocoa
Broccoli, cooked	
Collards, cooked	
Mustard greens, cooked	
Turnip greens, cooked	
Ice cream	

100 mg Purine Diet*	
Foods Highest in Purines	**Foods Moderately High in Purines**
Liver	Meats
Kidney	Fish
Sweetbreads	Asparagus
Mussels	Cauliflower
Goose	Lima and kidney
Anchovies	beans
Sardines	Lentils
Herring	Mushrooms
Salmon	Peas
Mackerel	Spinach
Scallops	One serving (3 oz)
Clams	may be chosen
Oysters	from the above
Shrimp	list
Tuna	
Fish roe	
Meats extracts, including bouillon, consommé, meat stock soups	
Yeast, baker's and brewer's	
Gravies	

Oxalate Content of Some Foods and Beverages†	
High	**Low**
Rhubarb	Meats
Spinach	Fish
Beet greens	Dairy products
Swiss chard	Eggs
Turnip greens	Cereals
Beets	Cabbage
Sorrel	Asparagus
Parsley	Cauliflower
Sweet potatoes	Peas
Dill	Turnips
Nuts	Lettuce
Unripe bananas	Radishes
Chocolate	Apples
Cocoa	Ripe bananas
Ovaltine	Apricots
Tea	Melons
Coffee	Peaches
Grapefruit juice	Pears
Orange juice	Pineapples
Cranberry juice	Plums
Grape juice	Raspberries
Draft beer	Margarine
Pepper	

*Adapted from Wainer L, Resnick V, Resnick M. Nutritional aspects of stone disease, in Pak C (ed). Renal Stone Disease: Pathogenesis, Prevention, and Treatment. Boston, Martinus-Nijhoff, 1987, pp 91 and 113.
†From Insogna K, Broadus A. Nephrolithiasis, in Felig P, Baxter J, Broadus A, et al. (eds). Endocrinology and Metabolism, ed 2. New York, McGraw-Hill Book Company, 1987, p 1555, with permission.

Table 24–7. Drug Therapy of Urolithiasis

Drug	Starting Dose	Cost* (US $/Month)
Hydrochlorothiazide (HCTZ)	25 mg b.i.d.	1.00
HCTZ/amiloride (Moduretic)	25/2.5 mg b.i.d.	9.00
Milk of magnesia	1 tablet t.i.d.	3.00
Neutral orthophosphate (Neutra-Phos)	500 mg t.i.d.	2.00
Cellulose sodium phosphate (Calcibind)	2.5 g t.i.d.	41.00
Potassium citrate	20 mEq t.i.d.	9.00
Acetohydroxamic acid	250 mg t.i.d.	45.00
Allopurinol	100 mg t.i.d.	8.00

*Average wholesale price to pharmacy. From American Druggist (Blue Book). New York, Hearst Corporation, 1987–88. The cost to the patient is higher.

to maintain urine volume at 2.5 to 3.0 L/day is the cornerstone of therapy for any patient with urolithiasis. Studies suggest that only 10 to 15% of patients with recurrent stone disease have been properly instructed on the importance of fluid intake. Fluid intake should be distributed throughout the day, especially 2 to 3 hours after meals and at bedtime. The bulk of ingested fluids should be water; dairy products increase calcium excretion, and teas, coffee, and certain juices are high in oxalate.

CALCIUM STONES

The first step in therapy consists of adequate fluid intake and dietary instruction. A moderately restricted calcium diet of approximately 600 mg/day can be achieved by eliminating milk and other dairy products, fortified cereals, chocolate, smoked fish, and canned meats. Because a high intake of dietary sodium increases urinary calcium excretion and may reduce urinary citrate excretion, patients should restrict their sodium intake to 80 mEq (about 2 g of sodium) per day. Diets high in animal protein have been associated with calcium stone formation, and it is advisable to reduce animal protein intake. Lower calcium intake potentially allows for greater oxalate absorption; thus, patients with calcium oxalate stones may benefit from a modest reduction in dietary oxalate. This can be achieved by avoiding certain leafy vegetables and plant products such as spinach, rhubarb, beets, chocolate, cocoa, tea, coffee, draft beer, and nuts. Patients with major problems of oxalate absorption and excretion may require a very low

oxalate diet. (See Table 24–6 for a summary of potential dietary changes.) Eight weeks after therapy is initiated, patients should be re-evaluated with a 24-hour urine collection (to measure sodium, calcium, and creatinine levels and volume) and a KUB roentgenogram. If urinary volume is low or urinary sodium level is high, the patient should be reinstructed on the importance of adequate fluid intake and low salt intake. Continued hypercalciuria requires dietary instruction by a nutritionist. The presence of either hypercalciuria or continued stone formation requires the initiation of drug therapy. If the calcium excretion normalizes or there is no evidence of increased stone formation, the patient should be continued on the same regimen and re-evaluated in 1 year.

Primary drug therapy for idiopathic hypercalciuria is a thiazide diuretic such as hydrochlorothiazide, 25 to 50 mg twice a day. Thiazides reduce excretion of urinary calcium by an average of 150 mg/day and have an additional beneficial effect by reducing urinary oxalate. One week after thiazide therapy is initiated, the patient should be re-evaluated for hypokalemia. This particular side effect of thiazides may cause symptoms of dizziness and weakness and may impair urinary citrate excretion. The combined use of thiazides with amiloride may be preferable to thiazides alone. This combination causes a greater hypocalciuric effect and less hypokalemia and hypocitraturia than thiazides alone. Urinary calcium should be rechecked 4 to 8 weeks after thiazide therapy is started.

If a patient continues to form stones or if hypercalciuria persists after thiazide therapy, neutral orthophosphate therapy (Neutra-Phos) may be tried. This agent provides an absorbable source of phosphate that reportedly works by increasing the level of pyrophosphate, an inhibitor of calcium phosphate and calcium oxalate crystallization in the urine, and by decreasing urinary calcium excretion. Diarrhea, a common side effect of therapy, is minimized by taking the tablets before meals and by starting at low doses. Soft tissue calcification is a potentially serious side effect, and orthophosphates are contraindicated in patients with urinary tract infections, infection stones, and medullary sponge kidney because phosphaturia may contribute to the growth of struvite and calcium phosphate stones.

Magnesium is an inhibitor of calcium oxalate and phosphate crystallization in the urine and has been shown to reduce the passage of calcium stones. Magnesium hydroxide or magnesium oxide may cause diarrhea and is contraindicated in patients with renal failure or chronic urinary tract infections.

Cellulose sodium phosphate, a nonabsorbable ion exchange resin, decreases calcium absorption by "binding" calcium in the intestinal lumen. This agent should be used only after absorptive hypercalciuria has been diagnosed. The action of cellulose sodium phosphate to decrease hypercalciuria is potentially negated by its actions of increasing phosphate and oxalate excretion and decreasing urinary magnesium. Therefore, patients require a low oxalate diet and magnesium supplementation to avoid stone recurrence. This agent should be used cautiously for patients with congestive heart failure and ascites because the exchangeable sodium content is 35 to 48 mEq/15 g of cellulose sodium phosphate.

Potassium citrate is frequently useful for patients with chronic diarrhea, renal tubular acidosis, or hypokalemia from thiazide diuretics. By providing ingested alkali, this agent increases urinary pH and promotes citrate excretion. The usual starting dose of 20 mEq three times a day is titrated until urinary citrate levels reach normal levels (400 to 700 mg/day). Side effects from the tablet preparation are minor and are generally related to gastrointestinal distress.

Parathyroidectomy is the primary therapy in patients with hyperparathyroidism. If the patient is not a surgical candidate or if surgery must be delayed, orthophosphate therapy may be used. In postmenopausal women, replacement estrogen is an alternative medical treatment.

Phosphate Stones

Patients with pure calcium phosphate stones should have the underlying cause of stone formation treated if possible. Patients with distal renal tubular acidosis can be effectively treated with potassium citrate in quantities sufficient to normalize the serum bicarbonate concentration.

Infection stones of the renal pelvis and bladder are particularly difficult to treat medically because it is virtually impossible to eradicate bacteria in the presence of a foreign body. Removal of stones, either by surgery or by lithotripsy, is the treatment of choice. Culture-specific parenteral antibiotics should be started 24 hours before surgery. The duration of postoperative antibiotic treatment is controver-

sial; prolonged (6 to 12 months), low dose antibiotics have successfully prevented recurrent stones, but recent studies suggest that shorter term treatment (2 to 3 weeks) is as effective. If the patient is not a surgical candidate, urinary phosphorus excretion should be kept below 450 mg/day by diet or by phosphate binders such as aluminum hydroxide (Amphojel 45 ml four times a day). Patients should limit intake of magnesium-containing antacids and cathartics. Acetohydroxamic acid (Lithostat), a urease inhibitor, decreases urine alkalinity and ammonia production even in the presence of persistent infection. This drug is considered to be adjunctive therapy and should not be used in place of surgery or culture-specific antibiotics. Prolonged use of this drug both prevents growth of new stones and promotes dissolution of pre-existing ones.

Uric Acid Stones

Uric acid stones can be treated with increased fluid intake, a low protein diet (50 to 60 g/day), and urinary alkalinization to a pH of 6.7 to 7.0. Sodium bicarbonate or citrate therapy may be complicated by the development of calcium phosphate or calcium oxalate stones; therefore, potassium citrate is the preferred agent to alkalinize urine. Therapy should start at 20 mEq three times a day, and patients should check their urinary pH three to four times a day with pH paper. Alkalinizing urine to a pH greater than 7.0 increases the possibility of calcium phosphate stones. If the above measures are ineffective, the addition of allopurinol, 300 mg/day, is usually effective.

Patients with calcium oxalate stones, normocalciuria, and hyperuricosuria may be treated with allopurinol, 300 mg/day, rather than a thiazide diuretic. Patients with both hyperuricosuria and hypercalciuria should be treated with a thiazide diuretic because allopurinol is not effective in the presence of hypercalciuria.

Cystine Stones

The mainstay of therapy for patients with cystine stones is hydration and alkalinization of the urine. The solubility of cystine between the pH of 4.5 to 7.0 is approximately 300 mg/L; therefore, urine output should be titrated to keep the cystine concentration at less than 300 mg/L. In patients who excrete more than 1000 mg of cystine daily, D-penicillamine or alpha-mercaptopropionylglycine (tiopronin) can enhance the solubility of cystine. The use of these agents is limited by potentially serious side effects.

Follow-up of Patients with Urolithiasis

Patients undergoing therapy for urolithiasis should be re-evaluated periodically. In general, 24-hour urine studies should be re-evaluated 8 weeks after any new treatment is initiated. Patients with persistent abnormalities of these analyses may require repeated instruction on the importance of medication, dietary compliance, and increased fluid intake. Normalization of biochemical parameters requires an annual re-evaluation.

Patients with retained stones should be followed every 6 to 12 months with a urinalysis and a KUB roentgenogram or ultrasound of the kidneys and bladder. Cystoscopy should be considered for persistent hematuria, especially in the elderly. Urine culture is necessary for pyuria. The presence of an infection requires consideration of either surgery or lithotripsy with prolonged antibiotic use. If radiography demonstrates increasing stone size or hydronephrosis, surgery or lithotripsy should be considered.

Bibliography

Coe F, Parks J. Recurrent renal calculi: causes and prevention. Hosp Pract 21:49–57, 1986.
> Using a case presentation format, the authors concisely discuss the clinical evaluation of recurrent calcium oxalate stones. Included in the paper is an extensive outpatient diagnostic protocol employed at the University of Chicago.

Consensus Conference. Prevention and treatment of kidney stones. JAMA 260:977–981, 1988.
> This concise review of nephrolithiasis advocates a more limited diagnostic evaluation (urinalysis, serum chemistries, plain radiographs, and IVP) for single-stone formers, and a more complete evaluation (including 24-hour urine chemistries) for patients with multiple stones or recurrent disease. The article discusses the utility of lithotripsy but stresses the importance of medical prevention of further stone formation.

Erickson S. When should the stone patient be evaluated? Med Clin North Am 68:461–468, 1984.
> The author argues that limited diagnostic evaluation is warranted for patients who have idiopathic calcium stone disease and form single stones.

Insogna K, Broadus A. Nephrolithiasis, in Felig P, Baxter J, Broadus A, et al. (eds). Endocrinology and Metabolism, ed 2. New York, McGraw-Hill Book Co., 1987, pp 1500–1577.
> This superb review details the physiology, pathophysiology, and clinical management of nephrolithiasis (235 references).

Pak C (ed). Renal Stone Disease: Pathogenesis, Prevention, and Treatment. Boston, Martinus Nijhoff Publishing, 1987.
> This clearly written, well-organized book thoroughly reviews urolithiasis.

Pak C. Urolithiasis: calcium stones, in Bayless T, Brain M, Cherniack R (eds). Current Therapy in Internal Medicine—2. Toronto, BC Decker, 1987, pp 1071–1073.
> This is a concise review of diagnostic evaluation and treatment of calcium stones. A table outlines the subtypes of hypercalciuria.

Pak C, Britton F, Peterson R, et al. Ambulatory evaluation of nephrolithiasis. Am J Med 69:19–30, 1980.
> An ambulatory protocol evaluated 241 consecutive patients seen in a specialized clinic. A physiologic disturbance was demonstrated in 90% of patients, and a definitive diagnosis was given to 95%.

Pak C, Sakhaee K, Crowther C, et al. Evidence justifying a high fluid intake in treatment of nephrolithiasis. Ann Intern Med 93:36–39, 1980.
> High fluid intake reduces the likelihood of calcium salt crystallization and increases the minimum saturation needed to elicit spontaneous nucleation of calcium oxalate.

Smith L. Urolithiasis, in Schrier R, Gottshalk C (eds). Diseases of the Kidney, ed 4. Boston, Little, Brown & Co., 1988, pp 785–813.
> This chapter is an excellent, detailed clinical review of urolithiasis (154 references).

25

Evaluation and Management of Vaginal Discharge

JACK D. McCUE, M.D.

Of office visits to primary care practitioners, 10% are for vulvovaginitis and account for as many as 10 million visits yearly. Topical vaginal antimicrobials are prescribed more commonly by physicians than are oral antimicrobials. Despite the limited number of infectious agents responsible for about 90% of vulvovaginitis, the diagnostic approach is often viewed as confusing, and relapsing or recurrent vaginitis is a particular source of frustration for physician and patient alike.

Normal Vaginal Secretions

The quantity and quality of normal secretions vary greatly with age, sexual activity, stage of menstrual cycle, degree of sexual arousal, use of contraceptive devices or drugs, emotional state, and frequency of douchings. Normal secretions derive primarily from cervical mucus and true transudation through the vaginal wall, which lacks mucous glands. Exfoliated cells and secretions are altered by bacteria, primarily anaerobic and facultatively anaerobic lactobacilli, to produce a modest amount of secretions that are acidic (pH 3.8 to 4.2), clear or white, homogeneous or somewhat flocculent, viscous, and essentially odorless, and that contain few polymorphonuclear neutrophils (PMNs).

Causes of Vulvovaginitis Symptoms

There are three well-described forms of vulvovaginitis: bacterial vaginosis (BV), *Trichomonas* vaginitis (TV), and *Candida* vulvovaginitis (CV). The proportion of each type seen in clinical practice varies greatly, depending on the type of practice and the numbers of sexual partners of the patients. BV and TV tend to be more common in reports from sexually transmitted disease clinics, TV is most common in women with other concurrent sexually transmitted diseases, and CV is most common in studies of middle-class primary care practices in which TV is relatively less common. A primary care practitioner with a middle- or working-class population of patients can expect to see about 45% CV, 35% BV, 10% TV, and 10% others/undiagnosable.

Other important causes of vulvovaginitis symptoms include trauma and bacterial infection in patients with estrogen-deficient (atrophic) vaginopathy and infectious cervicitis. The latter condition, usually caused by infection with *Neisseria gonorrhoeae, Chlamydia trachomatis,* or herpes simplex, is a most important and often overlooked cause of increased discharge or discomfort. Ovulation, increased sexual activity, frequent douching, use of oral contraceptives, pregnancy, and malignancies are other causes of increased vaginal discharge. Increased attention to normal secretions or so-called psychosomatic vaginitis occurs in fewer than 5% of patients with genitourinary complaints.

Candida Vulvovaginitis

Candida albicans accounts for about 90% of CV infections and the remainder are caused by *C. glabrata;* there are no clinical differences. These yeasts are part of our normal flora and may be cultured from the vaginas of 25 to 50% of normal, asymptomatic women. As is true of most opportunistic infections, in which a normally commensal organism causes infection, a predisposing factor is often present: diabetes, glycosuria, recent use of antibiotics (especially tetracyclines), obesity, pregnancy, debility, depressed cell-mediated immunity, or use of birth control pills, corticosteroids, and immunosuppressant drugs. If there are no predisposing drugs or conditions, tight clothing, warm weather, and menstruation predispose to CV. Some patients may be peculiarly susceptible to CV, perhaps because their epithelial cells permit adherence, germination, or invasion of *Candida* more readily. In addition, some strains of *Candida* may be especially virulent, and eradication of yeast colonization is required to prevent a relapse of infection in some patients.

CV is not a sexually transmitted disease. Although men may have a yeast infection and yeast may be cultured from men after their sexual contact with women who have a yeast infection, sexual transmission is of negligible importance.

Clinical Manifestations

Inflammation and irritation of the vulva and vagina typically result in complaints of itching or dyspareunia. Approximately half of women complain of increased or abnormal discharge. A changed or offensive odor is uncommon. The discharge is classically thrush-like: white clumps of discharge ("cottage cheese") adhere to inflamed mucosa, and satellite lesions are present. About half of women with CV have a thin, nondiagnostic discharge.

Laboratory Findings

The pH is normal (below 4.5), in contrast to TV and BV. Diagnosis is based on a positive result for one of three tests: (1) The 10% potassium hydroxide (KOH) preparation, which involves adding one or two drops of 10% KOH to a generous amount of discharge, stirring with the wooden end of a swab and applying a glass coverslip (warming gently until bubbling occurs is optional). This procedure dissolves epithelial cells and other debris that could obscure fungal forms. Sensitivity is approximately 70 to 80% for trained observers who examine 10 to 20 high-dry fields per slide. (2) A Gram's stain is more expensive and troublesome but increases sensitivity to 80 to 90%. In addition, unlike the 10% KOH prep-

aration, which cannot be used to diagnose other types of vaginitis, the Gram's stain may indicate features of TV or BV. (3) A yeast culture is the most sensitive method for detecting yeast, with a sensitivity exceeding 90%. It need not be done if the 10% KOH preparation or Gram's stain is positive. It is most helpful if all "bedside" diagnostic tests are nondiagnostic and the pH is below 4.5.

The specificity of 10% KOH, Gram's stain, and culture for the presence of yeast approaches 100%. The specificity for the diagnosis of CV, however, is unknown. Probably the 10% KOH, which requires large numbers of yeast to be positive, is most specific (?90% +) and the culture, which detects large numbers of asymptomatic carriers, is least specific (?60%). In other words, a positive culture in the absence of a characteristic clinical presentation should not be regarded as diagnostic of CV, only as a supportive test. Papanicolaou smears have poor sensitivity (< 50%) and unknown specificity for CV.

Treatment

Asymptomatic patients with positive cultures should not usually be treated. Table 25–1 shows alternative treatment regimens for symptomatic patients. Usual success rates are 80 to 90%, with nystatin and boric acid capsules being least effective. For intensely pruritic vulvitis, external application of antifungal cream may provide more rapid symptom relief than tablets alone. Precipitating factors should be systematically addressed.

Cultures should not be routinely done after treatment. About 25% of successfully treated patients have persistently positive cultures. Repeated recurrence of symptomatic CV has

Table 25–1. *Alternative Treatment Regimens for Vulvovaginal Candidiasis*

Drug	Regimen
Miconazole	500 mg tablet vaginally once
Clotrimazole	200 mg tablet vaginally every day × 3 days
	100 mg tablet vaginally every day × 7 days
	1 applicator of 2% vaginal cream every day × 7 days
Nystatin (Mycostatin)	100,000 U vaginal tablet/cream every day × 7–14 days
Ketoconazole*	400 mg every day × 3–7 days
Boric acid*	600 mg in gelatin capsule vaginally every day × 14 days

*Avoid during pregnancy.

been approached with three strategies (listed in the order in which they are usually tried): (1) self-diagnosis and treatment with short-course miconazole, clotrimazole, or ketoconazole by refillable prescription; (2) regular prophylaxis with 400 mg of ketoconazole or miconazole/clotrimazole for 5 days at the beginning of menses; (3) continuous prophylaxis with 100 mg of ketoconazole daily. Yogurt contains strains of lactobacilli that do not colonize the vagina and should not be prescribed as a dietary or topical treatment. Perineal drying with a hair dryer, cotton underwear, avoidance of trousers, and use of talcum powder (*not* cornstarch) are simple adjunctive measures that may help prevent relapses. Oral nystatin has been used unsuccessfully in an attempt to eliminate a presumed gastrointestinal reservoir of pathogenic fungi in women with recurrent vaginitis.

Bacterial Vaginosis

There is no simple etiologic explanation for BV. *Gardnerella vaginalis* is present in all cases, but it can also be cultured from 30 to 70% of healthy, asymptomatic women. There is a dramatic reduction of lactobacilli in BV to the point of near eradication. In addition, anaerobic organisms (*Peptococcus, Bacteroides,* and *Mobiluncus* species) increase in numbers up to 1000-fold. *Mycoplasma hominis* is nearly always present. BV is more common among women with multiple sexual partners, although it should not be considered a sexually transmitted disease. BV is not an invasive infection; it is a superficial mucosal infection of anaerobic organisms that is benign and essentially without serious medical sequelae.

Clinical Manifestations

A musty or fishy odor caused by production of two polyamines—putrescine and cadaverine—by anaerobic bacteria is the major and usually the only symptom. Irritation, inflammation, and increased discharge are atypical. The typical discharge is thin, adherent to the vaginal wall, scanty, yellow or gray, malodorous, and rarely frothy.

Laboratory Findings

The diagnosis of BV requires that three or four features are present. (1) A typical dis-

charge (described earlier) is found. (2) The pH (tested by dipping a piece of pH paper attached to forceps or clamps into the discharge while avoiding cervical mucus and menstrual blood, which are alkaline) is above 4.5. The higher the pH, the more likely is the diagnosis. (3) "Clue" cells are seen on a wet preparation, which consists of one drop of discharge and one or two drops of normal saline stirred and examined through a coverslip on high-dry magnification. The typical clue cell is an epithelial cell that has lost its sharp margins and has an unfocused granular appearance because of the adherence of bacteria over the entire cell surface. (4) A "sniff" test, which can be done as part of the 10% KOH preparation, is positive. When 10% KOH is added to the drop of discharge and stirred, volatile odoriferous amines with a characteristic fishy smell are released.

The first three observations have about 70 to 80% sensitivity and specificity. The sniff test may be positive in TV and is less sensitive as well; it is of dubious benefit for routine examinations. Gram's stain reveals no lactobacilli (large gram-positive bacilli), *Gardnerella* morphotypes (smaller gram-variable bacilli), and clue cells (epithelial cells with small gram-variable bacilli adhering to the cell surface). It is a very reliable method of diagnosing BV; sensitivity and specificity in one study were 100% in experienced hands. Cultures for *Gardnerella* add nothing and should not be done. A symptomatic woman with a typical discharge, an elevated pH, and clue cells present can be said to have BV with near certainty.

Treatment

Metronidazole is the best-studied antimicrobial used in the treatment of BV; depending on the dosing regimen, cure rates of higher than 90% can be expected. The standard regimen is 500 mg twice daily for a week, although equal cure rates were obtained in one large study with two single 2-g doses on days 1 and 3. Cure rates of about 65 to 85% have been recorded in several other studies of 2-g single-dose regimens. Metronidazole is not very active against *G. vaginalis* (its hydroxy metabolite is more active), but it is highly active against nearly all other anaerobes found in BV. It is also inactive against lactobacilli, which perhaps permits faster recolonization with the normal lactobacillus flora.

Ampicillin or amoxicillin 500 mg four times

daily for a week has given highly variable results but usually has a 10 to 20% lower cure rate than metronidazole. Tetracycline, erythromycin, and topical sulfa drugs are ineffective. Chloramphenicol or amoxicillin plus clavulanate might be effective but has not been as well studied. In an earlier study, intravaginal tetracycline was effective but regularly caused CV as a complication.

Routine treatment of sexual partners does not increase cure rates and should be reserved for relapsing or unusual cases; the dose is the same as that for BV. Metronidazole has been feared to be carcinogenic on the basis of rodent and bacterial studies, but human studies have not confirmed this possible risk. First-trimester use has been associated with a higher than expected incidence of fetal and perinatal death and spontaneous abortion; second- and third-trimester use of metronidazole has been found to be safe. Ampicillin or amoxicillin should be considered for initial treatment during pregnancy, with metronidazole as a second-line drug in the second or third trimester. High dose regimens of metronidazole are associated with nausea and dysgeusia in 10 to 20% of patients. Because it blocks alcohol metabolism, antabuse-like reactions may occur within 24 hours of the last dose of metronidazole.

Trichomonas Vaginitis

T. vaginalis is highly adapted to infecting the genitourinary tissue of men and women by attaching to and damaging the epithelial lining. It is a protozoan parasite with highly characteristic jerking motility from four polar flagella. Trichomonads are anaerobic, with metabolic enzyme systems similar to those of the obligate bacterial anaerobes found in increased concentrations in BV. There are different strains of *T. vaginalis* with various degrees of virulence and susceptibility to killing by metronidazole.

T. vaginalis is usually considered a sexually transmitted agent: The prevalence of TV correlates directly with the number of sexual partners in sexually active women, and it is the most common cause of vaginitis in sexually transmitted disease clinics. It should be seriously considered when a woman being treated for another sexually transmitted disease complains of a vaginal discharge; in addition, 25 to 35% of women with TV diagnosed in sexually transmitted disease clinics also have a chlamydial or gonorrheal infection. Hence, routine culturing for other veneral pathogens is justifiable in women with TV and multiple sexual partners.

Unlike traditional sexually transmissible pathogens, however, *T. vaginalis* has a predilection for older women and is a common cause of vaginitis in postmenopausal, institutionalized women. It is suspected that transfer of this relatively hardy organism by staff who do not wash their hands, by the use of a moist towel on more than one patient, or by urine spillage is responsible for cases seen in chronic care facilities.

Men may become infected with *T. vaginalis* or may transmit it without developing symptoms. When colonized with trichomonads, men tend to eliminate them quickly and nearly all have negative cultures after 2 to 4 weeks. It may be that strains of trichomonads, known to be highly fastidious about the type of cell to which they attach, do not adhere to male genitourinary epithelial cells as well as they do to female cells. Despite the development of cell-mediated and humoral immunity to *T. vaginalis,* which may prevent infection from extending beyond superficial genitourinary tissue, recurrent and relapsing infections are common.

Clinical Manifestations

Although up to half of women with trichomoniasis are asymptomatic, most eventually become symptomatic. A true asymptomatic carrier state is uncommon; when questioned carefully, most women have some mild symptoms of TV.

Increased, abnormal discharge is the major complaint. Irritation and vulvar inflammation, as in CV, may occur and may be acute and severe. Odor, as in BV, may also be present. A gray or yellow-green discharge in moderate to large amounts is seen; frothiness (CO_2 bubbles) and punctate hemorrhages of the cervix ("strawberry cervix") are uncommon. Symptoms may worsen during or after menstruation; abdominal pain, for unclear reasons, may be present.

Laboratory Findings

Clinical recognition of TV alone is neither specific nor sensitive. Diagnosis depends on the finding of motile trichomonads on a wet preparation (see earlier section on BV for

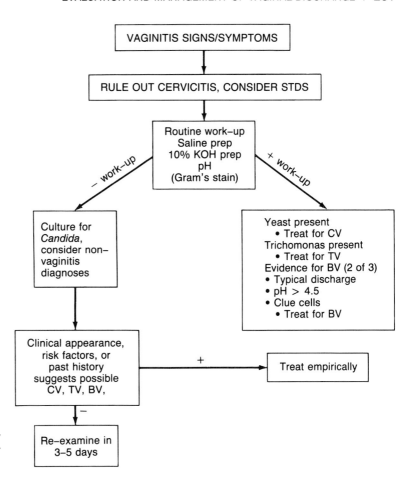

Figure 25–1. Decision analysis for diagnosis and treatment of vulvovaginitis.

methods). Gentle warming by the microscope substage light increases the typical jerking motility, and phase-contrast microscopy further aids recognition. The organisms are pear-shaped and intermediate in size between epithelial cells and PMNs; experienced observers can identify them by Gram's stain or with the assistance of acridine orange staining. Inexperienced observers find them hard to locate on Gram's-stained smears because of the tendency of PMNs to clump around them.

Sensitivity of the wet preparation is about 80% in women with TV; specificity is close to 100%. Papanicolaou smears are equally specific but less sensitive. Cultures are easy to perform but are not available at most laboratories; cultures are highly sensitive and 100% specific. Asymptomatic women have fewer organisms, and the sensitivity of all diagnostic tests for them falls to about 50% or less. Immunofluorescent antibody assays currently being tested suggest that previously cited sensitivity figures may be too high, but these data are as yet preliminary.

The pH is usually above 4.5 and the sniff test may be positive (see earlier section on BV for methods), which can cause misdiagnosis as BV. In addition, BV and TV may occur simultaneously.

Treatment

Metronidazole is highly active against more than 90% of trichomonads; relatively high levels of metronidazole resistance have been noted in trichomonads cultured from TV that did not respond to metronidazole treatment. A single 2-g dose gives cure rates in excess of 90% if male sexual partners are simultaneously treated to prevent reinfection. If sexual partners are not treated, the cure rate falls slightly to about 85%. A similarly high cure rate could be achieved by sexual abstinence or by use of a condom for 3 to 4 weeks. If the standard 250-mg three times daily or 500-mg twice daily regimens are used, it may be unnecessary to treat sexual partners. Small studies show that a 1.5-g single-dose regimen gives the same cure rate as a 2-g dose regimen, and as little as 1 g gives only slightly inferior cure rates. (See the BV section for comments on adverse reactions to metronidazole therapy.) Because the organisms are found in the urethra, bladder, and various glands, one would expect topical therapy to be relatively less effective, although topical therapy with clotrimazole may be helpful during the first trimester of pregnancy.

Treatment failure is usually due to reinfection. If resistant organisms are suspected, however, high dose regimens of 500 mg to 1.5 g twice daily for 7 to 14 days may be used. In difficult resistant cases, intravenous metronidazole has been used, although oral metronidazole is very well absorbed.

Diagnostic Approach

Clinical distinction among the three types of vaginitis is unreliable. Typical CV is easily recognized, but half of the cases of CV are atypical. BV and TV are not distinguishable in most cases and may occur as coinfection. Although treatments for BV and TV are similar, one's approach to treating sexual partners and looking for other sexually transmitted diseases is different.

Cervicitis, perhaps the most important nonvaginitis diagnosis to consider, is recognized by white or yellow cervical mucopus or the presence of 10 or more PMNs per high power field by Gram's stain of the cervical secretions (whether or not mucopus is visible). Symptoms suggesting endometritis or salpingitis should increase the suspicion that a vaginal discharge is the result of an upper genital tract infection.

The decision tree in Figure 25–1 is somewhat complicated because tests are done in a different order temporally. For example, the pH test is done at the time of the examination, although the result may not be used or may be used after microscopy to make a diagnosis of BV or justify empirical treatment for CV. The complex possibilities, therefore, do not fit a decision tree neatly.

What most clinicians do is treat on the basis of positive results of a wet preparation or 10% KOH preparation. If microscopic results are negative for TV or CV, a diagnosis of BV is attempted by considering pH, appearance and odor of discharge, and clue cells. If physicians are unable to make a diagnosis of BV, they make a clinical hunch and treat empirically for TV, BV, or CV based on all the clinical information, re-examine for sexually transmitted diseases, or reschedule the patient for re-evaluation after 3 to 5 days when the yeast culture and sexually transmitted disease cultures will have been reported.

Bibliography

Addison LA. The role of the office laboratory in the diagnosis of vaginitis. Primary Care 13:633–646, 1986.
  Detailed step-by-step illustrated explanations of the procedures that should be done as part of the routine office evaluation of vaginitis.
Ansel R, Totten PA, Spiegel CA, et al. Nonspecific vaginitis. Diagnostic criteria and microbial and epidemiologic associations. Am J Med 74:14–22, 1983.
  A careful innovative examination of the reliability of the diagnostic criteria for BV in 397 unselected symptomatic and asymptomatic university students. In this group, 25% met the criteria for BV, half of whom were asymptomatic.
Eschenbach DA, Hillier S, Critchlow C, et al. Diagnosis and clinical manifestations of bacterial vaginosis. Am J Obstet Gynecol 158:619–628, 1988.
  Trained observers found that Gram's stain predicted the presence of Gardnerella organisms better than standard criteria for BV. Elevated pH and positive sniff test were the least sensitive indicators of BV. BV may be a risk factor for pelvic inflammatory disease.
Hager WD, Brown ST, Kraus SJ, et al. Metronidazole for vaginal trichinosis. Seven-day vs single-dose regimens. JAMA 244:1219–1220, 1980.
  The cure rate was 86% in 93 women receiving a single 2-g dose compared with 91.6% in 83 women receiving the standard 7-day regimen.
Hill LV, Embil JA. Vaginitis. Current microbiologic and clinical concepts. Can Med Assoc J 134:321–331, 1986.
  A well-referenced review article summarizing accepted approaches to vaginitis.
Holmes KK, Mardh PA, Sparling PF, et al. (eds). Sexually Transmitted Diseases. New York, McGraw-Hill Book Co., 1984.
  A major textbook in infectious diseases that has several chapters dealing with vaginitis with extensive referencing and a pathophysiologic orientation.
Jerve F, Berdal TB, Bohman P, et al. Metronidazole in the treatment of non-specific vaginitis. Br J Vener Dis 60:171–174, 1984.
  Patients (429) with BV were given a variety of metronidazole regimens. The regimens with the best cure rates (94%) were with 2 g on days 1 and 3 and 1.2 g daily for 5 days.
Lossick JG, Muller M, Gorrell T. In vitro drug susceptibility and doses of metronidazole required for cure in cases of refractory vaginal trichinosis. J Infect Dis 153:948–955, 1986.
  Thirty-one patients with TV refractory to standard treatment were found to have resistant trichomonads. Cure required an average of 2.6 g metronidazole per day for 9 days.
Mandell GL, Douglas RG, Bennett JE (eds). Principles and Practice of Infectious Diseases. New York, John Wiley & Sons, 1985.
  A major textbook in infectious diseases that has several chapters dealing with vaginitis with extensive referencing and a pathophysiologic orientation.

McCue JD. Evaluation and management of vaginitis. An update for primary care practitioners. Arch Intern Med. In press.

A review of the material covered in this chapter, extensively referenced.

Paavonen J, Stamm WE. Lower genital tract infections in women. Infect Dis Clin 1:179–198, 1987.

A well-referenced review article summarizing accepted approaches to vaginitis.

Sobel J. Recurrent vulvovaginal candidiasis. A prospective study of the efficacy of maintenance ketoconazole therapy. N Engl J Med 315:1455–1458, 1986.

Continuous ketoconazole (100 mg daily) prevented recurrent CV best, although cyclic clotrimazole or ketoconazole also gave good results.

Spiegel CA, Amsel R, Holmes KK. Diagnosis of bacterial vaginosis by direct Gram stain or vaginal fluid. J Clin Microbiol 18:170–177, 1983.

In 60 women, 25 of whom had BV, the Gram's stain was 100% sensitive and specific.

Swedberg J, Steiner JF, Deiss F, et al. Comparison of single-dose vs one-week course of metronidazole for symptomatic bacterial vaginosis. JAMA 254:1046–1049, 1985.

Single-dose (2 g) metronidazole produced significantly inferior symptomatic cure results (47%) compared with 7 days of 500 mg twice daily (83%).

26

Diagnostic Evaluation and Treatment of Urinary Tract Infection in Men

BENJAMIN A. LIPSKY, M.D.

Overview and Epidemiology

Urinary tract infection (UTI) is usually considered to be mainly a problem of female populations. There are comparatively few data about the epidemiology, diagnosis, and treatment of UTIs in males, despite the fact that these infections are relatively common. For example, data from 1977 to 1978 for the United States show that there were 76 office visits annually per 1000 men for urogenital problems. Approximately 40% of these visits were for infectious problems: 10% for cystourethritis (nonvenereal), 25% for prostatitis (all types), and 5% for epididymitis and orchitis (of all causes). A greater number of these patients (48%) were seen by primary care physicians than by urologists (36%).

Bacteriuria in Neonates and Children. As shown in Figure 26–1, male infants have a higher rate of UTIs than female infants. This is probably largely attributable to the greater incidence of congenital anatomic genitourinary disorders in bacteriuric boys, which ranges from 40 to 85%. Other potential causes for this male predominance include a possible decreased resistance to infection, more frequent occurrence of incomplete bladder emptying, and increased exposure of the male infant urethral meatus to fecal contamination. Several studies have shown that uncircumcised male infants have a significantly higher rate of UTIs than those who are circumcised. With increasing age, the foreskin is more easily retracted, which results in improved penile hygiene. This may account for both the diminishing colony counts of periurethral aerobic flora and the decreasing incidence of UTI with

age in boys. After the neonatal period, the prevalence of bacteriuria in male populations remains quite low until late middle age. For unclear reasons, the characteristics of UTIs in young boys differ from those in girls: infections tend to occur at an earlier age, radiologic abnormalities are more frequent, and the overall morbidity is greater, especially from chronic pyelonephritis.

Bacteriuria in the Elderly. The incidence of UTIs increases progressively with age in men, such that after about age 65 it is similar to that in women. This dramatic rise in these infections in older men is undoubtedly related mainly to prostatic enlargement, which results in lower urinary tract obstruction. The residual urine remaining in the bladder after voiding serves as a good culture medium for any bacteria that gain entry to the urinary tract. This fact and a greatly increased incidence of use of urinary tract instrumentation (e.g., catheterization, cystoscopy) are considered to be the major contributors to high rates of bacteriuria in elderly men, especially those who are hospitalized or institutionalized. Because the prevalence of bacteriuria rises with both age and functional disability, it is not surprising that it occurs in 20 to 50% of both male and female nursing home residents. In a carefully studied group of elderly male veterans in a long-term care hospital, Nicolle and colleagues found that the prevalence of bacteriuria was 37%, whereas the incidence was 0.4 episodes per patient-year and the acquisition rate by nonbacteriuric patients was about 40% per year. Once asymptomatic bacteriuria developed in these men, it tended to persist or recur. Bacteriuria was somewhat more likely

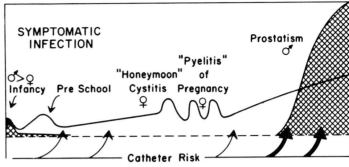

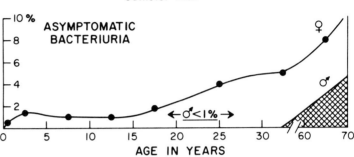

Figure 26–1. *Overview of the frequency of symptomatic UTIs and prevalence of bacteriuria according to age and gender. Modified from the original concept of Jawetz and reprinted with permission from Kunin CM. Detection, Prevention and Management of Urinary Tract Infections, ed 4. Philadelphia, Lea & Febiger, 1987.*

to be continuous (i.e., found on all cultures obtained over a period of years) than intermittent. Gross structural genitourinary abnormalities were not common in these men, but bacteriuria was significantly associated with confusion or dementia and with bowel or bladder incontinence. Of possible factors precipitating the initial acquisition of bacteriuria, the most frequently found was a concurrent illness. Table 26–1 shows the approximate prevalance of bacteriuria in various male (compared with similar female) populations.

Table 26–1. *Prevalence of Bacteriuria in Various Populations**

Population	Males	Females
Normal subjects (screening)		
Infants	1	0.5
School children	0.03	1.5
College students	< 0.01	5
Adults	0.05	10
Elderly		
65–85 yr old	5	15
> 85 yr old	15	25
Patients		
Adult medical clinic	4	6
Adult urology clinic	8	—
Adult inpatients		
< 70 yr old	7.5	30
> 70 yr old	25	30
Institutionalized elderly	> 30	> 30
After instrumentation		
Urethral catheterization	5	5
Transurethral procedures	20	40

*Percentages are approximations based on widely varying values from many studies in different settings.

Pathophysiology

The pathophysiology of UTIs in females is fairly well understood. In brief, micro-organisms resident in the rectal and perineal areas colonize the nearby vaginal introitus; some women appear to have a genetic predisposition to such colonization, and some bacteria (especially *Escherichia coli*) are particularly likely to become uropathogens. These colonizing bacteria then migrate to the urethral meatus, ascend the short (3 to 4 cm) urethra, and cause UTIs ranging from urethritis to pyelonephritis. The picture is not nearly so clear in men. First, the urethral meatus is a considerable distance from the perineum and anus (Fig. 26–2). Second, the meatus is surrounded by the squamous epithelium of the glans penis, a microbial environment very different from that of the mucous membrane of the vaginal vestibule. Third, the urethra is substantially longer (15 to 20 cm) in men, which makes successful ascent of potential uropathogens to the bladder more difficult.

Prostatic Hypertrophy. Perhaps the most important structure pathophysiologically, at least in older men, is the prostate gland. Most authorities believe that obstruction caused by prostatic enlargement leads to the residual bladder urine that invites UTIs in men. Equally critical is the role played by the prostate if it becomes infected, because it may serve as a focus for reinfection of the urinary tract. In fact, the predominant UTI problem

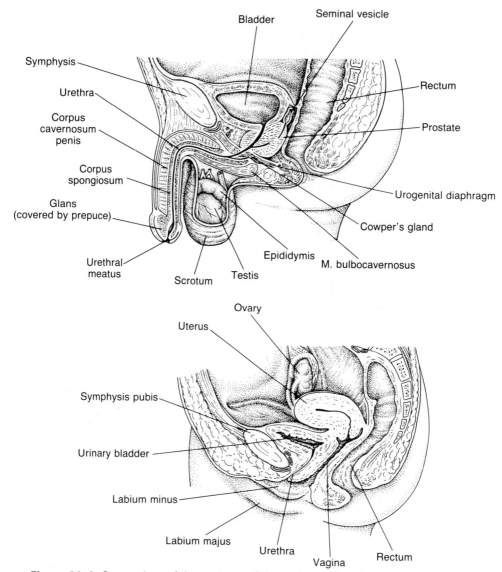

Figure 26–2. *Comparison of the anatomy of the male and female genitourinary tracts.*

in adult men is recurrent infections, and it is believed by most experts, although supportive evidence is meager, that chronic bacterial prostatitis is the predominant cause of this syndrome. How the prostate becomes infected is unknown, but presumably it occurs by retrograde migration of bacteria from the bladder through the ejaculatory ducts. Other potential methods of infection include hematogenous or lymphogenous spread of organisms from other sites. The frequent occurrence of prostatic calculi in older men also contributes both to the risk of developing an infection and to the difficulty of its eradication.

Genitourinary Abnormalities. Anatomic problems may also be seen in adult males. These are usually acquired rather than congenital disorders. Few efforts have been made to systematically compare similar groups of bacteriuric and nonbacteriuric men to determine which specific factors may predispose to infection. In one earlier study of hospitalized male veterans, prostatic hypertrophy, urogenital calculi, a history of urogenital instrumentation or surgery, and previous UTIs were all found more commonly among the bacteriuric men. There was no association of UTI with predisposing factors in men under age 40, but there was in those aged 40 to 70; over age 70 the prevalence of predisposing factors was so high as to preclude recognizing any association. A more recent study of elderly men found that certain features were significantly more common in the men who were bacteriuric: use of a urethral or condom catheter, urinary incontinence, and a history of a previous UTI.

Sexual Activity. Because of the association of sexual intercourse with UTIs in women, this has been considered a potential route of infection in bacteriuric men. Although there have been a few reported instances in which a UTI was almost certainly heterosexually acquired, this appears to be an uncommon event. A related issue is whether homosexually active men might be at increased risk for UTIs because insertive anal intercourse could predispose to infection by a mechanism analogous to that in heterosexually active women. Based on few data showing an increased risk of UTIs and epididymitis caused by *E. coli* in homosexually active men, it seems reasonable to conclude that they are probably at increased risk for urogenital infections caused by coliforms as well as other venereal pathogens.

Diagnosis

Symptoms. Symptoms of UTI in men can be roughly divided into those that are primarily irritative (e.g., dysuria, frequency, urgency, strangury) and those that are primarily obstructive (e.g., hesitancy, nocturia, slow stream, dribbling). The latter symptoms are presumed to reflect prostatic swelling caused by either infection or inflammation. Based on our experience at the Seattle VA Medical Center, about three quarters of men with primarily irritative symptoms and about one third of those with primarily obstructive symptoms have bacteriuria. Thus, although these symptoms are worth eliciting, they do not adequately include or exclude a diagnosis of UTI. Bacteriuria in men, in addition to predisposing to prostatitis, has the potential for causing infection of the epididymis, seminal vesicles, and testicles. These infections are usually readily diagnosed by history and physical examination. As with women, symptoms are generally unreliable for distinguishing lower UTIs from upper UTIs in men. UTIs must, of course, be distinguished from urethritis (gonococcal and nongonococcal) and noninfectious genitourinary disorders, some of which (e.g., nonbacterial prostatitis and obstructive uropathy) may have similar symptoms.

Physical Examination. A physical examination is of limited utility in diagnosing UTIs in men. Nevertheless, the examination should include a thorough inspection and palpation of the genitals, always including retraction of the foreskin of an uncircumcised man. Evidence of a urethral discharge, meatal erythema, inflammation of the glans, other penile lesions, an enlarged or tender epididymis or testicle, or inguinal lymphadenopathy should be specifically sought. The suprapubic and costovertebral areas should be palpated and percussed for evidence of tenderness, and a rectal examination should then be performed to palpate the prostate gland and, if possible, the seminal vesicles. In acute prostatitis, the gland is warm and tender; chronic prostatitis does not usually cause any characteristic palpatory changes. Except with concomitant acute prostatitis, epididymo-orchitis, or pyelonephritis, fever is unusual in men with a UTI.

Urine Culture

SPECIMEN COLLECTION: VOIDED URINE

The diagnosis of a UTI ultimately rests on the urine culture (Fig. 26–3*A*). To interpret the results of the culture correctly, however, it is critical that the specimen be properly obtained. Despite the plethora of investigations on how urine specimens should be obtained from women, very few studies have been performed on male populations. Because of their urogenital anatomy, women's voided urine specimens are easily contaminated with genitoperineal flora. This fact has led to the near-universal recommendation that these specimens be obtained only after cleansing the urethral meatus, and by a midstream-void procedure. The obvious differences in male anatomy should reduce the likelihood of contamination of a urine culture specimen. A few studies of young boys have shown that they can usually provide uncontaminated specimens, especially when supervised and if they are circumcised. One study of adult men found that voided specimens obtained under variable conditions in different practitioners' offices showed specimen contamination in fewer than 1% of cases.

Whether or not a clean-catch midstream-void procedure for obtaining urine cultures from men is necessary is worth considering. The process is time-consuming to explain and somewhat cumbersome to perform, especially for the elderly and disabled patients who con-

DIAGNOSIS

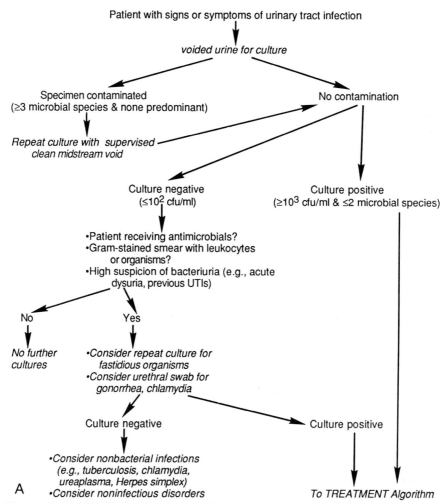

Figure 26–3. Algorithmic approach to diagnosis and treatment of bacteriuria in men.

stitute the majority of men with UTIs. In fact, my colleagues and I have shown that even after receiving instructions in the method, including the use of a graphic poster, many men could not perform the task properly. In two prospective randomized trials conducted among outpatients at our medical center, we have shown that neither meatal cleansing nor midstream sampling is usually necessary for obtaining urine specimens for culture, regardless of a man's circumcision status. Furthermore, in one study we compared the culture results of voided specimens with those of bladder specimens obtained by urethral catheterization or suprapubic bladder aspiration. We found that culture results of both the first-void and midstream-void samples correlated extremely well (r = 0.96) with the bladder speci-

mens, which proved the accuracy of the voided urine specimen in detecting true (i.e., bladder) bacteriuria. Thus, an initial-void specimen obtained without prior cleansing of the glans penis should be suitable in most situations in which a urine culture is needed for a man. This is particularly true in symptomatic subjects because the likelihood of a true positive culture is greater in this population than when screening for bacteriuria among asymptomatic subjects. If a culture result suggests that the specimen is contaminated (contains three or more different species with none being predominant [i.e., constituting > 80% of the growth], especially if one or more is usually not a uropathogen), a repeat culture of a midstream-void specimen collected under supervision should be performed.

TREATMENT

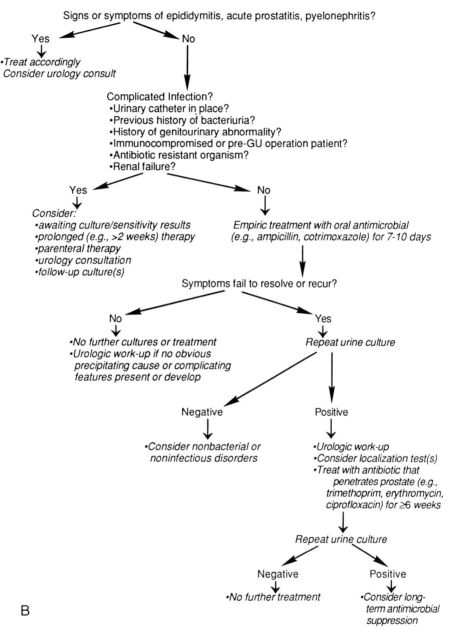

B

Figure 26–3 Continued

SPECIMEN COLLECTION: BLADDER URINE

Another important issue in diagnosing bacteriuria is when and how to obtain a bladder specimen. As mentioned above, we have found that voided urine accurately reflects bladder urine and suffices in most situations. For the occasional patient who cannot void at will or who has been unable to produce an uncontaminated specimen, it may be necessary to obtain

a bladder specimen. Bladder specimens are most often obtained by "in-and-out" urethral catheterization. There are a number of problems with this technique, in particular the small but definite risk of inducing bacteriuria or other genitourinary problems (e.g., meatal or urethral trauma). Our limited data and the much greater experience of Stamey and colleagues at Stanford University suggest that suprapubic aspiration is usually a preferable method for obtaining a bladder specimen (Fig. 26–4). For patients who have no coagulation disorders or abdominal wall defects, this technique is quite safe; it is also highly accurate, simple to perform, and, in the opinion of most patients who have experienced both, less traumatic than urethral catheterization.

SPECIMEN COLLECTION: CATHETERIZED PATIENTS

Obtaining a urine specimen that yields useful information is somewhat of a challenge in catheterized subjects. In those with indwelling urethral catheters, this may be performed by cleansing the side port of the catheter with povidone-iodine and aspirating urine with a sterile syringe. Of course, if the catheter has been in place for more than a few days the urine culture is almost invariably positive; in this instance the difficulty lies in interpreting the results, which must be based on the patient's clinical circumstances. Many elderly or institutionalized men who have urinary incontinence wear an external (condom) catheter urinary drainage system. Studies suggest that wearers of condom catheters may in fact be at increased risk for developing UTIs, especially when catheters are worn continuously or for prolonged periods, if the catheter drainage tubing becomes kinked or clogged, or if a continuous downward flow of urine from the catheter to the drainage bag is not ensured. Because this apparatus soon becomes bacterially colonized, however, it is difficult to obtain an uncontaminated urine specimen from these men. A recent study in male nursing home patients has shown that highly accurate cultures can be obtained from these men by using this simple standardized technique: a new (but not sterile) external catheter and drainage system is applied after the glans is cleaned with povidone-iodine, and the first-void specimen is collected from the drainage bag in 30 to 120 minutes.

BACTERIURIA SCREENING

Once a urine specimen has been appropriately collected, it must be properly processed by the microbiology laboratory. Here there would be expected to be few differences between specimens from male and female subjects, but again there are limited data for men. My colleagues and I have published our experience using the Gram-stained smear of urine in a male population and have shown that

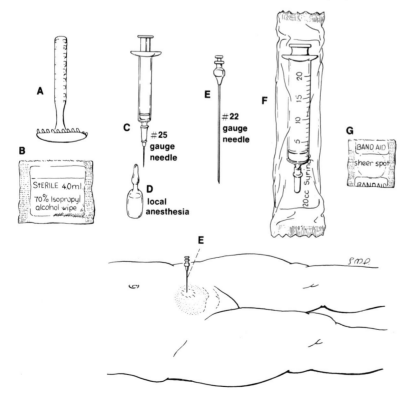

Figure 26–4. Technique of suprapubic aspiration of the bladder (SPA). From Stamey TA. Prevention of Recurrent Urinary Infections. New York, Science & Medicine Publishing Co., 1973, with permission.

it is comparable to most of the other new rapid diagnostic methods. The Gram-stained smear of unspun urine is considered positive when there are one or more micro-organisms or white blood cells per high power field (HPF) (100 ×); its sensitivity is about 0.85 and its specificity is about 0.60. The presence of pyuria (usually defined as $\geq$ 8 to 10 white blood cells/mm^3 of unspun urine) is known to correlate well with bacteriuria in women, but this finding has not been well studied in men. In our experience and in two other published studies, the presence of 10 or more white blood cells/mm^3 (or per HPF for centrifuged specimens) correlates with the presence of bacteriuria in men with a sensitivity and specificity of about 0.75.

Some have suggested that for women with the dysuria-pyuria syndrome, a urinalysis alone may be sufficient or even preferable as the initial diagnostic step. This is probably not an appropriate diagnostic strategy for men. As mentioned earlier, the accuracy of pyuria in predicting bacteriuria is less well studied in men, but it appears to be considerably lower. Furthermore, the micro-organisms causing UTIs in men are more diverse and less predictable than in women. Finally, men are usually not successfully treated with short courses of antibiotics. Therefore, symptomatic men (whether or not they have pyuria) should have a urine culture to determine if they are infected and with what micro-organism.

URINE CULTURE INTERPRETATION

Recently a major issue concerning interpretation of urine culture results has been the degree of bacteriuria in a voided specimen that should be considered to distinguish true bacteriuria from contamination. Studies of women suggest that 10^5 or more colony-forming units (cfu)/ml may be an appropriate level for asymptomatic women, but in acutely dysuric women with coliform infection, 10^2 or more cfu/ml is a more accurate cutoff. We have examined this issue in our population of male veterans by comparing voided specimens with bladder specimens as described earlier. Growth of 10^3 or more cfu/ml of a single or predominant species most accurately separated true bacteriuria from specimen contamination; this definition has both a sensitivity and a specificity of 0.97. Of importance is that only 3% of our bacteriuric men grew fewer than 10^3 cfu/ml; it is therefore unnecessary (as well as impractical) to detect such low concentra-

tions of bacteria on routine urine cultures from men. We therefore recommend that for men, growth of 10^3 or more cfu/ml of a single or predominant ($\geq$ 80% of the micro-organisms grown) species should be considered to be true bacteriuria, whereas growth of fewer than 10^3 cfu/ml or growth in any amount of three or more species with none being predominant should be considered to be specimen contamination. Our experience and that described in two other VA medical centers suggest that a single urine culture, when obtained from a cooperative man, is more than 95% reliable in establishing the diagnosis of bacteriuria, whether he is symptomatic or asymptomatic. Repeat cultures should be necessary only when results of the first specimen are nondiagnostic, i.e., are contaminated or contain fewer than 10^3 cfu/ml.

Localization Studies

Upper Versus Lower Tract. As with bacteriuric women, it may occasionally be necessary to determine whether a man with a UTI has an upper tract (i.e., renal) infection or a lower tract infection. This might be useful in determining whether to treat asymptomatic bacteriuria or to decide to prescribe suppressive treatment for recurrent bacteriuria. The gold standard test for this determination is a ureteral catheterization study, but this is tedious, expensive, and uncomfortable for the patient. The bladder washout test described by Fairley is a somewhat simpler method that can be used when it is not necessary to know which kidney is infected. Reports on the use of these procedures have mainly concerned female subjects, but there is no reason to believe that their accuracy is dependent on gender.

Antibody-Coated Bacteria. Another localization method, which has the appeal of being completely noninvasive, is the test for antibody coating of bacteria grown from urine. In general, patients with simple cystitis have a negative test, whereas those with complicated infections (e.g., hemorrhagic cystitis) or an upper tract infection have a positive result. The test is considered to be less reliable in children, and it is reported to be positive in some men with prostatitis. In one study with 59 asymptomatic bacteriuric men attending a urology clinic at Boston VA Medical Center, 76% were found to have a positive antibody-coated bacteria test. All 42 patients enrolled in the VA Cooperative study of recurrent UTI in men, only half of whom had a positive prostatic localization, had a positive antibody-coated bacteria test. Because there are problems with performing and interpreting this test and it is not generally available in clinical laboratories, I cannot recommend using it.

Prostatic Localization. One form of localization study often recommended for bacteriuric men is the prostatic localization, called the Stamey-Meares (after the authors who first described it) or four-glass (after the method) test. This procedure is considered the only reliable means of diagnosing chronic bacterial prostatitis. As shown in Table 26–2, it involves obtaining four specimens—three of urine, and (if possible) one of expressed prostatic secretions. A positive test is defined as one in which either the expressed prostatic secretion or voided bladder 3 specimen (prostatic specimen) has a substantially (usually 10-fold) greater colony count than the voided bladder 1 specimen (urethral specimen). If the specimens all yield 10^5 or more cfu/ml, it is not possible to interpret the test; in this instance the patient should be treated briefly with an antibiotic that attains therapeutic levels in the bladder but not the prostate gland (e.g., nitrofurantoin), and the test should be repeated.

Because there is no other standard against which to judge this procedure, it is unclear how often the test yields false-positive or false-negative results. In the absence of another method by which to judge the clinical usefulness of the prostatic localization test, we evaluated it in 136 men with bacteriuria or various other genitourinary problems. Although more than 80% of the men had a history of UTIs, only 33% were bacteriuric when the four-glass test was performed. Among the bacteriuric men, 18 (40%) had a positive localization. There were no statistically significant differences in present or past genitourinary history, physical examination, or laboratory tests between the men who had a positive localization test and those who did not. Our limited data

also suggest that the outcome of antibiotic treatment is similar for bacteriuric men with positive and negative localizations. Thus, the localization test does not appear to identify a clinically or microbiologically distinct group of men, and I see little reason to recommend it.

Etiologic Agents

Usual Micro-organisms. More than 80% of UTIs in women are caused by *E. coli,* with a smaller percentage attributable to *Staphylococcus saprophyticus* and less often to other aerobic gram-negative bacilli. The situation for males is somewhat different. Gram-negative bacilli are responsible for about three quarters of UTIs, but *E. coli* causes less than half of the infections in boys and only about a quarter of those in men. Other gram-negative bacilli, particularly *Proteus* and, to a lesser extent, *Providencia* species, are responsible for the remainder. Gram-positive species, especially enterococci and coagulase-negative staphylococci, account for about a fifth of infections in both boys and men. Patients who have been previously treated for UTIs, especially those who have been institutionalized, often have more unusual and antibiotic-resistant organisms. In most reported series, *S. saprophyticus* has not been specifically identified; where it has been sought, it is only occasionally found as a uropathogen in males.

Fastidious Micro-organisms. Unusual uropathogens are sometimes isolated from men. *Trichomonas vaginalis* is a rare cause of urethritis and prostatitis, usually in the consorts of women with vaginal infections. We have reported our serendipitous finding of eight cases of UTI in men caused by nontypable strains of *Haemophilus influenzae.* All but one of these men had functional or anatomic genitourinary disorders. By culturing all of the voided urine specimens from men that were submitted to our clinical microbiology labora-

Table 26–2. *Procedure for Localization of Infection in the Male Lower Urinary Tract by Use of Segmented Urine Cultures*

Specimen	Symbol	Description
Voided bladder 1	VB_1	Initial 5–10 ml of urinary stream
Voided bladder 2	VB_2	Midstream specimen
Expressed prostatic secretions	EPS	Secretions expressed from prostate by digital massage after midstream specimen
Voided bladder 3	VB_3	First 5–10 ml of urinary stream immediately after prostatic massage

From Krieger JN. Sex Transm Dis 11:103, 1984, with permission.

tory in a manner conducive to the growth of fastidious species (i.e., on chocolate agar incubated under 7% CO_2), we also showed that *Gardnerella vaginalis,* best known for its association with bacterial vaginosis in women, was present as the sole or predominant organism in colony counts of 10^3 or more in 3% of our male veterans. We postulate that this organism may be a sexually acquired colonizer of the urethra that may cause UTIs under certain circumstances. Clarke and colleagues have reported that 34% of urine specimens from adult men submitted to a British Public Health Laboratory yielded organisms on standard media, but a further 24% grew fastidious species (e.g., corynebacteria, anaerobes, lactobacilli) on special media. Although these and other fastidious organisms can occasionally cause UTIs, the routine use of special techniques to detect them is not justified. Such techniques may, however, be helpful in cases of sterile pyuria or in symptomatic men (especially those with genitourinary disorders) who have negative routine culture results.

Treatment

Cystitis

Very few studies have addressed the treatment of UTIs in male patients and those that report results for male patients separately have not usually defined the type of infection (i.e., simple cystitis versus prostatic, renal, or other complicated infections). Authorities have stated that UTIs in men are virtually always complicated infections and therefore require prolonged therapy. An uncontrolled study in 1965 reported that a 10-day course of sulfamethizole and methenamine mandelate cleared bacteriuria for 3 to 6 months in 59% of 44 hospitalized men. More recent reports on the efficacy of new antimicrobial agents in patients with UTIs often include some male subjects; in most cases, cure rates for men with a variety of antibiotics are similar to those for women. In light of these data and knowing the bacterial species usually found in bacteriuric men (see earlier section), I would suggest treating presumed cystitis empirically with either ampicillin (250 mg four times a day) or co-trimoxazole (trimethoprim/sulfamethoxazole, 160/800 mg twice daily) given orally for 7 to 10 days (Fig. 26–3B). When a Gram-stained smear is available, empiric treatment should be based on its results. For example,

Gram-positive cocci may represent enterococci, which would dictate use of ampicillin.

If empiric therapy is required in patients who are likely to be infected with antibiotic-resistant organisms (e.g., institutionalized men), an aminoglycoside (e.g., tobramycin) may be appropriate initial therapy. Alterations in treatment can then be considered, depending on the results of culture and sensitivity reports and the patient's clinical response. Expensive and broad-spectrum agents should be selected only when sensitivity results or a history of drug allergy justify their use (see Chap. 28). Parenteral therapy is needed only if the patient is seriously ill or unable to tolerate oral medications. Single-dose antibiotic treatment, which is successful in many bacteriuric women, has been tried in only a few men; in one study of bacteriuric men who were elderly or had catheter-related infections, the cure rates were 32% with co-trimoxazole and 8% with tobramycin. Therefore, pending additional studies, this is not appropriate therapy for men. In general, factors associated with a favorable prognosis in eradicating bacteriuria in men are growth of a single bacterial species (especially *E. coli*), absence of significant urinary tract obstruction, and absence of anatomic or functional genitourinary abnormalities.

Pyelonephritis is probably less common in bacteriuric men than women. One study employing ureteral catheterization found that only 38% of men, compared with 60% of women, had a renal source for their UTI. Men with pyelonephritis presumably should receive the same treatment as women: 2 weeks of an antibiotic that attains adequate renal tissue levels, such as ampicillin or co-trimoxazole, but not agents such as nitrofurantoin or methenamine mandelate.

Recurrent Bacteriuria

The major problem confronting the clinician treating bacteriuric men is recurrent bacteriuria, i.e., repeated infections usually occurring within a month of "successful" treatment. When appropriate bacteriologic identification is performed, these recurrences are usually shown to be relapsing infections, meaning that they are caused by the identical organism. The cause of this problem is generally thought to be a chronic infection in the prostate gland that has not been eradicated by standard courses of antimicrobial therapy. Two studies published in 1979 of a combined total of 62 men with recurrent infections compared prolonged treatment (6 or 12 weeks) with shorter treatment (10 or 14 days), with trimethoprim/sulfamethoxazole (160/800 mg twice daily). Overall treatment success was somewhat disappointing, but both studies showed that the longer course of treatment was more effective (about 65% cured) than the shorter (about 35% cured). Almost all of these subjects had a positive result on the antibody-coated bacteria test; in the one study in which localization tests were performed, about half of the men had evidence of prostatic infection.

Prostatitis

Acute bacterial prostatitis is an uncommon infection that is usually caused by the same organisms that cause cystitis or urethritis. Patients often are systemically ill and may require parenteral antibiotic treatment. Most antibiotics achieve high concentrations in the acutely inflamed gland, so penicillins, cephalosporins, aminoglycosides, and other agents may be given. To the contrary, treatment of chronic prostatic infections is hampered by poor penetration of most antibiotics into noninflamed prostatic tissue and secretions. Because it is assumed that many bacteriuric men have a prostatic focus for their infection, some clinicians treat them all with an antibiotic that is believed to achieve adequate levels in the prostate, i.e., trimethoprim, erythromycin, quinolones such as ciprofloxacin and ofloxacin, and, perhaps, doxycycline and aminoglycosides such as kanamycin. Carbenicillin indanyl sodium is recommended by some physicians, but there are few convincing data of its efficacy. Despite prolonged (6 to 12 weeks) administration of these agents, failure rates for treatment of chronic bacterial prostatitis are usually 30 to 40%. In some instances, repeated courses or chronic prophylaxis with antibiotics (see later on) is helpful; occasionally surgical extirpation of the prostate is necessary, especially if prostatic calculi are present.

Nonbacterial prostatitis is a far more common syndrome than proven chronic bacterial prostatitis. This entity is defined by evidence of prostatic inflammation (i.e., $\geq$ 10 leukocytes/HPF in expressed prostatic secretions) but negative urine and/or expressed prostatic secretions cultures in men with various genitourinary symptoms. The cause of this disorder is unknown, but because of speculation that at least some of these patients may have infec-

tions with *Mycoplasma* or *Chlamydia* species, many authorities empirically treat them with a course of tetracycline or erythromycin. Some men symptomatically improve, but because these organisms can now be detected by many clinical microbiology laboratories, therapy should be guided by evidence of infection.

Antimicrobial Prophylaxis

A study performed by the U.S. Public Health Service with 249 men with a history of chronic bacteriuria and evidence of "tissue infection" followed for up to 10 years evaluated the efficacy of continuous antimicrobial prophylaxis. Compared with a placebo, treatment with full therapeutic doses of any of the active drugs (sulfamethizole, nitrofurantoin, or methenamine mandelate) delayed recurrences of infections, decreased the frequency of acute clinical exacerbations (from 48 to 22%), and reduced the cumulative bacteriuria recurrence rate at 2 years (from about 70 to about 50%). All patients in this study initially received organism-specific antibiotic treatment; despite the high percentage who had mixed-organism infections and genitourinary structural abnormalities, a sterile urine was achieved in 85% after 48 to 72 hours. Furthermore, a quarter of the patients who received this single short course of therapy had no further recurrences, which demonstrated that prolonged or continuous therapy is certainly not necessary in all men with chronic or recurrent bacteriuria. Widespread clinical experience suggests that low doses of co-trimoxazole (one regular strength tablet a day) and probably other antimicrobials are also quite effective for long-term suppression.

Which men with recurrent bacteriuria should receive continuous suppressive therapy? The findings of the U.S. Public Health Service study and other evidence (see later on) suggest that chronic bacteriuria rarely results in renal failure, hypertension, or urosepsis. Furthermore, one must consider the potential for antibiotics to induce antibiotic-resistant bacteria and the expense and possible toxicity of drug therapy. Therefore, suppressive therapy is best only for patients with frequent (e.g., more than three or four per year) or severe (e.g., upper tract) acute clinical exacerbations of UTIs. In addition, men with various genitourinary problems or systemic disorders (see later on) are at particular risk for urosepsis and require prophylaxis.

Asymptomatic Bacteriuria

As shown in Table 26–1, asymptomatic bacteriuria is common in the elderly. Because they have neither genitourinary nor systemic symptoms, the need for treating these subjects is a matter of some debate. Recently several studies have suggested that asymptomatic bacteriuria may be associated with increased mortality in both young and elderly subjects, but other studies have disputed a causal link between asymptomatic bacteriuria and any serious sequelae. Two recent papers have demonstrated that bacteriuric men are more frequently confused, demented, and incontinent and have a higher prevalence of malignancies than nonbacteriuric men. At 5 to 10 years of follow-up, however, the mortality for the two groups is not significantly different. Furthermore, an investigation of the outcome of antibiotic treatment of asymptomatic bacteriuria in elderly institutionalized men found that although untreated men had a higher rate of bacteriuria, the proportion with infectious morbidity of any type and the mortality rate were similar in the treated and untreated men.

I believe that the available data do not support routinely treating all subjects with asymptomatic bacteriuria. Treatment is appropriate before performing any genitourinary instrumentation or for those who have one of the following additional conditions: a serious congenital or acquired abnormality of the urinary tract (e.g., polycystic kidney disease, ureteral reflux, urinary tract obstruction); a compromising medical condition (e.g., valvular heart disease, certain prosthetic devices, immunocompromising condition); or a microorganism with special morbidity (e.g., tuberculosis, invasive fungi, and perhaps urea-splitting organisms if the patient has developed urolithiasis).

Diagnostic Work-up

Localization Studies. As described earlier (Fig. 26–3*A*), it is only rarely necessary to determine whether a bacteriuric man has an upper tract infection or to discover which of the kidneys is the source of an infection. Empiric long-term therapy with antibiotics attaining high serum levels is the more prudent approach in men suspected of having a renal infection. Deciding when to perform the prostatic localization test is a more difficult matter. As previously mentioned, there is relatively

little evidence that prostatic infection is common in bacteriuric men or that it is actually defined by this test. At a minimum, it is time-consuming, relatively expensive (requiring four separate cultures), and often uncomfortable for the patient; furthermore, it is not widely known about by practicing physicians and not often performed even by those who understand its potential usefulness. I would recommend using it only when it would be important to prove a prostatic source of bacteriuria (e.g., before planning ablative prostatic surgery because of recurrent bacteriuria) or for research trials of prostatitis treatments.

Radiography. Studies of the need for a diagnostic evaluation of bacteriuric women have shown that only selected subgroups, e.g., young girls with recurrent bacteriuria, are benefited by procedures such as intravenous pyelography, retrograde cystography, or cystoscopy. The yield of these studies in most adult women does not justify their cost or potential risks. For men it has generally been suggested that even a single episode of bacteriuria indicates the need for these diagnostic procedures. This recommendation is based on the assumption that UTIs are sufficiently uncommon in men as to warrant searching for an anatomic or functional genitourinary abnormality. Indeed, 50 to 80% of the mostly elderly men who have recurrent bacteriuria have been found to have an abnormal intravenous pyelogram, about half of whom have an upper urinary tract defect. Even younger men without recurrent infections have been found to have abnormalities in a quarter to a third of cases. With more sensitive diagnostic tools, e.g., urodynamic pressure/flow videocystography, about 80% of bacteriuric men have been shown to have lower urinary tract disorders.

There is considerable debate, however, about the clinical and prognostic significance of abnormalities detected by various roentgenographic and urodynamic tests. Many of these defects, if not most, do not require surgical or other specific treatment. Potentially important urinary tract abnormalities are worth seeking in young boys but are probably not sufficiently common in older bacteriuric men to warrant consideration of diagnostic studies after their first UTI. This is especially true when there is an obvious precipitating cause of the infection, such as urinary tract instrumentation. Diagnostic studies are probably indicated for most men with recurrent or complicated infections. Invasive procedures should be performed only after treatment of the infection. Exactly which tests are necessary is unclear, but most authorities recommend an intravenous pyelogram and, in men beyond middle age, a cystoscopy. Videocystography is not generally available, but a simple flow meter may serve the purpose of detecting obstruction to voiding. Surgical correction of major (especially upper tract) abnormalities is likely to reduce the risk of acquisition and morbid consequences of UTIs, but whether improvement of prostatic obstruction does the same is a matter of controversy.

Bibliography

Booth CM, Whiteside CG, Milroy EJH, et al. Unheralded urinary tract infection in the male. A clinical and urodynamic assessment. Br J Urol 53:270–273, 1981.

This retrospective study of 50 consecutive men referred to a urology department because of UTIs in the absence of previous or persisting genitourinary symptoms found that although only 22% had abnormalities shown by standard intravenous urography or endoscopy, 80% had significant lower urinary tract abnormalities found with pressure/flow videocystography. These results were true even of men suffering their first episode of cystitis, and the prevalence of lower urinary tract disorders was significantly greater than that seen in women.

Clarke M, Pead L, Maskell R. Urinary infection in adult men: a laboratory perspective. Br J Urol 57:222–226, 1985.

During a 10-week period, 585 urine culture specimens were received at a public health laboratory in England, which suggests that symptoms of UTI among men are unexpectedly frequent. Standard overnight aerobic urine cultures were positive in only 34% of these specimens; by using special laboratory techniques, however, various fastidious organisms were isolated in an additional 26% of patients.

Freeman RB, Smith WM, Richardson JA, et al. Long-term therapy for chronic bacteriuria in men. U.S. Public Health Service cooperative study. Ann Intern Med 83:133–147, 1975.

This multicenter study followed 249 bacteriuric men for up to 10 years and demonstrated the effectiveness of continuous antimicrobial treatment in delaying recurrences of bacteriuria and reducing acute clinical exacerbations of infection. The study also defined characteristics associated with successful treatment of bacteriuria and the relatively benign long-term prognosis of chronic bacteriuria.

Gleckman R, Crowley M, Natsios GA. Therapy of recurrent invasive urinary tract infections of men. N Engl J Med 301:878–880, 1979.

Men with recurrent UTIs caused by Enterobacteriaceae who had a positive antibody-coated bacteria test had fewer relapses when treated with trimethoprim/sulfamethoxazole for 6 weeks compared with those treated for 2 weeks. Recurrences of infection were found to be relapses with the same micro-organism rather than reinfection with a new strain.

Krieger JN. Prostatitis syndromes: pathophysiology, differential diagnosis, and treatment. Sex Transm Dis 11:100–112, 1984.

The various inflammatory and infectious conditions that may affect the prostate gland are lucidly discussed in this comprehensive overview.

Lipsky BA. Urinary tract infections in men. Epidemiology, pathophysiology, diagnosis, and treatment. Ann Intern Med 110:138–150, 1989.

Lipsky BA, Inui TS, Plorde JJ, et al. Is the clean-catch midstream void procedure necessary for obtaining urine culture specimens from men? Am J Med 76:254–262, 1984.

This prospective study of 308 paired specimens from 254 men attending a urology clinic demonstrated that neither circumcision status nor meatal cleansing before specimen collection was significantly related to bacteriuria or contamination rates of urine cultures. Contamination rates were only slightly higher in initial compared with midstream-voided specimens. Therefore, the clean-catch midstream-void procedure is usually unnecessary for men.

Lipsky BA, Ireton RC, Fihn SD, et al. Diagnosis of bacteriuria in men: specimen collection and culture interpretation. J Infect Dis 155:847–854, 1987.

A comparison of 76 sets of urine specimens from 66 men showed that culture results of bladder specimens (obtained by urethral catheterization and/or suprapubic aspiration) showed excellent agreement with those of voided specimens, whether they were clean-catch midstream or uncleansed first-void specimens. The criterion for clean-catch midstream-void specimens that best differentiated sterile from infected urine was growth of $\geq 10^3$ cfu of one predominant species/ml.

Lipsky BA, Plorde JJ, Tenover FC, et al. Comparison of the AutoMicrobic System, acridine-orange stained smears, and Gram-stained smears in detecting bacteriuria. J Clin Microbiol 22:176–181, 1985.

This article demonstrates the usefulness of the Gram-stained smear in screening for bacteriuria in a male population.

Musher DM, Thorsteinsson SB, Airola VM II. Quantitative urinalysis. Diagnosing urinary tract infection in men. JAMA 236:2069–2072, 1976.

By using a hemocytometer chamber, it was shown with specimens from noncatheterized men with bacteriuria, hospitalized men with indwelling urinary catheters, and healthy male controls that uninfected urine usually contained $\leq 10^3$ white blood cells/ml, whereas infected urine regularly had $\geq 10^4$ white blood cells/ml.

Nicolle LE, Bjornson J, Harding GKM, et al. Bacteriuria in elderly institutionalized men. N Engl J Med 309:1420–1425, 1983.

Among 88 noncatheterized male residents of a long-term care ward, the prevalanece of bacteriuria was 33% and the incidence was 45 infections/100 patient-years. Single-dose therapy, with either trimethoprim/sulfamethoxazole or tobramycin, was successful in less than a quarter of the patients. Eradication of bacteriuria was not associated with a decrease in infectious morbidity or mortality.

Nicolle LE, Henderson E, Bjornson J, et al. The association of bacteriuria with resident characteristics in elderly institutionalized men. Ann Intern Med 106:682–686, 1987.

Subgroups among 91 elderly institutionalized men who were nonbacteriuric, intermittently bacteriuric, or continuously bacteriuric for 3 years had similar survival rates after 6 years of follow-up. Bacteriuric men were more frequently demented and incontinent, which demonstrated that bacteriuria was associated with higher functional disability but not with increased mortality.

Nordenstam GR, Brandberg CA, Oden AS, et al. Bacteriuria and mortality in an elderly population. N Engl J Med 314:1152–1156, 1986.

Study of a representative sample of 1966 70-year-old Swedish subjects revealed that fatal diseases associated with bacteriuria may explain the increase in mortality among elderly patients with bacteriuria. In particular, men with bacteriuria had an increased frequency of cancer, and this accounted for their increased mortality.

Ouslander JG, Greengold BA, Silverblatt FJ, et al. An accurate method to obtain urine for culture in men with external catheters. Arch Intern Med 147:286–288, 1987.

This article describes the technique for obtaining urine specimens from men wearing a condom catheter drainage system.

Pead L, Maskell R. Urinary tract infection in adult men. J Infect 3:71–78, 1981.

Among 999 men aged 15 to 50 years who presented to general practitioners with symptoms suggesting a UTI, only 22% had bacteriuria and 63% had sterile pyuria.

Reilly BM. Male genito-urinary infections, in Practical Strategies in Outpatient Medicine. Philadelphia, WB Saunders, 1984, pp 363–375.

This excellent chapter provides thoughtful and practical strategies for diagnosing and treating various genitourinary infections commonly seen in male outpatients.

Smith JW, Jones SR, Reed WP, et al. Recurrent urinary tract infections in men. Characteristics and response to therapy. Ann Intern Med 91:544–548, 1979.

In this VA cooperative study, men with recurrent UTIs randomized to treatment with trimethoprim/sulfamethoxazole for 12 weeks had a significantly higher cure rate than those treated for 10 days. All of the men had a positive antibody-coated bacteria test and 52% had evidence of prostate infection; recurrent infections were usually with the same organism and mostly occurred within 4 weeks of completing therapy.

Stamey TA. Pathogenesis and treatment of urinary tract infections. Baltimore, Williams & Wilkins, 1980, pp 1–51, 430–474.

This book is a comprehensive treatise on urinary infections from an author with extensive clinical and research experience with male and female subjects.

Wolfson SA, Kalmanson GM, Rubin ME, et al. Epidemiology of bacteriuria in a predominantly geriatric male population. Am J Med Sci 250:163–173, 1965.

This is one of the first epidemiologic studies of bacteriuria in men, performed with medical inpatients at a VA Medical Center. It defined the incidence of infection, etiologic agents, risk factors, and outcome of treatment.

27

✓ Adult Women with Acute Dysuria

ANTHONY L. KOMAROFF, M.D.

Women with acute dysuria and without symptoms or signs suggesting acute pyelonephritis are frequently seen in office practice. For 30 years the conventional view has been that (1) such patients have infection limited to the bladder; (2) the responsible micro-organisms are almost always gram-negative coliforms; (3) the most valuable test is a urine culture; (4) the diagnosis of urinary tract infection (UTI) is made by finding more than 100,000 bacteria/ml (positive culture results); and (5) patients with positive culture results should receive 7 to 14 days of antibacterial treatment. Recent evidence seriously challenges each of these five assumptions.

The following sections summarize this evidence and review a new scheme for categorizing women with acute dysuria, which has been presented elsewhere previously. The discussion that follows pertains only to nonpregnant adult women without clinical evidence of acute pyelonephritis; the comments are not applicable to children of either sex or to adult men.

Causes of Acute Dysuria

Acute Pyelonephritis

The symptoms and signs of acute pyelonephritis—dysuria, frequency and urgency in association with fever, flank pain, nausea and vomiting, rigors, and costovertebral angle tenderness—are well-known to clinicians. Urinalysis almost always reveals marked pyuria and bacteriuria. The urine culture colony count is usually greater than 100,000 organisms/ml of urine, although this may not initially be the case in 10 to 15% of patients. Hematuria and proteinuria may also be present for several days during the height of the inflammation. Depending on how sick and how frail the patient, outpatient treatment with an oral an-

248

tibacterial regimen or hospitalization with parenteral treatment may be indicated. As a general rule, I hospitalize patients with fevers of greater than 102°F, recurrent rigors, or marked dehydration, or any patients who are immunocompromised.

Subclinical Pyelonephritis

Thirty percent of patients in most primary care settings and 80% of patients in emergency rooms serving indigent populations have the clinical picture of lower UTI but actually have an upper tract infection. This has been demonstrated in studies with bilateral ureteral catheterization, the bladder washout technique, and the antibody-coated bacteria assay.

These patients with what is called subclinical pyelonephritis may have minimal symptoms that smolder for long periods. The infection may be difficult to eradicate. The optimal therapeutic regimen is unknown. Many patients are likely to require prolonged therapy (e.g., 6 weeks of full-dose therapy) to achieve eradication of a persistent renal focus of infection.

At the initial visit, the urinalysis typically displays pyuria and bacteriuria; hematuria and proteinuria may also be transiently present. A urine culture typically reveals more than 100,000 organisms/ml of urine.

Lower Urinary Tract Bacterial Infection

During the past 15 years, it has become apparent that many women with symptoms of lower UTIs have so-called negative culture results: fewer than 100,000 bacteria/ml of urine. Until recently, it had been conventional to say that patients with a positive culture had cystitis, whereas patients with a negative culture had infection limited to the urethra: the acute urethral syndrome.

It now appears that this distinction is unjustified and that the traditional criterion of a positive culture (greater than 100,000 bacteria/ml) is not useful in *symptomatic* women. Instead, as Stamm and his colleagues have shown, the symptomatic woman with pyuria on urinalysis and a colony count of greater than only 100 bacteria/ml should be regarded as having a lower urinary tract bacterial infection. Treatment of this entity, even when the culture is negative, is demonstrably effective (alternative treatment approaches are discussed later).

Chlamydial Urethritis

Urethral infection with *Chlamydia trachomatis* accounts for some fraction of cases of acute dysuria in women. Urinalysis typically reveals pyuria but not bacteriuria; hematuria is very unusual, as is proteinuria. A urine culture typically is sterile: the chlamydiae do not grow on the media used for urine bacterial cultures. Treatment with tetracycline hydrochloride or erythromycin for at least 7 days is effective.

Other Urethral Infections

Occasionally urethritis may be caused by *Neisseria gonorrhoeae, Trichomonas vaginalis, Candida albicans,* or herpes simplex. All of these forms of urethritis except candidal urethritis typically produce pyuria. Urine cultures for the traditional bacteria typically are sterile or contain few organisms of various types. Standard treatment regimens are available and effective for each entity.

No Recognized Pathogen

Even after vigorous attempts are made to isolate many different bacterial, viral, fungal, chlamydial, and protozoal infectious agents, a substantial fraction of women with dysuria have no recognized pathogen, have no pyuria, and do not respond to antimicrobial treatment. The absence of pyuria in these patients is useful because it indicates to the clinician that antimicrobial treatment is probably unnecessary. The cause of the dysuria may be a ure-

thral inflammation from trauma, dessicating agents, or other noninfectious factors.

Vaginitis

Patients with vaginitis may have a chief complaint of dysuria and not of vaginal discharge or irritation, although these latter symptoms almost always are elicited by the clinician in patients with vaginitis. In some settings, vaginal infections are actually more frequent causes of the presenting complaint of dysuria than are urinary infections. Typically, except when a trichomonal infection involves the urethra as well as the vagina, pyuria is absent.

The Dysuria-Pyuria Syndrome

In the woman with dysuria, the presence of pyuria strongly suggests the presence of any of several treatable entities: acute pyelonephritis, subclinical pyelonephritis, lower urinary tract bacterial infection, chlamydial urethritis, and other urethritis. Conversely, pyuria is usually absent in patients in whom no recognized pathogen can be found; these patients also do not respond to antibacterial treatment. Pyuria is also usually absent in patients with vaginal infection, who are typically treated with antimicrobials different from those used for UTIs.

Therefore, patients with acute dysuria and pyuria have a syndrome (called the dysuria-pyuria syndrome) that almost always can benefit from immediate antibacterial treatment, and patients without pyuria do not. However, because each possible cause of dysuria and pyuria requires a different therapy, the finding of pyuria does not indicate *what* the treatment should be. The judgment is made on the basis of other data.

Thus, the finding of pyuria on urinalysis not only is more readily available than a urine culture result but also appears to be a better predictor of treatable infection than is the result of a culture.

Diagnostic Tests

Urinalysis

The urinalysis is valuable in the diagnosis of UTI in the otherwise healthy adult woman for several reasons. First and foremost, as described earlier, the presence or absence of *pyuria* is of great importance. Second, the presence of *hematuria* has value in tending to rule out chlamydial and other forms of urethritis as well as vaginitis; probably the same is true of *proteinuria*. When seen, *white blood cell casts* clearly indicate an upper tract infection. Urine *glucose* has value in suggesting previously unrecognized diabetes mellitus, which in turn raises the possibility of papillary necrosis and (possibly) perinephric abscess in the patient with symptoms and signs of acute pyelonephritis.

The value of pyuria has been established primarily by the work of Stamm and his colleagues, who defined pyuria as being eight or more leukocytes/cm^3 in uncentrifuged urine; this corresponds to approximately two to five leukocytes per high power field in centrifuged urine sediment.

Leukocyte Esterase Test

The leukocyte esterase test, available on urine dip sticks, appears to be a quite specific measure of pyuria (specificity ranging from 93 to 98%) but is relatively less sensitive (sensitivity ranging from 74 to 96%). However, one loses potentially valuable information in forgoing microscopic examination (casts, hematuria, bacteriuria) of the urine sediment.

Urine Culture

As is apparent from earlier comments, the urine culture is less valuable for women with acute dysuria than is the urinalysis. It does have some role, as will be discussed in the management strategy proposed later. Its most important role may be in the follow-up of patients rather than as part of an initial diagnostic test battery.

Proposed Management Strategy

Consider Vaginitis

As shown in Figure 27–1, the patient first should always be asked about symptoms of vaginal discharge and irritation; if such symptoms are present, a pelvic examination should be performed and appropriate therapy should be given for vaginitis (and possibly concomitant urethritis). A urinalysis and urine culture

probably are unnecessary, although urinary and vaginal infections occasionally can coexist.

Consider Subclinical Pyelonephritis

Second (Fig. 27–1), risk factors suggestive of subclinical pyelonephritis should be sought: known underlying urinary tract pathology, diabetes mellitus or other conditions or therapies producing an immunocompromised state, urinary infections in childhood, documented relapse in the past, symptoms for 7 to 10 days before seeking care (this also suggests chlamydial urethritis), or three or more previous urinary infections or acute pyelonephritis in the past year. Subclinical pyelonephritis may also be more likely in indigent, inner-city residents.

Although there are few data to support this policy, I would recommend (Fig. 27–1) treating patients with any one of these risk factors in the following manner. I would obtain a urinalysis and urine culture for all such patients. For patients with pyuria, I would recommend immediately initiating 10 days of treatment with one of the standard antimicrobial agents (e.g., ampicillin, 250 mg four times a day) before the culture result returns.

Every effort should be made to obtain a follow-up culture 2 to 4 days after the end of therapy because patients with subclinical pyelonephritis may be particularly prone to relapse. I would treat patients who then are shown to have relapsing infection for 6 weeks. For patients who relapse after a 6-week course of therapy, I would order diagnostic studies to look for a cause of the persistent infection (e.g., intravenous pyelogram [IVP] and retrograde studies).

Consider Chlamydial and Gonococcal Urethritis

As summarized in Figure 27–2, chlamydial urethritis is suggested by (1) a sexual partner with recent urethritis; (2) a new recent sexual partner; (3) the stuttering onset of symptoms over a period of days rather than abruptly; and (4) the absence of hematuria. Gonococcal urethritis is also likely in patients whose recent sexual partners have urethritis and in patients with a past history of gonorrhea. It is also more likely in indigent, inner-city women. I believe that patients with any one of these risk factors for chlamydial or gonococcal urethritis

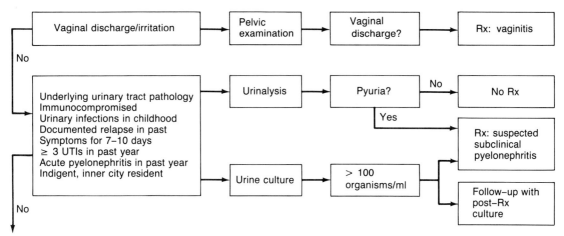

Figure 27–1. *Approach to immediate diagnosis and treatment: first, assess the possibility of vaginitis; second, assess the possibility of subclinical pyelonephritis.*

should have a pelvic examination and urinalysis (Fig. 27–2). Purulent discharge from the urethral (or cervical) os should be Gram stained. A positive Gram's stain is a reliable indicator of gonorrhea and should lead to immediate treatment. A mucopurulent discharge from the cervical or urethral os that demonstrates leukocytes but no organisms probably raises the likelihood of chlamydial infection and is sufficient grounds for immediate treatment.

Chlamydial urethritis is often seen in combination with chlamydial cervicitis, an entity characterized by mucopurulent cervical discharge and edematous areas on the exocervix, which is responsive to the same therapeutic regimen. Probable chlamydial cervicitis should be treated promptly (Fig. 27–2).

In patients with risk factors for chlamydial or gonococcal urethritis and pyuria without bacteriuria, treatment sufficient to cover chlamydial or gonococcal urethritis should be instituted, even if the pelvic examination is normal. Finally (Fig. 27–2), when a patient has a history of gonorrhea or a history of recent exposure, a gonorrhea culture from the urethral and cervical os should be obtained even in the absence of a purulent discharge by using a calcium-alginate-tip swab.

Consider Lower Tract Bacterial Infection

In 60 to 70% of patients, none of the above categories applies. As shown in Figure 27–3,

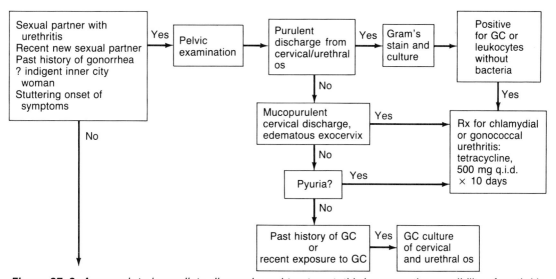

Figure 27–2. *Approach to immediate diagnosis and treatment: third, assess the possibility of urethritis.*

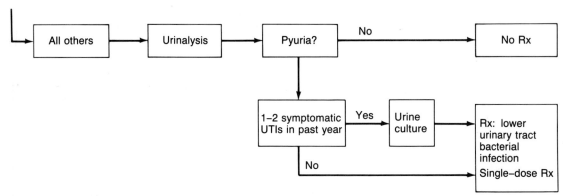

Figure 27–3. *Approach to immediate diagnosis and treatment: fourth, assess the possibility of lower urinary tract bacterial infection; fifth, assess the possibility of no infection.*

for such patients, I would obtain a urinalysis and treat those patients who have pyuria with one of the efficacious single-dose regimens: trimethoprim/sulfamethoxazole, 160/800 mg; amoxicillin, 2 to 3 g; sulfisoxazole, 1 g. I would not obtain a urine culture at the initial visit for this group of patients, except in those patients with one or two previous symptomatic urinary infections during the past year.

Diagnostic and Therapeutic Issues in Recurrent Infection

As shown in Figure 27–4, women who develop recurrent infections with the *same* organism may well have an uneradicated upper tract infection and should have an IVP and cystoscopic examination. The role of these two diagnostic studies is harder to define when patients have had three or more infections in the past year with *different* organisms (reinfections). In three studies, IVP revealed a surgically correctable lesion in fewer than 1% of patients, and cystoscopy revealed a correctable lesion (e.g., urethral diverticulum) in up to 4% of patients. On this basis, I recommend cystoscopy in patients with three or more reinfections in a year, but I avoid obtaining an IVP unless there are five or more reinfections in a year. When the bacteriology is such that one cannot clearly tell whether the patient is suffering from reinfection or persistent infection—unfortunately a common situation—it probably is wisest to obtain both the IVP and cystoscopic examination.

I recommend antimicrobial prophylaxis with trimethoprim/sulfamethoxazole, 40/200 mg

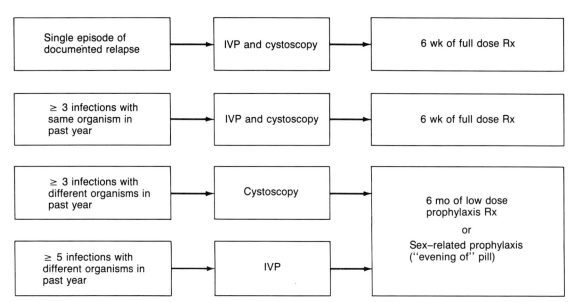

Figure 27–4. *Approach to diagnosis and treatment in recurrent infection.*

each day, in a woman who has had three or more bacterial infections in a year; a reasonable duration of prophylaxis is 6 months.

Bibliography

Brunham RC, Kuo C, Stevens CE, et al. Therapy of cervical chlamydial infection. Ann Intern Med 97:216–219, 1982.
Study of therapeutic approaches to cervical chlamydial infection.

Buckwold FJ, Ludwig P, Harding GKM, et al. Therapy for acute cystitis in adult woman: randomized comparison of single-dose sulfisoxazole vs trimethoprim-sulfamethoxazole. JAMA 247:1839–1842, 1982.
Randomized trial demonstrating the efficacy of single-dose therapy.

Chernow B, Zaloga GP, Soldano S, et al. Measurement of urinary leukocyte esterase activity: a screening test for urinary tract infections. Ann Emerg Med 13:150–154, 1984.
Study of the accuracy of a dipstick assay for pyuria.

Fairley KF, Carson NE, Gutch RC, et al. Site of infection in acute urinary-tract infection in general practice. Lancet 2:615–618, 1971.
Early study demonstrating the importance of low-count bacteriuria and the acute urethral syndrome.

Fang LST, Tolkoff-Rubin NE, Rubin RH. Efficacy of single-dose and conventional amoxicillin therapy in urinary-tract infection localized by the antibody-coated bacteria technic. N Engl J Med 298:413–416, 1978.
Controlled study of single-dose therapy and demonstration of the difficulties in treating subclinical pyelonephritis.

Fowler JE, Pulaski ET. Excretory urography, cystography, and cystoscopy in the evaluation of women with urinary-tract infection: a prospective study. N Engl J Med 304:462–465, 1981.
Evaluation of the yield of various diagnostic tests in women with recurrent urinary infection.

Grover SA, Komaroff AL, Weisberg M, et al. The characteristics and hospital course of patients admitted for presumed acute pyelonephritis. J Gen Intern Med 2:5–10, 1987.
Retrospective review of clinical and laboratory findings in patients hospitalized for presumed acute pyelonephritis.

Kass EH. Asymptomatic infections of the urinary tract. Trans Assoc Am Physicians 69:56–63, 1956.
Landmark article on the quantification of bacteriuria.

Komaroff AL. Acute dysuria in women. N Engl J Med 310:368–375, 1984.
Review of the various causes of acute dysuria in women and management of the different entities.

Komaroff AL. Urinalysis and urine culture in women with dysuria. Ann Intern Med 104:212–218, 1986.
Review focusing on the contributions of urinalysis and urine culture in the diagnosis of dysuria.

Komaroff AL, Friedland G. The dysuria-pyuria syndrome. N Engl J Med 303:452–454, 1980.
Essay summarizing the importance of pyuria in the management of patients with dysuria.

Komaroff AL, Pass TM, McCue JD, et al. Management strategies for urinary and vaginal infections. Arch Intern Med 138:1069–1073, 1978.
Study of the predictive value of different clinical and laboratory findings in diagnosis of different causes of dysuria. First study to highlight importance of vaginal infections in producing dysuria.

Ronald AR, Boutros P, Mourtada H. Bacteriuria localization and response to single-dose therapy in women. JAMA 235:1854–1856, 1976.
Demonstration of the entity of subclinical pyelonephritis and the efficacy of single-dose therapy.

Rothenberg RB, Simon R, Chipperfield E, et al. Efficacy of selected diagnostic tests for sexually transmitted diseases. JAMA 235:49–51, 1976.
Study highlighting the value of Gram's stain in diagnosing gonococcal infections in women.

Rubin RH, Fang LST, Jones SR, et al. Single-dose amoxicillin therapy for urinary tract infection: multicenter trial using antibody-coated bacteria localization technique. JAMA 244:561–564, 1980.
Large study demontrating the efficacy of single-dose therapy.

Savard-Fenton M, Fenton BW, Reller LB, et al. Single-dose amoxicillin therapy with follow-up urine culture. Am J Med 73:808–813, 1982.
Demonstration of the effectiveness of single-dose therapy.

Stamm WE, Counts GW, McKevitt M, et al. Urinary prophylaxis with trimethoprim and trimethoprim-sulfamethoxazole: efficacy, influence on the natural history of recurrent bacteriuria, and cost control. Rev Infect Dis 4:450–455, 1982.
Detailed review of the value of prophylaxis in women with recurrent infections.

Stamm WE, Counts GW, Running KR, et al. Diagnosis of coliform infection in acutely dysuric women. N Engl J Med 307:463–468, 1982.
Study confirming the importance of low-count bacteriuria.

Stamm WE, Counts GW, Wagner KF, et al. Antimicrobial prophylaxis of recurrent urinary tract infections: a double-blind, placebo-controlled trial. Ann Intern Med 92:770–775, 1980.
Demonstration of the value of prophylaxis in women with recurrent urinary infections.

Stamm WE, Running K, McKevitt M, et al. Treatment of the acute urethral syndrome. N Engl J Med 304:956–958, 1981.
Demonstration of the efficacy of treatment for low-count bacteriuria and chlamydial urethritis.

Stamm WE, Wagner KF, Amsel R, et al. Causes of the acute urethral syndrome in women. N Engl J Med 303:409–415, 1980.
Landmark study demonstrating the importance of low-count bacteriuria and chlamydial urethritis.

Stansfield JM. The measurement and meaning of pyuria. Arch Dis Child 37:257–262, 1962.
Detailed analysis of alternative methods for measuring pyuria.

28

Management of Patients with Chronic Urinary Catheters

RICHARD A. MORIN, M.D.
RICHARD GARIBALDI, M.D.

Introduction

In his classic editorial published in 1958 entitled The Case Against the Catheter, Beeson pointed out the potential hazards of urinary drainage by indwelling catheters and advised physicians to use these devices only when absolutely necessary. This admonition remains true to this day. Nonetheless, the use of urinary catheters is now an accepted adjunct to medical care for selected patients. Temporary bladder drainage is frequently required for surgical patients who have received general or spinal anesthesias and patients with debilitating medical illnesses. Long-term catheterization is frequently used for patients with spinal cord injuries, impaired bladder function, or decubitus ulcers caused by incontinence, immobility, and malnutrition. Indwelling urethral catheters are indicated for severely incapacitated and terminally ill patients who cannot be managed effectively with behavioral training, drugs, skilled nursing care, surgery, special clothing, or urinary collection devices. Sometimes, for these patients, the benefits of patient comfort and expeditious nursing outweigh the potential risks of catheterization. In most skilled care nursing homes today, between 2 and 10% of patients are treated by long-term urethral catheterization.

Many of the principles for managing patients with chronic indwelling urethral catheters have been derived from studies of patients who have undergone short-term catheterization in acute care hospitals. Unfortunately, relatively few data regarding prevention and treatment are available for chronically catheterized patients who reside in long-term care facilities or at home. As yet, there are no prospective, randomized, controlled clinical trials comparing chronic catheterization with alternative techniques of urinary bladder drainage. Therefore, much of the information that is contained in this chapter is subjective. Nonetheless, it reflects present thinking on the epidemiology and control of infection in chronically catheterized patients and presents a practical approach to their management.

Pathophysiology of Catheter-Associated Urinary Infection

The sterility of bladder urine is maintained by a variety of intrinsic mechanisms that prevent the influx of urethral bacteria into the bladder and inhibit the growth of organisms that attempt to colonize bladder urine. These defenses include the long urethra and bacteriostatic properties of prostatic secretions in men, urine acidity and osmolality, and intrinsic antimicrobial bladder mucosal factors that are poorly characterized. The insertion of a urethral catheter, however, bypasses many of these defenses and provides an access route for bacteria to colonize and infect bladder urine. In catheterized patients, bacteria may migrate into the bladder in urethral mucus outside the catheter or in the column of urine within the catheter. The indwelling catheter also acts as a foreign body that can cause irritation and inflammation in the mucosa of the bladder wall. This mucosal disruption allows bacterial invasion to occur more readily. The presence of the catheter eliminates the periodic flushing of urethral bacteria that usually occurs with micturition and distorts the anatomy of the bladder. This results in incomplete emptying of bladder urine and a loss of integrity of the vesicoureteral antireflux valves. The catheter may also serve as a nidus for encrustations of protein, calcium, mucin, and struvite crystals. These concretions are ecologic hiding places for potential bladder pathogens.

Definition of Catheter-Associated Urinary Tract Infection

The diagnosis of catheter-associated urinary tract infection must be based on clinical judgment. Objective criteria alone, such as urine microbiology, bacterial colony counts, or findings on urinalysis, do not establish the diagnosis of infection. The presence of 10^5 or more colony-forming units (cfu)/ml urine may reflect either bladder colonization or infection. These entities must be distinguished on clinical grounds. Colonization is defined as asymptomatic bacteriuria, whereas infection is defined by symptoms or signs of inflammation. Catheter-urine cultures with 10^2 or 10^3 cfu/ml urine are sometimes responsible for clinically significant infection. On the other hand, colony counts of 10^5 or more cfu/ml urine are often associated with asymptomatic colonization. In addition, parameters such as pyuria and hematuria that are used so frequently to define infection in noncatheterized patients cannot be relied on for a diagnosis of infection in the catheterized patient. These microscopic findings may be traumatic consequences of catheter-associated mucosal injury.

Characteristic clinical symptoms of urinary infection may be absent, atypical, or unobtainable in the chronically catheterized patient. The presence of the catheter precludes symptoms such as dysuria and urinary frequency. Chronically catheterized patients often suffer from other conditions that impair their ability to communicate such symptoms as back pain or suprapubic pain. Frequently, the clinician must base the diagnosis of urinary tract infection on the clinical finding of fever and the absence of other focal sources of infection. It is worth noting that in a prospective study by Warren and coworkers of fevers in chronically catheterized patients, only 2 of 98 patients with febrile episodes of possible urinary origin had signs or symptoms localized to the urinary tract. Occasionally, fever may also be absent. In these cases, a change in mental status, unexplained tachycardia, or increased respiratory rate may be the only clues for urinary tract infection and impending urosepsis.

Epidemiology and Natural History of Bacteriuria in Chronically Catheterized Patients

The insertion of a urethral catheter immediately predisposes the patient to an increased risk of bacteriuria and infection. Between 1 and 20% of patients exposed to a single, in-and-out catheterization develop bacteriuria; the risk is greatest in patients who are most debilitated. The rate of acquired bacteriuria for patients with indwelling catheters is between 2 and 5% per day during the first week of catheterization. By the end of 1 week, between 20 and 40% of catheterized patients are bacteriuric; after 1 month, virtually 100% are colonized. Chronically catheterized patients are usually colonized with two or more bacterial species (Table 28–1). Many of these organisms are resistant to commonly prescribed antibiotics. Organisms that colonize the urine are in a constant state of flux, even without the selection pressure of antibiotics. Some organisms, particularly *Providencia stuartii,* persist for several weeks, whereas other isolates, such as enterococci and certain Enterobacteriaceae, colonize bladder urine for shorter periods. The relative persistence of colonization with *P. stuartii* may be due to unique properties of this organism to adhere to catheter material or bladder mucosa cells.

These observations have practical implications for clinicians caring for chronically catheterized patients. Many microbiology laboratories do not routinely identify or perform antimicrobial sensitivity tests on urine specimens that contain two or more isolates. This policy is appropriate for noncatheterized patients because the recovery of multiple isolates from urine frequently represents urethral contamination. However, this practice may delay

Table 28–1. *Common Isolates Identified in Urine Specimens of Patients with Chronic Indwelling Catheters*

Gram Positive
Enterococci
Coagulase-negative *Staphylococcus* species
Corynebacterium species
Gram Negative
Escherichia coli
Proteus mirabilis
Providencia stuartii
Pseudomonas aeruginosa
Morganella morganii
Klebsiella pneumoniae
Yeast
Candida albicans

the diagnosis and choice of optimal antibiotic treatment of chronically catheterized patients with urosepsis. The laboratory must be instructed to identify and test all isolates from the infected catheterized patient. Furthermore, the dynamic state of urinary colonization precludes the value of surveillance cultures to predict the cause of infection in chronically catheterized patients who become septic. Definitive therapy must be based on sensitivity test results of isolates that are recovered from the urine at the time of symptomatic infection. Treatment based on isolates collected from an asymptomatic period may be misleading and delay the initiation of effective therapy.

The clinical significance of asymptomatic bacteriuria in the chronically catheterized patient has not been well delineated. There does not appear to be a predictable progression from asymptomatic colonization to symptomatic infection, bacteremia, and death. Even though indwelling catheters are frequently cited as a major risk factor for gram-negative bacteremia, the actual incidence of symptomatic infection among chronically catheterized patients is quite low. Warren and coworkers observed an incidence of approximately one febrile episode per 100 days of catheterization, and these episodes could not always be attributed to a urinary source of infection. The majority of the observed febrile episodes were low grade fevers, which were of short duration and which resolved without antibiotic intervention. The specific factors that precipitate the transition from asymptomatic bacteriuria to symptomatic infection are incompletely understood. Transient obstruction, catheter manipulation, catheter-associated trauma, change in colonization pattern, and reduction in urine

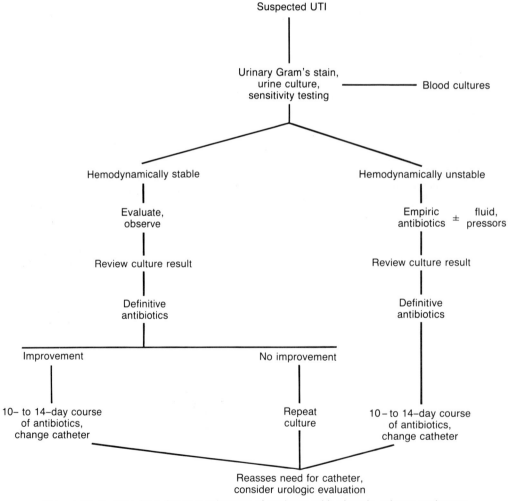

Figure 28-1. Algorithm for management of patients with chronic urinary catheters.

Table 28–2. Cost of Antibiotics Commonly Used in Treating Urinary Tract Infections Based on a 10-Day Course of Therapy

Antibiotic	Dose	Frequency (Hourly Interval)	Cost* (US $)
ORAL ANTIBIOTICS			
Ampicillin, generic	500 mg	6	5.20
Polycillin (Bristol)			13.80
Cephalexin, generic	500 mg	6	31.36
Keflex (Lilly)			60.10
Cefadroxil			
Duracef (MJ)	500 mg	12	36.25
Norfloxacin			
Noroxin (Merck)	400 mg	12	40.50
Sulfisoxazole, generic	500 mg	6	1.09
Gantrisin (Roche)			5.14
Trimethoprim/ sulfamethoxazole, generic	160/800 mg	12	2.50
Bactrim (Roche)			12.88
Septra (Burrows Wellcome)			12.88
PARENTERAL ANTIBIOTICS			
Ampicillin, generic	1 g	4	75.00
Polycillin (Bristol)			288.00
Aztreonam			
Azactam (Squibb)	1 g	8	356.25
Cefazolin, generic	1 g	6	202.40
Kefzol (Lilly)			262.00
Gentamicin, generic	80 mg	8	49.50
Garamycin (Schering)			114.60
Mezlocillin			
Mezlin (Miles)	3 g	8	340.35
Tobramycin			
Nebcin (Lilly)	80 mg	8	200.53

*Cost to pharmacist based on the average wholesale price in Drug Topics Red Book 1988; cost to patient is higher.

flow have been suggested, but not proved, as possible predisposing factors. Finally, the long-term consequences of catheter-associated bacteriuria are also not well defined. Some investigators have suggested that chronically colonized patients are at an increased risk for hypertension, pyelonephritis, renal failure, or premature death. However, these associations remain controversial and await further, long-term epidemiologic confirmation.

Treatment of Catheter-Associated Infections

Most clinicians agree that patients with chronic indwelling catheters and asymptomatic bacteriuria should not be treated with antibiotics. Attempts to eradicate asymptomatic bacteriuria result in the propagation of multi–antibiotic-resistant organisms without any sig-

nificant long-term decrease in bacteriuria. Systemic antibiotics should be reserved for those patients with symptomatic infections.

When a patient with a chronic indwelling catheter has signs or symptoms indicative of infection, it is imperative that the physician examine the patient and obtain appropriate laboratory tests to investigate the possible sources of infection. Although urinary tract infection is always a consideration, other possibilities include meningitis, pneumonia, diverticulitis, appendicitis, cholecystitis, soft tissue abscesses, infected decubitus ulcers, adverse drug reactions, and iatrogenic causes. These are but a few of the many explanations that can be responsible for a clinical picture of sepsis in an elderly, chronically catheterized patient.

Once it has been determined that the source of infection is the urinary tract, the physician must consider the current clinical status of the patient in guiding further diagnostic tests and treatment (Fig. 28–1). If the patient has a low grade temperature, is hemodynamically stable, and appears to be nontoxic, the physician should arrange for a urine culture and sensitivity testing of all isolates. The choice of appropriate antibiotic therapy (Table 28–2) should be guided by the results of sensitivity testing.

The tempo of diagnosis and treatment differs considerably in the case of the patient who has a high fever (temperature greater than 38.8°C), is hemodynamically unstable, or has a toxic appearance. In such a clinical situation of sepsis, diagnosis and treatment must be instituted simultaneously. Diagnostic tests should include a Gram's stain of the urine, urine culture with sensitivities of all isolates, and blood cultures. The Gram's stain of the urine can provide a direction for selecting empiric antibiotic therapy (Table 28–3). Additional

Table 28–3. Empiric Antibiotics for Urosepsis Based on Gram's Stain Findings*

Gram's Stain	Empiric Parenteral Antibiotics
Gram-positive cocci	(1) Ampicillin and gentamicin (2) Vancomycin and gentamicin
Gram-negative rods	(1) Mezlocillin or piperacillin and tobramycin or amikacin (2) Aztreonam (3) Ceftazidime (4) Imipenem
Yeast	(1) Amphotericin B

*Doses and dosing intervals must be adjusted based on renal status.

Table 28–4. *Cost of Diagnostic Tests*

Test	Cost* (US $)
Gram's stain of urine	9.25
Quantitative urine culture with sensitivity testing	31.00; 15.00 (per isolate)
Urinalysis	9.25
Blood cultures	33.50 (per set)
Blood urea nitrogen	7.50
Creatinine	8.50

*Costs cited are representative. Actual costs to the patient may vary considerably from clinical laboratory to clinical laboratory.

laboratory studies should include renal studies (blood urea nitrogen and serum creatinine levels) (Table 28–4), especially if the use of potential nephrotoxic antibiotics is anticipated.

Treatment of the septic patient must be started immediately. Initially, all possible efforts must be directed at restoring intravascular volume and regaining a normotensive status. This is usually accomplished with fluid resuscitation and the utilization of vasopressor agents such as dopamine or dobutamine. Only after hemodynamic resuscitation efforts have been started should empiric antibiotics be added. After the antibiotic sensitivity test results of the urine isolate are available, therapy should be tailored to treat the pathogens that have been identified.

In patients with chronic indwelling catheters who are receiving treatment for symptomatic infections, antibiotic therapy should be limited to a course of 10 to 14 days. If the patient's symptoms do not resolve or if they relapse soon after the antibiotics are discontinued, a re-evaluation is warranted. The re-evaluation should include repeating the urine culture and sensitivity studies. In some situations, urologic evaluation is necessary to identify anatomic abnormalities, stones, or incomplete bladder drainage. Every effort must be made to exclude the possibility of extraurinary explanations for the symptoms.

In all patients with chronic indwelling catheters who require treatment of urinary tract infections, the current need for the catheter and alternatives to continued catheterization should be carefully considered. If it is determined that there is no other option but catheterization, the present catheter should be changed before completion of the antibiotic course.

Candiduria and fungal urinary tract infections require special mention. Cutaneous candidal infections involving periurethral mucosal surfaces are common in catheterized patients.

These infections respond well to topical antifungal therapy. No treatment is required for the patient with asymptomatic candidal urinary colonization. Bladder irrigation with amphotericin B, 100 mg/500 ml sterile distilled water infused into the bladder through a three-way catheter, is recommended for symptomatic, uncomplicated, catheter-associated candidal cystitis. In patients with upper urinary tract or systemic candidal infection, intravenous amphotericin B is required.

Prevention of Infection

For patients who need chronic urethral catheterization, the following strategies have been strongly recommended to minimize the risk of acquiring catheter-associated infection:

- Catheterize only when necessary.
- Emphasize washing of hands.
- Educate personnel in the correct techniques of catheter insertion and care.
- Insert catheter by using aseptic technique and sterile equipment.
- Secure catheter properly.
- Maintain closed sterile drainage.
- When irrigation is necessary, use intermittent method.
- Obtain urine samples aseptically.
- Maintain unobstructed urine flow.

Unfortunately, no single approach has been proved to prevent infections in chronically catheterized patients, and most interventions add significant costs to care. Most experts agree that health care workers must be carefully educated on how to prevent bacterial contamination of catheter urine. This education should emphasize the importance of the patient's personal hygiene. Good perineal care is recommended to prevent fecal bacteria from contaminating the periurethral surface and colonizing bladder urine. Personnel caring for the catheterized patient should wash their hands before manipulating the catheter or drainage bag.

Catheters should be inserted as atraumatically and aseptically as possible. Closed sterile drainage is essential; this means that the catheter tubing junction is not opened unless aseptic precautions are maintained and that the spout on the drainage bag is not contaminated when urine is drained. The bag should be positioned off the floor but at a level no higher than the urinary bladder to prevent reflux.

Drainage bags with air vents, antireflux valves, or ports for the instillation of hydrogen peroxide, povidone-iodine, or chlorhexidine have not been shown to be efficacious in decreasing rates of bacteriuria or infection. There are no convincing data to suggest that silicone catheters are more effective than latex catheters in preventing infection. Catheters made of new synthetic materials, impregnated with silver ions and other antibacterial substances, are being studied in ongoing clinical trials. Forceful bladder irrigation with saline solution is not routinely recommended. This should be done only when obstruction by a clot or cellular debris is compromising urinary flow. In situations such as this, measures are usually taken to increase urine flow and to change the entire catheter and drainage bag system.

Other strategies for infection control are aimed at preventing bacteria from entering the bladder on the outside of the catheter in urethral mucus. The use of topical antibiotic ointments and other antibacterial substances to cleanse the catheter-urethral interface have not been shown to be efficacious in controlled trials. Twice daily meatal cleansing with povidone-iodine or neomycin-polymyxin ointments are no more effective in decreasing urinary colonization than green soap. On the other hand, the cost of twice daily treatments, approximately $2 per day, adds up to tens of millions of dollars per year when multiplied by the total number of patients with indwelling catheters.

Efforts should be made to maintain the natural antibacterial defenses of the urinary tract. Whenever possible, mechanical problems such as stones, anatomic defects, or ureteral reflux should be corrected to allow more complete bladder emptying. Urine flow and acidity also help to inhibit the growth of colonizing bacteria. The instillation of antibacterial solutions such as neomycin-polymyxin solution or acetic acid directly into the bladder has not been proved to be effective in preventing bacteriuria. In fact, the use of antibiotic solutions predisposes to colonization with resistant organisms. The possible beneficial effects of antibacterial infusions are negated by the more frequent openings of the closed drainage system, with subsequent contamination of bladder urine. Long-term use of systemic antibacterial agents, such as nitrofurantoin, trimethoprim-sulfamethoxazole, methenamine mandelate, and methenamine hippurate, have also not been proved to be efficacious in preventing bacteriuria. The lack of effectiveness of methenamine is partially explained by its relatively long reaction time and difficulties in acidifying urine to the pH needed to hydrolyze it to its active compound, formaldehyde. The use of systemic antibiotics predisposes to colonization and infection with resistant organisms.

Whenever possible, urinary catheters should be avoided. Several alternatives to catheterization have been suggested to have less risk of urinary tract infection than chronic catheterization. These alternatives include disposable diapers, intermittent catheterization, and condom or Texas catheters. However, the assumption of lower infection rates with these devices has not yet been proved in controlled, prospective clinical trials. In fact, each of these alternatives is associated with its own side effects and may not be as appropriate as chronic catheterization for certain patients. For instance, patients with urinary retention secondary to prostatic obstruction cannot be drained effectively with any of these techniques. Diapers require frequent changing to avoid skin maceration and breakdown. Condom catheters also require frequent nursing attention; they often cause phimosis, penile edema, ulcerations, and superficial infection, which may in turn infect bladder urine. Intermittent catheterization is a more useful approach for patients who can be trained to catheterize themselves. It is less practical for patients who are noncooperative because it requires frequent nursing attention with regularly scheduled catheterizations and additional monitoring for bladder distention.

Summary

The management of patients with chronic indwelling urinary catheters is a difficult challenge for clinicians. Virtually all patients with long-term urethral catheters have polymicrobic bacteriuria and evidence of bladder inflammation. There is no clear-cut infection control strategy to prevent these patients from developing symptomatic infection. The clinician must be alert to the subtle ways in which infection can appear in these patients. Only symptomatic infections should be treated with antibiotics. The choice of a particular antibiotic regimen should be based on the results of cultures and sensitivity tests performed on organisms isolated at the time of appearance of acute symptoms.

Bibliography

Eddeland A, Hedelin H. Bacterial colonization of the lower urinary tract in women with long-term indwelling urethral catheter. Scand J Infect Dis 15:361–365, 1983.
A longitudinal study of the correlation between bacterial colonization in the urethra of 16 patients with long-term indwelling urethral catheters and bacterial colonization of the bladder urine.

Epstein SE. Cost-effective application of the Centers for Disease Control Guideline for Prevention of Catheter-associated Urinary Tract Infections. Am J Infect Control 13:272–275, 1985.
A review of the Centers for Disease Control guidelines with emphasis on effective and cost-efficient application to the clinical setting.

Garibaldi RA, Burke JP, Dickman ML, et al. Factors predisposing to bacteriuria during indwelling urethral catheterization. N Engl J Med 291:215–219, 1974.
A study of 405 patients with temporary urethral catheters. Risks identified included female gender, old age, critical illness, breaks in the closed urinary drainage system, and improper care of the drainage bag.

Gillespie WA. Antibiotics in catheterized patients. J Antimicrob Chemother 18:149–151, 1986.
A review of the indications for antibiotics for prophylaxis and for treatment of urinary infection in the catheterized patient.

Gleckman R, Blagg N, Hibert D, et al. Catheter-associated urosepsis in the elderly. J Am Geriatr Soc 33:479–482, 1985.
A prospective study of 13 elderly patients with long-term urethral catheters who required hospitalization because of urosepsis. Distinguishing factors included a traumatic catheter-related event, polymicrobial bacteriuria, and bacterial resistance to commonly prescribed antibiotics used in the treatment of community-acquired urinary infections.

Kunin CM. Care of the catheter, in Detection, Prevention and Management of Urinary Tract Infections, ed 4. Philadelphia, Lea & Febiger, 1987, pp 245–297.
A comprehensive review of current catheter care methods including alternatives to chronic urethral catheterization.

Kunin CM, Chin QF, Chambers S. Indwelling urinary catheters in the elderly. Am J Med 82:405–411, 1987.
A study investigating the formation of catheter encrustations in patients with and without blocked catheters.

Lundeberg T. Prevention of catheter-associated urinary-tract infections by the use of silver-impregnated catheter. Lancet 2:1031, 1986.
A randomized prospective study of 102 patients investigating the effectiveness of silver-impregnated catheters in the reduction of incidence of bacteriuria in short-term urinary catheterization.

Nix DE, Durrence CW, May JR. Amphotericin B bladder irrigations. Drug Intell Clin Pharm 19:299–300, 1985.
An article providing a detailed account of the various methods of performing amphotericin B bladder irrigation.

Ouslander JG, Greengold B, Chen S. Complications of chronic indwelling urinary catheters among male nursing home patients: a prospective study. J Urol 138:1191–1195, 1987.
A prospective study of the incidence of symptomatic urinary tract infections among male nursing home residents with long-term indwelling urinary catheters.

Schaeffer AJ. Catheter-associated bacteriuria. Urol Clin North Am 13:735–747, 1986.
An extensive review of catheter-associated bacteriuria with an excellent discussion of the pathophysiology and a detailed analysis of risk factors predisposing the patient to catheter-associated bacteriuria.

Steward DK, Wood GL, Cohen RL, et al. Failure of the urinalysis and quantitative urine culture in diagnosing urinary tract infections in patients with long-term urinary catheters. Am J Infect Control 13:154–160, 1985.
A prospective study investigating the diagnostic value of sequential urinalysis and quantitative urine culture. The data reveal that both tests are poor predictors of urinary infection.

Warren JW. Catheters and catheter care. Clin Geriatr Med 2:857–881, 1986.
An extensive review of the complications of long-term urinary catheterization.

Warren JW, Tenney JH, Hoopes JM, et al. A prospective microbiologic study of bacteriuria in patients with chronic indwelling urethral catheters. J Infect Dis 146:719–723, 1982.
A prospective study of the micro-organisms isolated from the urine of patients with long-term urethral catheters.

Warren JW, Damron D, Tenney JH, et al. Fever, bacteremia and death as complications of bacteriuria in women with long-term urethral catheters. J Infect Dis 155:1151–1157, 1987.
A prospective study of the natural history of female patients with long-term catheterization. Data include the incidence of febrile episodes associated with catheter-related urinary tract infection.

Wong ES. Guidelines for the prevention of catheter-associated urinary tract infection. Infect Control 2:125–130, 1981.
The Centers for Disease Control guidelines for the prevention of catheter-associated urinary tract infections.

PART SIX

Geriatrics

29

Evaluation of Falls in Elderly Persons

LAURENCE Z. RUBENSTEIN, M.D., M.P.H.
ALAN S. ROBBINS, M.D.

Falls and instability are among the most serious problems facing the older population. They are major causes of mortality, morbidity, immobility, and premature placement in a nursing home. Many etiologies and risk factors predispose to falls. A fall may be defined as an unexpected event resulting in a person inadvertently coming to rest on a lower surface. There must be a systematic and individualized diagnostic and therapeutic approach to patients who have fallen. Attention should also be paid to identifying and reducing risk factors to prevent falls among frail older persons.

Epidemiologic Considerations

Both the incidence of falls in adults and the severity of complications rise steadily after middle age. Accidents are the fifth leading cause of death in people over age 65, and falls constitute two thirds of these accidental deaths. About three fourths of deaths resulting from falls in the United States occur in the 12% of the population age 65 and older. Approximately one third of this age group living at home fall each year, and about 1 in 40 of them is hospitalized. Of those admitted to a hospital after a fall, only about half are alive a year later. Repeated falls are a common reason for admission of previously independent elderly persons to long-term care institutions: at least two studies of patients admitted to nursing homes indicated that serious or frequent falling was the most common precipitating reason for the institutionalization (associated with more than one third of admissions). Moreover, fear of falling has been shown to be a major reason for the use of wheelchairs and other restrictions of mobility.

One of the most serious consequences of a fall, hip fractures, assumes epidemic proportions in old people—172,000 occurred in 1985. The cumulative lifetime incidence of hip fracture in the United States for those reaching age 90 is 32% for women and 17% for men. In 1984, the annual cost of hip fractures in the United States was estimated at 7 billion dollars.

Many population-based studies have described the epidemiology of falls in different settings, and rates are quite variable. Lowest rates (0.2 to 0.6 per person annually; a mean of 0.3) are reported among community-living, generally healthy elderly. Most of these falls result in no serious injury, with 5% or less producing a fracture or requiring hospitalization. As would be expected, persons living in long-term care institutions have the highest rates (0.6 to 3.6 per bed annually; a mean of 1.7), and persons in hospitals have an intermediate rate (0.6 to 2.9 per bed annually; a mean of 1.5). Falls among elderly in institutions also tend to result in more serious complications, with 10 to 25% of such falls resulting in a fracture or laceration. In most studies, older women have somewhat higher rates of falls and of fractures than men, which are probably related to the higher number of older women living alone, osteoporosis, and gait instability.

The real problem of falls in the elderly is not simply one of a high incidence because young children and athletes certainly have a higher incidence of falls than all but the frailest elderly. Rather, it is a combination of a high incidence together with a high susceptibility to injury. The propensity for injury is due to a high prevalence of clinical diseases (e.g., osteoporosis) and age-related physiologic changes (e.g., slowed protective reflexes) that make even a relatively mild fall particularly dangerous.

The U.S. Public Health Service has estimated that two thirds of deaths caused by falls are potentially preventable. This might be accomplished in several ways. Identifying and eliminating environmental risks in homes or institutions could prevent many falls related primarily to environmental causes. Adequate medical evaluation and treatment for underlying medical conditions might prevent many medically related falls. Finally, many patients who have irreversible medical problems causing their falls could still benefit from learning adaptive behavior to minimize the severity of falls. This chapter presents a systematic approach for determining why an elderly person falls and for minimizing the chances of recurrence.

Causes of Falls

Table 29–1 lists the major causes of falls and their relative frequencies based on the major published studies. The relative frequencies of etiologies differ depending on the populations studied. Frail, high risk populations have higher rates of medically related falls and higher incidences of falls of all types than do healthier populations. Nonetheless, Table 29–1 provides some useful ranges.

Accidents are the most common cause of falls, accounting for 30 to 50% in most series. However, many falls attributed to accidents really stem from the interaction between identifiable environmental hazards and increased

Table 29–1. Causes of Falls in the Elderly: Summary of Eight Studies That Included Careful Work-ups

Cause	Percentage	Range (%)
Accident or related to environment	37	12–53
Gait problems or weakness	12	3–30
Drop attack	11	1–25
Dizziness/vertigo	8	3–19
Postural hypotension	5	2–24
Syncope	1	0–13
Other specified causes*	18	6–37
Unknown	8	5–21

Adapted with permission from the American Geriatric Society, Falls and instability in the elderly, by Rubenstein LZ, Robbins AS, Schulman BL, et al., J Am Geriatr Soc 36:266–278, 1988.
*This category includes central nervous system disturbances, acute illness, confusion, poor eyesight, drugs, alcohol, and falling out of bed.

individual susceptibility to hazards from accumulated effects of age. Older people have stiffer, less coordinated gaits that are a greater hazard than those of younger people. Posture control, body-orienting reflexes, muscle strength and tone, and height of stepping all decrease with aging and impair ability to avoid a fall after an unexpected trip. Impairments of vision, hearing, and memory, also associated with aging, tend to increase the number of trips and stumbles. In addition to the increased vulnerability of elderly people, avoidable environmental dangers are frequent. Elderly people who live at home usually face many hazards that can be ameliorated:

- Unstable furniture and appliances
- Creaky stairs with poor rails
- Throw rugs and frayed carpets
- Poor lighting
- Low beds and toilets
- Pets
- Objects on floor
- Medications (psychoactive or hypotensive)

Similarly, for the 5% of those who live in institutions, many correctable environmental factors have been associated with falls (Table 29–2).

After accidents, the broad category of gait problems and weakness is the next most common cause for falls. The etiology of gait problems and weakness is clearly multifactorial. In addition to the age-related changes in gait and balance mentioned earlier, gait problems can stem from dysfunctions of the nervous, muscular, skeletal, circulatory, and respiratory systems as well as from simple deconditioning after a period of inactivity. Muscle weakness is an extremely common finding among the aged population. Although there is general agreement that reduction in muscle strength accompanies the aging process, much of this stems from disease and inactivity rather than aging per se. Regardless of the precise etiologies, several case-control studies have clearly shown an increased risk for falls and fractures among individuals with gait and muscle dysfunctions.

Drop attacks are defined as sudden falls without loss of consciousness and without dizziness. A sudden change in head position is often a precipitating event. This syndrome has been attributed to transient vertebrobasilar insufficiency, although it is probably due to more diverse pathophysiologic mechanisms. Patients often experience associated leg weakness, which is usually transient but can persist for hours. Tone and strength sometimes can be restored more rapidly if patients push their feet against a solid object. Although drop attacks are to be considered an important etiology of falls, recent data suggest that they cause substantially fewer than the 11% indicated in Table 29–1.

The sensation of dizziness is an extremely common complaint of elderly patients who fall. This complaint requires a careful history because the description of dizziness means different things to different people and can arise from very different etiologies. True vertigo, a sensation of rotational movement, may indicate a disorder of the vestibular apparatus, e.g., benign positional vertigo, acute labyrinthitis, or Ménière's disease. Symptoms described as imbalance on walking often reflect a gait disorder. Many patients describe a vague lightheadedness that may reflect cardiovascular problems, hyperventilation, orthostasis, drug side effect, anxiety, or depression.

Orthostatic hypotension, defined as a decrease of more than 20 mm of systolic blood pressure between lying and standing positions, has a 10 to 30% incidence among otherwise healthy elderly people living at home. It can stem from several factors, including autonomic dysfunction (frequently related to age, diabetes, or central nervous system damage), hypovolemia, low cardiac output, parkinsonism, metabolic and endocrine disorders, and medications (particularly sedative, antihypertensive, and antidepressant drugs). The orthostatic decrease in blood pressure may be more pronounced on arising in the morning because the baroceptor response is diminished after prolonged recumbency. Orthostatic hypotension may also be exacerbated by certain activities and after meals.

Syncope, or sudden loss of consciousness with spontaneous recovery, results from decreased cerebral blood flow or occasionally from metabolic causes such as hypoglycemia or hypoxia. The most frequent etiologies in elderly persons are cardiac arrhythmias (especially ventricular tachycardia and sick sinus syndrome), orthostatic hypotension, situational causes (e.g., micturition and defecation), and syncope of unknown cause. Less common causes are vasodepressor-vasovagal reactions, transient ischemic attacks, and seizures (see Chap. 2). A history of syncope may be difficult to obtain because many patients do not remember exactly what occurred during

the fall, and drop attacks or dizziness may be confused by the patient with syncope.

Other specified causes of falls include disorders of the central nervous system, cognitive deficits, poor vision, side effects of drugs, alcohol intake, and acute illness. Diseases of the central nervous system (e.g., cerebrovascular disease, dementia, normal pressure hydrocephalus, parkinsonism) often result in falls by causing dizziness, orthostatic hypotension, and gait disorders. Drugs frequently have side effects that result in impairment of mentation, stability, and gait. Especially important are agents with sedative, antidepressant, and antihypertensive effects, particularly diuretics, vasodilators, and beta blockers. Alcohol use is an under-reported but common problem in the elderly. Patients should be specifically questioned about this because alcohol is an occult cause of instability, falls, and serious injury. Other less common causes of falls include anemia, hypothyroidism, unstable joints, foot problems, and severe osteoporosis with spontaneous fracture.

Because most elderly individuals have more than one identifiable age-related change or medical condition that constitutes risk factors predisposing to falls, the exact cause is frequently difficult to determine and requires keeping these many possibilities in mind. The relevant risk factors can be better identified, however, if care is taken to link specific symptoms with specific possible causes, as will be discussed later. Several case-control studies have quantified the relative risk of various factors associated with falls in institutional settings. These are given in Table 29–2.

Diagnostic Approach

Table 29–3 outlines a general approach for a physician treating an older person who has fallen. After stabilization of any acute problems brought on by the fall, such as a head injury or fractures, a systematic search for the underlying cause of the fall should be undertaken.

A careful and well-directed history is the most helpful part of the diagnostic process. Obtaining a full report of the circumstances and symptoms surrounding the fall is crucial. However, as the patient may have poor recollection of these events, reports from witnesses are often of great importance. Historic factors that can point to a specific etiology or

Table 29–2. Factors Associated with Increased Risk of Falls Among Elderly Persons in Institutions

Category of Factor	Factor
Medical	Acute medical illness
	Multiple chronic disorders
	Decreased functional status
	Previous history of falls
	Multiple medications
	Impaired mobility
	Disordered balance and gait
	Decreased muscle strength
	Impaired mental status
	Depression
Environmental	Recent admission or transfer
	Hazardous furniture
	Slick, hard floors
	Unsupervised activities
	Insufficient number of nurses
	Meal times

narrow the differential diagnosis include a sudden rise from a lying or sitting position (orthostatic hypotension), trip or slip (gait, balance, or vision disturbance or an environmental hazard), unexplained drop attack without loss of consciousness (vertebrobasilar insufficiency), looking up or sideways (arterial or carotid sinus compression), and loss of consciousness (syncope or seizure). Symptoms experienced near the time of falling may also point to a potential cause: dizziness or giddiness (orthostatic hypotension, vestibular problem, hypoglycemia, arrhythmia, side effect of a drug), palpitations (arrhythmia), incontinence or tongue biting (seizure), asymmetric weakness (cerebrovascular disease), chest pain (myocardial infarction or coronary insufficiency), or loss of consciousness (any cause of syncope). Medications and the existence of concomitant medical problems may be important contributory factors. Other questions to ask during the

Table 29–3. Approach to the Patient Who Has Fallen

Assess and treat injury
Determine probable cause of fall
  History
  Physical examination (See Table 29–4)
  Laboratory and other tests (e.g., complete blood count, serum electrolyte studies, electrocardiography, Holter monitor)
Prevent recurrence
  Treat underlying illness
  Reduce accompanying risk factors (e.g., visual problems, orthostasis)
  Reduce environmental hazards (e.g., home assessment)
  Teach adaptive behavior (e.g., slow rising, gait training, use of cane or walker)

history that might be helpful in directing further work-up and planning of care include: How long was the patient on the ground? What effect did the fall have on patient confidence, fear of further falls, and activity? Are there any effects on caregiver expectations, fears, and plans for future activities?

Table 29–4 outlines important findings to look for during the physical examination. Especially pertinent are orthostatic changes in pulse and blood pressure, the presence of arrhythmias, carotid bruits, nystagmus, focal neurologic signs, musculoskeletal abnormalities, visual loss, and gait disturbances. Careful examinations of mental and neurologic status are often crucial. Even if risk factors are discovered that did not cause the fall in question, their identification and treatment can probably reduce the likelihood of subsequent falls.

It is often useful to attempt (under carefully monitored conditions) to reproduce the circumstances that might have precipitated the fall, such as positional changes, head turning, urination, or carotid pressure. Gait and stability should be assessed by close observation of how the patient rises from a chair, stands with eyes open and closed, walks, turns, and sits down. One should take particular note of gait velocity and rhythm, stride length, double support time (the time spent with both feet on the floor), height of stepping, use of assistive devices, and degree of sway. Imbalance observed during head turning or flexion is an important finding associated with vestibular or vertebrobasilar pathology and indicates a significant increased risk of falling.

The laboratory evaluation need not be extensive, but should include several key tests when the cause is not obvious: complete blood count to search for anemia or infection; serum chemistry analyses, especially sodium, potassium, calcium, glucose, and creatinine; electrocardiography to document arrhythmia; and thyroid function tests because occult thyroid disease may be difficult to diagnose clinically. Even then, the clinical evaluation and initial laboratory tests may not detect an intermittent problem that may have been the cause of the fall (e.g., orthostatic changes, arrhythmias, or electrolyte disturbances).

An ambulatory cardiac (Holter) monitor is advisable when a transient arrhythmia is suspected by history, in cases of otherwise unexplained syncope, or when the patient with unexplained falls has a history of cardiac disease and has been given cardiac medication. The likelihood of finding suggestive abnormal-

Table 29–4. Key Findings to Note on Physical Examination

Area of Investigation	Finding
Vital signs	Postural pulse and blood pressure changes
	Fever or hypothermia
Head, eyes, ears, nose, throat	Nystagmus
	Visual impairment
	Ear pathology
	Hearing impairment
Neck	Bruit
	Motion limitation
	Motion-induced imbalance
Chest	Rales (congestive heart failure or pneumonia)
Heart	Arrhythmia
	Murmur
Extremities	Arthritic changes
	Motion limitations
	Deformities
	Fractures
	Podiatric problems
Neurologic	Altered mental status (dementia, confused state)
	Focal deficits
	Peripheral neuropathy
	Muscle weakness
	Rigidity
	Tremor
	Gait or balance abnormality

ities by Holter monitoring in elderly patients who fall is particularly high. In one small series, 32% of patients who had fallen had arrhythmias documented by Holter monitoring that were thought to be responsible for the falls. Only one fourth of these patients with arrhythmias had evidence of the arrhythmia on the initial resting electrocardiogram. However, because transient arrhythmias are so prevalent among the elderly, it is often unclear whether a monitored abnormality is related to the fall unless corresponding symptoms are noted during the monitoring process. Therefore, it is essential that the patient is instructed to keep a careful diary of symptoms during Holter monitoring. It must be kept in mind that the sensitivity, specificity, and predictive values of Holter monitoring for assessment of falls have yet to be completely determined.

In high risk elderly patients (see Table 29–2) even without a history of falls, a thorough examination may be helpful in identifying potentially correctable problems (e.g., decreased vision, postural hypotension, diminished strength, and impaired gait). Although the efficacy of screening a low risk elderly population has not been evaluated, the following periodic assessments done in connection with routine medical visits might help prevent falls: postural blood pressure measurement, visual acuity testing, balance and gait evaluation, mental status check, and review of medication and environmental risks.

Therapy and Prevention

The purpose of the diagnostic approach outlined for the patient who has fallen is to uncover direct or contributing causes for the fall that are amenable to medical therapy or other corrective interventions. Among the more obvious examples, cardiac dysrhythmias clearly related to a fall should be treated with antiarrhythmic drugs or a pacemaker, or both. Hypovolemia related to hemorrhage or dehydration calls for treatment directed toward restoring hemodynamic stability. Parkinsonism usually responds to specific therapy, at least for a while; in advanced cases, however, safe ambulation can require extensive supervision and use of assistive devices. Discontinuing medication that causes postural hypotension or undue sedation is often adequate to prevent further falls in a frail elderly person.

For patients with gait and balance disturbances, specific assistive devices are often helpful. These devices include walkers, crutches, canes, and even modifications of shoes. Because the assistive device must be tailored to the patient, it should be prescribed in consultation with a physiatrist or physical therapist.

Many such patients (e.g., those with stroke, hip fracture, arthritis, or parkinsonism) can also benefit from a program of gait training under supervision of a physical therapist.

Several techniques may aid patients with persistent orthostatic hypotension resulting from autonomic dysfunction: sleeping in a bed with the head raised to minimize a sudden drop in blood pressure on rising; wearing elastic stockings to minimize venous pooling in the legs; rising slowly or sitting on the side of the bed for several minutes before standing up; and avoiding heavy meals and activity during hot weather. If conservative mechanical measures are ineffective, circulating blood volume can be increased by liberalizing dietary salt, provided that associated medical conditions do not preclude this. If disabling postural hypotension persists, mineralocorticoid therapy can be initiated with low doses of fludrocortisone acetate (Florinef Acetate), beginning at 0.1 to 0.2 mg/day. Extreme caution must be used to prevent precipitating congestive heart failure, fluid overload, hypokalemia, and hypertension.

Persons subject to drop attacks from vertebrobasilar insufficiency associated with head motion may be helped by use of a cervical collar. The collar should be prescribed in consultation with a neurologist or physiatrist for proper fit because an ill-fitting collar theoretically could cause carotid compression.

More difficult are managing and preventing recurrent falls in patients for whom a specific cause cannot be identified or in patients who have multiple or irreversible causes of falls. A careful search for and correction of other risk factors that predispose to falling (such as visual and hearing deficits) are essential. For disabilities that do not properly resolve with treatment of the underlying medical disorder (e.g., hemiparesis, ataxia, persistent weakness, or joint deformities), a trial of short-term rehabilitation in consultation with a physiatrist or physical therapist may improve safety and diminish long-term disability. When irreversible problems exist, residual limitations should be explained and coping methods should be developed.

Physicians should caution patients to eliminate home hazards such as loose or frayed rugs, trailing electrical cords, and furniture that is unstable or that obstructs movement. Patients and their families should be advised of the importance of specific environmental improvements: adequate lighting, bathroom grab rails and a raised toilet seat, secure stairway banisters, raising or lowering the bed, and an easily accessible alarm system. Sometimes, furniture can be rearranged to provide support to an unstable patient for ambulation to the bathroom. A home evaluation can be performed by a visiting nurse or other experienced person qualified to suggest modifications. Table 29–5 summarizes recommendations of several authors as to what to check during a home evaluation. Indirect data support the value of such home modification, as suggested by stud-

Table 29–5. Home Safety Checklist: Summary of the Most Important Items from Several Published Lists

Area of Home	Recommendation
All living spaces	Remove throw rugs
	Secure carpet edges
	Remove low-lying furniture and objects on floor
	Reduce clutter
	Remove cords and wires on floor
	Check lighting for adequate illumination at night (especially bathroom pathway)
	Secure carpet or treads on stairs
	Eliminate furniture that is too low to sit in
	Avoid waxing floors
	Ensure that telephone is reachable from floor
Bathroom	Install grab bars in tub and shower and near toilet
	Use rubber mats in tub and shower
	Remove floor mats when not using tub and shower
	Install raised toilet seat if seat is too low
Outside	Repair cracked sidewalks
	Install handrails on stairs and steps
	Keep shrubbery trimmed back on access path to house
	Install adequate lighting outside doors and in walkways leading to doors

ies of institutions that were especially designed to meet the needs and vulnerabilities of the elderly. Such institutions have substantially lower accident rates than those without such special attention.

In addition to the work-up and focused interventions to prevent further falls for the patient who has fallen, older individuals who have not fallen can probably benefit from an abbreviated fall prevention program. Such a program could be performed in the office setting as part of a periodic health maintenance program. Such an abbreviated fall prevention program should include (1) a discussion with patient (and caregiver where appropriate) of the nature of the problem, (2) a focused history and physical examination (Table 29–4) to determine risk factors, (3) discussion of home hazards and distribution of a home health hazards checklist (see Table 29–5 and Bibliography); and (4) advice on exercise to improve gait and activities, with appropriate cautions about overexertion.

In conclusion, the majority (or at least a large proportion) of falls in elderly people are probably preventable with careful medical and environmental evaluation and intervention. Therefore, a vigorous diagnostic, therapeutic, and preventive approach is appropriate for all older patients who fall, and as well as for those simply at high risk of falling. Any intervention that can make inroads on the fifth leading cause of death in the elderly will clearly have major impact.

Bibliography

Gordon M, Huang M, Gryfe CI. An evaluation of falls, syncope, and dizziness by prolonged ambulatory cardiographic monitoring in a geriatric institutional setting. J Am Geriatr Soc 30:6–12, 1982.

This paper describes the usefulness of Holter monitoring in selected patients who fall. In the series of 59 subjects who fell, cardiac arrhythmia played a role in 12, only 2 of which detected on the routine resting electrocardiogram.

Hogue C. Injury in late life: I. Epidemiology. II. Prevention. J Am Geriatr Soc 30:183–190, 276–280, 1982.

This is a careful epidemiologic review.

Kellog International Work Group on Prevention of Falls in the Elderly. The prevention of falls in later life. Dan Med Bull 34(Suppl 4):1–24, 1987.

This is an excellent, fact-filled consensus paper and literature review on falls and their prevention in older people.

Robbins AS, Rubenstein LZ. Postural hypotension in the elderly. J Am Geriatr Soc 32:769, 774, 1984.

This is a review of the epidemiology, causes, and treatment approaches.

Rubenstein LZ, Robbins AS, Schulman BL, et al. Falls and instability in the elderly. J Am Geriatr Soc 36:266–278, 1988.

Two case presentations are followed by detailed discussions of the epidemiology of falls, etiologic factors, muscle weakness, gait and balance dysfunction, and environmental assessment.

Sudarsky L, Ronthal M. Gait disorders among elderly patients. A survey study of 50 patients. Arch Neurol 40:740–743, 1983.

This study found that a single diagnosis could be made in the majority of elderly patients examined for an undiagnosed gait disorder.

Tinetti EM, Williams TF, Mayewski R. Fall risk index for elderly patients based on number of chronic disabilities. Am J Med 80:429–434, 1986.

This study prospectively identified known risk factors for falls and concluded that the risk of falling increases as the number of chronic disabilities increased. A scored assessment form was also introduced that may be of great value in other studies.

U.S. Consumer Product Safety Commission. Home Safety Checklist for Older Consumers. Washington, DC, U.S. Consumer Product Safety Commission, 1985.

This is a helpful guide for older persons for "accident- and fall-proofing" their homes.

Whipple RH, Wolfson LI, Amerman PM. The relationship of knee and ankle weakness to falls in nursing home residents: an isokinetic study. J Am Geriatr Soc 35:13–20, 1987.

This case-control study reports a significant relationship between lower extremity weakness and falls.

30

Evaluation and Care of the Demented Patient

RICHARD F. UHLMANN, M.D., M.P.H.
ERIC B. LARSON, M.D., M.P.H.

Introduction

Dementia is a common, serious health problem, particularly in the elderly, and has substantial social and economic impacts for the demented individuals themselves, their families, and society. These impacts are likely to increase markedly in the United States and other industrialized nations during the next 50 years as an increasing number and proportion of individuals become aged.

Dementia is a syndrome characterized by global loss of intellect sufficient to impair social or occupational functioning without diminished consciousness (Table 30–1). Some loss of intellect, however, is a normal consequence of aging. For example, composite norms for immediate recall and learning on the Wechsler Memory Scale are 20 to 50% lower in individuals in their 70's compared with individuals in their 20's and 30's. To diagnose dementia, one must consider not only patients' absolute cognitive functioning but also their function relative to baseline. For example, average cognition in a highly educated professional may indicate significant loss of function.

Primary manifestations of dementia, such as confusion, forgetfulness, and disorientation, may also occur in other organic brain syndromes such as delirium, schizophrenia, and depression. In contrast, delirium is characterized primarily by an acute confusional state with heightened awareness; schizophrenia by psychotic symptoms; and depression by affective disturbances (although this may vary in the elderly, as discussed later). However, dementia may coexist with other organic brain syndromes.

Table 30–1. Diagnostic Criteria for Dementia

A. Demonstrable evidence of impairment in short- and long-term memory. Impairment in short-term memory (inability to learn new information) may be indicated by inability to remember three objects after 5 minutes. Long-term memory impairment (inability to remember information that was known in the past) may be indicated by inability to remember past personal information (e.g., what happened yesterday, birthplace, occupation) or facts of common knowledge (e.g., past presidents, well-known dates).

B. At least one of the following:
1. Impairment in abstract thinking, as indicated by inability to find similarities and differences between related words, difficulty in defining words and concepts, and other similar tasks.
2. Impaired judgment, as indicated by inability to make reasonable plans to deal with interpersonal, family, and job-related problems and issues.
3. Other disturbances of higher cortical function, such as aphasia (disorder of language), apraxia (inability to carry out motor activities despite intact comprehension and motor function), agnosia (failure to recognize or identify objects despite intact sensory function), and "constructional difficulty" (e.g., inability to copy three-dimensional figures, assemble blocks, or arrange sticks in specific designs).
4. Personality change, i.e., alteration or accentuation of premorbid traits.

C. The disturbance in A and B significantly interferes with work or usual social activities or relationships with others.

D. Not occurring exclusively during the course of delirium.

E. Either 1 or 2:
1. There is evidence from the history, physical examination, or laboratory tests of a specific organic factor (or factors) judged to be etiologically related to the disturbance.
2. In the absence of such evidence, an etiologic organic factor can be presumed if the disturbance cannot be accounted for by any nonorganic mental disorder, e.g., major depression accounting for cognitive impairment.

From Diagnostic and Statistical Manual of Mental Disorders (DSM-III R), ed 3 revised. Washington, DC, American Psychiatric Association, 1987, p 107, with permission.

Epidemiology

The prevalence of dementia increases with age, reflecting both an age-related physiologic decline in cognitive functioning and the increased prevalence of dementing illnesses in the elderly. Dementia is primarily a disease of the "old old." Estimates of its incidence in younger individuals vary widely; however, it is probably less than 0.1% in individuals less than 60 years of age and less than 2% in individuals 60 to 65 years of age. Crude estimates of the incidence of dementia in the general population of the United States are 5% among individuals 65 years of age or older and 20% in those 80 years of age or older. Thus, currently 1.5 million Americans 65 years of age or older are thought to be demented. An equal number of persons over 65 years of age exhibit mild cognitive impairment but do not meet clinical criteria for dementia. The incidence of dementia also varies according to setting and, notably, is markedly higher in residents of long-term care institutions, in which it has been estimated to be 50% or more.

The prevalence of Alzheimer's disease, the most common cause of dementia, also increases with age. Its etiology is unknown, and it may, in fact, represent a common neuropathologic end point of several genetic and environmental diseases. As a genetic disorder, Alzheimer's disease can occur in familial aggregations, including some in which a defect has been localized to chromosome 21. It is also common in persons with Down's syndrome who survive to age 30. In support of an environmental etiology, it is interesting to note that young individuals with dementia pugilistica exhibit neurofibrillary tangles characteristic of Alzheimer's disease. Certain hypotheses propose that aluminum, other metallic ions, viral agents, and various other factors are involved in the etiology of Alzheimer's disease.

Alzheimer's disease is by far the most common cause of dementia. The frequencies of other causes of dementia vary according to the population studied. Multi-infarct dementia, dementia associated with alcoholism, depression that mimics dementia, side effects of medications, and hypothyroidism have each been noted in 2 to 5% of community-based populations (Table 30–2). In inpatients admitted for acute or subacute dementia, however, a tumor, normal pressure hydrocephalus, and Huntington's disease have also been present in several percent or more (Table 30–3).

Because of age-related physiologic changes and loss of homeostatic capacity, elderly persons generally have diminished cognitive reserve and, as a result, are more susceptible to confusion with superimposed illness. Many in-

Table 30–2. Illnesses or Conditions Causing Dementia in 200 Patients

Cause of Dementia	Number of Patients (%)
Alzheimer's-type condition	149 (74.5)*
Drugs	19 (9.5)
Alcohol	8 (4.0)
Hypothyroidism	6 (3.0)
Multi-infarcts	3 (1.5)
Other metabolic diseases	
Hyperparathyroidism	2 (1.0)
Hyponatremia	2 (1.0)
Hypoglycemia	1 (0.5)
Other (cause known)	8 (4.0)
Cause unknown	7 (3.5)
Benign senescent forgetfulness	3 (1.5)
Not demented	15 (7.5)

Modified from Larson EB, Reifler BV, Sumi SM, et al. Arch Intern Med 1986, 146:1918, Copyright 1986, American Medical Association.
*Twelve of these patients also had Parkinson's disease.

dividuals who become demented with superimposed illness eventually develop fixed dementia. Thus, superimposed illness may function as a "stress test" for underlying cognitive dysfunction and as a predictor of dementia.

A large number of diseases may cause dementia (Table 30–4). Many of these dementias are potentially reversible by virtue of the treatability of the underlying disorder, but most patients do not have complete resolution of dementia with treatment. The majority, however, show short-term improvement after the initial medical evaluation because of treatment of the dementing illness or the associated med-

Table 30–3. Summary of Four Studies of Dementia Among Inpatients

Cause of Dementia	Number of Patients (%)
Potentially reversible causes	82 (20.2)
Pseudodementia	29 (7.1)
Normal pressure hydrocephalus	22 (5.4)
Resectable mass lesions	15 (3.7)
Drug toxicity	8 (2.0)
Other reversible causes	8 (2.0)
Probably irreversible causes	324 (79.8)
Alzheimer's type	197 (48.5)
Alcoholism	43 (10.6)
Multi-infarcts	39 (9.6)
Huntington's chorea	15 (3.7)
Others	30 (7.4)
Total	406 (100)

From Benson DF, in Beck JC (moderator). Ann Intern Med 97:231–241, 1982 with permission. Adapted from Wells CE. Chronic brain disease: an overview. Am J Psychiatry 135:1–12, 1978; Smith JS. The investigation of dementia: results in 200 consecutive admissions. Lancet 1:824–827, 1981.

Table 30–4. Illness That Can Cause Dementia in Geriatric Patients

---

I. Illnesses associated with dementia that is usually progressive or irreversible
   A. Common
      Alzheimer's disease
      Multi-infarct dementia
      Alcohol-related encephalopathy
      Parkinson's disease
   B. Uncommon
      Anoxic encephalopathy
      Post-traumatic encephalopathy
      Pick's disease
      Huntington's disease
      Jakob-Creutzfeldt's disease
      Progressive supranuclear palsy
      Spinocerebellar degeneration
II. Causes of potentially reversible dementia
   A. Common
      Medication
      Hypothyroidism
      Other metabolic derangements
         Hyponatremia
         Hypoglycemia (usually in a treated diabetic)
         Hypercalcemia
   B. Uncommon
      1. Normal-pressure hydrocephalus
      2. Other neurologic syndromes
         Subdural hematoma
         Occlusive cerebrovascular disease with transient ischemic attacks
         Mass lesions (brain tumor and abscess)
      3. Nutritional deficiencies
         Wernicke-Korsakoff's syndrome
         Vitamin B_{12} deficiency
         Pellagra
      4. Toxins
         Alcohol
         Heavy metals (lead, mercury, manganese)
         Organic compounds
         Bromide
         Carbon monoxide
      5. Infections
         Neurosyphilis
         Chronic fungal or bacterial meningitis
      6. Inflammatory illnesses with vasculitis
         Giant cell arteritis
         Rheumatoid arthritis
         Polyarteritis nodosa
      7. Other metabolic abnormalities
         Wilson's disease
         Chronic renal failure
            Uremia
            Dialysis dementia
         Chronic hepatic failure
         Hypopituitarism
         Thyrotoxicosis
         Cushing's syndrome
         Adrenal insufficiency
         Hyperglycemia

From Larson EB, Lo B, Williams ME. J Gen Intern Med 1:116–126, 1986, with permission.

ical problems. Nevertheless, after 1 year only approximately 10 to 20% of patients show sustained signs of improvement.

Evaluation of Dementia

In most instances the diagnosis of dementia may be established on the basis of a careful history and examination of mental status. Brief, standardized mental status examinations, such as Folstein's Mini-Mental State and Pfeiffer's Short Portable Mental Status Examination (Table 30–5) are purportedly valid tests for dementia or delirium but do not distinguish between the two. The sensitivity and specificity of the Folstein test are higher than 80%, but it also has a high false-positive rate in poorly educated individuals. The Pfeiffer test has been standardized for educational attainment. Thus, such instruments are useful clinical adjuncts but should not be considered definitive tests for dementia. Serial examinations or more sensitive neuropsychologic testing may also be needed, especially in mild dementia and for individuals with high baseline cognitive functioning.

Despite the obvious importance of the history of present illness in dementia, by definition, demented patients are impaired in their ability to provide it. Primary care providers, therefore, should encourage family members or others who are familiar with the patient's history to be present when eliciting the history of present illness.

Potentially reversible dementias are likely to be shorter (usually less than 2 years) and less severe than irreversible dementias. Degenerative dementias, such as Alzheimer's disease, Parkinson's disease, and Pick's disease, typically have an insidious onset and progressive course. Patients with Pick's disease are said to exhibit personality changes, particularly disinhibition, but patients with other diseases, including Alzheimer's disease, can show these same changes. Multi-infarct dementia is characterized by a stepwise course reflective of multiple strokes. The suspicion of multi-infarct dementia may also be increased by evidence of cerebrovascular disease or associated risk factors, such as hypertension. A predictive clinical index, the Hachinski scale, has been developed to predict the likelihood of multi-infarct dementia (Table 30–6). The Hachinski scale appears to have high negative predictive value but low positive predictive value. A family history of dementia may be helpful for

Table 30–5. Short Portable Mental Status Questionnaire

Pertinent Questions	Scoring
1. What is the date today (month/day/year)? 2. What day of the week is it? 3. What is the name of this place? 4. What is your telephone number? (If no telephone, what is your street address?) 5. When were you born (month/day/year)? 7. Who is the current president of the United States? 8. Who was the president just before him? 9. What was your mother's maiden name? 10. Subtract 3 from 20 and keep subtracting 3 from each new number all the way down.	0–2 errors = intact 3–4 errors = mild intellectual impairment 5–7 errors = moderate intellectual impairment 8–10 errors = severe intellectual impairment Allow one more error if subject had no grade school education. Allow one fewer error if subject had education beyond high school.

From Kane RL (ed). Essentials of Clinical Geriatrics. New York, McGraw-Hill Book Co., 1984, with permission. After Multidimensional Functional Assessment: The OARS Methodology, ed 2. Durham, NC, Duke University Center for the Study of Aging and Human Development, 1978.

the clinical diagnosis of Alzheimer's-type dementia and Huntington's disease.

Other historical clues regarding causes of dementia should be sought, particularly depression, side effects of medication, alcohol abuse, and thyroid disease. Depression coexists in about one quarter to one third of demented patients and may itself cause impaired cognition as a caricature of dementia, so-called pseudodementia. Dysphoria is a less frequent complaint and vegetative symptoms are more frequent complaints in older patients than in younger patients. Many prescription drugs, including sedative/hypnotics, antipsychotics, antidepressants, narcotic analgesics, histamine 2 receptor antagonists, digoxin, beta blockers, steroids, and nonsteroidal anti-inflammatory drugs, may induce dementia, especially in the elderly (Table 30–7). Many widely used over-the-counter drugs may affect cognitive functioning, notably anticholinergics, decongestants, and antihistamines. In addition, the cognitive deficits of Parkinson's disease or Alzheimer's disease may be exacerbated by anticholinergic, dopaminergic, and other drugs used to treat associated movement disorders. The elderly are far more likely than younger individuals to exhibit neuropsychiatric drug side effects because of a loss of cognitive reserve as well as age-related changes in pharmacokinetics, especially drug distribution and metabolism.

Other important aspects of the demented patient's history include recent (subdural hematoma) or remote (post-traumatic encephalopathy) head trauma. A fluctuating level of consciousness may be seen in dementing illnesses associated with increased intracranial pressure. In addition, a history of acute cerebral anoxia related to cardiovascular events or chronic anoxia related to chronic lung disease, heart failure, or anemia should be sought. Some illnesses, such as congestive heart failure

Table 30–6. Hachinski Ischemic Scale

Feature	Score*
Abrupt onset	2
Stepwise deterioration	1
Fluctuating course	2
Nocturnal confusion	1
Relative preservation of personality	1
Depression	1
Somatic complaints	1
Emotional incontinence	1
History of hypertension	1
History of strokes	2
Evidence of associated atherosclerosis	1
Focal neurologic symptoms	2
Focal neurologic signs	2

From Larson EB, Featherstone HJ, Reifler BV, et al. Dev Neuropsychol 1:145–171, 1985, with permission.
*If ≥ 7, multi-infarct dementia; if ≤ 4, primary degenerative dementia.

Table 30–7. Medication Groups That Commonly Cause Intellectual Dysfunction in the Elderly

I. Direct central nervous system effects
   Sedative-hypnotic agents
   Antihypertensives
   Analgesics
   H_2 histamine antagonists (e.g., cimetidine)
   Digitalis preparations
   L-Dopa
   Anticholinergics
   Anticonvulsants
   Psychotropic agents
   Antiarrhythmics
   Anti-inflammatory agents (including corticosteroids)
II. Secondary metabolic central nervous system
   Diuretics
   Hypoglycemic agents
   Antibiotics
   Analgesics
   Corticosteroids

From Larson EB, Featherstone HJ, Reifler BV, et al. Dev Neuropsychol 1:145–171, 1985, with permission.

and chronic lung disease, are unlikely to present as dementia but may cause it. An acute onset of fixed dementia in the context of alcohol withdrawal may suggest Wernicke-Korsakoff's syndrome. History of exposure to heavy metals, organic compounds, and other toxins at home or work should be elicited.

Incontinence is common in demented patients and is frequently due to functional causes (e.g., impaired orientation or mobility) or associated urologic problems. However, a small percentage of demented patients are thought to suffer from normal pressure hydrocephalus, the diagnosis of which rests on the clinical triad of urinary incontinence, gait ataxia, and dementia. In these cases, the gait abnormality and incontinence are usually prominent and the dementia is mild in contrast to late stage Alzheimer's disease in which dementia predominates.

Demented patients often have unrecognized general medical problems, in part because of a diminished awareness and reporting of symptoms. Many of these problems may themselves contribute to excess cognitive and other types of morbidity. For example, untreated or improperly treated vision or hearing impairment may result in reduced orientation. In addition, hearing impairment may result in social isolation with attendant depression and cognitive dysfunction.

Human immunodeficiency virus (HIV) encephalitis may cause dementia, even in the absence of other manifestations of acquired immunodeficiency syndrome. Thus, HIV dementia should be considered in demented patients who are HIV seropositive or untested but are at risk for acquired immunodeficiency syndrome, even if other clinical evidence of immunodeficiency is lacking. HIV-positive patients are also at risk for coexistent central nervous system infections (such as with *Cryptococcus neoformans, Toxoplasma gondii,* and cytomegalovirus) and tumors (such as Kaposi's sarcoma and lymphoma), which may further exacerbate cognitive dysfunction.

The physical examination is most useful in identifying coexisting but previously unrecognized medical problems. It occasionally offers direct clues as to the cause of dementia. Structural lesions such as stroke and tumor usually produce focal neurologic abnormalities; however, there may be an absence of focal findings. In addition, patients with Alzheimer's-type dementia may have focal findings late in the disease. So-called subcortical dementias such as Parkinson's disease, Wilson's disease, and Huntington's disease may produce extrapyramidal signs such as tremor, festinating gait, rigidity, bradykinesia, and masked facies. Parkinson's disease and Alzheimer's disease frequently coexist clinically and neuropathologically. Heavy metal poisoning, alcoholism, vitamin B_{12} deficiency, and hypothyroidism may be associated with peripheral neuropathy. Although a lack of vibratory sensation may increase suspicion for these conditions, it is a nonspecific finding, especially in older patients.

Although neurosyphilis is uncommon in community-based geriatric populations, demented elderly should be examined for signs consistent with tabes dorsalis, paresis, and meningovascular syphilis. The presence of neck stiffness in the elderly, however, has low predictive value for meningitis, given the high prevalence of degenerative arthritis.

A task force of the National Institute on Aging has suggested use of a panel of ancillary laboratory assays for the evaluation of demented patients. These tests include ones directed specifically at diagnosing the cause of dementia as well as others directed toward promotion of general health and disease prevention. In view of the prevalence of various causes of dementia and the accuracy and costs of various tests (Tables 30–8 and 30–9), we recommend that only a few tests should routinely be ordered in evaluating dementia. These include a blood chemistry panel to identify metabolic abnormalities such as hypercalcemia, hyperglycemia, hypoglycemia, and uremia. In addition, we recommend determination of thyroxine level to rule out hypothyroidism, a relatively common and treatable cause of dementia in the elderly. A test for thyroid-stimulating hormone level may increase the sensitivity for detecting incipient hypothyroidism because the level of this hormone, in the presence of an intact hypothalamic-pituitary axis, would become elevated to compensate for dwindling production of thyroxine by the thyroid. In such instances, low normal thyroxine levels would be found in the context of an elevated level of thyroid-stimulating hormone.

In addition, complete blood count, smear, and red blood cell indices are useful in screening for nutritional anemias. Dementia related to vitamin B_{12} deficiency in the absence of anemia or evidence of megaloblastosis is thought to be extremely rare. Thus, it is probably safe to screen for vitamin B_{12}–associated dementia on the basis of complete blood count, smear, and mean corpuscular volume. How-

Table 30–8. Results of Routine Blood Tests in the Dementia Work-up*

| | Percentage of 200 Patients | | |
| | Abnormal | | |
	LEADING TO DIAGNOSIS OF POTENTIAL THERAPEUTIC IMPORTANCE	OF NO KNOWN CLINICAL CONSEQUENCE	Normal
Complete blood cell count†	5.7	9.3	85.1
Serum cyanocobalamin	1.0	0.5	96.5
Serum folate	5.7	2.1	92.3
ESR	0.0	14.5	85.5
VDRL	0.0	1.1	98.9
Chemistry battery (SMA-12)†	9.9‡	24.0	66.1
Glucose, electrolytes	1.6	12.0	86.5
Creatinine serum urea nitrogen	6.8	0.0	93.2
Calcium	1.6	5.7	92.7
Bilirubin, alkaline phosphatase	0.0	6.8	93.2
Albumin, total protein	0.0	7.3	97.7
Serum phosphate	1.7	14.8	83.5
Hepatic enzymes (AST, ALT)	0.0	5.1	94.9
Serum T_4 by RIA	1.5	2.1	96.4
T_3 resin uptake	1.5	0.5	98.4
Thyrotropin†	3.1	15.5	81.3

Modified from Larson EB, Reifler BV, Sumi SM, et al. Ann Intern Med 1986, 146:1919, Copyright 1986, American Medical Association.
*ESR indicates erythrocyte sedimentation rate; AST, aspartate aminotransferase; ALT, alanine aminotransferase; T_4, thyroxine; RIA, radioimmunoassay; T_3, tri-iodothyronine; VDRL, Veneral Disease Research Laboratories.
†Likely to be of value as a screening test.
‡Includes 13 patients with chronic renal failure.

ever, should clinical suspicion of vitamin B_{12} deficiency exist because of peripheral neuropathy, possible malabsorption, or inadequate nutritional intake, the level should be checked. Folate deficiency is common in demented, chronically diseased individuals because they are at increased risk for inadequate nutritional intake, but this deficiency probably does not cause dementia.

If indicated by clinical suspicion, blood levels of medications associated with dementia may be determined. Patients in high risk groups for acquired immunodeficiency syndrome should receive HIV antibody testing.

Identification of individuals who should be screened for neurosyphilis and the choice of methods for doing so are controversial. Demented patients who are young, have a history of sexual promiscuity or known exposure to syphilis, or have signs of tabes dorsalis or meningovascular syphilis clearly should be screened. The serum fluorescent treponemal antibody absorption (FTA-ABS) test is highly sensitive in detecting syphilis and thus is useful in ruling it out if results are negative. Neurosyphilis, however, very uncommonly presents as dementia in the elderly. Given this, the positive predictive value of FTA-ABS is likely to be low in the elderly (i.e., most positive tests are false positives). The Venereal Disease

Research Laboratory test is more specific but less sensitive than FTA in diagnosing syphilis and it should be ordered if the serum FTA-ABS test is positive to reduce the number of false positives.

Lumbar puncture appears to have an extremely low yield in determining the etiology of dementia except in patients less than 55 years of age or those with a subacute or acute course, history of fever, meningismus, history of syphilis, or positive syphilis serologic results.

Computerized tomographic (CT) and magnetic resonance imaging (MRI) brain scans may seem useful for diagnostic and prognostic purposes but rarely affect patient management. Frequently they are interpreted too liberally, particularly for atrophy and lucency. CT evidence of brain atrophy is a nonspecific, age-related finding that has little correlation with cognitive functioning. These imaging techniques have the highest predictive value in patients who, by virtue of their history or neurologic findings (as discussed earlier), have a relatively high a priori likelihood of structural lesions such as multi-infarct dementia, tumor, subdural hemorrhage, or normal pressure hydrocephalus.

Lack of structural lesions on CT or MRI scans in combination with typical clinical features of Alzheimer's disease probably en-

Table 30–9. *Different Tests Used in the Dementia Work-up and Their Costs*

Test*	1984 University Hospital Charge ($)
CBC	15.75
ESR	11.00
VDRL	9.50
FTA	6.00
Serum folate level	41.00
Serum vitamin B_{12} level	50.50
RBC folate level	82.00
SMA-12	34.75
SMA-7†	22.00
SGOT	18.00
Serum phosphate	11.50
Thyroid screen (T_4-RIA, T_3RU)	20.25
Urinalysis	10.00
TSH level	38.25
ACTH stimulation	43.00
Chest x-ray	71.25
Skull x-ray (limited)	63.75
CT scan	356.00
EEG (standard)	224.00
ECG	37.00
Cost per patient	$1,165.50

From Larson EB, Featherstone HJ, Reifler BV, et al. Dev Neuropsychol 1:145–171, 1985, with permission.
*CBC indicates complete blood count; ESR, erythrocyte sedimentation rate; VDRL, Veneral Disease Research Laboratories; FTA, fluorescent treponemal antibody; RBC, red blood cell; SGOT, serum glutamic-oxaloacetic transaminase; T_4, thyroxine; T_3, tri-iodothyronine; RIA, radioimmunoassay; TSH, thyroid-stimulating hormone; ACTH, adrenocorticotropin; CT, computed tomography; EEG, electroencephalogram; ECG, electrocardiogram.
†SMA-7 = BUN, creatinine, glucose, sodium, potassium, chloride, bicarbonate.

hances the ante mortem diagnostic accuracy of this entity. Nevertheless, the diagnostic yield of CT or MRI brain scans in such individuals is likely to be low. In such instances, CT or MRI scans are primarily useful to reassure both family and physician that potentially reversible lesions have not been missed and, in so doing, better define the patient's prognosis. Such information may be invaluable in planning future care.

All demented patients under the age of 50 should probably receive a brain CT scan because the prevalence of Alzheimer's disease is much lower, and that of other causes, such as tumor, is much higher.

The accuracy of clinical diagnosis of Alzheimer's disease has not been rigorously validated but is probably around 80%. The clinical diagnosis of Alzheimer's disease is largely a diagnosis of exclusion. Standardized criteria for clinical diagnosis of probable or possible Alzheimer's disease have been proposed by a Work Group on the Diagnosis of Alzheimer's Disease on the National Institute of Neurological and Communicative Disorders and Stroke (NINCDS), and the Alzheimer's Disease and Related Disorders Association (ADRDA) (Table 30–10). The validity of clinical diagnostic criteria such as these is currently being investigated. The gold standard for diagnosis remains tissue diagnosis. Thus, autopsy with histopathologic examination of brain tissue should be offered for individuals in whom a definitive clinical diagnosis was not made, particularly those with suspected Alzheimer's disease. Despite the expense, the autopsy may be useful to progeny who might be genetically predisposed to Alzheimer's disease.

Management Issues

As in many chronic diseases, the management of patients with dementia rests upon a triad of (1) treating the primary illness, (2) identifying and treating comorbidity, and (3) enhancing the patient's support system.

Pharmacologic treatment of the cognitive deficits of Alzheimer's-type dementia is, unfortunately, highly limited at present. Ergoloid mesylates have been shown in most clinical trials to result in modest improvements, in aggregate, in various cognitive, affective, and behavioral symptoms. Although the optimum dose and duration of therapy are unknown, a trial of at least 3 and perhaps 6 months may be necessary for a therapeutic effect. Available information suggests that the minimum effective daily dose is probably 3 to 6 mg. This drug was initially marketed as a cerebral vasodilator, but its mechanism of action in Alzheimer's-type dementia is unknown.

Because the brain in Alzheimer's disease is characterized by a deficit of acetylcholine, much research and development is currently focused on orally administered, centrally acting cholinergic drugs. At least one of these drugs, tetrahydroaminoacridine, has produced significant short-term cognitive improvement in Alzheimer's-type dementia in one study. No cholinomimetics, however, have yet received approval for treatment of Alzheimer's-type dementia in the United States.

Demented patients also frequently develop other neuropsychiatric symptoms such as depression, agitation, and psychosis. Simple measures, including reassurance and environmental modifications to enhance patient safety and orientation, are often sufficient to manage such problems. Antidepressant, antipsychotic,

Table 30–10. *NINCDS-ADRDA Work Group Criteria for Clinical Diagnosis of Alzheimer's Disease*

I. The criteria for the clinical diagnosis of PROBABLE Alzheimer's disease include:

    dementia established by clinical examination and documented by the Mini-Mental Test, Blessed Dementia Scale, or some similar examination, and confirmed by neuropsychologic tests;

    deficits in two or more areas of cognition;

    progressive worsening of memory and other cognitive functions;

    no disturbance of consciousness;

    onset between ages 40 and 90, most often after age 65; and

    absence of systemic disorders or other brain diseases that in and of themselves could account for the progressive deficits in memory and cognition.

II. The diagnosis of PROBABLE Alzheimer's disease is supported by:

    progressive deterioration of specific cognitive functions such as language (aphasia), motor skills (apraxia), and perception (agnosis);

    impaired activities of daily living and altered patterns of behavior;

    family history of similar disorders, particularly if confirmed neuropathologically; and

    laboratory results of:

        normal lumbar puncture as evaluated by standard techniques.

        normal pattern of nonspecific changes in EEG, such as increased slow-wave activity, and

        evidence of cerebral atrophy on CT with progression documented by serial observation.

III. Other clinical features consistent with the diagnosis of PROBABLE Alzheimer's disease, after exclusion of causes of dementia other than Alzheimer's disease, include:

    plateaus in the course of progression of the illness;

    associated symptoms of depression, insomnia, incontinence, delusions, illusions, hallucinations, catastrophic verbal, emotional, or physical outbursts, sexual disorders, and weight loss;

    other neurologic abnormalities in some patients, especially with more advanced disease and including motor signs such as increased muscle tone, myoclonus, or gait disorder;

    seizures in advanced disease; and

    CT normal for age.

IV. Features that make the diagnosis of PROBABLE Alzheimer's disease uncertain or unlikely include:

    sudden, apoplectic onset;

    focal neurologic findings such as hemiparesis, sensory loss, visual field deficits, and incoordination early in the course of the illness; and

    seizures or gait disturbances at the onset or very early in the course of the illness.

V. Clinical diagnosis of POSSIBLE Alzheimer's disease:

    may be made on the basis of the dementia syndrome, in the absence of other neurologic, psychiatric, or systemic disorders sufficient to cause dementia, and in the presence of variations in the onset, in the presentation, or in the clinical course;

    may be made in the presence of a second systemic or brain disorder sufficient to produce dementia, which is not considered to be *the* cause of the dementia; and

    should be used in research studies when a single, gradually progressive severe cognitive deficit is identified in the absence of other identifiable cause.

VI. Criteria for diagnosis of DEFINITE Alzheimer's disease are:

    the clinical criteria for probable Alzheimer's disease and

    histopathologic evidence obtained from a biopsy or autopsy.

VII. Classification of Alzheimer's disease for research purposes should specify features that may differentiate subtypes of the disorders, such as:

    familial occurrence;

    onset before age 65;

    presence of trisomy-21; and

    coexistence of other relevant conditions such as Parkinson's disease.

From McKhann G, Drachman D, Folstein M, et al. Neurology 34:939–944, 1984, with permission.

and sedative/hypnotic drugs may themselves cause cognitive dysfunction as well as may increase the risk of falls and should be used with caution only after less risky treatments have proved inadequate. If these drugs are used, low doses should initially be chosen and the patient should be closely monitored for side effects. Within classes of drugs, those that are less sedating and anticholinergic should be considered. For example, antidepressants vary considerably in these side effects (Table 30–11). When administered at bedtime, sedatives, antipsychotics, and antidepressants may be less likely to cause daytime falls, sedation, or confusion. For agitation, shorter-acting benzodiazepines are preferred; longer-acting benzodiazepines are generally contraindicated in demented patients. Neuroleptics, however,

Table 30–11. Antidepressant Drug Treatment in Dementia*

Drug	Dosage			Comment
	Begin	**Increase by**	**Up to**	
Desipramine	10 mg/day	10 mg/3–5 days	150 mg/day	Relatively few anticholinergic side effects according to clinical reports; no controlled research data in elderly.
Doxepin	10 mg/day	10 mg/3–5 days	150 mg/day	Sedative action, minimal orthostatic hypotensive effects reported in nondemented, relatively healthy depressed patients (controversial).
Nortriptyline	10 mg/day	10 mg/5–7 days	60 mg/day	Minimal orthostatic hypotensive effects (controversial); blood levels recommended because of postulated therapeutic window in younger patients (50–150 ng/ml).
Trazodone	25 mg/day	25 mg/3–5 days	300 mg/day	No demonstrable anticholinergic activity, occasional priapism, sedation, cardiovascular toxicity reported, especially in overdose.
Monoamine oxidase inhibitors (e.g., phenelzine)	15 mg/day	15 mg/5–7 days	60 mg/day	Reported effective in depressed elderly and depressed demented patients; hypotensive effects; dietary and medication monitoring by responsible caregivers to prevent hypertensive crises with tyramine-containing foods or adrenergic decongestants.
Neuroleptics				Widely used, but practically no controlled data on efficacy in treating depressed demented patients; anticholinergic and extrapyramidal side effects; should be reserved for use in psychotically depressed and/or demented patients, short-term only because of tardive dyskinesia.

Reprinted with permission from the American Geriatric Society, Physician management of the demented patient, by Winograd CH, Jarvik LF. J Am Geriatr Soc 34:295–308, 1986.
*In general: begin with lowest possible dose; maintain at dosage level giving some improvement; use divided doses; electrocardiographic monitoring is recommended for patients given tricyclic antidepressants.

Table 30–12. Medical Diagnoses in Elderly Patients Evaluated for Dementia (n = 200)

Diagnosis	Percentage of Patients with Newly Recognized Diagnosis (n = 92 Diagnoses)	Percentage of Patients with Diagnosis (n = 248 Diagnoses)
Hypertension	1.0	23.0
Osteoarthritis	2.5	13.5
Depression without Alzheimer-type dementia	7.5	10.5
Chronic obstructive pulmonary disease	0.5	10.0
Cerebrovascular accident	4.0	7.0
Congestive heart failure	1.0	6.0
Low serum folate level	5.5	5.5
Peptic ulcer disease	1.0	5.5
Parkinson's disease without Alzheimer-type dementia	3.0	4.0
Diabetes mellitus	0.0	4.0
Ischemic heart disease without congestive failure	1.0	3.0
Urinary tract infection	2.5	2.5
Transient ischemic attacks	1.0	2.5
Symptomatic peripheral vascular disease	0.0	1.5
Iron-deficiency anemia	1.5	1.5
Rheumatoid arthritis	0.5	1.5
Vitamin B_{12} deficiency	1.0	1.5
Hyperparathyroidism	1.5	1.5
Other miscellaneous diagnoses	11.0	19.5

From Larson EB, Lo B, Williams ME. J Gen Intern Med 1:116, 1986, with permission. Adapted from Larson EB, Reifler BV, Sumi SM, et al. Arch Intern Med 1986, 146:1917, Copyright 1986, American Medical Association.

have a more clearly documented efficacy. The efficacy of propranolol, carbamazepine, and lithium in demented patients have not been documented in placebo-controlled studies.

Well-controlled studies of the impact of cerebrospinal fluid shunting in normal pressure hydrocephalus are lacking. Available evidence suggests, however, that shunts are most likely to benefit individuals with prominent gait disturbance and mild dementia.

Although multi-infarct dementia is irreversible, risk factors for future strokes, such as hypertension and smoking, should be ameliorated through appropriate intervention. In addition, low dose aspirin should be administered prophylactically, especially for males with carotid bruits. Some recovery is usually seen after each stepwise deterioration, which reflects normal physiologic and psychologic adaptation after a cerebrovascular accident.

Given the high prevalence of unrecognized medical problems in the demented elderly (Table 30–12), detection and treatment of associated comorbidity may result in significant clinical improvement. For example, treatment of congestive heart failure, chronic lung disease, or anemia may enhance patients' functional capacity. In addition, patients' orientation can frequently be enhanced by appropriate treatment of hearing and vision impairment. The risk of falls can be reduced by elimination of unneeded medications as well as by environmental modifications. As in other elderly populations, demented elderly persons are likely to have undetected dental and podiatric problems. Treatment of these problems may also enhance health and functional status.

Demented elderly are typically incapable of providing for their basic nutritional needs. When coupled with the impaired thirst mechanism of the elderly, their functional deficits result in a higher risk of dehydration. Opportunities to engage in physical activities may also be limited in demented elderly. Exercise should be encouraged to maintain basic muscle strength and tone, coordination, cardiovascular conditioning, orthostatic mechanisms, gastrointestinal motility, other physiologic functions, and self-image.

Perhaps the major risk factor for institutionalization among demented elderly is the resilience of the patient's support system. Notably, elderly persons often cite institutionalization as their greatest fear. Caring for a demented individual has been aptly described as a "36-hour day." In addition to providing educational and emotional support for the patient's family and other caregivers, physicians and other health care professionals can significantly prolong the patient's ability to reside at home by facilitating in-home logistical support. Respite care to relieve the caregiver of constant responsibility is essential and is becoming increasingly available through formal community day-care and other programs. In addition, peer support groups, chore services, home-delivered meal programs, and visiting nurse services are available in many communities. Moreover, psychopathology, including depression and abusive behavior, and physical illness often occur among caregivers and should be monitored by physicians.

Bibliography

Beck JC, Benson DF, Scheibel AB, et al. Dementia in the elderly: the silent epidemic. Ann Intern Med 97:231–241, 1982.
  Somewhat dated but well-written review. Provides especially useful summaries of pathophysiology of Alzheimer's disease and studies of dementia among inpatients.
Dans PE, Cafferty L, Otter SE, et al. Inappropriate use of the cerebrospinal fluid venereal disease research laboratory (VDRL) test to exclude neurosyphilis. Ann Intern Med 104:86–89, 1986.
  An interesting empiric study and discussion of diagnosis of neurosyphilis.
Editorial. Cholinergic treatment in Alzheimer's disease: encouraging results. Lancet 1:139–141, 1987.
  A brief critical review of clinical trials of cholinomimetics for improving cognitive functioning in Alzheimer's-type dementia.
Hollister LE, Yesavage J. Ergoloid mesylates for senile dementias: unanswered questions. Ann Intern Med 100:894–898, 1984.
  A critical review of clinical studies of this potentially useful but often overlooked drug.
Larson EB, Reifler BV, Fetherstone HJ, et al. Dementia in elderly outpatients: a prospective study. Ann Intern Med 100:417–423, 1984.
  Clinically oriented, descriptive study of epidemiology of dementia in the setting where it most commonly is seen: the clinic.
National Institutes of Health Consensus Development Conference Statement. Differential diagnosis of dementing diseases. Alzheimer Dis Assoc Dis 2:4–15, 1988.
  Consensus conference addressing a variety of issues in dementia: definition, differential diagnosis, appropriate diagnostic evaluation, and future research avenues. Commentaries by various investigators follow this article (pages 16–28).
Navia BA, Jordan BD, Price RW. The AIDS dementia complex: I. Clinical features. Ann Neurol 19:517–524, 1986.
  Descriptive study of clinical features of AIDS dementia.

Rabins PV, Mace NL, Lucas MJ. The impact of dementia on the family. JAMA 248:333–335, 1982.

A small study providing useful information for primary care providers on the impact of dementia on family caregivers.

Rango N. The nursing home resident with dementia. Ann Intern Med 102:835–841, 1985.

Review of ethical principles of medical decision-making in this particularly challenging subset of demented patients.

Risse SC, Barnes R. Pharmacologic treatment of agitation associated with dementia. J Am Geriatr Soc 34:368–376, 1986.

Useful critical review of a difficult management issue in the care of demented patients.

Vernadakis A. The aging brain. Clin Geriatr Med 1:61–94, 1985.

Well-written, detailed review of neurobiology of aging.

Winograd CH, Jarvik LF. Physician management of the demented patient. J Am Geriatr Soc 34:295–308, 1986.

Excellent overview of primary care approach to management of dementia. Provides detailed sections on identification and intervention of medical, behavioral, social, and psychiatric manifestations of dementia.

31

Diagnosis and Treatment of Urinary Incontinence

FITZHUGH C. PANNILL, M.D.

Urinary incontinence is a very significant health problem for millions of older adults and has serious medical, social, and economic implications for patients and their families. Although as many as 50% of elderly women have rare episodes of incontinence, 5 to 10% of community living elderly men and women have more significant incontinence that results in social disability. Patients who have acute medical illnesses or who live in long-term care institutions have a much higher prevalence of incontinence. The annual cost of incontinence in the community is estimated to be more than 6 billion dollars.

Some surveys show that elders view incontinence as a normal accompaniment of aging. However, frequent incontinence is inconvenient and causes social isolation and depression—substantial psychologic and social burdens. Both nurses and physicians rarely ask patients about incontinence and tend to ignore this problem. Patients, adopting this disinterest, rarely volunteer information or seek medical help specifically for urinary incontinence. Thus, despite evidence that cure, control, or significant amelioration of incontinence is possible, patients tend to suffer in silence, both in the community and in institutions.

The initial step in the diagnosis and treatment of incontinence is identifying the problem. All older patients should be asked directly and nonjudgmentally about incontinence. Many authorities recommend an open-ended question such as, "Do you have any trouble losing your urine and getting wet?"

In this chapter I discuss normal bladder function and causes of incontinence, the evaluation of incontinence, and a proposed algorithm for therapy.

Physiology and Pathophysiology of Bladder and Urethral Function

Under central nervous system control, the bladder and urethra act in concert to allow urinary storage and release. The bladder muscle, or detrusor, relaxes slowly as urinary volume increases. With this increasing volume, proprioceptive receptors in the bladder wall send an increasing number of impulses through the spinal cord to the midpons micturition control center. At a certain level of activity, neurons in this center discharge, causing a cholinergically mediated neuronal discharge in the detrusor wall, contraction of the detrusor muscle, increase in detrusor pressure, and release of urine. This activity can be inhibited by the central nervous system under both unconscious and conscious control. "Uninhibited" bladder contractions occur when this inhibition fails and the bladder contracts at low urine volumes, seemingly without control. Incontinence is inevitable when such contractions increase bladder pressure to a level greater than urethral pressure. Cholinergic agonists or any irritative foci in the bladder increase detrusor contractions. Conversely, anticholinergic agents can suppress bladder contractions to variable degrees and cause significant urinary retention.

The urethra is a smooth muscle organ that maintains constant tension under alpha-adrenergic stimulation. By impairing urethral pressure, alpha antagonists decrease resistance to urine flow. In women, an equally important component of urethral resistance is the normal pelvic anatomy that allows increases of intraabdominal pressure to be transmitted not only to the bladder but to the urethra. This transmission increases urethral pressure to counteract abdominal pressure surges caused by coughing, sneezing, or exercise. Aging and menopause cause laxity of the pelvic floor muscles with resultant decreased pressure transmission and urinary leakage related to increased abdominal pressure.

Bladder pressure, volume, sensation of filling, normal and abnormal detrusor contractions, and urine flow rates can all be measured directly by urodynamic testing. Quantification of urinary flow rates during voiding can indicate an obstruction of the outlet or impaired contractility. Values less than the normal range of 10 ml/s may be useful for screening, especially in men. During urodynamic testing, the bladder is slowly filled with carbon dioxide or sterile saline, and the changes in pressure are directly measured. A normal response to increasing volume is a slow gradual rise in pressure. The slow accumulation of fluid in the bladder is usually imperceptible to the patient until a volume of about 200 ml is reached. Maximal bladder capacity, or the volume that can be comfortably held, varies between 250 and 500 ml. Normal voiding begins when a contraction overcomes inhibition, bladder pressure rises, and urethral resistance drops.

Urodynamic testing detects detrusor instability by measuring sharp detrusor muscle contractions that the patient cannot voluntarily inhibit. An atonic bladder fails to generate adequate detrusor contractions, even at extremely high bladder volumes (more than 500 ml). A small amount (25 to 50 ml) of postvoid residual urine is common in older people, but amounts more than 150 ml are abnormal and indicate either obstruction or poor contractility. All of these parameters are easily documented by cystometry, although standing posture and coughing may be needed to demonstrate uninhibited contractions. Although urethral pressure can be measured directly, the overlap in normal and abnormal values makes these measurements less clinically useful. Occasionally, other more specialized examinations may be necessary, including cystoscopy (for suspicion of obstruction), sphincter electromyography (to examine sphincter relaxation), and videocystourethrography (to examine urethral mechanics during voiding).

Bladder capacity, voiding volume, urinary leakage with stress, and postvoid residual volumes can be easily measured in the office. This is discussed later in this chapter.

Although incontinence is not a normal accompaniment of aging, several physiological changes that occur in the bladder and urinary system with age predispose to difficulty with urinary control. For example, bladder capacity and compliance, urethral length and closure pressure, and urinary flow rate all decrease, whereas postvoid residual volumes and the frequency of uninhibited bladder contractions increase. Elderly persons also develop higher nocturnal rates of water and electrolyte excretion than younger people, which explains the common symptom of nocturia. The sum of all of these changes, however, is insufficient to cause incontinence, and continence is normally maintained even at advanced ages.

Causes and Treatment of Incontinence

Most authorities distinguish established from transient incontinence. Any implication that "transient" causes do not result in chronic incontinence is not true. However, the distinction is helpful as transient suggests nonurologic causes, usually coexisting medical diseases, that can be treated and either improved or cured by standard medical therapy. Etiologies of transient causes have been summarized by Resnick in a mnemonic DIAPPERS (Table 31–1). Changes in mental status from both organic disease (i.e., hypoxia, hyponatremia, delirium, dementia, cerebrovascular disease) or psychiatric illnesses (psychoses, depression) can cause incontinence as the patient may not respond to normal bladder cues. Later stages of Alzheimer's disease frequently cause incontinence because of apraxia of learned toileting skills, confusion, or an uninhibited bladder from structural brain abnormalities. Urinary tract infections, vaginal infections or inflammation, and fecal impactions can produce bladder irritation resulting in incontinence. Hyperglycemia, hypercalcemia, and diabetes insipidus increase urine volume and can overwhelm bladder capacity. Patients who are

Table 31–1. Transient Causes of Incontinence

D	—Delirium (confusional state)
I	—Infection, urinary tract (symptomatic)
A	—Atrophic urethritis or vaginitis
P	—Pharmaceuticals
P	—Psychologic disorders, especially depression
E	—Endocrine disorders (hypercalcemia or hyperglycemia)
R	—Restricted mobility
S	—Stool impaction

From Resnick N. Hosp Pract 21:80E, 1986, with permission.

restrained or unable to more quickly may lose urine before reaching the toilet.

A wide variety of drugs can cause incontinence by various mechanisms (Table 31–2). Drugs with anticholinergic side effects are common offenders. These include a wide variety of prescribed and over-the-counter medications. Drugs in the latter category, such as antidiarrheals and antihistamines, may be easily overlooked unless asked about specifically.

Established incontinence is due to urologic pathology or abnormalities of the bladder, urethra, or nervous system control (Table 31–3).

Urge incontinence, which is the most common type, is caused by the loss of central nervous system inhibition over reflex detrusor contractions (detrusor instability) or by local bladder irritation. Some cases are idiopathic. Patients typically complain of urinary urgency or spasm, followed by the loss of *large* amounts of urine as the bladder contracts and empties suddenly. Other symptoms include nocturia, loss of urine without warning, and severe urinary frequency (more than five or six times per day). Causes of urge incontinence include neurologic conditions (Alzheimer's disease, other dementias, brain tumors, Parkinson's disease, stroke, and cervical spondylosis or other spinal cord disease), and local irritative lesions in the bladder (infections, tumors, interstitial cystitis, and outlet obstruction). The diagnosis of detrusor instability can be made when cystometry demonstrates sharp, dramatic increases in pressure (more than 15 cm H_2O) at normal urine volume. Cystometry may just show a small, noncomplaint bladder. Idiopathic cases may be due to deconditioned voiding reflexes with chronic, frequent, low volume voiding, which decreases bladder volume and increases detrusor tone and irritability over time. Both neurotic personality traits and fears of urinary accidents may be responsible for this cycle.

Therapy for detrusor instability must initially be directed to a reversible cause. Thus, a careful search on examination should be made for any signs of spinal cord compression, Parkinson's disease, other neurologic disease, tumors, infections, or outlet obstruction. In patients with no reversible causes, anticholinergic therapy (flavoxate 100 mg three to four times a day; oxybutynin 5 mg two to four times a day; imipramine 25 mg two to four times a day) may help decrease bladder contractions. At higher doses, these drugs can cause urinary retention, confusion, and orthostatic hypotension. Bladder training, toileting regimens, and biofeedback have all been used with success rates as high as 85%, especially in idiopathic cases, but require special expertise usually beyond that of the generalist. Although palliative measures such as pads and undergarments are useful, neither indwelling catheters nor condom catheters are recommended because of the high incidence of infections.

Stress incontinence is identified clinically by the observation of small of amounts of urinary leakage that occur with increasing abdominal pressure (coughing, sneezing, running). The incontinence is usually associated with stress or upright posture, occurs predominantly in the daytime, and is not associated with nocturia, urgency, frequency, or other urinary symptoms. In most patients (predominantly women), pelvic floor laxity causes the urethra to tilt posteriorly and allows increases in abdominal pressure to force urine out. Certain

Table 31–2. Medications That Can Affect Continence

Type of Medication	Potential Effects on Continence
Diuretics	Polyuria, frequency, and urgency
Anticholinergics	Urinary retention, overflow incontinence, and fecal impaction
Psychotropic drugs	
Antidepressants	Anticholinergic actions and sedation
Antipsychotics	Anticholinergic actions, sedation, rigidity, and immobility
Sedatives/hypnotics	Sedation, delirium, and muscle relaxation
Narcotic analgesics	Urinary retention, fecal impaction, sedation, and delirium
Alpha-adrenergic blockers	Urethral relaxation
Alpha-adrenergic agonists	Urinary retention
Beta-adrenergic agonists	Urinary retention
Alcohol	Polyuria, frequency, urgency, sedation, delirium, and immobility

From Ouslander JB. Clin Geriatr Med 2:715–730, 1986, with permission.

Table 31–3. Summary of Established Incontinence

Incontinence Type	Etiology	Prevalence*	Symptoms	Signs	Voiding Parameters	Urodynamics	Treatment
Urge	1. Defects in central nervous system inhibition (detrusor instability) 2. Bladder irritation 3. Idiopathic deconditioning	Com: 30% NH: 60%	Urgency, frequency, nocturia, loss of large amounts of urine	Underlying central nervous system disorder Urinary tract infection or vaginitis as irritative lesions	Loss of large urine volumes (> 50 ml) Small bladder capacity with frequent losses	Uninhibited contractions Small bladder capacity Normal postvoid residual	Anticholinergic medications Treat source of irritation Biofeedback Habit retraining
Stress	1. Pelvic muscle laxity 2. Neuropathy 3. Urologic surgery	Com: 60% (mostly women) NH: 25%	Loss with exercise, coughing	Leakage of small amounts with coughing Atrophic vaginitis	Loss of small urine volumes Daytime incontinence (correlates with exercise)	Normal	Surgery Estrogens (women), alpha agonists Pelvic strengthening exercises
Overflow	1. Detrusor inadequacy 2. Outlet obstruction 3. Impaired bladder sensation	Com: 10% NH: 15%	Hesitancy, straining, incomplete emptying, frequent small voidings	Palpable bladder Prostate enlargement Difficult catheterization	Nocturia Frequent loss of small (10–50 ml) amounts of urine Poor stream	Poor bladder contractions Bladder capacity > 500 ml Large postvoid residual (> 150 ml)	Surgery Prazosin Intermittent catheterization

*Com indicates living in the community; NH indicates living in a nursing home.

patients may have stress-induced detrusor instability (leakage is delayed several seconds after the stress) or neurologic abnormalities of the sphincter. Stress incontinence is infrequent in men; for example, incontinence that occurs after prostate surgery is most likely due to detrusor instability.

The clinical examination in patients with stress incontinence is usually normal, but large cystoceles, rectoceles, or urethral prolapse can contribute to incontinence by distorting pelvic anatomy. Pelvic laxity is hard to judge and correlates poorly with clinical signs of atrophic vaginitis. Urethritis and atrophic vaginitis may contribute independently to stress incontinence. Postvoid residual and bladder function during cystometry are normal.

Therapy is multidimensional and aimed at restoring normal pelvic geometry. Large cystoceles, prolapse, or signs of urethral prolapse should be evaluated by a urologist or gynecologist. If done properly and practiced carefully, pelvic floor (Kegel) exercises are effectve in restoring pelvic floor strength and continence (Table 31–4). Topical estrogen cream and alpha-adrenergic agonists (phenylpropanolamine 25 mg two to four times a day) are also useful. Surgery to correct the laxity can be recommended if urodynamic test results are normal (to exclude coexisting detrusor instability) and if the patient is a good surgical risk. Pessaries and weight loss are useful adjunctive measures. Patients may rarely require the surgical placement of an artificial sphincter.

Table 31–4. *Treatment Schedule for Stress Incontinence*

I Modified Kegel exercise; pelvic floor muscle exercise
  A. While voiding, actively stop flow—repeat several times during each voiding session
  B. When completely aware of which muscles are being contracted—then consciously contract these muscles three or four times a day, intermittently, for 10 min*
II Estrogen vaginal cream
  Apply ½ applicator daily for 1 week, then every other day (Premarin Vaginal Cream)
III Oral estrogens (Premarin, 0.650 mg daily)
IV When you feel the need or urge to void (urine or stool) do it then, before pressures increase
V If after 4–6 months this therapy fails, then we will consider other diagnostic and therapeutic procedures

Reprinted with permission from the American Geriatric Society, Stress urinary incontinence: a simple and practical approach to diagnosis and treatment, by Mohr JA, et al. J Am Geriatr Soc 31:476–478, 1983.
*If lower abdominal or back pain begins with or after exercise, then you are contracting the wrong muscles and you must start over with actively stopping urine flow while voiding.

Overflow incontinence, a third and less common cause of established incontinence, occurs when detrusor contractions are inadequate to overcome urethral resistance except at very high urine volume. The pathogenesis is either low pressure detrusor contractions (atonic bladder) or an abnormally high urethral resistance related to obstruction. Patients usually leak frequently, have hesitancy and decreased urine flow, have to strain to void, and sense the presence of postvoid residual. A few patients are unaware of bladder fullness because of poor sensation. Occasionally, the bladder can be palpated. The postvoid residual is usually greater than 150 ml. Sacral spinal cord function can be abnormal if a neurologic problem is involved. An atonic bladder can be seen in diabetics and in alcoholics with sacral nerve damage. Obstructions are usually due to an enlarged prostate or urethral stricture. Most, if not all, of these patients need a urologic evaluation to discover treatable obstructions. In the absence of surgically correctable lesions, Credé voiding or intermittent self-catheterization may be helpful. Prazosin (1 to 3 mg three times a day) is an alpha-adrenergic antagonist that may reduce outlet resistance by relaxing the internal bladder sphincter. Bethanecol is less effective in increasing bladder contractions and may have significant cholinergic side effects.

Combinations of different types of incontinence (mixed incontinence) are frequent. Accurate figures are unavailable, but in one study 50% of the institutionalized patients with stress incontinence also had detrusor instability. Detrusor-urethral sphincter dyssynergia (simultaneous contraction of both bladder and urethral muscles) can simulate obstruction and destrusor instability but is usually seen only in patients with complex neurologic conditions (multiple sclerosis, Parkinson's disease). Detrusor hyperactivity in combination with impaired contractility was documented by one investigator in 33% of incontinent nursing home residents. This condition—an overactive bladder that empties ineffectively—has been only recently identified by Resnick. These patients suffer from unimpaired contractions but are left with a high residual urine volume, which is indicative of poor bladder emptying. Studies of community living elderly women have identified mixed diagnoses in about 20% of the population. The exact significance of these mixed diagnoses must await further information, but the mixed types are probably more common in institutionalized patients and those with chronic illness.

Evaluation and Assessment of the Incontinent Patient

The evaluation of incontinence in ambulatory practice should focus on determining and ameliorating the causes of incontinence. The determination by a generalist of a cause of established incontinence is possible but may require a urologic referral. Although all patients need a complete history and physical examination, the history should focus on urinary symptoms and characterization of the incontinence and associated symptoms. Information on diabetes, neurologic conditions, previous surgery, and medications is also important (Table 31–5).

The incontinence chart (Fig. 31–1) is a record of incontinence frequency, timing, volume, and frequency of normal voidings and nocturnal events that the patient or family should maintain for 3 to 7 days. This chart allows the frequency of incontinence to be quantitated both before and after therapy; it can be used to estimate bladder capacity and may indicate etiology.

The physical examination should identify associated neurologic and genitourinary diseases, with special attention paid to abdominal, neurologic, and pelvic/rectal examinations. Most important, an effort should be made to reproduce stress-induced leakage. This is most easily done by having the patient hold tissue paper over the urethral opening and, with a full bladder, cough vigorously several times to precipitate leakage. Any leakage is absorbed on the tissue and easily identified. The test should be scored as a negative (no leakage) or positive (any leakage). This maneuver must be done with a full bladder. The patient should then void for urinalysis and culture, and the voided urine should be collected and measured. Sterile bladder catheterization should then be performed to measure the postvoid residual. The sum of voided volume and postvoid residual volume approximates bladder capacity. Catheterization is easily done in women during a pelvic examination. Catheterization in men does carry some risk of precipitating obstruction, but most authorities believe that this risk is minimal. Any difficulty in passing the catheter should be noted and the catheter should not be forced. Laboratory examinations should include urinalysis, urine culture, and measurement of levels of electrolytes, glucose, calcium, and blood urea nitrogen.

Identified causes of transient incontinence need to be recorded and treated. It may be difficult to specifically identify the role of any one of these factors in a particular patient. The factors are also additive. For example, an elderly woman with significant arthritis of the hip and consequent poor mobility may have little trouble getting to the toilet until she begins taking a diuretic for treatment of hypertension. The elimination of transient causes requires careful therapy of infections, depression, fecal impaction, and arthritis, and changing as many problematic drugs as possible. Multiple problems may need to be ranked by priority, based on their likelihood of contribution and ease of therapy, and each problem should be treated in turn.

Although there is a paucity of data, better information is becoming available to determine the sensitivity and specificity of incontinent symptoms for established incontinence. The

Table 31–5. Clinical Evaluation

History

Urinary symptoms (frequency, dysuria, straining, decreased stream, incomplete emptying, nocturia)

Incontinence symptoms (urgency, stress, amount, timing, duration, associations with medications, sleep, exercise)

Fluid intake and voiding patterns (bedtime drink?, caffeinated beverage)

Active medical problems (diabetes, neurologic disease, heart failure, genitourinary surgery, arthritis, mobility, recent acute illnesses, pelvic irradiation)

Medications (prescription, nonprescription)

Environmental factors (location of bathrooms, ease of access, restraints)

Incontinence chart

Physical

Orthostatic blood pressure

Test for stress leakage with full bladder

Neurologic (mental status, upper motor neuron signs, peripheral sensation, motor strength, perineal sensation, sacral reflexes, anal tone)

Palpable bladder after voiding

Pelvic examination (vaginitis, atrophy, pelvic floor laxity, prolapse, cystoceles, masses)

Rectal examination (prostate size, impaction, masses)

Postvoid residual volume by catheterization

Laboratory

Urine analysis and culture; measured volumes of urine

Blood analyses (electrolytes, glucose, urea nitrogen, calcium)

```
┌─────────────────────────────────────────────────────────────┐
│                    │ INCONTINENCE CHART │                    │
│                                                               │
│  CODE                                                         │
│  Please Record for Each Time Slot Daily:                     │
│  DRY—Patient was dry                                          │
│  WET—Patient lost urine                                       │
│  BR—Patient used bathroom                                     │
└─────────────────────────────────────────────────────────────┘
```

TIME	DATE	DATE	DATE	DATE	DATE	DATE	DATE	COMMENTS
6 a.m. to 10 a.m.								
10 a.m. to 2 p.m.								
2 p.m. to 6 p.m.								
6 p.m. to 10 p.m.								
10 p.m. to 2 a.m.								
2 a.m. to 6 a.m.								

Figure 31–1. *Urinary incontinence chart. From Pannill FC. Clin Rep Aging 1(3):12, 1987, with permission.*

mixture of diagnoses, lack of data for men, and the commonality of symptoms to many different diagnoses impair this approach, however. Better data are available for women, and the data in Table 31–6 can be used as a guide to decision-making for these patients. Frequency of urination and urgency are sensitive but nonspecific symptoms for urge incontinence; upper motor neuron signs, although more specific, do not have a higher predictive value. For stress incontinence, the usefulness of most symptoms or signs is not great, although some authorities believe that if stress incontinence exists as an isolated symptom, the likelihood of sphincter weakness incontinence is high. There are few data available on

Table 31–6. *Operating Characteristics in Women*

Disease (Prevalence)	Symptoms or Signs	Sensitivity (%)	Specificity (%)	Positive Predictive Value (%)	Negative Predictive Value (%)
Urge incontinence (40%)	Frequency	69	34	41	62
	Urgency with incontinence	77	36	45	71
	Nocturia	56	54	44	65
	Upper motor neuron signs	31	91	67	66
Stress incontinence (35%)	Incontinence with stress (symptom)	57	58	43	72
	Vaginitis	45	67	42	70
	Stress leakage on examination	92	93	87	95
Overflow incontinence (12%)	Straining	43	95	55	92
	Decreased stream	71	77	31	96
	Incomplete emptying	36	79	18	90
	Palpable bladder	62	99	87	95

From Pannill FC, Mushlin AE, Urinary incontinence, in Griner PF, et al. (eds). Clinical Diagnosis and the Laboratory. 1986, Chicago, Year Book Medical Publishers, reproduced with permission.

this point. The actual demonstration by stress maneuvers of incontinence is highly sensitive and specific for the diagnosis, however. Patients who do not show any symptoms of straining, decreased stream, or incomplete emptying are unlikely to have overflow incontinence (high negative predictive value).

Again, the incontinence chart (Fig. 31–1) can provide helpful clues to etiology and therapy. As examples, patients with primarily morning incontinence may take their diuretics or antihypertensive medication before each accident. Predominantly nocturnal incontinence may be related to sleeping medications or postural reabsorption of pedal edema. Wide swings in timing between accidents usually point to activity-related incontinence. A loss of small amounts of urine during daytime activities but none at night points to sphincter weakness. Patients who lose large amounts of urine at regular intervals during the day usually have detrusor instability.

Ouslander has developed an algorithm (Fig. 31–2) for assessing urinary incontinence. This algorithm has not been validated for large numbers of patients and thus should be used only as a guide to decision-making. It aims to (1) identify reversible conditions; (2) identify patients who need a referral for further urologic evaluation; and (3) diagnose and treat patients with uncomplicated incontinence without a urologic referral (patients who do not improve need a referral).

Patients with urinary tract infections, glycosuria from diabetes mellitus, fecal impactions, or vaginitis should be treated for these conditions first and then re-evaluated. Medications that could contribute to the incontinence should be stopped if possible. Patients who are immobile or otherwise restrained from having easy access to toileting facilities need to have their underlying problem investigated and treated. For example, a stroke patient may need rehabilitation and a bedside commode. Patients with multiple genitourinary surgeries or a history of pelvic irradiation probably need a referral to a urologist before therapy is attempted. If the examination raises a suspicion of spinal cord compression, a neurologist should be consulted immediately.

A clinical evaluation revealing bladder distention, an enlarged or nodular prostate, hematuria (in the absence of infection), or significant pelvic prolapse should prompt a referral to a urologist or gynecologist. Patients who have a postvoid residual urine volume of more than 100 ml, a difficult catheterization, or severe hesitancy also need a urologic referral for evaluation of possible obstruction. Patients with very small bladder capacities (under 100 ml) as measured at voiding are also very difficult to treat without urologic assistance. These above restrictions apply to a minority of patients but identify patients who have conditions that could progress or cause problems with treatment.

Patients who have objective evidence of stress incontinence can be treated safely with pelvic floor exercises (Table 31–4) and topical estrogen or alpha-adrenergic agonists if there are no contraindications to these drugs. As this regimen is relatively free from side effects, it should be started in all patients with stress incontinence unless surgery for the condition is planned. Surgical candidates should have urodynamic testing to eliminate coexisting detrusor instability.

Patients who do not have overflow symptoms, stress incontinence, or other problems have a high likelihood of either detrusor instability or a normal but small capacity bladder. Some authorities recommend that these patients should be treated empirically with low dose anticholinergic medications (oxybutynin) and bladder-retraining exercises. Treatment without further testing is likely to improve a high percentage of patients, but anticholinergics should not be used for patients with overflow incontinence or anatomic obstructions. Patients with a higher probability of overflow incontinence may have symptoms such straining, decreased stream, or incomplete emptying, or a postvoid residual close to or more than 150 ml. Patients with partial outlet obstruction causing detrusor instability may be particularly difficult to identify without cystoscopy. Therefore, patients given anticholinergics should be examined regularly for evidence of increasing postvoid residual volumes. Orthostatic hypotension and other anticholinergic side effects should also be monitored. Patients whose symptoms do not improve after a few weeks or who have adverse side effects should be referred for a urologic evaluation.

This approach should allow therapy to be started in more than half of the patients whom a generalist is likely to see in the office. The remainder and those who do not improve need further evaluation, but this approach should reduce the number of necessary referrals. With increasing knowledge, diagnostic approaches and medications are improving, and almost all patients should be able to overcome incontinence.

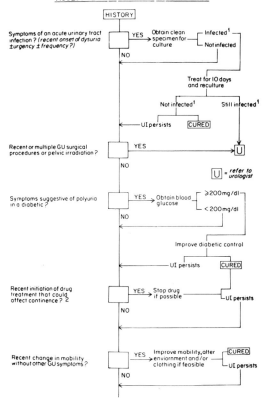

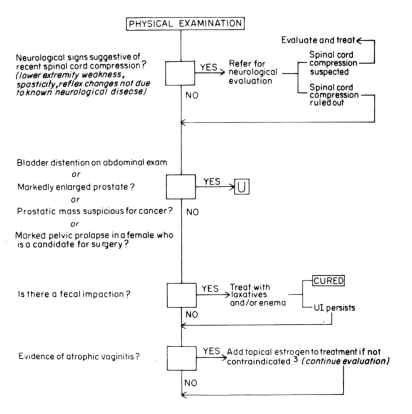

Figure 31–2. Algorithm developed by Ouslander, which uses a set of simplified diagnostic tests of bladder function. The algorithm and diagnostic tests are being tested in prospective studies. From Ouslander JG. Clin Geriatr Med 2:726, 727, 1986, with permission.

Illustration continued on following page

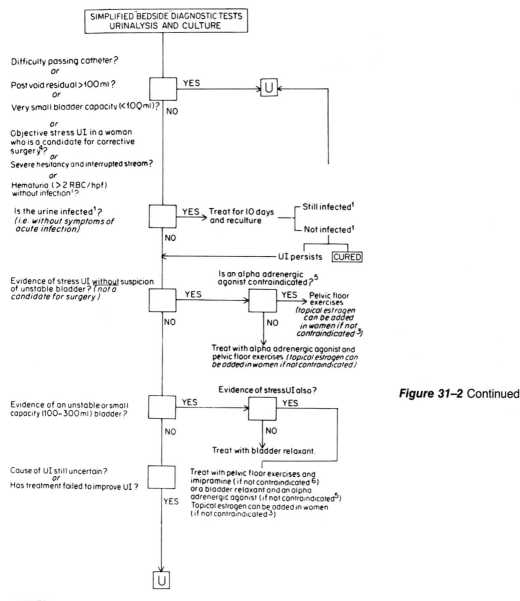

Figure 31-2 Continued

SIMPLIFIED BEDSIDE DIAGNOSTIC TESTS
URINALYSIS AND CULTURE

Difficulty passing catheter?
or
Post void residual >100ml?
or
Very small bladder capacity (<100ml)?
or
Objective stress UI in a woman
who is a candidate for corrective
surgery[4]?
or
Severe hesitancy and interrupted stream?
or
Hematuria (>2 RBC/hpf)
without infection[1]?

Is the urine infected[1]?
(i.e. without symptoms of
acute infection)

YES → Treat for 10 days and reculture ┌ Still infected[1]
                                        └ Not infected[1]

UI persists   [CURED]

Evidence of stress UI without suspicion
of unstable bladder? (not a
candidate for surgery)

Is an alpha adrenergic agonist contraindicated?[5]

YES → Pelvic floor exercises
(topical estrogen can be added in women if not contraindicated[3])

Treat with alpha adrenergic agonist and pelvic floor exercises (topical estrogen can be added in women if not contraindicated)

Evidence of an unstable or small capacity (100-300ml) bladder?

Evidence of stress UI also?

Treat with bladder relaxant.

Cause of UI still uncertain?
or
Has treatment failed to improve UI?

Treat with pelvic floor exercises and imipramine (if not contraindicated[6]) or a bladder relaxant and an alpha adrenergic agonist (if not contraindicated[5]) Topical estrogen can be added in women (if not contraindicated[3])

[U]

NOTES

1. Infected defined as growth of 10^5 colonies per milliliter of a pathogenic organism.

2. Drugs that can affect continence include diuretics, psychotropics, anticholinergics and other agents with autonomic effects

3. Contraindications to estrogen treatment include history of breast cancer, thromboembolic disease, poorly controlled hypertension

4. Severe symptoms and/or failed medical therapy in past; willing to and medically capable of undergoing surgery

5. Contraindications to alpha adrenergic agonists include poorly controlled hypertension, symptomatic heart or peripheral vascular disease, hyperthyroidism

6. Contraindications to impramine include cardiac conduction defects, symptomatic heart disease (angina, congestive heart failure), closed angle glaucoma

ABBREVIATIONS

[U] = REFER TO UROLOGIST
UI = URINARY INCONTINENCE
mg/dl = MILLIGRAMS PER DECILITER
ml = MILLITERS
RBC = RED BLOOD CELLS
hpf = HIGH POWER FIELD

Several national organizations are available to provide patients and families with advice, support, and information. Patients can be referred to Help for Incontinent People (HIP) Inc., P.O. Box 544, Union, SC 23379, 803–585–8789 or The Simon Foundation, P.O. Box 815, Wilmette, IL 60091, 803–23–SIMON for patients, 312–864–3913 for physicians. These organizations provide helpful newsletters and information on bulk purchase of incontinent aids and the latest forms of therapy.

Bibliography

Burgio KL, Whitehead WE, Engel BT. Urinary incontinence in the elderly: bladder sphincter biofeedback and toileting skills training. Ann Intern Med 104:507–515, 1985.
Reports first comprehensive study of biofeedback and related therapies; success rates of 82 to 94% were achieved

Diorono AC, Wells TJ, Brink CA, et al. Urinary incontinence in elderly women: urodynamic evaluation. J Am Geriatr Soc 35:943–946, 1987.
Study of symptoms, signs, and urodynamics in 200 community living incontinent women.

Hadley EC. Bladder training and related therapies for urinary incontinence in older people. JAMA 256:372–379, 1986.
Comprehensive review of bladder training, habit retraining, timed and prompted voiding, and biofeedback.

Mohr JA, Rogers J Jr, Brown TN, et al. Stress urinary incontinence: a simple and practical approach to diagnosis and treatment. J Am Geriatr Soc 31:476–478, 1983.
Studies 46 elderly women who were successfully evaluated and treated for stress incontinence with estrogens and pelvic exercises.

Ouslander JG. Technologies for managing urinary incontinence. (Health Technology Case Study 33.) Washington DC, U.S. Congress Office of Technology Assessment, OTH HCS-33, July 1985.
Review of all available methods of treatment and management, including garment pads and appliances.

Ouslander JG (ed). Urinary incontinence. Clin Geriatr Med 2:639–886, 1986.
Fifteen chapters in entire issue review prevalence; psychosocial and economic aspects; physiology; evaluation; and all methods of treatment; includes algorithm.

Ouslander JG, Hepps K, Ras S, et al. Genitourinary dysfunction in a geriatric outpatient population. J Am Geriatr Soc 34:507–514, 1986.
Comprehensive evaluation of 264 elderly subjects with detailed analysis of clinical characteristics, urodynamics, and treatment results.

Pannill FC, Mushlin AE. Urinary incontinence, in Griner PF, et al. (eds). Clinical Diagnosis and the Laboratory. Chicago, Year Book Medical Publishers, 1986, pp 337–397.
Discussion of sensitivity, specificity, and operating characteristics of symptoms, signs, and laboratory tests in incontinent women.

Pannill FC, Williams TF, Davis R. Evaluation and treatment of urinary incontinence in long term care. J Am Geriatr Soc 36:902–910, 1988.
Results of comprehensive evaluation and treatment of 48 incontinent patients. Fifty-five percent of patients treated improved at least 30%.

Resnick NM, Yalla SV. Management of urinary incontinence in the elderly. N Engl J Med 313:800–805, 1985.
Review of incontinence with emphasis on diagnosis.

Resnick NM, Yalla SV. Detrusor hyperactivity with impaired contractile function. JAMA 257:3076–3081, 1987.
Evidence of a previously unrecognized problem causing incontinence in elderly nursing home residents.

Sier H, Ouslander J, Olerzech S. Urinary incontinence among geriatric patients in an acute-care hospital. JAMA 257:1767–1771, 1987.
Incontinence, present in 35% of hospitalized patients, usually preceded hospitalization but was rarely evaluated by the physicians or staff.

Wells TJ, Brink CA, Diokno AC, et al. Urinary incontinence in elderly women: clinical findings. J Am Geriatr Soc 35:933–939, 1987.
Study of symptoms, signs, and urodynamics in 200 community living incontinent women.

Williams ME, Pannill FC. Urinary incontinence in the elderly: physiology, pathophysiology, diagnosis and treatment. Ann Intern Med 97:895–907, 1982.
A comprehensive review of the subject.

32

Care of the Nursing Home Patient

PATRICK W. IRVINE, M.D.
KENNETH D. ENGBERG, M.D.

With aging of the population and the resulting increased prevalence of chronic illness and disability, a greater proportion of internal medicine practice is likely to shift into nursing homes. At present, there are 1.3 nursing home beds for each acute care hospital bed in the United States. This number is expected to increase, as will the intensity of medical services provided in nursing homes. The nursing home environment, however, is very different from the hospital-based and clinic-based settings where internists have traditionally trained and with which they are most familiar.

Compared with acute care, long-term care is characterized by more private ownership. Investor-owned nursing homes substantially outnumber governmental and nonprofit facilities. Generally underfunded and understaffed, the nursing home industry is regulated more closely by the government than the acute care system. This may have evolved in response to previous neglect in long-term care facilities, although it is unclear whether increased regulation has been responsible for improved quality of care. According to a recent Institute of Medicine report, significant deficiencies in quality persist despite these regulations. Although most of these quality issues are not physician related, there is a tremendous need for physicians to improve clinical practice within nursing homes.

Unique Character of the Nursing Home

To practice effectively in the nursing home, the physician must learn to use the system to greatest advantage. There are several important characteristics distinctive to nursing homes.

Nursing homes are much more "process driven" than most other health care organizations. State and federal government regulations tightly control staff/resident ratios, hours of training for staff, intervals between physician visits, and countless other variables. Because each nursing home is surveyed annually by inspectors who carefully review records in detail, the nursing home staff may appear preoccupied with regulation compliance and documentation. With the new federal surveys there is somewhat more attention given to "outcomes" as measured by resident care and by interviews with residents and family members. Nevertheless, an emphasis remains on audits of data pertaining to process and structure. Because adverse findings of such surveys may result in decertification from the federal Medicaid and Medicare programs as well as in fines or revocation of licensure, nursing homes continue to require strict physician compliance with regulations.

Primary emphasis in long-term care is devoted to the resident's quality of life and functional independence. This is reflected in the comprehensive care plan that is completed shortly after admission and reviewed periodically for each resident. Medical, psychologic, and social concerns are incorporated into one overall plan that is followed by the nursing home multidisciplinary team. Because many residents live the remainder of their lives in the facility, it is important to maintain a home-like environment and to promote individual autonomy. Whenever possible, residents are given choices in day-to-day living (such as roommate, food menu, clothing options, and activities) and may participate on resident councils to influence overall policies. The autonomy and dignity of each resident must also be considered in making ethical decisions such as advanced directives for limited treatment.

For physicians, the nursing home requires a shift in medical attitudes and practice styles to avoid overmedicalizing the home-like setting. Major emphasis should be devoted to maximization of independent function and delay of progressive deterioration of residents, rather than to inappropriate extensive medical intervention. By their nature, however, nursing homes present multiple incentives to actually encourage dependency among frail residents. Any observed decline in a resident's functional independence may be inappropriately viewed by professional staff and family members as a natural adjustment to nursing home living. Because less staff effort and time are required to perform activities of daily living for residents than to assist or encourage the individuals to perform these activities on their own, professionals must be careful not to inadvertently promote greater dependency. Although in the short-run, providing all care may be more cost effective with respect to nursing and physical therapy, the long-term effects of learned helplessness are clearly detrimental and more costly. For individuals who enter nursing homes planning to go home, prevention of learned dependency is of paramount importance.

Nursing home residents are uniquely vulnerable to abuse from individuals providing their care. Such vulnerability is characterized by major dependency on the caregiver and, when abused, the inability to voice complaints—for physical and/or mental reasons—and an associated fear of reprisal by the abusing caregiver. Many nursing home residents are severely impaired and do not have family members or others to serve as advocates for them. Physical and psychologic abuse of dependent elderly persons is prone to arise because of these conditions.

Attempts to create a home-like environment and to promote functional independence and autonomy are challenged today as nursing homes increasingly become sites for short-term transitional and posthospital care. Rapid discharges of sicker patients from hospitals force the nursing home to provide more complex nursing care and increasingly "medical" services. The added problems of rapid patient turnover and complex technology present substantial stresses for professional staff in these homes. Nurses in long-term care have traditionally been relatively isolated from frequent physician interactions and are often poorly prepared—technically and psychologically—to manage sicker patients. Nursing assistants provide 90% of the hands-on care but often lack sufficient experience and training needed to work with these patients. Physicians may be frustrated by a system unable to provide the higher intensity of care needed for their patients.

Finally, nursing homes are chronically underfunded. Rather than being reimbursed based on diagnosis or diagnosis-related groupings, nursing homes are generally reimbursed according to each resident's medical and nursing needs. Under a financing system that is gradually being phased out, the intensity of nursing home care has been classified according to skilled or intermediate levels. (These are sometimes called ICF and SNF for intermediate care facility and skilled nursing facility, respectively.) Each nursing home defines specific factors (usually dependency in daily living activities and other functions) and special nursing requirements that are used to classify each resident according to categories of skilled and intermediate level of care. The physician, however, must certify that the specific level of care is appropriate. In this role, the physician then becomes the arbiter of long-term care financing, the professional who determines how much the individual or government pays for the services of the nursing home.

Under a new system of long-term care financing established in many states, resource utilization groups (RUGS) are used to determine reimbursement. This system clusters residents into groups according to types of services. Reimbursement under this system—sometimes called the case-mix system—corresponds better to the actual care needs of individual residents. The amount of reimbursement is dependent on the accuracy of nursing records and to some degree on physician records. Unless care needs are documented well in progress notes, the nursing home may be underpaid. Such systems—where the level of payment is determined by the completeness of nursing and physician records—cause nursing homes to place major emphasis on record-keeping or "charting for dollars" rather than on the more traditional clinical and administrative functions of the medical record. These case-mix systems, which vary from state to state, may also provide an inappropriate financial incentive for nursing homes to encourage dependency and thereby increase reimbursement. Under some case-mix systems, successful rehabilitation is paradoxically rewarded with lower reimbursement!

Organizational Structure of the Nursing Home

Several members of the nursing home staff provide unique functions to assist attending physicians. These individuals and their roles in the nursing home are outlined in Table 32–1. In addition, several physicians on the staff participate in formulating policies on medical care within nursing homes. Most key committees (outlined in Table 32–2) have physician members to address concerns about clinical practice. Primary care physicians who attend patients living within the home are usually organized according to an open model medical staff, whereby any physician may attend patients, or a closed model, whereby attending physician privileges are controlled and limited. Regardless of the medical staff structure, a medical practice agreement or physician by-laws may be used to delineate responsibilities of the attending physician, authorize certain activities of the medical director (for example, the quality assurance program), and encourage physician participation and accountability.

Clinical Practice in the Nursing Home

Clinical practice in the nursing home is quite distinct from that in other settings. Table 32–3 outlines certain strengths and weaknesses of the nursing home setting with respect to clinical monitoring, medication compliance, nutrition, staffing, and the availability of laboratory and x-ray services.

The general approach to medical evaluation and treatment is also specific for the long-term care setting, particularly with the medically unstable patient. In the nursing home, serious illness commonly presents in a nonspecific manner. Such presentations may be related to cognitive dysfunction, other disorders of communication, or masking of symptoms in this population. The first indicator of serious illness may be an observation of weight loss, delirium, incontinence, frequent falls, or simply an increased respiratory rate. Subtle signs and symptoms must therefore be evaluated carefully. Pneumonia without a cough, myocardial infarction without pain, and urinary tract infection without dysuria are all relatively common.

Accurate diagnosis may be made more difficult by inaccurate assessments performed by nursing staff, inappropriate attempts to evaluate acute events by telephone, and inconsistent availability of reliable and valid laboratory tests and x-rays. Certain studies done in the nursing home may be less sensitive and specific than similar studies performed in a hospital (e.g., portable chest and bone x-rays). Although there is currently little financial incentive for physicians to evaluate and manage subacute problems in the nursing home, on-

Table 32–1. Key Staff of the Nursing Home Associated with Medical Care

Staff Position	Responsibilities
Medical Director	A physician, usually with training or interest in geriatric medicine, who functions to ensure that medical care is appropriate within the home. He or she acts as a liaison between attending physicians and provides education for nurses and other staff and primary medical input for medically related administrative decisions. The medical director is often called on to interpret the actions of physicians for staff.
Director of Nurses	A registered nurse who is responsible for all nursing operations within the facility. In addition to being responsible for nursing personnel and policies, his or her personal philosophy of nursing is often implemented throughout the facility.
Consulting Pharmacist	A pharmacist who reviews each resident's record on a monthly basis to evaluate prescription of medications. Most pharmacists follow guidelines developed by the Health Care Financing Administration. These include items such as timeliness of serum potassium levels for residents given diuretics, availability of serum digoxin levels for residents given digoxin, use of no more than one medication of any drug family, orders for an excessive number of medications overall, and the presence of a diagnosis for each medication. Physicians must put their recommendations into proper clinical context before implementation.
Infection Control Nurse	A registered nurse of the facility who is usually charged with responsibility for implementing the infection control program. She or he develops policies and procedures, educates other staff, and conducts surveillance for infections.
Administrator	The individual who is responsible for overall operation of the facility, including staff, financing, maintenance of the facility, and the philosophy of care.

Table 32–2. *Typical Nursing Home Committees*

Name of Committee	Composition	Responsibilities
Utilization Review/Medical Practice	Medical director, other physicians from the staff, administrator, director of nursing, others.	• Primary point for physician input about policies associated with clinical practice. • Determines level of care for reimbursement purposes. • Conducts quality assurance audits relevant to medical care.
Infection Control	Medical director and/or physician with expertise in infectious diseases; infection control nurse; representatives from nursing, housekeeping, dietary, laundry, pharmacy, and other departments.	• Develops policies and procedures concerning infection control practices in the facility. • Common areas of activity include tuberculosis control, general isolation practices, influenza prevention programs, surveillance of contagious diseases in the facility, in-service education, and aspects of employee health relevant to infections. • Usually responsible for environmental sanitation within the facility.
Pharmacy	Medical director and/or other physicians, consulting pharmacist, administrator, director of nursing, and others.	• Develops policies and procedures for use of medications within the facility. • Includes determining the composition of emergency medication supplies, reviewing consultant pharmacy activities, reviewing medication errors and adverse drug reactions, and conducting medication audits.
Safety	Medical director, safety director, administrator, director of nursing, and others.	• Ensure that the environment is safe for resident care and staff employment. • Matters pertaining to medical care, e.g., falls and serious incidents, are reviewed to prevent them in the future.
Quality Assurance	Medical director, administrator, director of nursing, and others	• Provides a systematic program to monitor, evaluate, and improve the quality of health care and quality of life for residents of the nursing home.
Ethics	Medical director, director of nursing, administrator, chaplain, attorney, resident representative, family representative, and others.	• Develops policies and procedures that address ethical issues in the nursing home, such as advanced directives for limited treatment. • Provides educational opportunities for physicians, staff, and residents about ethical issues. • Serves as a resource for patients, families, and professionals on ethical dilemmas regarding clinical care in the facility.

site evalutions can reduce unnecessary emergency room visits and hospitalizations. Nurse practitioners trained in geriatrics can also effectively assess and manage many acute medical problems. Of course, any decision to actively treat an acute illness must be made with careful consideration of the intervention's impact on quality of life. Diagnostic studies that do not change the treatment are usually not justified.

The goals for the routine physician visit to nursing home patients differ from those of a typical clinic or hospital visit. In the nursing home, the physician often spends less time on concerns of a strictly medical nature and directs more attention to psychosocial issues, functional capacity, regulatory compliance, education and counseling, and advocacy for quality care. More observational data are available for the physician. Nurses and other professional staff benefit from extra educational efforts to properly implement orders. This educational role for attending physicians becomes even more important as nursing homes accept

Table 32–3. Clinical Advantages to Care
in the Nursing Home

Twenty-four-hour nursing observation occurs for early
    detection, evaluation and assessment, and monitoring
    of clinical events.
Compliance problems with medications are nearly
    eliminated.
Sound nutrition is provided and therapeutic diets are
    monitored.
Daily functional capacity is observed.
Activities, physical therapy, and occupational therapy
    provide rehabilitation and additional monitoring of
    functional status.
Companionship and emotional support are available.
Systematic accident prevention is practiced.
Laboratory and x-ray services are usually available.

patients who require more complex nursing
care. Patient education and family conferences
are also appropriate and are time-consuming,
especially when ethical issues are discussed.
Careful development of advanced directives
for limiting treatment, however, is essential to
good nursing home practice. Sometimes, visits
with patients who are stable can appropriately
be considered social calls, although they actually provide an excellent opportunity to address psychosocial concerns. For the lonely
elderly widow with no surviving relatives or
friends—and for most patients—such unstruc-
tured visits are truly reassuring and therapeutic.

Finally, one of the most important functions
for the routine visit is to advocate for quality
care. The physician is often in the best position
to judge the appropriateness and quality of
care provided in any given nursing home.
When problems do develop with staffing or
morale, the physician is often the first to see
adverse consequences such as the development
of pressure sores, contractures, dehydration,
and depression.

Strategy for Nursing Home Visits

The strategy that each physician follows for
nursing home visits is highly variable. There
are, however, some basic components to visits
that appear to enhance effectiveness, as follows.

1. With respect to the frequency of visits,
more frequent visits may be needed when the
patient is unstable or during certain high-risk
periods. These include the period shortly after
admission (or readmission from the hospital),
or whenever the patient is grieving or recovering from an acute illness. Although patients
who are medically stable can be placed on

alternate visit schedules, this should be
avoided unless they are truly stable. Visits to
private pay patients are required only every 6
months, but patients should be seen more
frequently (e.g., each 2 months) until they
have adapted to the nursing home and they
are clearly medically stable. In most states,
physicians must visit Medicaid patients receiving skilled care or rehabilitation services every
30 days.

2. Regular visits to patients who are stable
may be brief, but they should include a systematic assessment of current status. Any recent
changes in medical condition, functional status, affect, or response to medications should
be reviewed with the nursing staff. A change
in weight is particularly important as it may
indicate an underlying illness.

3. Orders of the physician should be reviewed, updated, and renewed. Medication
orders (regular and as-needed drugs) should
be evaluated at every visit with the goal to
reduce the number of medications and eliminate unnecessary drugs whenever possible.
Each order should have a stop date to prevent
treatment after the condition is resolved.

4. Physicians also monitor the progress of
patients receiving physical and/or occupational
therapy by observations of patient function on
the ward and discussions with rehabilitation
staff and nursing staff on the patients' floor.
Particular attention should be directed to the
appropriateness of continued therapy (restorative or maintenance) and the potential for
discharge from treatment. In facilities where
therapies are particularly aggressive and tend
to be overutilized, the floor nurses are often
good judges of true progress in function.

5. Family members may have significant observations or concerns relevant to care, and
these should be discussed before, during, or
after the visit whenever possible.

6. After data have been reviewed and progress has been discussed with nursing staff, the
physician should interview and examine the
patient. A complete examination with the patient disrobed is usually not necessary or practical on routine visits. When preparatory data
indicate that a problem may exist, however, a
complete examination relative to the problem
is necessary. In general, functional capacity,
cognition, hydration, and skin condition
should be evaluated in all patients.

7. At least biannually, the comprehensive
care plan prepared by the multidisciplinary
team should be reviewed and contributions
should be made as appropriate. This plan,

developed in a care conference, lists specific problems, goals for each problem, and the approach the team will take to reach the goal. Medical input is important to this process to ensure its medical appropriateness and also to make certain that there are no overlooked treatable conditions underlying the problems.

8. The progress note for each visit should document the patient's current status with subjective and objective information, information, an assessment, and plans for subsequent care. Although many physicians consider the nursing home record to be of limited clinical value, it is invaluable as a means to reconstruct the logic of previous clinical decisions and guide future planning. Current records are also important for the on-call physician who may not know the patient and for nursing staff and other members of the interdisciplinary team.

9. Some families appreciate receiving a telephone call from the physician after nursing home visits to report on progress. Caregiving does not stop when loved ones enter nursing homes. In some instances, the feelings of frustration, worry, and guilt experienced by family members actually increase. Every effort should be made to facilitate open communication with families.

10. At the conclusion of each visit, the physician should be sure that the patient has a current problem list, clear delineation of limited treatment plans, and a clinical plan in the progress notes.

Telephone Communication

When a problem arises between nursing home visits that is managed by telephone, the situation must be handled cautiously. A clear history must be available from the nurse; this should include measurements of vital signs, current medications, changes in functional status, and physical examination findings. Other important baseline information such as current medical problems and clinical plan should be available from the chart. By using these data, most minor problems can be managed over the telephone, especially when one is familiar with the patient and the nurse. If the physician is uncomfortable about the clinical situation, regardless of the presence or absence of a limited treatment plan, a visit to the nursing home or transfer to the hospital emergency room is appropriate. Communication with the physician in the emergency room facilitates an appropriate evaluation. A physician's exami-

nation is usually the most critical element needed to diagnose and treat the illness properly. Such action is particularly important if the nurse appears hesitant, uncomfortable, or incompetent.

There are situations when a visit to the nursing home is preferable to telephone management, such as during the terminal care period for cancer patients. The physician's presence at the bedside assures patients that supportive care will be continued, reassures them that they are not being abandoned, and provides psychologic support for the family and nursing home staff.

Standing Orders

Standing orders should not serve as a means to minimize "unnecessary" communication with physicians when patients become ill. If such orders are used at all, purely administrative and trivial clinical issues such as "regular diet for holidays," "leave from the nursing home with family," and other simple instructions are appropriate. A sample of appropriate standing orders is included in Table 32–4.

Clinical events that may herald more serious

Table 32–4. Example of Model Standing Orders*

1. Resident may leave on a pass with the family as desired. Send medications with resident after instruction of resident and/or family member. Notify physician if there is any question regarding medication compliance.
2. Resident may have limited amounts of alcoholic beverages as he or she requests.
3. Notify physician of all falls within a reasonable period—according to nursing judgment—after the fall occurs.
4. Diet of choice on holidays and other special occasions as determined by resident.
5. Patient may see podiatrist or dentist as necessary.
6. Glycerine suppository (one) each day when necessary for constipation.
7. Acetaminophen 650 mg every 6 hours as needed for minor pain. Call physician if there is no relief, or if more than two doses are given in a 48-hour period. Do not give for fever or abdominal pain unless specified by physician.
8. Milk of magnesia 30 ml each day as needed for constipation.
9. For diarrhea, check for impaction and fever, then change diet to clear liquids and avoid dairy products for 24 hours. Call physician if:
   Symptoms persist for longer than 24 hours
   Diarrhea is severe or fever is present
   Significant abdominal pain is present

*Appropriateness of specific orders may vary by individual nursing home and state.

medical problems should not be addressed by standing orders. Examples of inappropriate standing orders include the use of antipyretics for fever, antitussives for cough, and medications for diarrhea. These symptoms may be the first important clue to a more serious illness that requires vigorous diagnosis and treatment. Many authorities believe that substantial morbidity and mortality might be prevented in nursing homes by early detection and treatment.

Restraint management is another matter that should not be routinely addressed on standing orders. Restraint orders need to specify consent of the patient's family, periodic release practices, and duration of application. In many cases, the delirium that necessitates the use of restraints should be evaluated medically concurrent with the application of the devices.

Comprehensive Appraisals

At admission and periodically thereafter, some type of comprehensive appraisal of health status should occur. The components of this appraisal are somewhat controversial. Although the traditional history and physical examination is unlikely to identify subclinical problems among nursing home patients for whom early detection is likely to make a difference in outcome, there are other important reasons to perform such examinations. These include patient expectations, the prevention of iatrogenic events, and the opportunity to review known medical problems and update plans for treatment; in some communities and nursing homes, they may also represent a "standard of care." Table 32–5 provides an outline of options for the periodic appraisal, which should be individualized according to standards of care, patient wishes, and other indications of appropriateness. Ideally on admission, physicians develop plans for future periodic appraisals in accord with each patient's individual needs.

With the health appraisal, the comprehensive functional assessment should be reviewed. Results of this should be compared with previous assessments to give a clear picture of change over time, prognosis, and effectiveness of the current care plan. A structured mental status instrument, such as the Mini-Mental State or Short Portable Mental Status Questionnaire, should be utilized in this assessment. The functional assessment should also focus

Table 32–5. Possible Components of Periodic Health Appraisals*

Functional assessment (need not be performed by physician)
  Toileting/incontinence of bowel and bladder
  Mobility and gait
  Dressing
  Feeding
  Bathing
  Hearing
  Vision
  Mental status and affect
  Behavioral problems
Medical evaluation/health maintenance
  Breast examination
  Pelvic examination
  Pap test
  Mammography
  Rectal examination
  Stool hemoccult test
  Proctosigmoidoscopy
  Laboratory studies:
    Hemogram
    Serum chemistry analyses
    Urinalysis
    Thyroid function tests
    Glycosylated hemoglobin analysis
    Drug levels (e.g., digoxin, phenytoin)
Immunizations/skin tests
  Pneumococcal infection
  Influenza
  Tetanus/diphtheria
  Tuberculin (two-step)
  Skin test controls
Oral/dental evaluation
Advanced directives for limited treatment
  Do not resuscitate
  Do not intubate
  Avoid hospitalization
  Supportive care
  Avoid artificial fluids and nutrition
  Avoid other specific diagnostic or treatment modalities such as antibiotics

*Evaluations should be highly personalized.

on gait and prevention of falls, vision, and psychologic function. Periodic case finding for hearing loss through audiometry is commonly promoted among nursing home residents. Although there is a high prevalence of significant hearing loss, the number of patients appropriate for hearing aides is often small. Such institutional programs are indicated only when emphasis is on comprehensive aural rehabilitation rather than on identification of candidates for purchase of electronic hearing devices. Periodic oral assessments are also important in this population. These examinations should include a careful evaluation of the mouth, teeth, and dentures. A dentist performs these examinations best; however, a physician can screen patients when a dentist is not available.

Several studies have now demonstrated the

lack of utility for broad panels of laboratory screening tests in the nursing home. For individual patients with a past history of certain illnesses, periodic laboratory studies may be appropriate. In most cases, however, the utility of such endeavors is low, particularly when careful attention has been devoted to regular physical examinations and pursuit of symptoms. On the other hand, in situations where physicians have been underattentive to hands-on patient care, the utility of screening examinations may be higher.

Immunizations should be reviewed and updated as appropriate. Most nursing home patients should have a current tetanus/diphtheria immunization (every 10 years after the primary series), pneumococcal vaccine (currently recommended once in a person's lifetime), and annual influenza immunizations. In addition, each patient should be reviewed for appropriateness of providing low dose amantadine during influenza A outbreaks.

The periodic appraisal should also include a careful review of plans to limit treatment. Advanced directives are always subject to change according to the wishes of each patient and/or proxy. In accord with this, periodic review and documentation of that review are appropriate. The plans should be discussed with the nursing staff to make sure there is common understanding of the patient's wishes.

Nurse Practitioners

Many physicians have found nurse practitioners to be especially helpful in the nursing home. Acting partly as physician extenders and partly as professionals providing primary care, these individuals are well suited to bridge the gap between medicine and nursing functions. Many simple problems, e.g., urinary tract infections, can be treated by nurse practitioners via algorithms or protocols. The nurse practitioner can extend the capabilities of the physician by organizing routine visits and spending more time with families, nursing staff, and rehabilitative staff. The nurse practitioner also effectively conducts quality assurance activities and presents in-service educational programs.

Organizing Attending Care in Nursing Homes

Many experts in nursing home practice believe that it is critically important for physicians to establish a clear working relationship with staff members of the nursing home and a working knowledge of each nursing home in which one practices. According to this approach, it is difficult for an attending physician to provide quality clinical services where that physician cares for only a few patients; familiarity never develops with the staff or the operations of that particular home. On the other hand, if physicians limit their practice to only a few nursing homes but have more patients in each home, there is greater opportunity to develop a working relationship with nurses, understand the strengths and weaknesses of rehabilitation programs, appreciate the proclivity for medication errors, and become familiar with the capabilities of the social work staff. Such working knowledge presents major advantages in achieving high quality care. This strategy, for physicians to limit the number of nursing homes and increase the activity level within each home, is also consistent with the trend to encourage more participation of physicians in nursing home care.

Special Clinical Problems

Certain clinical problems are more commonly encountered in nursing home practice than in office practice. Many of these, such as delirium, weight loss, incontinence, and falls, are discussed in other chapters in this book. General strategies for nursing home management of infections, weight loss, problem behavior, medications, and constipation are presented here. An approach to managing pressure sores is given in Table 32–6.

Infection Strategy

Pneumonia and urinary tract and skin and soft tissue infections are the most prevalent types of nursing home infections. Although standard approaches to measuring infections in nursing homes have not been recognized to date, prevalence surveys have found from 8 to 18% of patients infected or given antibiotic therapy at any time. Infections have also been reported as a disproportionate cause of hospital admissions among nursing home patients. Infections in this population often present with nonspecific symptoms and signs such as confusion, falls, and tachypnea. The presence of fever in elderly nursing home patients has special significance and requires aggressive

Table 32–6. Treatment of Pressure Sores

Shea's Classification of Pressure Sores*	Suggested Treatment
Grade I ulcer (superficial breakdown with loss of epidermis)	Relieve pressure (turn every two hours, static air or eggcrate mattress) Keep skin meticulously clean and dry Maintain nutritional status
Grade II ulcer (shallow ulcer extending to but not involving subcutaneous fat)	Relieve pressure (as above) Debride necrotic tissue Consider occlusive dressing (DuoDerm, Op Site) for clean, shallow, noninfected ulcer Wet-to-dry saline dressings for deeper, more necrotic ulcers
Grade III ulcer (full thickness wound extending into subcutaneous fat)	Relieve pressure (consider air-fluidized or low-air-loss therapy if cannot position off ulcer and nonhealing on regular bed) Debride necrotic tissue surgically Wet-to-dry saline dressings or whirlpool Consider surgery: primary closure, grafting, or rotation of skin flap Observe for osteomyelitis or infection
Grade IV ulcer (penetration to deep fascia with muscle or bone exposed)	Relieve pressure (as with grade III) Extensive surgical debridement of necrotic tissue Saline dressing packed in wound or whirlpool treatments Surgical procedures required (as above) Observe for osteomyelitis or sepsis

*Shea JD. Clin Orthop 112:89–100, 1975.

evaluation for bacterial infections. Because diagnostic studies may not be readily available among these debilitated patients, empiric treatment with antibiotics is sometimes appropriate; one such approach is provided in Table 32–7. Whenever possible, however, treatment with adequate diagnostic information is encouraged. Asymptomatic bacteriuria is a common condition among this population and usually does not require treatment. Immunizations for influenza, pneumococcal infections, and tetanus/diphtheria remain the mainstay of primary prevention. The long-term utility of pneumococcal vaccine among nursing home patients has yet to be demonstrated; the relatively close nursing home environment may select for colonization by pneumococci of the nonvaccine capsular types.

Because outbreaks of tuberculosis occur with relative frequency among nursing home patients, the disease must be considered in any suspicious clinical situation. Thus the tuberculin skin test status of each nursing home resident must be clearly established. Recent publications have suggested that the nursing home population serves as an inapparent reservoir for the disease in the United States. It is particularly important because of the major potential for transfer to fellow patients, staff, and the community. A two-step tuberculin skin test is highly recommended among these patients because of waning immune function. Decisions to treat tuberculin positive elderly patients are complex and each must be made on an individual basis.

Infection control programs in nursing homes have not developed to the modern level of sophistication typical of hospitals. In most

Table 32–7. Empiric Antibiotic Therapy in the Nursing Home*

Type of Infection	Clinically Stable	Clinically Unstable†
Pneumonia	Oral amoxicillin, trimethoprim/sulfamethoxazole, first- or second-generation cephalosporin	Parenteral cephalosporin and aminoglycoside
Urinary tract	Oral amoxicillin, trimethoprim/sulfamethoxazole, cephalosporin, or quinolone	Parenteral cephalosporin or ampicillin, and aminoglycoside
Cellulitis	Dicloxacillin, first-generation cephalosporin	Parenteral broad spectrum coverage

*Empiric therapy is discouraged unless it is clearly the only approach available.
†Unless a limited treatment plan is established that specifically addresses serious infection, unstable patients would usually be hospitalized for definitive diagnosis and treatment.

homes, little effort is devoted to these activities and designated staff are poorly trained, lack direction and resources, and perform the function part-time. Potential admission of patients with acquired immunodeficiency syndrome has prompted many nursing homes to enhance infection control activities.

Medication Strategy

Polypharmacy remains a common problem in long-term care facilities, with most residents receiving three or more drugs daily. Laxatives and analgesics are the most frequently ordered, followed by psychotropic, diuretic, and cardiac agents. Increased drug use in this setting is related to the high frequency of chronic diseases, empiric use of medications (especially as needed drugs), and too often, inappropriate prescribing by the attending physician. The resulting adverse side effects and drug interactions affect physical and mental functioning as well as the quality of life of nursing home residents.

Strategies for reducing drug use in the nursing home must begin with more rational pharmacotherapy by physicians. Medication should be given only when necessary and the effects should be monitored carefully. In general, initiation with low doses and careful upward titration under observation may reduce side effects. Some conditions common in this population, such as asymptomatic bacteriuria, systolic hypertension, and dependent leg edema, may not require drug therapy. Drug profiles need to be reviewed during each physician's visit, with the number of drugs and drug dosage reduced whenever possible. Because nursing home patients can be closely monitored, changing drug regimens is safer in this population. Inappropriate use of as needed orders for drugs such as aspirin should be avoided. Clinical pharmacists conduct drug reviews on each patient monthly and their recommendations may be helpful. Guidelines for appropriate use of medications commonly used in nursing homes are presented in Table 32–8.

Evaluation of Weight Loss

Weight loss, one of the cardinal indicators of illness in the elderly, is associated with special implications among this patient group. In many cases, the problem is artifactual because of an inaccurate scale. When weight loss is real, however, its cause may be subtle and requires additional investigation. Compared with an independent-living population, nursing home residents are more likely to lose weight from behavior-associated problems—such as those related to dementia, delirium, and depression—than from other pathophysiologic causes. Psychotropic medications that cause subtle cognitive dysfunction, anticholinergic side effects, or gastrointestinal symptoms may also be associated with weight loss.

Management of Problem Behavior

The prevalence of mental illness has been estimated at 60 to 90% among nursing home residents. The most frequent serious behavior problems are verbal disturbances, physical resistance to care, and physical aggression.

The underlying cause for the behavioral disturbance should be sought in the physical, psychologic, and environmental domains. An acute medical illness or adverse medication effects must always be considered. When found, the cause of the problem should be corrected to the degree possible. Particular attention needs to be given to the nursing milieu and patient-patient relationships. When developed in a skilled and coordinated team fashion, behavioral interventions by nursing staff are often effective and appropriate. Assistance from a knowledgeable psychologist may be invaluable to guide staff interventions.

Medication is occasionally necessary to control maladaptive behavior; however, it is rarely effective if employed as an isolated treatment. Drug treatment should not be expected to abolish disturbed behavior but rather to attenuate its frequency and effects to a point where nursing measures become effective. Among patients with cognitive dysfunction, the choice of the psychotropic drug should depend on the nature of the disturbance. When the disturbance is associated with agitative symptoms, an antipsychotic agent with sedating properties (such as thioridazine) or a short-acting benzodiazepine (such as oxazepam) is most effective; when psychotic symptoms such as hallucinations are the problem, a less-sedating antipsychotic agent such as haloperidol is most appropriate. In most cases, the appropriate dose of these agents is miniscule compared with usual doses administered to patients with schizophrenia. When necessary in acute episodes, the antipsychotic drugs can be supplemented with short-acting sedating agents such as ben-

Table 32–8. Guidelines for Use of Medications in the Nursing Home

Drug	Comments/Recommendations
Analgesics	Avoid prescribing analgesics on an as needed basis. Acetaminophen is safe and effective for noninflammatory conditions. Codeine is effective but aggravates constipation.
Diuretics	Monitor for hypokalemia, orthostatic hypotension, dehydration, incontinence. Are not appropriate for mild dependent edema. May be withdrawn in stable patients (with close monitoring). May be "held" during acute illness expected to be associated with dehydration.
Digoxin	Signs of toxicity may be subtle. Monitor blood levels. Many elderly persons with sinus rhythm and no heart failure may not need digoxin.
Antihypertensives	Orthostatic hypotension and central nervous system effects are common. Monitor orthostatic blood pressure. Avoid overtreatment, especially systolic hypertension.
Antidepressants	May cause sedation, postural hypotension, and anticholinergic side effects. Use agent with least adverse effects first (such as trazodone, nortriptyline, desipramine).
Sedatives and hypnotics	Insomnia is common among institutionalized elderly. Use nonpharmacologic measures for sleep disorders if possible. Avoid long-acting benzodiazepines (such as diazepam or flurazepam).
Antipsychotics	Seek underlying cause for behavioral problem before starting antipsychotic drugs. Include orders to monitor orthostatic blood pressure, sedation, and extrapyramidal side effects. Watch for drug accumulation. Use small doses.

zodiazepines or hydroxyzine. Changes in the antipsychotic component should not be made until sufficient time has elapsed to see beneficial effects; sometimes this is a matter of weeks. After a period of acceptable behavior control, the medication should be gradually withdrawn.

Management of Constipation

Constipation refers to infrequent passage of hard, dry stools and is extremely common among nursing home residents. Contributing factors include prolonged inactivity, inadequate hydration, poor dietary and toilet habits, laxative abuse, and medications. Demented bedridden patients may develop severe constipation with fecal impactions, fecal incontinence, and other complications. A therapeutic approach to constipation in the nursing home should include education and diet as well as medication.

The alert resident should be reassured that irregular or infrequent stools do not indicate constipation or poor health. Adequate exercise (walking), proper body positioning during toileting, and the timing and setting of toileting all need to be considered by nursing staff. The ideal diet to prevent constipation includes adequate fluid, fiber, and laxative foods. Unfortunately, many nursing home residents refuse high roughage foods, find bran supplements unpalatable, or may even require special diets low in fiber.

Bulking agents such as psyllium (Metamucil, Effersylium) are extremely useful for patients with inadequate intake of dietary fiber. However, these agents must be used in sufficient quantity and with adequate fluid intake to be effective. They are also contraindicated where fecal impaction is present or suspected. Patients who strain during defecation may benefit from a stool softener such as docusate sodium (Colace). For patients resistant to bulking agents, a stimulant suppository (Dulcolax) can be given each morning and a colonic irritant such as senna (Senokot, Perdiem) at bedtime. Milk of magnesia may be used for relief of acute constipation but should be avoided by patients with renal failure. Lactulose syrup is quite expensive but well tolerated and can be titrated to regulate stools in patients not responding to other agents.

BIBLIOGRAPHY

Elliot DL, Watts WJ, Grand DE. Constipation: mechanism and management of a common clinical problem. Postgrad Med 74:143–149, 1983.
An excellent overview and approach to the problem are provided.

Fawler EM. Equipment and products used in management and treatment of pressure ulcers. Nurs Clin North Am 22:449–462, 1987.
This is a practical guide to current therapeutic options available for pressure sore treatment.

Irvine PW, Carlson K, Adcock M, et al. The value of annual medical examinations in the nursing home. J Am Geriatr Soc 32:540–545, 1984.
This study demonstrated a very low yield (less than 2% of examinations yielded important findings) for a standard annual physical examination among a nursing home population. It points out the need to individualize annual medical appraisals in the nursing home.

Lamy PP. Prescribing for the elderly. Littleton, MA, PSG Publishing Co., 1986.
A general resource presents a parsimonious approach to medication management in elderly persons.

Norman DC, Castle SC, Cantrell M. Infections in the nursing home. J Am Geriatr Soc 35:796–805, 1987.
This article reviews common infections in the nursing home as to etiology, diagnosis, and treatment.

Reuler OB, Cooney TG. The pressure sore: pathophysiology and principles of management. Ann Intern Med 94:661–666, 1981.
This article gives a basic review of the pathophysiology, diagnosis, and fundamental aspects of treatment for these preventable lesions.

Salzman C. Clinical Geriatric Psycho-pharmacology. New York, McGraw-Hill Book Co., 1984.
This resource concentrates on psychotropic medications.

Stead WW, Lofgren JP, Warren E, et al. Tuberculosis as an endemic and nosocomial infection among the elderly in nursing homes. N Engl J Med 312:1483–1487, 1985.
This investigation emphasized the importance of clear delineation of purified protein derivative status among all nursing home residents in view of suggestions that significant spread of tuberculosis occurs in nursing homes.

Uhlmann RF, Clark H, Pearlman RA, et al. Medical management decisions in nursing home patients: principles and policy recommendations. Ann Intern Med 106:879–885, 1987.
This paper outlines the unique aspects of decisions to limit treatment among nursing home patients who have major functional impairment and questionable quality of life.

Zweibel NR, Cassel CK (eds). Clinical and policy issues in the care of the nursing home patient. Clin Geriatr Med 4:471–690, 1988.
This entire issue is devoted to the nursing home patient.

PART SEVEN

Hematology/Oncology

33

Long-term Anticoagulation: Indications and Management

BARRY M. STULTS, M.D.
WILLARD H. DERE, M.D.
THOMAS H. CAINE, M.D.

Nearly 500,000 outpatients in the United States receive anticoagulants annually for treatment and prophylaxis of thromboembolic disorders. Because both the untreated thromboembolic disorder and anticoagulant therapy may be associated with considerable morbidity and some mortality, the decision to use anticoagulants with a particular patient is frequently complex. The physician must consider several variables:

1. The risk of thromboembolism and its associated morbidity and mortality without anticoagulation.

2. The expected reduction in thromboembolic risk with anticoagulation.

3. The risk of anticoagulant-induced complications, especially hemorrhage, which may vary significantly among patients.

4. The effect of anticoagulant therapy on the patient's quality of life, including the economic costs of medications and laboratory monitoring, required changes in lifestyle or occupation, and the anxiety that may be generated in some patients who take anticoagulants.

5. The age and life expectancy of the patient.

Unfortunately, for many thromboembolic disorders, available studies do not provide sufficient data concerning these variables. For certain patients, it may be difficult for physicians to adequately quantify the relative benefit/risk ratio for anticoagulant therapy. In view of this uncertainty, several groups of experts have recently reviewed the available evidence on the indications for and complications associated with anticoagulant therapy. In this chapter, we will summarize their conclusions and also consider the basic pharmacologic effects of anticoagulants and techniques to optimize their administration.

Pharmacology and Laboratory Monitoring of Anticoagulants

Warfarin, the most utilized outpatient anticoagulant, is a vitamin K antagonist that leads to the synthesis of biologically inactive forms of clotting factors II, VII, IX, and X. The serum half-life of these clotting factors varies from 4 to 6 hours for factor VII to 2 to 3 days for factors II and X. The effects of warfarin are usually monitored by the one-stage prothrombin time (PT), which is sensitive to three of the four vitamin K–dependent factors. It is useful to express the PT as the prothrombin time ratio (PTR): patient's prothrombin time in seconds divided by normal control prothrombin time in seconds. Although warfarin therapy may significantly increase the PTR within 24 hours because of suppression of factor VII, maximal depression of the activity of clotting factors with longer half-lives (and therefore maximal antithrombotic effect) is delayed up to 5 to 7 days. Warfarin also inhibits the synthesis of the anticoagulant proteins C and S, which are important in preventing thrombosis on the vascular endothelium. Because protein C has a short half-life similar to that of factor VII, the first few days of warfarin therapy could theoretically produce a hypercoagulable state, as the anticoagulant activity of protein C would decrease before the levels of clotting factors II, IX, and X. These events may relate to the pathophysiology of the rare complication of warfarin-induced skin necrosis, discussed later in the chapter.

Considerable confusion has resulted from the use of different thromboplastins for the measurement of the PTR. Thromboplastins derived from rabbit brain are used in most centers in North America, whereas human brain thromboplastins have been used in Europe. The latter are more responsive to the reduction in vitamin K–dependent factors, resulting in a significantly greater PTR compared with the same plasma sample tested with rabbit brain thromboplastin. To minimize confusion, the World Health Organization suggests that all PTR measurements undergo a standardized correction and be expressed as the International Normalized Ratio (INR). This ratio is the PTR that would be observed if the plasma sample were tested with the international reference material derived from human brain. PTRs of 1.3 to 1.5, 1.5 to 2.0, and 2.0 to 2.5, with rabbit brain thromboplastins, correspond to INRs of 2.0 to 3.0, 3.0 to 4.5, and 4.5 to 7.0, respectively. Most North American laboratories do not yet express PTRs as the INR, and subsequent PTRs in this chapter refer to the uncorrected measurements with rabbit brain thromboplastin.

Subcutaneous heparin may be used as an alternative to warfarin for outpatient anticoagulation of selected patients with venous thromboembolism and for pregnant women with prosthetic heart valves. Heparin exerts its major anticoagulant effect by augmenting antithrombin III inhibition of several activated coagulation factors; it has no effect on the production of these factors. Therefore, in contrast to warfarin, its antithrombotic effects occur immediately and are also dissipated 8 to 12 hours after cessation of subcutaneous administration. Heparin therapy is usually monitored by measuring the activated partial thromboplastin time.

Anticoagulant Therapy for Specific Thromboembolic Disorders

A task force sponsored by the American College of Chest Physicians (ACCP) and the National Heart, Lung, and Blood Institute (NHLBI) has recently published recommendations on anticoagulant therapy for thromboembolic disorders, including indications for use and suggested intensity and duration of therapy, together with an estimate of the relative strength of the scientific evidence supporting each recommendation (Table 33–1). Of special note are their recommendations on the intensity of warfarin therapy. The task force suggested the use of low intensity warfarin therapy to a PTR of 1.3 to 1.5 (a PT of 15 to 18 seconds) for all thromboembolic disorders except mechanical prosthetic heart valves and recurrent systemic embolism. For these two disorders they recommended conventional warfarin therapy to a PTR of 1.5 to 2.0 (a PT of 18 to 24 seconds). There is good evidence from randomized clinical trials supporting the efficacy of low intensity warfarin therapy for prevention and treatment of venous thromboembolism and for primary prevention of cerebral embolism in patients with acute myocardial infarction and in patients with bioprosthetic heart valves. In contrast, the evidence supporting the other recommendations for either low intensity or conventional warfarin therapy is considerably weaker, coming from nonrandomized trials and/or case studies. Further studies are needed to better delineate the optimal therapeutic range of warfarin therapy for these other thromboembolic disorders.

Venous Thromboembolism: Deep Vein Thrombosis and Pulmonary Embolism

Without a course of outpatient anticoagulation after inpatient heparin therapy, the recurrence rate of proximal (popliteal vein and above) deep vein thrombosis over the next 3 months is nearly 50% compared with 2 to 4% for patients given therapeutic anticoagulation. A recent controlled study has demonstrated that low intensity warfarin (PTR = 1.3 to 1.5) is as effective as conventional warfarin (PTR = 1.5 to 2.0) in preventing recurrent venous thromboembolism, but it is associated with a four-fold lower rate of hemorrhagic complications (5 versus 20%). Low intensity warfarin is therefore the treatment of choice to prevent recurrence of deep vein thrombosis or pulmonary embolism, or both. An equally effective and safe (but somewhat more expensive and inconvenient) regimen is the administration of subcutaneous heparin every 12 hours in a dose sufficient to prolong the activated partial thromboplastin time to 1.5 times the control value 6 hours after a dose. This regimen of adjusted dose subcutaneous heparin is useful for patients with certain contraindications to warfarin, including pregnancy (warfarin is a

Table 33–1. Recommendations for Long-Term Anticoagulation

Thromboembolic Disorder	Recommended PTR	Duration of Therapy	Level of Evidence*	Comments
1. Venous thromboembolism				More prolonged or lifetime anticoagulation may be required for recurrences or ongoing risk factors.
a. Proximal deep vein thrombosis/pulmonary embolism	1.3–1.5	3 mo for first episode	Strong	
b. Isolated calf deep vein thrombosis	1.3–1.5	6 wk for first episode	Weak	
2. Chronic atrial fibrillation (AF)				Indications for anticoagulation of chronic AF without coexisting heart disease are uncertain; patients over age 60 with lone AF have increased risk of stroke.
a. With cardioembolic stroke	1.5–2.0	Lifetime	Weak	
b. With valvular or nonvalvular heart disease	1.3–1.5	Lifetme	Weak	
c. With thyrotoxicosis	1.3–1.5	From diagnosis until euthyroid state and sinus rhythm re-established for 4 wk	Weak	
3. Cardioversion of AF	1.3–1.5	3 wk before and 4 wk after cardioversion	Weak	Anticoagulation not required for cardioversion of other atrial arrhythmias.
4. Valvular heart disease				Anticoagulation not required for uncomplicated mitral valve prolapse or aortic bioprosthetic heart valves in presence of sinus rhythm. Addition of dipyridamole is optional for patients with mechanical prostheses and is indicated if systemic embolism recurs despite adequate warfarin therapy.
a. Mitral regurgitation or stenosis				
i. With cardioembolic stroke	1.5–2.0	Lifetime	Weak	
ii. With chronic or paroxysmal AF	1.3–1.5	Lifetime	Weak	
iii. With enlarged left atrium (diameter > 55 mm) and sinus rhythm	1.3–1.5	Lifetime	Weak	
b. Mitral valve prolapse				
i. With cardioembolic stroke	1.5–2.0	Lifetime	Weak	
ii. With AF or recurrent transient cerebral ischemia refractory to aspirin therapy	1.3–1.5	Lifetime	Weak	
c. Mechanical prosthetic heart valves	1.5–2.0	Lifetime	Weak	
d. Bioprosthetic heart valves				
i. Mitral position, sinus rhythm	1.3–1.5	For first 3 mo after replacement	Strong	
ii. Mitral position with AF or left atrial thrombi	1.3–1.5, or 1.5–2.0	Lifetime	Weak	
5. Acute myocardial infarction (AMI)				Indications for anticoagulation beyond 3 mo are uncertain.
a. Transmural anterior AMI or large inferior AMI with heart failure or AF	1.3–1.5 1.3–1.5	For 3 mo after AMI For 3 mo after AMI	Strong Weak	
b. Post-AMI with severe heart failure, AF, or prior venous thromboembolism	1.3–1.5	Lifetime	Weak	
6. Idiopathic dilated cardiomyopathy	1.3–1.5	Lifetime	Weak	
7. Prevention of recurrent cardioembolism	1.5–2.0	Lifetime	Weak	

Modified from ACCP-NHLBI recommendations: Dalen JE, Hirsh J. Chest 89:1S–106S, 1986, with permission.
*Strong = supporting evidence from randomized trials; weak = suggestive evidence from nonrandomized trials or uncontrolled case studies.

teratogen), warfarin allergy, a history of war-farin-induced skin necrosis, or inability of the patient to have regular monitoring of the PTR.

The optimal duration of anticoagulation for proximal deep vein thrombosis and pulmonary embolism is unknown. Recommendations vary from 1 to 12 months. The most common practice is to use anticoagulants for patients with either no or transient risk factors for venous thromboembolism (e.g., postoperative state, immobilization, estrogen therapy) for 3 months after the initial episode. The subsequent recurrence rate for the next year after cessation of anticoagulation is between 4 and 12%. Patients with permanent risk factors, particularly malignancies and hereditary hypercoagulable states, should receive lifetime anticoagulation. For patients with recurrent venous thromboembolism but no apparent ongoing risk factors, some clinical experts recommend 1 year of anticoagulation for a first recurrence and lifetime anticoagulation for any subsequent recurrences.

The management of isolated calf vein thrombosis is controversial. The risk of pulmonary embolism is low, but 20 to 30% of calf vein thromboses extend proximally (usually within the first week after onset of symptoms), which increases the risk of pulmonary embolism and chronic venous insufficiency. Some experts recommend that patients with venographically confirmed calf vein thrombosis, especially if they have either limited cardiopulmonary reserve or ongoing risk factors for venous thromboembolism, should receive intravenous heparin for 7 days followed by low intensity warfarin or adjusted dose subcutaneous heparin for 6 weeks. Alternatively, serial impedance plethysmography, if available and of locally validated accuracy, may be used to detect proximal extension of calf vein thrombi and guide treatment decisions in patients with clinically suspected deep vein thrombosis. Anticoagulation is not required for patients with clinically suspected deep vein thrombosis if the initial and serial follow-up plethysmographic examinations on days 2, 5, and 10 show no evidence of proximal extension. Several large prospective studies have confirmed the efficacy of this approach.

Atrial Fibrillation

About 15% of all ischemic strokes are associated with atrial fibrillation (AF), and in the age group over 75 years old, this fraction increases to nearly 40%. Between 60 and 70% of AF-associated strokes are presumed to be cardioembolic in origin; coexistent cerebrovascular disease is the cause of the remainder. Fifty per cent of these strokes result in death or major disability. Prior stroke, both valvular and nonvalvular heart disease, age over 60 at the onset of AF, and possibly thyrotoxicosis increase the risk of stroke. In contrast, patients with AF not associated with coexisting heart disease (i.e., lone AF) and who are below age 60 appear to have a low risk of stroke that does not differ significantly from that of age- and sex-matched controls. The risk of stroke may be two- to three-fold higher in the first year after the onset of AF. Table 33–2, derived from several studies, gives estimates of the annual stroke risk for different patient groups with AF.

Controlled trials assessing the benefit/risk ratio for anticoagulation of different patient groups with chronic AF have not been conducted. Retrospective studies strongly support long-term anticoagulation of patients with mitral stenosis and AF. Prospective trials of anticoagulation for patients with nonvalvular AF are now in progress in the United States and Europe. Pending results of these studies, therapeutic decisions must be individualized. Currently, in the absence of contraindications, long-term anticoagulation with warfarin should be strongly considered for AF patients with (1) prior systemic embolism; (2) mitral valve disease, including patients with paroxysmal AF; (3) cardiomyopathy of any etiology; (4) thyrotoxicosis, until a euthyroid state and sinus rhythm have been restored for 4 weeks. Some clinicians also recommend anticoagulation for patients with AF and the bradycardia-tachycardia syndrome. There is no consensus about anticoagulation of patients with chronic lone AF. Based on existing information, anticoagulation may be considered for patients with onset of lone AF after age 60; however, careful

Table 33–2. Annual Stroke Risk in Patient Groups with Chronic AF

Patient Group	% Annual Stroke Risk
Prior stroke	10–20
Rheumatic valvular disease	4–5
Nonvalvular AF*	1.5–4
Lone AF, age over 60	2.6
Lone AF, age under 60	0.1

*A majority of these patients have structural heart disease related to hypertension, coronary artery disease, or other causes.

review of the individual benefits and risks of anticoagulation in this elderly population is critical. Pending further studies, the ACCP-NHLBI task force recommends that patients with a prior systemic embolism receive anticoagulation therapy to a PTR of 1.5 to 2.0 and the other patient groups to a PTR of 1.3 to 1.5.

Cardioversion

Without anticoagulation, the incidence of systemic embolism after electrical or chemical cardioversion of AF is 1 to 5%. There is limited evidence that prior anticoagulation with low intensity warfarin therapy may reduce the incidence to below 1%. The time in AF necessary for a thrombus to form within the left atrium is unknown; some clinicians recommend anticoagulation before cardioversion if AF has been present 3 or more days, whereas others believe that the period of low embolic risk is up to 7 days unless there is coexistent mitral valve disease. Anticoagulation with low intensity warfarin is recommended for 3 weeks before cardioversion to allow any thrombus present to adhere to the atrial wall. Despite restoration of sinus rhythm, emboli may appear up to 3 weeks after cardioversion because of a delay in resumption of mechanical atrial contraction. Therefore, anticoagulation should be continued for 4 weeks after cardioversion. Emboli are rare after cardioversion of other atrial tachyarrhythmias, and prophylactic anticoagulation is generally not indicated.

Valvular Heart Disease

MITRAL AND AORTIC VALVE DISEASE

The annual incidence of systemic embolism is 1 to 5% for patients with mitral stenosis and 1 to 3% for patients with severe chronic mitral regurgitation. The risk of embolism increases with coexistent chronic or paroxysmal AF, advancing age, and a prior history of embolism. Left atrial size is not an independent risk factor; however, patients with marked left atrial enlargement (> 55 mm diameter by M-mode echocardiography) are at high risk for AF, and therefore, for systemic embolism. There is considerable evidence that anticoagulation prevents recurrent embolism in these patients; by extension, it may prevent initial embolism as well. Patients with prior embolism

should receive anticoagulants to a PTR of 1.5 to 2.0, whereas those with chronic or paroxysmal AF alone can receive low intensity warfarin. Some clinicians also advocate low intensity warfarin anticoagulation for mitral stenosis patients in sinus rhythm if the left atrial diameter is greater than 55 mm or if the patient is over age 35. Anticoagulation is not required in the absence of these risk factors.

In patients with mitral valve prolapse, there is a very low incidence of transient ischemic attacks and stroke of 1/6000 per year. Asymptomatic mitral valve prolapse patients in sinus rhythm therefore require no treatment. Prolapse patients with otherwise unexplained transient ischemic attacks may be treated with aspirin, 1 g/day, or if aspirin is ineffective, with low intensity warfarin. Long-term anticoagulation is indicated for mitral valve prolapse patients with chronic or paroxysmal AF (PTR = 1.3 to 1.5) and for those with prior stroke (PTR = 1.5 to 2.0).

Patients with isolated aortic valve disease in sinus rhythm are at low risk for embolism and do not require long-term anticoagulation.

PROSTHETIC HEART VALVES

The risk of thromboembolism with prosthetic heart valves depends on the type of valve and is also increased in the presence of AF, left atrial thrombus, and previous emboli. The risk is also greater in the first 3 months and possibly the first 12 months after surgery. Without anticoagulation, all mechanical heart valves have a high incidence of systemic embolism (5 to 25% per year) and valve thrombosis, which is reduced by long-term conventional warfarin therapy (PTR = 1.5 to 2.0) to 1.5 to 3.0% per year. The combination of warfarin and dipyridamole, 400 mg/day or 5 to 6 mg/kg/day, may further reduce embolic risk and is clearly indicated for patients who experience emboli despite therapeutic warfarin. For patients with bleeding complications with conventional warfarin therapy, an alternative regimen combines low intensity warfarin and dipyridamole. The utility of low intensity warfarin alone is unknown but is currently under investigation.

Bioprosthetic valves have a lower incidence of systemic embolism than mechanical valves in the absence of anticoagulation. Mitral bioprostheses carry the greatest risk, which without anticoagulation ranges from 1% per year for patients in sinus rhythm to 5% per year for patients with chronic AF or a left atrial thrombus noted at surgery. About 25% of the emboli occur in the first 3 months after surgery. Controlled trials of anticoagulation in this setting have not yet been performed. Most experts recommend that all patients with mitral bioprostheses, and optionally those with aortic bioprostheses, receive warfarin for the first 3 months after surgery. Both low intensity and conventional warfarin regimens have been suggested. Thereafter, patients with chronic AF or left atrial thrombi should continue warfarin treatment indefinitely. Patients in sinus rhythm without left atrial thrombi do not require long-term anticoagulation; however, a single study suggests that long-term therapy with aspirin, 0.5 g/day, may lower the incidence of thromboembolism in these patients.

Acute Myocardial Infarction

The primary theoretical reasons to use anticoagulants for these patients are to prevent recurrent infarctions, venous thromboembolism, and systemic embolism from left ventricular mural thrombi. Most studies have found that long-term oral anticoagulation does not significantly reduce the incidence of recurrent myocardial infarctions or death. Subcutaneous heparin, 5000 units every 12 hours until the patient is ambulatory, adequately prevents venous thromboembolism in most patients after infarction.

Long-term oral anticoagulation does reduce the incidence of systemic embolism in survivors of an acute myocardial infarction. Systemic emboli, 75% of which are cerebral, occur in 2 to 4% of infarction patients not receiving anticoagulants. Nearly 70% of these emboli occur in the first month after infarction. Embolic risk peaks at the end of the first week and in most patients declines to very low levels by 8 to 12 weeks after infarction. The vast majority of patients with systemic embolism have had transmural anterior acute myocardial infarction associated with apical wall dyskinesis or akinesis; coexisting heart failure, AF, and possibly the morphologic appearance of the source left ventricular mural thrombus (e.g., mobile thrombi with protruding or pedunculated edges) may further increase the risk of embolism. Patients with uncomplicated inferior infarctions or nontransmural anterior infarctions are at low risk for embolism. Randomized and nonrandomized studies have demonstrated that anticoagulation therapy initiated shortly after hospital admission with full doses of

intravenous heparin and followed by low intensity warfarin for 1 to 3 months reduces the incidence of systemic embolism by 25 to 75%. In the absence of contraindications, this anticoagulant regimen should be strongly considered for patients with transmural anterior infarctions and possibly for large inferior infarctions complicated by heart failure or AF. The decision to use anticoagulants is best determined by these clinical criteria rather than evidence of the presence or absence of a mural thrombus on two-dimensional echocardiogram. Echocardiography performed in the first few days after infarction does not detect the majority of mural thrombi, which develop after 3 days; on the other hand, if echocardiography and anticoagulation are delayed until 7 to 10 days after infarction, it is too late to prevent emboli that occur during the first week. Finally, up to 20% of echocardiograms may be technically inadequate in this situation.

Very little is known about the embolic risk or efficacy of anticoagulant therapy for left ventricular thrombi persisting beyond the first 3 months after infarction. In different retrospective and small prospective studies, the incidence of stroke varies from less than 1 to 10 to 15% during follow-up periods of 2 years. No firm recommendations about anticoagulation can be made for these patients at the current time.

Cardiomyopathies

Without anticoagulation, patients with idiopathic dilated cardiomyopathy have a 10 to 20% lifetime incidence of systemic embolism and a 5 to 10% incidence of pulmonary embolism. A significant proportion of systemic emboli occur in the first year after diagnosis. Cardiac rhythm (sinus rhythm versus AF), hemodynamic status, and evidence of the presence or absence of ventricular mural thrombi on an echocardiogram do *not* clearly influence the risk of systemic embolism. There are no prospective studies documenting the benefit/risk ratio for prophylactic anticoagulation of these patients. Limited retrospective data suggest a significant reduction in the incidence of both systemic and venous thromboembolism when warfarin therapy is initiated shortly after diagnosis. Low intensity warfarin is recommended for patients with no prior history of systemic embolism.

Patients with hypertrophic cardiomyopathy and paroxysmal or chronic AF have a significant risk of systemic embolism and should receive low intensity warfarin. The incidence of systemic embolism and the indications for anticoagulation in patients with ischemic cardiomyopathy are unknown.

Cerebral Ischemia

Anticoagulant therapy does not clearly reduce and possibly increases morbidity and mortality after both transient ischemic attacks and completed thrombotic stroke. In contrast, antiplatelet therapy with aspirin, 1 g/day, reduces the incidence of subsequent stroke and death in both patient groups. If aspirin therapy or carotid endarterectomy is ineffective or contraindicated for patients with recurrent transient ischemic attacks, some neurologists recommend carefully monitored oral anticoagulation for 3 to 6 months.

The management of acute cardioembolic stroke is complex and controversial and beyond the scope of this chapter; it is thoroughly reviewed in the ACCP-NHLBI monograph edited by Dalen and Hirsh and in a recent editorial review by Yatsu and colleagues. Patients with a prior cardioembolic stroke should receive long-term warfarin anticoagulation to a PTR of 1.5 to 2.0.

Management of Chronic Anticoagulation in the Perioperative Period

For surgical procedures, the risk of bleeding with continued anticoagulation must be balanced against the risk of thromboembolism if anticoagulants are stopped. Minor surgical procedures involving superficial structures (e.g., dental extraction, inguinal herniorrhaphy) carry a low risk of bleeding even if therapeutic anticoagulation is continued. In contrast, with major invasive surgery, the incidence of significant perioperative bleeding is 13 to 45% in anticoagulated patients; however, the risk of bleeding is not increased if the PT at surgery is prolonged no more than 20% above the control value. For most chronically anticoagulated patients—except those with mechanical heart valves and/or prior systemic embolism—the risk of a thromboembolic event is low if warfarin is discontinued 2 to 3 days preoperatively and restarted at the usual dose 1 to 2 days after surgery. The PT at surgery

should be normal or prolonged at most only 2 to 3 seconds. Patients with mechanical heart valves, particularly those with mitral prostheses or prior embolism, may be at higher risk of systemic embolism (5 to 20%) if perioperative anticoagulation is totally discontinued. Warfarin should be stopped 3 to 5 days before surgery with substitution of therapeutic intravenous heparin until 6 hours before surgery. Intravenous heparin and warfarin may be restarted 36 to 48 hours after surgery, with heparin continued for several days until the PTR is again therapeutic. Patients with isolated mechanical aortic protheses and no history of embolism may simply have warfarin stopped 3 days before surgery and restarted 1 to 2 days postoperatively; some clinicians recommend the addition of low molecular weight dextran in these patients for the first 2 to 3 days after surgery.

Anticoagulants in Pregnancy

The primary indications for anticoagulation during pregnancy include treatment and prophylaxis of venous thromboembolism and prevention of systemic embolism and valve thrombosis in patients with artificial heart valves. Effective anticoagulation would reduce maternal mortality and morbidity without harming the fetus or neonate. Unfortunately, there are few controlled data evaluating the efficacy and morbidity of anticoagulant therapy in pregnancy and no consensus as to optimal management.

Warfarin crosses the placenta freely and is a teratogen in the first trimester (8 to 30% incidence of embryopathy) and, more controversially, in the second trimester (0 to 16% incidence of embryopathy). Warfarin increases the risk of fetal intracranial hemorrhage in the third trimester and at delivery, as well as the risk of severe maternal hemorrhage in the event of unexpected obstetric complications such as abruptio placentae or urgent cesarean section. In contrast, heparin does not cross the placenta. Most current evidence suggests that it does not increase fetal or maternal morbidity and mortality, although some experts disagree. Prolonged heparin therapy in pregnancy does carry a low risk of symptomatic osteoporosis and a poorly quantified risk of subclinical bone demineralization, the prognosis of which is unknown.

Intravenous heparin is recommended to

treat acute venous thromboembolism in pregnancy. The regimens for long-term anticoagulation of these patients and for patients with artificial heart valves are more controversial. Several groups recommend use of heparin throughout pregnancy. Adjusted dose subcutaneous heparin (maintaining the middosing interval activated partial thromboplastin time at 1.5 to 2.0 times control) may be used until 1 week before delivery, when the patient is admitted and treated with intravenous heparin until induction of labor. Adjusted dose subcutaneous heparin and warfarin are started immediately after delivery, and the heparin is discontinued after 5 to 7 days when the desired PTR is attained. Other investigators believe that the teratogenic effects of warfarin in the second trimester have been greatly overestimated and note that the efficacy of adjusted dose heparin has not yet been demonstrated in this setting. They recommend adjusted dose heparin in the first trimester and again after the 35th week of gestation; warfarin is used from the 13th to 36th weeks.

Whether and how to treat women with a prior history of venous thromboembolism are also controversial. One of the regimens described earlier is frequently used for women with multiple previous episodes of venous thromboembolism or when a single episode occurred during the previous pregnancy. Women with a single prior episode unrelated to pregnancy are at lower risk of recurrence and may not require prophylactic anticoagulation until the postpartum period, when adjusted dose subcutaneous heparin or low intensity warfarin may be administered for 6 to 8 weeks.

Nursing mothers may safely use warfarin, which does not reach significant levels in breast milk. Some clinicians recommend obtaining a single, confirmatory PTR from the infant once the mother's PTR is therapeutic. Heparin is also not excreted in breast milk. There are rare case reports of heparin-induced osteoporosis in lactating women.

Physicians should counsel women with thromboembolic disorders about the maternal and fetal risks of pregnancy. For women receiving long-term warfarin therapy, pregnancy should be planned in advance so that this teratogenic drug can be discontinued and substituted with heparin *before* conception. These women should also be advised to contact their physician if expected menses is delayed more than 2 or 3 days.

Complications of Anticoagulant Therapy

Hemorrhage

Hemorrhage is the most common and important complication of anticoagulant therapy. The gastrointestinal and genitourinary systems and surgical wounds are the most frequent sites of hemorrhage, although bleeding may also occur from nasal, soft tissue, pulmonary, retroperitoneal, intracerebral, and other sources. The incidence of hemorrhage differs considerably in available investigations in part because of variable definitions and study populations. Table 33–3 gives the cumulative incidence of fatal, major (requiring hospitalization and/or transfusion or resulting in death), and minor anticoagulant-induced hemorrhage for different thromboembolic disorders, as pooled from several studies. A recent investigation of hospitalized patients initiating long-term anticoagulant therapy with warfarin found that major and minor bleeding developed before discharge from the hospital in 5 and 6% of patients, respectively.

Risk factors for hemorrhage have not been fully characterized but may include the variables in Table 33–4. Patients with risk-increasing comorbid conditions or concomitant drug therapy that cannot be eliminated should receive long-term anticoagulation only after careful assessment and frequent reassessment of the benefit/risk ratio of therapy. These patients should be monitored at frequent intervals for clinical evidence of bleeding.

Excessive anticoagulation clearly increases the risk of major hemorrhage. However, 50% or more of all bleeding episodes occur with the PTR in the therapeutic range. Compared with conventional warfarin therapy (PTR = 1.5 to 2.0), low intensity warfarin and adjusted dose subcutaneous heparin have two- to fourfold lower rates of hemorrhage, although thus far this has been documented only in patients with venous thromboembolism and bioprosthetic heart valves. The risk of hemorrhage also varies with different thromboembolic disorders and is greatest in patients with ischemic cerebrovascular disease and venous thromboembolism (Table 33–3). A multivariate discriminant analysis of hospitalized patients beginning long-term anticoagulation found several independent risk factors for major bleeding before discharge from the hospital: intensity of anticoagulation; concurrent use of intravenous heparin in patients over age 60;

Table 33–3. Anticoagulant-Induced Hemorrhage in Various Thromboembolic Disorders (Pooled Rates)

Thromboembolic Disorders	Total Bleeding (%)	Fatal Bleeding (%)	Major Bleeding* (%)	Minor Bleeding (%)
Ischemic cerebrovascular disease	28.7	4.8	7.0	21.8
Venous thromboembolism	22.6	0	8.1	14.4
Ischemic heart disease	19.1	1.0	4.7	10.5
Atrial fibrillation	15.2	0.0003†	0.01†	14.2
Mechanical prosthetic heart valves	5.7	1.7	2.4	3.2

Modified from Dalen JE, Hirsh J. Chest 89:1S–106S, 1986, with permission.
*Resulting in hospitalization, transfusion, and/or mortality.
†These rates may not be reliable estimates.

certain comorbid conditions (severe anemia, malignancy, or renal, hepatic, or cardiac dysfunction); and worsening hepatic dysfunction.

Concomitant drug therapy may contribute to 30% of bleeding episodes in patients receiving anticoagulants. Even small doses of aspirin (500 to 1000 mg/day) increase the rate of hemorrhage (primarily gastrointestinal) fourfold in patients taking warfarin. Other nonsteroidal anti-inflammatory drugs may also increase the risk of bleeding, either by prolongation of the PTR (phenylbutazone and piroxicam) or by direct gastrointestinal irritation, or both; these drugs should be avoided, if possible. Many drugs regularly alter the effects of warfarin (Table 33–5). If these drugs must be initiated or discontinued, the warfarin dose should be adjusted by one third in the appropriate direction with serial monitoring of the PTR every 3 to 7 days for several weeks. The PTR should also be monitored more frequently when any other drug is added or discontinued.

Poor medication compliance and failure to monitor the PTR regularly may also predispose patients to hemorrhage. Patients should be carefully screened for chronic alcoholism before initiation of therapy. Thorough patient education and incorporation of patients into a regularly scheduled anticoagulation clinic with prompt telephone follow-up of missed appointments may facilitate monitoring and reduce complications.

The management of hemorrhage or warfarin overdose depends on the severity or risk of bleeding and on the degree of prolongation of the PTR. A management scheme is suggested in Table 33–6. Vitamin K_1 (phytonadione), 5 to 10 mg subcutaneously, reduces the PTR within 6 to 12 hours in most patients and generally does not make the patient refractory to subsequent warfarin therapy. Because warfarin has a longer half-life, vitamin K_1 may need to be readministered within 24 hours for patients with serious hemorrhage. If long-term anticoagulation is still required after stabiliza-

Table 33–4. Possible Risk Factors for Anticoagulant-Induced Hemorrhage

Intensity of anticoagulation
Specific thromboembolic disorder requiring anticoagulation (see Table 33–3)
Comorbid conditions
  Severe anemia (hematocrit of less than 30%)
  Malignancy
  Renal, hepatic, or cardiac dysfunction
  Coagulopathy (especially thrombocytopenia)
  Recent surgery or trauma
  Gastrointestinal lesions
  Severe, uncontrolled hypertension
  Gait instability (risk of falls)
Concomitant drug therapy
  Heparin (especially in patients over age 60)
  Aspirin
  Nonsteroidal anti-inflammatory agents
  Multiple drug therapy
Poor patient compliance
Inadequate physician supervision

Table 33–5. Drug Interactions with Warfarin*

Increase Warfarin Effect	Decrease Warfarin Effect
Allopurinol	Barbiturates
Anabolic steroids	Carbamazepine
Antiarrhythmics	Cholestyramine
Amiodarone	Estrogens
Quinidine	Griseofulvin
Antibiotics	Phenytoin
Cefmandole	Rifampin
Cefoperazone	Vitamin K (contained in
Ketoconazole	some multiple vitamin
Moxalactam	and enteral nutrition
Neomycin	products)
Trimethoprim-sulfamethoxazole	
Cimetidine	
Clofibrate	
Disulfiram	
Phenylbutazone	
Piroxicam	
Sulfinpyrazone	
Sulfonylurea oral hypoglycemics	

*A large number of other drugs may also alter the warfarin effect on occasion.

Table 33–6. Management of Warfarin-Associated Hemorrhage and/or Warfarin Overdose

Indication	Treatment
Life-threatening hemorrhage (active central nervous system or major gastrointestinal bleeding)	1. Volume replacement as needed 2. 2–8 U plasma 3. Vitamin K_1, 5–10 mg, subcutaneously; repeat as needed
Hemorrhage controlled, PTR ≥ 3.0, or high risk of hemorrhage,* PTR ≥ 3.0	1. Vitamin K_1, 5–10 mg, subcutaneously 2. Monitor carefully
No bleeding, PTR ≥ 3.0–4.0	1. Omit one or more warfarin doses 2. Consider vitamin K_1, 1–3 mg, orally or subcutaneously

*For example, active central nervous system disease or active peptic ulcer.

tion (e.g., patients with mechanical heart valves or recurrent thromboembolism), any underlying cause of hemorrhage should be treated and the PTR maintained at the lower limits of the desired therapeutic range with careful follow-up for recurrence of hemorrhage. Patients rendered transiently refractory to warfarin by large doses of vitamin K_1 may be temporarily treated with adjusted dose subcutaneous heparin.

Only a few studies have evaluated the etiologies of gross and microscopic bleeding in the gastrointestinal and genitourinary tracts in patients receiving anticoagulants. Patients with gross gastrointestinal bleeding obviously require thorough evaluation regardless of the degree of PTR prolongation. In two recent studies of patients with therapeutic PTRs, evaluation of occult gastrointestinal bleeding (positive stool guaiac tests) revealed significant lesions (exclusive of diverticula and hemorrhoids) in one third of the patients; more than 50% of these were neoplasms. Evaluation of gross hematuria in patients with therapeutic PTRs has revealed lesions (exclusive of prostate enlargement) in about 50%; one third of these lesions were malignancies. There are very few data concerning the significance of microscopic hematuria or gross hematuria associated with excessive PTR prolongation. Pending further studies, physicians may evaluate these patients immediately, or at the least, follow them closely with complete evaluation if hematuria persists or recurs.

Nonhemorrhagic Complications

Warfarin-induced skin necrosis is a rare complication caused by occlusion of cutaneous capillaries and venules and subcutaneous veins. About 75% of cases occur in women. This complication usually starts in the first 10 days of therapy as a discrete, painful, maculopapular eruption in areas of abundant adipose tissue (e.g., buttocks, breasts, anterior thighs, abdominal wall) and may progress to extensive necrosis of soft tissue and muscle and even death. The pathophysiology of this complication is poorly understood but may relate to a transient hypercoagulable state induced by early depletion of anticoagulant proteins before suppression of procoagulants; some patients prove to have absolute or functional protein C deficiency. Treatment consists of cessation of warfarin, local wound care, and possibly administration of heparin. During the first 10 days of warfarin therapy, patients and their physicians should frequently examine at-risk areas for evidence of erythema and tenderness.

The purple toes syndrome is another rare complication of warfarin. It usually occurs in the first 2 months of therapy in elderly patients with extensive aortic atherosclerotic disease. These patients have bilateral, painful, purplish discoloration of the plantar and lateral sides of the toes, which fades with local pressure or elevation and waxes and wanes with time. The lesions are caused by cholesterol microembolization from ulcerated atherosclerotic plaques in the aorta and large arteries. Early recognition and cessation of warfarin are important because progressive cholesterol embolization can involve the renal and cerebral circulations resulting in renal failure, stroke, and death.

Nonhemorrhagic complications of heparin therapy include thrombocytopenia, osteoporosis, hyperkalemia, and a variety of cutaneous lesions. The incidence of these complications in outpatients treated with adjusted dose subcutaneous heparin is unknown, although it is probably low. Heparin-induced thrombocytopenia may be mild, transient, and asymptomatic, or rarely, severe and associated with hemorrhage or arterial thromboembolism. The value of regular screening for thrombocytopenia has not been documented, and firm guidelines cannot be proposed. Severe osteoporosis with fractures occurs infrequently and has been observed primarily in patients receiving more than 20,000 units of heparin daily for more than 6 months; subclinical demineralization may be more common, but its clinical significance and potential reversibility are unknown. Careful review of the benefit/risk ratio is necessary before using adjusted dose heparin for longer than 6 months. The few patients developing hyperkalemia while treated with heparin have had moderate renal dysfunction, and retrospectively, concurrent hypoaldosteronism. Cutaneous lesions resulting from subcutaneous heparin include local ecchymosis and hematoma, urticarial-type reactions, large indurated and erythematous plaques, and rarely, skin necrosis similar to that induced by warfarin.

Administration of Anticoagulants

Because its maximal antithrombotic effect is delayed up to 4 to 7 days, warfarin should be used together with therapeutic doses of heparin for at least this time when treating acute thromboembolism; this overlap may also help prevent the rare cases of warfarin-induced skin necrosis. Although there are no studies of other disorders, for venous thromboembolism early initiation of warfarin within 1 to 3 days of starting a 7- to 10-day course of heparin is safe and cost effective and significantly shortens the length of hospitalization. When the activated partial thromboplastin time is therapeutic at 1.5 to 2.0 times control, heparin directly prolongs the PT by only 1 to 2 seconds in most patients; however, about 20% of patients have a 3- to 5-second prolongation. Because of this unpredictable change, the PTR should be repeated after heparin is stopped. In addition, if a low intensity warfarin regimen is desired, a PTR of 1.5 should be obtained during concurrent heparin therapy; a decrease to 1.3 to 1.4 when heparin is stopped may be expected.

Warfarin is a difficult drug to prescribe. There is a 10- to 20-fold variation in the appropriate maintenance dose, which cannot be adequately predicted for individual patients before initiation of therapy. As a result, early overanticoagulation or excessive time required to reach a therapeutic PTR are common. Most

physicians initiate warfarin therapy with a dose of 5.0 to 10.0 mg/day for 2 to 3 days; large loading doses of warfarin (>15 mg/day) should be avoided because they do not hasten the onset of effective anticoagulation but do increase bleeding risk. The PTR is monitored daily with adjustment of the warfarin dose to approximate a maintenance dose. Unfortunately, there are no simple rules to assist this estimate, and considerable experience is required to do it with relative accuracy. In general, with an induction regimen of 10 mg/day for 3 days, patients whose PT increases to 15 to 18 seconds within the first 24 to 48 hours metabolize warfarin slowly and often require maintenance doses of less than 5 mg/day, whereas those with no change in PTR after 3 days may require maintenance doses of 7.5 to 10 mg or higher per day. Tabular and computer-assisted methods (e.g., as suggested by Fennerty and colleagues and White and colleagues) for early dose adjustment and prediction of maintenance dose may be helpful to physicians with less experience in initiating warfarin therapy. The average maintenance dose is about 5.0 to 6.0 mg/day for conventional warfarin and 4.0 to 5.0 mg/day for low intensity warfarin, although as noted, there is tremendous variability. Once the PTR is in the desired range for 3 successive days, it may be measured two or three times in the subsequent week, then weekly for several weeks, and if stable, on a monthly basis thereafter. Many patients, especially in the early months of therapy, may require more frequent monitoring. Particularly during the first 2 months of therapy, physicians should repeatedly screen their patients for clinical evidence of bleeding.

During long-term follow-up, PTRs frequently fall outside the desired therapeutic range because of one or more reasons: (1) inaccurate laboratory measurement; (2) poor patient compliance (medication error or missed dose); (3) drug interactions; (4) major alterations in dietary vitamin K (Table 33–7); (5) concurrent illness affecting liver function; (6) otherwise unexplained alterations in warfarin pharmacology; and (7) a change in the brand formulation of warfarin used by the patient. PTRs significantly outside the desired range should be promptly repeated, and for very high PTRs patients should also withhold warfarin pending repeat test results. If the repeat PTR is similarly out of range, the possible causes noted should be investigated and the dose of warfarin adjusted appropriately, with a repeat PTR measurement within 2 to 4

Table 33–7. Patient Education for Outpatient Anticoagulation

Note symptoms and signs of
  Bleeding (including retroperitoneal)
  Recurrent thromboembolism
  Skin necrosis and purple toe syndrome in warfarin-treated patients
Advise use of measures to prevent bleeding complications
  Avoid aspirin; use acetaminophen for mild analgesia
  Avoid additional prescription or over-the-counter medications without prior physician notification
  Avoid alcohol or limit its use to 3 oz/day
  Minimize injury: avoid contact sports, climbing, and power tools; use electric razor for shaving and soft toothbrush;
    increase bathtub safety with floor mats and grab bars; use gloves with gardening; wear shoes at all times
Advise avoidance of major increments in vitamin K consumption if warfarin is used
  Vitamin-nutrient supplements containing vitamin K
  Continuous daily intake of green tea, broccoli, cauliflower, Brussels sprouts
Plan monitoring system of anticoagulant therapy
  Maintain calendar of warfarin doses
  Take warfarin at same time daily, preferably in the evening
  Notify physician of all missed or improper doses
  Avoid extra doses to compensate for missed doses
  Have PTR checked at least monthly unless otherwise directed by physician; contact physician for results of all PTR
    measurements within 24 hours
  Keep patient address and telephone number current with physician
Advise carrying of Medic-alert bracelet, necklace, or wallet card at all times
Advise notification of other physicians and dentists of anticoagulant therapy
Advise fertile women of teratogenic risk of warfarin: contact physician immediately if menses delayed more than 2–3
  days
Advise heparin-treated patients of osteoporosis risk

days, according to the circumstances. For PTRs close to the desired range, dosage changes for undesirable trends should not exceed 10%, so as to avoid wide fluctuations in PTR.

There are three brand formulations of warfarin in the United States: Coumadin (Du Pont), Panwarfin (Abbott), and Sofarin (Lemmon). Only one formulation should be used in any individual patient, as a recent case series noted a significant alteration in anticoagulant control when substitutions were made. Warfarin is available in several tablet sizes (2, 2.5, 5, 7.5, and 10 mg). To minimize errors, only a single tablet size should be prescribed; scored 5 and 2 mg tablets are useful for conventional and low intensity warfarin therapy, respectively. To reach an appropriate maintenance dose, many patients must alternate doses, e.g., 5.0 mg alternating with 7.5 mg, or 5.0 mg for 2 days and 7.5 mg every third day. To decrease errors, these patients should utilize a calendar with each day's dose prerecorded.

Adjusted dose subcutaneous heparin is generally administered every 12 hours (every 8 hours by some clinicians) in a dose sufficient to prolong the midinterval activated partial thromboplastin time to 1.5 to 2.0 times control. The maximal response of the activated partial thromboplastin time occurs 4 to 6 hours after subcutaneous injection, and a sustained anticoagulant effect persists throughout the injection period. Therapy may be initiated with a dose of 7500 to 10,000 units every 12 hours and titrated daily for 3 to 4 days until the desired activated partial thromboplastin time is reached. In patients already receiving therapeutic intravenous heparin, (activated partial thromboplastin time = 1.5 to 2.0 times control), the dose to be administered every 12 hours is approximately one third of the total 24-hour dose of intravenous heparin. In one study, the mean effective dose for long-term anticoagulation of patients with venous thromboembolism was 10,000 units every 12 hours. For nonpregnant patients, the required dose of heparin appears to be stable over time, and subsequent monitoring of the activated partial thromboplastin time may not be necessary. However, pregnant patients have progressively increasing heparin requirements until delivery and should be monitored at least monthly, and more frequently in the third trimester. The heparin is administered with a deep subcutaneous, intrafat injection with rotation of sites over the entire abdominal wall, remaining 2 inches or more away from the umbilicus. The patient grasps a 1- to 2-inch layer of fat between the fingers, holds it away from the deeper tissues, injects with a ½- or ⅝-in, 25- or 26-gauge needle attached to an insulin syringe, and applies pressure (not massage) to the site for 30 seconds. Sodium heparin at a concentration of 20,000 or 40,000 units/ml and calcium heparin at a concentration of 25,000 units/ml are most convenient. Although calcium heparin may have a more prompt anticoagulant effect, this is probably of little importance in long-term outpatient anticoagulation. Porcine sources of heparin are preferred to bovine sources because of a lower incidence of thrombocytopenia.

Anticoagulation clinics can facilitate more efficient outpatient anticoagulant therapy and may reduce the frequency of complications. Anticoagulation clinics may be hospital based with patient referrals from primary care physicians and staffed by a trained registered nurse or physician's assistant with appropriate supervision from a designated physician. Alternatively, within a single practice, all patients receiving anticoagulants may be scheduled on a given day each month to see the office nurse. At each visit, the clinic professional measures the PTR, seeks adverse reactions and complications, and repeats patient education. A hematocrit, urine dipstick test for heme, and stool guaiac analyses may also be performed at 6-month intervals. Patients are informed of the PTR results and any necessary dose changes within 24 hours. All test results and drug doses are recorded on flow sheets. Patients missing their appointments may be promptly contacted by phone or letter, which makes it more difficult for them to be lost from follow-up within a busy practice. Recent reports from centers using anticoagulation clinics document very low rates of major hemorrhage.

Patient Education

Although not rigorously demonstrated to reduce the frequency of hemorrhagic complications, physicians should provide patients with thorough oral and written instructions and should periodically review the patient's understanding of this information. Table 33–7 lists important concepts to transmit to the patient.

Bibliography

Brand FN, Abbott RD, Kannel HB, et al. Characteristics and prognosis of lone atrial fibrillation: 30-year follow-up in the Framingham study. JAMA 254:3449–3453, 1985.
> *The prospective data from Framingham reviewed indicate that elderly persons over age 60 with lone AF have a four-fold increased risk of stroke compared with age-matched controls. In contrast, the retrospec-*

tive data from the Mayo Clinic (see article by Kopecky and colleagues) found no increase in stroke risk in younger persons under age 60 with lone AF.

Charney R, Leddomado E, Rose DN, et al. Anticoagulation clinics and the monitoring of anticoagulant therapy. Int J Cardiol 18:197–206, 1988.
> *This article describes recent experience with hospital-based anticoagulation clinics. No major hemorrhage occurred during 922 patient-treatment months.*

Cuttino JT, Clark RL, Feaster SH. The evaluation of gross hematuria in anticoagulated patients: efficacy of IV urography and cystoscopy. AJR 149:527–528, 1987.
> *The importance of thorough diagnostic evaluation of genitourinary bleeding in anticoagulated patients is documented. About one half of these patients proved to have significant, previously unrecognized pathology, including neoplasms.*

Dalen JE, Hirsh J (eds). American College of Chest Physicians and the National Heart, Lung, and Blood Institute National Conference on Antithrombotic Therapy. Chest 89:1S–106S, 1986.
> *This is an excellent, comprehensive review of the indications for and complications associated with anticoagulant therapy for different thromboembolic disorders.*

DeSwiet M. Prescribing in pregnancy: anticoagulants. Br Med J 294:428–430, 1987.
> *This is a current review of the indications for and use of anticoagulants during pregnancy. See also pages 41–56B in Fuster and Chesebro for another excellent discussion of this problem.*

Dixon JE. Pregnancies complicated by previous thromboembolic disease. Br J Hosp Med 37:449–452, 1987.
> *This article is a current review of the indications for and use of anticoagulants during pregnancy.*

Errichetti AM, Holden A, Ansell J. Management of oral anticoagulant therapy: experience with an anticoagulation clinic. Arch Intern Med 144:1966–1968, 1984.
> *Recent experience with hospital-based anticoagulation clinics is described.*

Fennerty A, Dulber J, Thomas P, et al. Flexible induction dose regimen for warfarin and prediction of maintenance dose. Br Med J 288:1268–1270, 1984.
> *A simple tabular scheme for initiating low intensity warfarin therapy in heparinized patients is based on the PTR response to warfarin for days 1–4. Because human brain thromboplastin was used, the scheme cannot be directly applied in most North American hospitals.*

Fuster V, Chesebro JA (eds). Symposium on thrombosis and antithrombotic therapy—1986. J Am Coll Cardiol 8(Suppl B):1B–167B, 1986.
> *This is an excellent, comprehensive review of the indications for and complications associated with anticoagulant therapy for different thromboembolic disorders.*

Gallus A, Jackman J, Tillet J, et al. Safety and efficacy of warfarin started early after submassive venous thrombosis or pulmonary embolism. Lancet 2:1293–1296, 1986.
> *This reference provides evidence that warfarin initiated in the first 3 days of heparin therapy for acute venous thromboembolism is cost effective and safe.*

Hansten PD. Oral anticoagulant drug interactions, in Drug Interactions, ed 5. Philadelphia, Lea & Febiger, 1985, pp 66–114.
> *This chapter is an excellent review of definite, probable, and possible drug interactions with warfarin.*

Hirsh J, Levine MN (eds). A critical appraisal of the use of anticoagulant therapy: effectiveness, monitoring, and complications. Semin Thromb Hemost 12:11–71, 1986.

An excellent, comprehensive review of the indications for and complications associated with anticoagulant therapy for different thromboembolic disorders is provided.

Hirsh J, Levine MN. The optimal intensity of oral anticoagulant therapy. JAMA 258:2723–2726, 1987.

The ACCP/NHLBI recommendations for dosage and laboratory monitoring of oral anticoagulants are summarized concisely.

Hyman BT, Landas SK, Ashman RF, et al. Warfarin-related purple toes syndrome and cholesterol microembolization. Am J Med 82:1233–1237, 1987.

This article gives case reports and a review of a rare but dangerous complication of warfarin.

Jaffin BW, Bliss CM, Lamont JT. Significance of occult gastrointestinal bleeding during anticoagulation therapy. Am J Med 83:269–272, 1987.

This reference documents the importance of thorough diagnostic evaluation of occult gastrointestinal bleeding in anticoagulated patients. About one third of these patients proved to have significant, previously unrecognized pathology, including neoplasms.

Kewenter J, Svanvik T, Svensson C, et al. The diagnostic value of the Hemoccult as a screening test in patients taking anticoagulants. Cancer 54:3054–3058, 1984.

A thorough diagnostic evaluation of occult gastrointestinal bleeding in anticoagulated patients is important. About one third of these patients proved to have significant, previously unrecognized pathology, including neoplasms.

Kopecky SL, Gersh BJ, McGoon MD, et al. The natural history of lone atrial fibrillation: a population-based study over three decades. N Engl J Med 317:669–674, 1987.

The prospective data from the Framingham study reviewed by Brand and colleagues indicate that elderly persons over age 60 with lone AF have a four-fold increased risk of stroke compared with age-matched controls. In contrast, the retrospective data from the Mayo Clinic in this reference found no increase in stroke risk in younger persons under age 60 with lone AF.

Landefeld CS, Cook EF, Flatley M, et al. Identification and preliminary validation of predictors of major bleeding in hospitalized patients starting anticoagulant therapy. Am J Med 82:703–713, 1987.

A careful, retrospective study of in-hospital bleeding events during the initiation of long-term anticoagulant therapy. Multivariate discriminant analysis identified four independent risk factors for major bleeding: (1) comorbid conditions of cardiac, hepatic, and renal dysfunction and severe anemia; (2) concurrent heparin therapy in patients over age 60; (3) excessive anticoagulation; (4) worsening liver dysfunction during therapy.

Lutomski DM, Djuric PE, Draeger RW. Warfarin therapy: the effect of heparin on prothrombin time. Arch Intern Med 147:432–433, 1987.

Although therapeutic continuous intravenous heparin increases the PT only 1 to 2 seconds in most patients, the increment may be up to 3 to 5 seconds in 20% of patients.

Oakley C. Valve prostheses and pregnancy. Br Heart J 58:303–305, 1987.

This is a current review of the use of anticoagulants during pregnancy for women with valve prostheses.

Richton-Hewett S, Foster E, Apstein CS. Medical and economic consequences of a blinded oral anticoagulant brand change at a municipal hospital. Arch Intern Med 148:806–808, 1988.

This retrospective case series demonstrates a significant alteration in anticoagulant control after a warfarin brand change.

Rosiello RA, Chan CK, Teneza F, et al. Timing of oral anticoagulant therapy in the treatment of angiographically proven acute pulmonary embolism. Arch Intern Med 147:1469–1473, 1987.

Evidence is provided that warfarin initiated in the first 3 days of heparin therapy for acute venous thromboembolism is cost effective and safe.

Schuster GA, Lewis GA. Clinical significance of hematuria in patients on anticoagulant therapy. J Urol 137:923–925, 1987.

A thorough diagnostic evaluation of genitourinary bleeding in anticoagulated patients is important. About one half of these patients proved to have significant, previously unrecognized pathology, including neoplasms.

Stratton JR, Resnick RD. Increased embolic risk in patients with left ventricular thrombi. Circulation 75:1004–1011, 1987.

This small prospective study of patients with postmyocardial infarction left ventricular thrombi suggests that significant embolic risk persists for at least several years after the acute infarction.

Wessler S, Becker CG, Nemerson Y (eds). The new dimensions of warfarin prophylaxis. Adv Exp Med Biol 214:1–329, 1987.

This reference is an excellent, comprehensive review of the indications for and complications associated with warfarin therapy for different thromboembolic disorders.

White RH, Hong R, Venook AP, et al. Initiation of warfarin therapy: comparison of physician dosing with computer-assisted dosing. J Gen Intern Med 2:141–148, 1987.

This prospective study of the initiation of warfarin therapy demonstrates that a computer-assisted dosing regimen (Warfcalc) outperformed physicians who were not highly skilled anticoagulation experts; the computer regimen achieved a stable, therapeutic PTR earlier and with fewer episodes of overanticoagulation.

Yatsu FM, Hart RG, Mohr JP, et al. Anticoagulation of embolic strokes of cardiac origin: an update. Neurology 38:314–316, 1988.

This article is an editorial review of this controversial topic. Pending more definitive clinical trials, the authors make eight specific recommendations about anticoagulant therapy for cardioembolic stroke.

PART EIGHT

Allergy/Infectious Diseases

34

Chronic Rhinitis: Diagnosis and Management

HAROLD S. NELSON, M.D.

Anatomy and Physiology of the Nose

The nose contributes nearly 50% of the resistance to breathing. In return for this major expenditure of energy, the nose performs several critical functions in modifying the inspired air in a manner to protect the lower respiratory tract. During passage through the nose, the air is conditioned toward body temperature, almost completely if the ambient temperature is not too extreme and even under the most adverse conditions to within 10°C of body temperature. Whatever temperature is attained, sufficient water vapor is added to bring the air to 100% humidity. The turbulence and changes in airstream direction that occur in the nasal passages promote impaction of particulate matter. Particles larger than 10 μm are removed completely, and a major proportion of even submicrometric particles is also removed. Because of the proximity of the airstream to the nasal mucus blanket (never more than a few millimeters), foreign gases are efficiently absorbed and water-soluble gases such as SO_2 and formaldehyde are completely removed at any concentration likely to be encountered.

Blood flow in the nasal mucosa is controlled by resistance vessels, whereas the volume of blood in the nasal mucosa is controlled by large capacitance vessels. The latter, resembling those found in erectile tissue elsewhere in the body, determine the degree of nasal mucosal congestion, and hence their dilation results in increased nasal airway resistance. These capacitance vessels are constricted by alpha-adrenergic stimulation; therefore, sympathetic innervation and drugs have the greatest effect on nasal airway patency and nasal airway resistance. Parasympathetic stimulation, on the other hand, in addition to dilating the resistance vessels, which increases mucosal blood flow, stimulates secretion from nasal submucosal glands.

There is a cyclic variation in engorgement of the capacitance vessels of the nose such that the greatest part of respiration is normally through one nostril at a time. This state of congestion cycles from side to side every 3 to 8 hours.

Chronic Rhinitis

The symptoms of chronic rhinitis merge almost imperceptably into an awareness of normal nasal function; therefore, some criteria must be set for the presence of a disease state. It has been suggested that chronic rhinitis may be considered to be present if there are periods of nasal discharge, sneezing, or congestion persisting for an average of 0.5 to 1 hour/day on most days, or if the patient experiences abnormal responses to certain exposures or has periodic symptoms of sufficient severity to require therapy.

Incidence

Estimates of the incidence of chronic rhinitis vary and indeed probably differ with the age, genetic make-up, and exposure of the population. A survey of a midwestern U.S. town 25 years ago indicated that about 10% of the population had symptoms consistent with seasonal or perennial allergic rhinitis alone; if those who also had asthma were included, about 14% gave a history consistent with allergic rhinitis. Surveys of college student populations have yielded estimates slightly higher, and no survey reported cases of rhinitis whose symptoms did not suggest allergy. Therefore, it is likely that the incidence of chronic rhinitis of all types in the United States is at least 20% of the population.

Classification (Table 34–1)

ATOPIC RHINITIS

Atopic rhinitis is the nasal equivalent of bronchial asthma and eczema. All have in common a tendency to cluster in individuals and families and a close but not invariable association with allergy (the tendency to become sensitized as a result of normal environmental exposures). The unifying features that identify atopic rhinitis are a strong but not invariable hereditary pattern; a frequent association with bronchial asthma and eczema; a common picture characterized by tissue infiltration with plasma cells, lymphocytes, and eosinophils in descending order of frequency; and prominence of eosinophils in the nasal secretions.

Seasonal rhinitis is usually synonymous with allergic rhinitis or hay fever. An occasional patient, however, confuses certain periods of many viral respiratory infections with a true seasonal pattern of rhinitis. Even less commonly, patients have a summer seasonal rhinitis, and all attempts to demonstrate their sensitivity to seasonal aeroallergens are unsuccessful.

It is less clear how often perennial rhinitis is explained entirely on the basis of allergy. Certainly there is no evidence that seasonal sensitivities can cause perennial symptoms except in warmer climates where these aeroallergens are present throughout the year. The determination of the role of allergy is more difficult when skin tests are positive to house dust mite, indoor molds, or animal danders. In many parts of the country, it is impossible to preclude perennial exposure to these allergens. However, allergists practicing in semiarid regions, where mites and molds do not constitute a significant exposure and exposure to animal dander can be excluded by history, are impressed with the frequency with which patients who have allergic rhinitis during pollen seasons have persistent nasal symptoms throughout the year when they have no allergen exposures.

The occurrence of chronic rhinitis, often with nasal and ocular symptoms suggesting histamine release, profuse eosinophilia of the nasal secretions, and entirely negative skin tests, has been appreciated for half a century. In recent years, this entity has been rediscovered and given a number of names. As noted earlier, there are many arguments for considering this to be the nasal equivalent of nonallergic bronchial asthma or nonallergic atopic eczema and referring to it as nonallergic atopic rhinitis. This is a very common form of perennial rhinitis and constituted 30 to 50% of the rhinitis in several studies. Even this probably underestimates the true incidence because the authors of these studies performed only single nasal smears or disregarded small but abnormal numbers of eosinophils in nasal secretions.

Because the atopic state is systemic, although usually clinically most prominent in one of the potential target organs, atopic rhinitis is frequently accompanied by evidence of widespread involvement of other tissues of the respiratory tract. In perennial atopic rhinitis, evidence of hypertrophy of the mucous membranes of the paranasal sinuses can be identified by x-ray in approximately 40 to 50%. Nasal polyps, arising from the maxillary and ethmoidal sinuses, are frequently present, particularly in patients over age 40. These sinus mucous membranes and resulting polyps show the typical atopic histologic picture of plasma cell, lymphocyte, and eosinophil infiltration. Bronchial asthma is also a frequent accompan-

Table 34–1. Classification of Chronic Rhinitis

1. Atopic rhinitis
   a. Seasonal allergic rhinitis
   b. Perennial rhinitis
      i. With allergic triggers
      ii. Nonallergic
2. Infectious rhinitis
   a. Viral respiratory infections
   b. Chronic purulent rhinosinusitis
3. Other recognized types of rhinitis
   a. Rhinitis medicamentosa
      i. Topical
      ii. Systemic
   b. Hormonal
      i. Pregnancy
      ii. Hypothyroidism
   c. Mechanical obstruction
      i. Nasal septal deviation
      ii. Neoplasm
      iii. Foreign body
      iv. Enlarged adenoids
   d. Unknown etiology
      i. Wegener's granulomatosis
      ii. Atrophic
4. Chronic rhinitis without known cause or mechanism
   a. Idiopathic nonallergic rhinitis

iment of atopic rhinitis, and even more common are mild symptoms of cough (especially a prolonged cough after respiratory infections) and bronchial hyper-responsiveness to methacholine or histamine. A smaller number of these patients manifest idiosyncratic reactions to aspirin, such as asthma or naso-ocular symptoms such as congestion, sneezing, rhinorrhea, and conjunctival injection.

INFECTIOUS RHINITIS

Infectious rhinitis can occur as an acute viral respiratory infection, which may clear rapidly, but may also result in some lingering symptoms. Indeed, it has been shown that the impaired mucociliary clearance after a viral infection may persist for 2 to 6 weeks. More significant is chronic purulent rhinosinusitis, which is characterized by a predominance of neutrophils in the nasal secretions, presumably caused by bacterial infection in the paranasal sinuses. Chronic bacterial sinusitis can also lead to polyp formation. These polyps, characterized by neutrophilic infiltration, constitute approximately 10% of polyps in adults, whereas the eosinophilic polyps associated with atopic rhinitis constitute approximately 90%.

Chronic purulent rhinosinusitis can occur as a complication of the tissue changes and, more importantly, of the obstruction to sinus drainage caused by atopic rhinitis. Other causes include obstruction to the drainage of sinuses from any cause, cystic fibrosis, abnormal ciliary function, immune deficiency, and cleft palate. A characteristic feature in patients with ciliary dyskinesia is a persistent rhinorrhea that requires nose blowing every 0.5 to 2 hours and that is refractory to all treatment.

OTHER TYPES OF RHINITIS

Rhinitis medicamentosa may be caused by topical application of vasoconstrictors or ingestion of systemic medication for treatment of hypertension and depression. Commonly implicated topical medications causing chronic obstructive symptoms include all forms of topical decongestants as well as recreational use of cocaine. A clue to the latter is the presence of a red friable mucous membrane and failure to respond to all forms of treatment. Cholinergic eye drops employed for the treatment of glaucoma have been implicated in causing a watery nasal discharge. Systemically employed drugs commonly causing nasal congestion include the antihypertensive drugs reserpine, methyldopa, hydralazine, prazosin, clonidine, and guanethidine, and the antipsychotic agents chlorpromazine (Thorazine) and perphenazine. Rhinitis medicamentosa has not been reported after the use of oral decongestants; however, evidence of this has not been specifically sought. Chronic use of oral decongestants has been shown to reduce the response of peripheral vessels to alpha-adrenergic stimulation, presumably by down-regulation of alpha-adrenergic receptors. Because this is the same mechanism underlying rhinitis medicamentosa caused by topical decongestants, the possibility is suggested that mild, not easily recognized, and perhaps clinically insignificant degrees of rhinitis medicamentosa could result from chronic use of oral decongestants.

Approximately 20% of women develop symptoms of nasal congestion during pregnancy that remit with delivery. A hormonal basis is suspected, but the mechanism is not established. It appears probable that some women experience the same symptoms with oral contraceptives. Hypothyroidism is a recognized but rare cause of nasal congestion.

Mechanical obstruction to airflow, most frequently secondary to deviation of the nasal septum, can cause not only inspiratory difficulty but also a mild rhinorrhea.

Atrophic rhinitis occurs due to unknown causes in older people. Despite widely patent nasal passages, these patients complain of nasal congestion.

Idiopathic nonallergic rhinitis is preferred to the term vasomotor rhinitis. The latter term suggests that this is a homogeneous condition (which it probably is not), that the cause is known (which it certainly is not), and that the exaggerated reaction to changes in temperature, odors, and irritants is unique to this condition (which it is not because it characterizes patients with atopic rhinitis as well). These patients complain predominantly of nasal congestion and postnasal drainage, with a conspicuous absence of ocular symptoms, sneezing, and pruritus. They typically have no abnormal cellularity of nasal secretions or scrapings, no polyps, and normal sinus x-rays. They also tend to respond poorly to all medication, including topical corticosteroids. Many of the subjects formerly given a diagnosis of vasomotor rhinitis solely on the basis of negative skin tests actually had atopic rhinitis.

Diagnosis

A problem in establishing a specific diagnosis of rhinitis is presented by the similarity of the symptoms in all these conditions because the response of the nose is limited to itching and sneezing caused by stimulation of epithelial nerves, obstruction related to engorgement of the capacitance vessels, and increased secretions caused by increased output from the mucous glands. A useful distinction has been suggested between "sneezers" and "blockers" in relation to their likelihood of response to therapy. The former would be patients whose symptoms suggest histamine release not only by sneezing but also by nasal and ocular pruritus and watery rhinorrhea. These symptoms are usually seen in seasonal allergic rhinitis, but they can occur in any form of atopic rhinitis. Patients with these symptoms typically respond better than blockers not only to antihistamines but also to topical corticosteroids.

A number of secondary symptoms can occur with any form of rhinitis. Thus, patients may experience irritability, lassitude, and fatigue secondary to interference with sleep; loss of appetite because of interference with the sense of taste and smell; sore and irritated throat on arising related to mouth breathing during the night caused by nasal obstruction; night-time cough caused by postnasal drainage; and pain over the cheeks and bridge of the nose secondary to sinus congestion.

Physical findings are also of limited value in differentiating types of rhinitis. Patients with symptoms suggesting histamine release often present with injected conjunctiva, swollen and pale nasal mucosa, and thin nasal secretions. Those complaining only of obstruction and postnasal drainage, on the other hand, may exhibit only thick secretions and little obvious mucosal swelling. The possibility of a mechanical obstruction should be evaluated by careful examination of the nasal septum; if symptoms are intractable, a topical decongestant should be used to determine the degree to which symptoms of obstruction are reversible. The ready availability of fiberoptic rhinolaryngoscopy allows its use to evaluate patients for whom concerns remain regarding the possible presence of mechanical obstruction.

Laboratory Studies

The most useful studies in the evaluation of patients with nasal complaints are nasal cytologic smears and x-rays of the paranasal sinuses.

Nasal smears may be performed on specimens blown into wax paper, wiped with a swab, or scraped with a curette (a disposable plastic curette, the Rhinoprobe, is commercially available). For evaluation of eosinophils, only an eosin and methylene blue stain is required and may be performed in one or separate steps (Hansel's stain). This procedure may easily be performed in the physician's office and yields useful information within a few minutes. Although some studies have designated 25% eosinophils as abnormal, it is likely that the presence of 5 to 10% eosinophils represents a significant finding. Nasal smears for eosinophils are usually positive but are generally unnecessary for the evaluation of seasonal allergic rhinitis. They are useful in establishing the diagnosis of atopic (eosinophilic) perennial rhinitis, which implies a more favorable response to pharmacotherapy as well as a need to consider a possible allergic etiology. A nasal smear for eosinophils is sometimes helpful in differentiating between an allergic and a viral etiology of an acute episode of rhinitis. The presence of neutrophils on a nasal smear in the absence of an acute respiratory infection may indicate the need to evaluate the patient for the presence of unsuspected sinusitis.

Customarily three or four views constitute a sinus series; however, the Water's view is particularly useful for evaluating disease of the maxillary sinuses, and significant disease is rarely present in the other sinuses without involvement of the maxillary. Therefore, the Water's view alone is a useful and cost-effective screening study for the presence of significant involvement of the paranasal sinuses. Sinus x-rays should be performed as a baseline in patients with serious perennial rhinitis or perennial asthma. If the presence of sinusitis is established, subsequent treatment may be based on the occurrence of symptoms, fever, and purulent nasal secretions without need to repeat the x-rays unless there is a suspicion of complication such as osteomyelitis or a failure to respond to antibiotic therapy. Abnormalities noted on sinus x-rays, of course, do not necessarily indicate infection because as noted earlier, hypertrophic sinusitis is a frequent accompaniment of atopic rhinitis.

The possibility of ciliary dyskinesia may be a consideration in patients with severe sinopulmonary disease. A screening test that has been suggested is to place a few particles of saccharin 1 cm posterior to the tip of the inferior turbinate. The patient should be cautioned not to sniff, sneeze, cough, eat, or drink. A sweet taste should occur in the mouth within 60 minutes if mucociliary clearance is not impaired. There are a number of causes of impaired mucociliary clearance; therefore, an abnormal test is only an indication for the need for a more complete evaluation.

Additional studies that may sometimes be indicated are analysis of serum immunoglobulin levels for patients with repeated purulent infections, especially if there have also been repeated pneumonias and systemic infections, and audiometry and tympanometry in patients with a history of recurrent otitis.

Mechanisms of Allergic Rhinitis

Basophils and Mast Cells

There appear to be at least three types of mediator-containing metachromatic cells in the nose. Two types of mast cells have been described with different properties. One is a typical connective tissue mast cell that remains largely localized to the lamina propria of the nasal mucosa. The second, an atypical mast cell, is also found in the lamina propria but is the predominant mast cell of the epithelial cell layer. The third mediator-containing cell is the blood basophil, which is not normally found in large numbers in the nasal tissue but has been described as the predominant mediator-containing cell in nasal secretions. Nasal challenge with antigen has been reported to increase the number of basophils in the nasal secretions within 1 to 2 hours but to not change the number of mast cells in the epithelium. Studies of patients with allergic rhinitis indicate a seasonal increase in both basophils in nasal secretions and epithelial mast cells. The former migrate from the blood; the latter either migrate from the lamina propria or proliferate locally. It has been demonstrated that these two groups of metachromatic cells contain sufficient histamine to account for the allergic reaction without a need for antigen to be absorbed through the epithelium.

Antigen challenge followed by nasal washing has demonstrated the release of a number of mediators: histamine, tosyl-L-arginine methylester (TAME) esterase, kinins, prostaglandin D_2, and leukotrienes C_4, D_4, and E_4. Three to 8 hours after this immediate reaction there is a second release of mediators and a recurrence of symptoms. In this late nasal response, the same mediators are again released without need for reintroduction of allergen. A difference between the immediate and late reactions is the failure of prostaglandin D_2 to appear in the latter. This has led to speculation that the basophil might be important in mediating the late response because it, as opposed to the mast cell, does not release prostaglandin D_2.

Histamine released in the immediate reaction can account for most of the clinical symptoms of allergic rhinitis. The symptoms are produced by both direct and reflex mechanisms. The direct effect of histamine is on the blood vessels to produce dilation, which results in nasal obstruction. This response is thought to be mediated by both H_1 and H_2 receptors, accounting for the failure of conventional antihistamines to relieve this symptom. Histamine-induced increased permeability may also allow antigen penetration of the epithelium. The remaining results of histamine are mediated by stimulation of H_1 receptors on nerve endings in the epithelium. These effects include pruritus and sneezing and increased secretion, the latter mediated through cholinergic reflex pathways. It has been shown that there is virtually no direct effect of histamine on the release of glandular secretions. Two characteristic features of the allergic reaction are not produced by histamine: eosinophilia and increased nasal reactivity. It is likely that these responses are produced by other mediators.

Nasal Hyper-responsiveness

A major difficulty with the concept of vasomotor rhinitis is that its distinguishing characterisitic is said to be nasal hyper-responsiveness to nonimmunologic stimuli, such as weather and temperature changes, odors, and irritants, yet this same hyper-responsiveness equally characterizes atopic rhinitis. Heightened responsiveness has been demonstrated to both histamine and methacholine in perennial atopic rhinitis, and patients with seasonal allergic rhinitis have been shown to develop increased sensitivity to histamine and methacholine during their pollen seasons. Although the mechanisms of this hyper-responsiveness are not understood, it is a widespread phenomenon. There is an increased direct response of blood vessels to histamine and of the glands to methacholine, and there is an increase in reflex sneezing and histamine-induced secretions. Studies of the nasal mucosa have revealed an increased number of cholinergic receptors and decreased number of adrenergic receptors.

Therapy of Rhinitis

In considering the therapy of rhinitis, measures that are directed toward allergens—avoidance and immunotherapy—are appropriate only for patients in whom a significant allergic component has been demonstrated. Usually, however, treatment of rhinitis also includes a major component of pharmacotherapy, and the drugs employed are the same, whether or not an allergic component has been demonstrated.

Avoidance

The first consideration in the treatment of allergic rhinitis should be an attempt to avoid completely or decrease the exposure to offending allergens. Although complete elimination is seldom possible (except for family pets), a substantial reduction in exposure can often be accomplished. Most pollens and many mold spores peak during the midday or early afternoon. Counts are considerably reduced indoors, particularly if there is air conditioning and closed windows and doors. Therefore, patients with seasonal allergic rhinitis can often avoid excessive symptoms by not undertaking outdoor recreational activities during the times of highest pollen and spore counts. The spores, which become prevalent during periods of dampness and rain, are especially numerous during the early morning hours. If they are suspected of causing allergic problems, closing windows at night would be expected to effect a major reduction in exposure.

The most important contributors to perennial allergy—and the major components of house dust—are animal danders and allergens derived from the house dust mite. The latter is ubiquitous except in the drier portions of the United States such as the Rocky Mountains and the Southwest. Because house dust mites tend to accumulate in bedding, upholstered furniture, and adjacent carpeting, some degree of control is possible. Where this has been undertaken in a thorough manner, significant improvement in symptoms of asthma in children has been reported. The role of air-filtering devices in the avoidance of house dust mite allergen is not as clear because the allergen occurs predominantly in relatively large fecal pellets, which would be expected to fall rapidly in the air by gravity. Thus local sources, such as pillows, mattresses, and bed covers, appear more likely to be important than the allergen floating in the air and should be the target of environmental control measures, by frequent laundering or encasing in plasticized covers as appropriate.

Dander from pets, particularly cats and dogs, is a major perennial allergen. Clearly, complete avoidance should be possible, but emotional ties or the presence of pets in the homes of friends and relatives often frustrate avoidance measures. It should certainly be possible to "animal proof" the bedroom by completely excluding the pet from this room and keeping the door and heating ducts closed. No data yet indicate whether under these circumstances the use of a room air-filtering device in the bedroom would be a worthwhile additional measure. There is evidence that with the continued access of the pet to the bedroom, the concentration of allergen in the furnishings would negate any impact of the use of air filtration on total allergen load. If complete avoidance of the family pet is not possible, the more restricted the area in which the animal is allowed and the less furniture and carpeting to which it has access, the better.

The role of indoor mold allergy in producing allergic rhinitis is unclear. Damp areas in the house that cause symptoms should be dehumidified or avoided, and if humidifiers are employed elsewhere in the house, care should be taken that they are cleaned regularly and do not become a source of spore aerosols.

Nonimmunologic irritants are a problem for all patients with rhinitis. Some irritants can be avoided, and tobacco smoking within the home or workplace should be eliminated. It should also be possible, at least within the family, to avoid the use of strongly scented toiletries and cleaning products.

Pharmacotherapy

ANTIHISTAMINES

Competitive antagonists of the H_1 receptor have been the basic treatment for allergic and nonallergic rhinitis. The older preparations have been grouped into six categories with the expectation that changing from one class to another might evade the tolerance that develops to this group of drugs. It has been recently recognized that the tolerance is probably related to the histamine receptor and is not specific for the class of agent that induced it.

It has been suggested that patients be provided with multiple samples to determine which drug they find most effective. However, several studies employing representatives from each of the classes have confirmed a general pattern: the ethanolamines represented by chlorpheniramine and brompheniramine are preferred by the largest number of subjects; hydroxyzine in doses commonly employed appears to be slightly more effective than chlorpheniramine but also causes more side effects, which makes it less satisfactory. A limited number of studies suggest that azatadine may also cause relatively few side effects.

The side effects of the traditional antihistamines are primarily of two types. There are direct central nervous system effects, which sometimes include stimulation, restlessness, and nervousness but more often drowsiness and incoordination. The second major type of side effect is related to anticholinergic properties and include dryness of the mouth, urinary retention, impotence, and blurring of vision. Tolerance to the central nervous system side effects develops rapidly, and by 4 to 10 days the incidence of drowsiness is similar to that found with use of a placebo. Tolerance to the desired antihistaminic properties also develops over the first few weeks, but this does not appear to be as profound as the central tolerance, effectively improving the therapeutic ratio for these drugs. Recently antihistamines have been developed that are nonsedating because they do not cross the blood–brain barrier. Furthermore, these drugs are free of anticholinergic action, thus avoiding some of the other side effects of the traditional antihistamines. Of this group, only terfenadine is currently approved for use in the United States, but approval of astemizole appears likely in the near future.

Antihistamines reduce some but not all of the symptoms of allergic rhinitis. They effectively relieve pruritus, sneezing, and rhinorrhea, whereas they are largely ineffective for nasal congestion. Among the reasons offered for the latter is the demonstration that vasodilation is mediated by both H_1 and H_2 receptors. It has been suggested that combined treatment with H_1 and H_2 antagonists might enhance symptom relief and, indeed, the effectiveness of this combined treatment has been demonstrated both with nasal allergen challenge and in the course of seasonal allergic rhinitis. The combination has not achieved popularity, probably because of the availability of highly effective alternatives such as topical corticosteroids. The decision whether to try antihistamine treatment is best based on the type of symptoms experienced rather than on the perception of whether the symptoms are of allergic origin.

Pharmacokinetic studies of adults have uncovered unexpectedly long serum half-lives for a number of antihistamines. Hydroxyzine, chlorpheniramine, and brompheniramine all have half-lives of approximately 24 hours, which suggests that once-daily dosing at bedtime with nonsustained release formulations should provide effective relief of symptoms, particularly because symptoms of rhinitis tend to be worse on arising. This dosing schedule has the added advantage that maximum serum levels and therefore potential sedation occur while the patient is asleep. The use of single bedtime dosing, plus a gradual build-up of the dose over 1 to 2 weeks (such as chlorpheniramine 8 mg at bedtime, increasing if needed and sedation permitting to 16 mg after 3 to 7 days, and adding 8 mg in the morning after another 3 to 7 days if needed and symptoms permit), may allow use of inexpensive medications effectively with minimal side effects. In children, the serum half-lives of these same drugs are about 12 hours, perhaps accounting for the relatively larger doses of antihistamines employed in children but also making single daily dose therapy in children impractical. The new, nonsedating antihistamine terfenadine has a half-life somewhat shorter than the other preparations given, and twice-daily dosing appears appropriate. Astemizole, on the other hand, possesses pharmacologic properties of quite a different order, with a calculated half-life of 104 hours, and with suppression of skin tests persisting for several months after discontinuation of therapy.

In comparative trials, usually only 1 or 2 weeks long, terfenadine has produced control of symptoms equal to chlorpheniramine in doses of 6 to 16 mg/day but with a lower incidence of side effects. It has not been demonstrated by adequate controlled trials that the equal effectiveness and the reduced side effects continue with prolonged therapy. In one study comparing terfenadine and astemizole for several months in the treatment of seasonal allergic rhinitis, there appeared to be a complete loss of effectiveness of terfenadine after the first few weeks. Clearly, more long-term, controlled studies of terfenadine are needed, especially considering the marked cost differential between terfenadine and conventional antihistamines such as chlorpheniramine (Table 34–2).

It is frequently stated that antihistamines are

Table 34–2. Drugs Used for Rhinitis, Their Daily Dose, and Their Daily Cost

Generic/Proprietary Name	Daily Dose	Daily Cost* (US $)
Antihistamines		
Chlorpheniramine		
Chlortrimeton (12 mg)	12–24 mg/day	0.16–0.31
Generic (4 mg)		0.19–0.37
Hydroxyzine		
Atarax (25 mg)	75 mg	1.08
Terfenadine		
Seldane (60 mg)	120 mg	1.08
Decongestants		
Pseudoephedrine		
Sudafed (30 mg)	120 mg	0.33
Generic		0.28
Combination		
Dimetapp	2 tablets	0.42
12 mg brompheniramine		
72 mg phenylpropanolamine		
Drixoral	2 tablets	0.41
6 mg dexbrompheniramine		
120 mg pseudoephedrine		
Cromolyn		
Nasal		
Nasalcrom	12 sprays	1.25
Ocular		
Opticrom	12 drops	0.97
Corticosteroids		
Beclomethasone		
Beconase Nasal Inhaler	8 sprays	0.73
Vancenase Nasal Inhaler	8 sprays	0.62
Flunisolide		
Nasalide Solution	8–12 sprays	0.70–1.05

*Costs are based on a Denver Colorado supermarket, May 1987.

more effective when administered on a regular basis rather than taken as needed for relief of already existing symptoms. Because these drugs are competitive antagonists this seems reasonable. However, patients taking a single dose of chlorpheniramine achieved the same level of symptom control after 2 hours that was experienced by the group that had been taking the drug on a regular basis for several days. Another argument for regular use of the older preparations is that tolerance develops to the central nervous system side effects, which improves their therapeutic ratio.

DECONGESTANTS

The drugs employed as decongestants are nonselective alpha-adrenergic agonists capable of constricting blood vessels elsewhere in the body as well. For that reason, the preferred route of administration is topically to the nasal mucosa. Long-acting preparations for this pur-

pose are available and are recommended for treatment of nasal congestion associated with viral respiratory infections, to promote drainage with acute infections of the paranasal sinuses and middle ears, and during the first few days of topical corticosteroid therapy in patients with marked obstruction. The limitation to their use is the well-recognized development of rebound obstruction, probably related to down-regulation of the alpha-adrenergic receptors. The regular use of topical decongestants should be limited to 3 or 4 days unless topical corticosteroids are employed as well. Corticosteroids probably up-regulate the number of alpha-adrenergic receptors, which would delay the development of rhinitis medicamentosa. Therefore, continued use of topical decongestants in conjunction with corticosteroids is probably safe for 7 to 10 days.

Oral alpha-adrenergic agonists are also available, to be used both alone and in combination with antihistamines. They possess well-recognized side effects of tremor, restlessness, and agitation and can cause hypertension and urinary retention. Hypertension has been reported particularly with phenylpropanolamine, which appears to have a very narrow therapeutic range. Pseudoephedrine, the other commonly employed agent, has been less frequently implicated. A recent review concluded that there were inadequate studies to ensure the safety of their use in patients with hypertension. Because any effect of oral decongestants on blood pressure would be maximal during the first week of therapy, several random blood pressure determinations during the first 1 to 2 weeks may be sufficient to detect an adverse effect of these agents on blood pressure. There are also few studies addressing the effectiveness of these drugs as decongestants during the course of chronic administration when some degree of alpha-adrenergic tolerance may be presumed to have developed. A reduction in nasal airway resistance was demonstrated after a dose of 60 mg of rapidly absorbed pseudoephedrine, but it persisted for only 2 hours. The sympathomimetics have, however, one advantage: their side effects tend to be directly opposed to those of the older antihistamines, which makes the combination attractive from the standpoint of reduction in side effects.

CROMOLYN SODIUM

A nasal solution of 4% cromolyn sodium, administered four to six times daily, has been demonstrated to provide moderate relief of the symptoms of seasonal allergic rhinitis. As would be anticipated, it does not alleviate eye symptoms. Cromolyn nasal solution has also been tested in patients with perennial rhinitis; it produced a modest reduction of symptoms in patients with positive skin test but no better results than a placebo in patients with negative skin tests, even in those who had profuse nasal eosinophilia. The topical steroid sprays have consistently demonstrated marked superiority over cromolyn in comparative trials and would appear to be the preferred treatment except for patients with significant local side effects from the topical steroid preparations or with marked steroidphobia. Antihistamines have been demonstrated to be as effective as cromolyn and have the advantage of less frequent dosing, control of eye symptoms, and usually less cost. Therefore, in patients tolerating antihistamines they would appear to be the preferred initial treatment.

Cromolyn is also available as a 2% solution for use in the eyes. Again there is the inconvenience of use six times daily, but this preparation has good control of ocular symptoms as well as some effect on nasal symptoms and thus may compliment topical nasal steroids in the treatment of seasonal allergic rhinitis in patients whose ocular symptoms are prominent.

CORTICOSTEROIDS

Corticosteroids are the most effective pharmacologic agents, especially for atopic rhinitis. Their efficacy is probably attributable to their reversal of many of the pathophysiologic mechanisms of atopic rhinitis, including normalization of the number of epithelial mast cells, the response of the glands to cholinergic stimulation, the response to reflex stimulation, the sympathetic tone of the capacitance vessels, and epithelial and endothelial permeability.

Two nasal steroids are available: beclomethasone dipropionate as a micronized powder in a Freon-propelled vehicle or as an aqueous solution and flunisolide as a propylene glycol solution delivered by a pump spray. The initial dosage of the former is usually two to four discharges into each nostril daily, and these can be delivered as one spray four times daily or two twice daily without affecting efficacy. Flunisolide has frequently been initiated with two sprays into each nostril three times daily, but the dose may be decreased to twice daily without loss of benefit. In these dosage regimens, the two topical corticosteroids appear to be of similar efficacy. With both preparations, once symptoms are optimally controlled, a gradual tapering to the minimum effective dose is indicated. Both preparations have some tendency to cause mucosal bleeding, but a particular problem with flunisolide for some patients is nasal burning caused by the propylene glycol vehicle, which is sufficient in a few patients to cause them to discontinue use of the medication.

Both agents are very effective for seasonal allergic rhinitis, although symptom control is seldom complete. They do not relieve eye symptoms. Furthermore, there is a delay of several days for maximum effect. If marked nasal obstruction is present, they may be ineffective because of a lack of access to the nasal mucosa. Initiation of therapy with 3 to 5 days of prednisone 15 to 25 mg/day or use of a topical decongestant spray before each dose of corticosteroid for the same period may be necessary. Several studies suggest that antihistamines and topical corticosteroids are complimentary; there are no similar data for cromolyn and topical corticosteroids.

It is quite clear that the topical corticosteroids are more effective in atopic rhinitis than in rhinitis that is not related to the atopic diseases. Thus, a positive family history for atopic diseases, positive skin tests, pale and swollen appearance of the mucosa, and presence of eosinophils in the nasal secretions all have been found to be predictors of a favorable response to topical corticosteroids. Absence of these markers indicates perhaps at best a 25% chance of improvement. Despite this unpromising prospect for a response, these latter patients have usually failed to respond to other medications, and therefore, a 2-week carefully evaluated trial is indicated.

In patients with recurrent sinusitis or nasal polyps, treatment of the associated nasal symptoms with topical corticosteroids has been reported to diminish recurrences.

Rhinitis medicamentosa is treated by discontinuing the implicated drug. In addition, topical corticosteroids, by up-regulating the alpha-adrenergic receptors, often rapidly reverse the persistent obstruction that is the primary symptom of this condition.

MISCELLANEOUS TREATMENTS

The vehicle of the flunisolide spray (propylene glycol) and saline nasal sprays and washes have been reported to diminish symptoms of perennial rhinitis, and in some cases this has been accompanied by improvement in the histopathology.

The anticholinergic properties of the older antihistamines were thought to contribute to their efficacy by exerting a drying effect. Ipratropium bromide, a recently introduced anticholinergic, has been tried in selected cases of nonallergic perennial rhinitis characterized by marked rhinorrhea with some decrease in symptoms.

In patients failing to respond to any of the outlined therapies, the usual symptom is one of chronic nasal obstruction. A form of therapy that is occasionally helpful, although for no obvious reason, is the use of warm saline nasal washes at least several times daily. In addition, for patients in whom the persistent obstruction interferes with sleep it has been suggested that they employ topical decongestants at bedtime only. If the latter is resorted to, the possible development of rhinitis medicamentosa may be circumvented by accompanying the topical decongestant with a topical corticosteroid spray for reasons mentioned earlier.

WHICH AGENT FIRST?

For patients whose symptoms are predominantly itching, sneezing, or rhinorrhea, antihistamines are usually the drug of first choice, especially if there are accompanying ocular symptoms. If obstruction is an additional symptom, the addition of oral decongestants may be employed. Corticosteroids are usually employed first if the symptoms are predominantly obstructive. Corticosteroids would also be used in the event of failure to tolerate antihistamines or failure to obtain adequate relief. In the latter case, the combination of an antihistamine with the corticosteroids may be helpful in controlling ocular symptoms and secretions.

Immunotherapy

Immunotherapy is reserved for last because that is its proper role in the treatment of allergic rhinitis. This is not a reflection of lack of efficacy. Placebo-controlled studies have clearly demonstrated that injections of extracts of pollens, animal danders, and house dust mite produce not only a decrease in clinical symptoms on natural exposure but also immunologic changes that include a progressive decline in levels of immunoglobulin E specific

for the substances being injected. Thus, unlike the other treatment modalities mentioned, allergy immunotherapy offers the promise of actually reversing the allergic state.

Why then is the use of allergy immunotherapy deferred until other forms of therapy have first been tried and have failed? The reason is the rigorous requirements placed on the physician and the patient if allergy immunotherapy is to succeed. First, the physician must determine that the symptoms are truly allergic—that the nature and timing of symptoms, the patient's exposure, and the patient's degree of sensitivity strongly suggest a causal relationship. Next, the allergen must be specifically identified—this is often possible with pollens but often impossible with molds. Finally, potent extracts of these substances must be injected ultimately at high concentrations, which carry with them the danger of serious or rarely even fatal reactions. The requirement on the patient's part is an investment of time and money over several years if lasting results are to be obtained. Under present circumstances, allergy immunotherapy should be reserved for clear-cut allergy to well-defined allergens in patients who respond poorly to symptomatic therapy and have a prolonged season or perennial symptoms.

Bibliography

Dickson DJ, Cruickshank JM. Comparison of flunisolide nasal spray and terfenadine tablets in hay fever. Br J Clin Prac 38:416–420, 1984.
This is a comparative study of a new nonsedating antihistamine and a topical steroid in the treatment of seasonal allergic rhinitis.

Empey DW, Bye C, Hodder M, et al. A double-blind crossover trial of pseudoephedrine and triprolidine, alone and in combination, for the treatment of allergenic rhinitis. Ann Allergy 34:41–46, 1975.
This is one of the few published studies addressing the effectiveness of oral decongestants administered on a regular basis.

Hillas J, Booth RJ, Somerfield S, et al. A comparative trial of intra-nasal beclomethasone dipropionate and sodium cromoglycate in patients with chronic perennial rhinitis. Clin Allergy 10:253–258, 1980.
This study places in perspective the relative effectiveness of cromolyn sodium and topical corticosteroids in the treatment of perennial rhinitis.

Howarth PH, Holgate ST. Comparative trial of two nonsedative H_1 antihistamines, terfenadine and astemizole, for hay fever. Thorax 39:668–672, 1984.
This study raises questions regarding the effectiveness of terfenadine when employed on a chronic basis.

Incaudo GA. Diagnosis and treatment of rhinitis during pregnancy and lactation. Clin Rev Allergy 5:325–337, 1987.

Kray KT, Squire EN Jr, Tipton WR, et al. Cromolyn

sodium in seasonal allergic conjunctivitis. J Allergy Clin Immunol 76:623–627, 1985.

This is a placebo controlled study demonstrating the effectiveness of cromolyn sodium eye drops in treating the ocular symptoms of seasonal pollen allergy.

Long WF, Taylor RJ, Wagner CJ, et al. Skin test suppression by antihistamines and the development of subsensitivity. J Allergy Clin Immunol 76:113–117, 1985.

This study demonstrates the degree of loss of the effect of antihistamines that occurs with their chronic use. It also demonstrates clearly that the loss of effect is not limited to the class of agent that induced it but that it is a receptor phenomenon and applies equally to all classes of antihistamines.

Munch EP, Søborg M, Nørreslet TT, et al. A comparative study of dexchlorpheniramine maleate sustained release tablets and budesonide nasal spray in seasonal allergic rhinitis. Allergy 38:517–524, 1983.

This study demonstrates the relative merits of the two major forms of therapy for seasonal allergic rhinitis.

Murray AB, Ferguson AC. Dust-free bedrooms in the treatment of asthmatic children with house dust or house dust mite allergy: a controlled trial. Pediatrics 71:418–422, 1983.

This study demonstrates the effectiveness of environmental control measures in relieving the symptoms of asthmatic children sensitive to house dust mite.

Mygind N. Clinical investigations of allergic rhinitis and allied conditions. Allergy 34:195–208, 1979.

This is a useful summary of the classification and evaluation of patients with rhinitis.

Mygind N, Pederson CB, Prytz S, et al. Treatment of nasal polyps with intranasal beclomethasone dipropionate aerosol. Clin Allergy 5:159–164, 1975.

This study demonstrates the effect of topical corticosteroids in the treatment of nasal polyps.

Nelson HS. What is atopy? Sidestepping semantics. Postgrad Med 76:118–120, 123–129, 1984.

This paper discusses the atopic diseases and their underlying immunologic, cellular, and autonomic abnormalities.

Reinberg A, Gervais P, Levi F, et al. Circadian and circannual rhythms of allergic rhinitis: an epidemiologic study involving chronobiologic methods. J Allergy Clin Immunol 81:51–62, 1988.

Turkeltaub PC, Norman PS, Johnson JD, et al. Treatment of seasonal and perennial rhinitis with intranasal flunisolide. Allergy 37:303–311, 1982.

This study examines the degree of response as well as the type of patients who best respond to topical corticosteroid therapy.

Welsh PW, Stricker WE, Chu C-P, et al. Efficacy of beclomethasone nasal solution, flunisolide, and cromolyn in relieving symptoms of ragweed allergy. Mayo Clin Proc 62:125–134, 1987.

This study places in perspective the relative effectiveness of nasal cromolyn and nasal corticosteroids in seasonal allergic rhinitis.

35

Sore Throat in Adult Patients

ANTHONY L. KOMAROFF, M.D.

Streptococcal Pharyngitis

Diagnosis

Pharyngeal infection with group A beta-hemolytic streptococci constitutes the major form of pharyngitis for which curative treatment has been shown to be effective. Several studies have demonstrated that group A streptococci are isolated from a throat culture in 9 to 15% of adult patients seeking primary care for a sore throat. The frequency may be as high as 35% in children.

A history and physical examination can help raise or lower the probability of streptococcal pharyngitis in the individual patient. Table 35–1 presents a useful combination of findings to help the clinician estimate the probability of streptococcal pharyngitis. Table 35–2 presents a slightly more accurate "strep score" for estimating the probability of streptococcal pharyngitis, which should be used in conjunction with a nomogram (Fig. 35–1).

Laboratory tests have some utility in helping to make the diagnosis of streptococcal pharyngitis. The results of a *throat culture* and of the *rapid antigen detection tests* are useful but imperfect. On the one hand, these tests can

be *false positive*: some patients with a positive culture may be uninfected streptococcal carriers who do not exhibit a four-fold increase in antistreptococcal antibodies. Studies by our group of adults and studies of children indicate that among patients seeking care for a sore throat, only about 40% of those with a throat culture positive for group A streptococci exhibit serologic evidence of infection. This estimate of the frequency of the false-positive rate (the carrier state) may be somewhat high because treatment with penicillin can reduce the magnitude and the rate of antibody increase. On the other hand, a single-swab throat culture or rapid antigen test may be *false negative* in approximately 10% of patients, as defined by isolation of group A streptococci on a second swab.

A *white blood cell count* has limited value. Although leukocytosis has some correlation with streptococcal pharyngitis, it has no independent predictive value. (On the other hand, atypical lymphocytosis can be a valuable finding in suggesting a new Epstein-Barr virus infection.) Our studies of adult patients suggest that the *C-reactive protein test* does not provide significant additional predictive information (Komaroff AL, unpublished data). There is

Table 35–1. *Probability of Isolation of Streptococci from Adults with Different Combinations of Findings*

Clinical Findings		Probability of Isolation (%)	Recommended Action

Temperature less than 100°F
  no tonsillar exudate
  no anterior cervical adenitis
	and
	and
		1–3	No culture, no treatment: a false-positive culture could lead to unnecessary and potentially risky treatment

Temperature greater than 100°F
  tonsillar exudate
  anterior cervical adenitis
	or
	or
		14	Culture, and treat patients with positive culture results

Temperature greater than 100°F
  tonsillar exudate
  anterior cervical adenitis
	and
	and
		42	Treat immediately: a false-negative culture could prevent necessary treatment

From Komaroff AL, et al. J Gen Intern Med 1:1–7, 1986, with permission.
*Isolation of group A streptococci, not other streptococci, irrespective of antistreptococcal antibody response.

Table 35–2. *The Strep Score: A Linear Discriminant Model*

Parameter	Numerical Score
Marked tonsillar exudate	+2
Pinpoint tonsillar exudate	+1
Enlarged tonsils	+1
Tender anterior cervical adenopathy	+1
Myalgias	+1
Positive throat culture in past year	+1
Itchy eyes	−1

From Komaroff AL, et al. J Gen Intern Med 1:1–7, 1986, with permission.

some evidence that it may be more useful for children.

Several studies indicate that a *Gram's stain* of material from the area of maximal erythema or exudate may be of value. The best study of this question defined a Gram-stained smear as positive if spherical gram-positive cocci occurring singly and in pairs were found in association with disrupted polymorphonuclear cells (cells that demonstrated a loss of cytoplasmic integrity and cellular outlines). This study found that the Gram-stained smear had a sensitivity of 73%, a specificity of 96%, and a predictive value of 71%. This degree of accuracy is greater than that reported with any individual clinical finding (history or physician examination) or with any combination of clinical findings. The test adds both cost and time to the encounter with the patient and requires a trained observer.

Treatment

Treatment of streptococcal pharyngitis probably speeds the resolution of symptoms and signs in the sickest patients but not in the average patient. Treatment probably reduces the likelihood of streptococcal spread to close contacts, of suppurative infections (e.g., peritonsillar abscess, otitis, osteomyelitis of the skull), and of rheumatic fever, although the frequency of the latter two complications is extremely small. Treatment may reduce the probability of subsequent acute glomerulonephritis, although this has not been proved in sporadic streptococcal infections.

Acceptable treatment regimens and a follow-up plan are shown in Table 35–3.

Other Potentially Treatable Forms of Pharyngitis

Table 35–4 summarizes several potentially treatable bacterial forms of pharyngitis. Some are well established but infrequent; others are not yet well established but may be surprisingly frequent.

Among the latter group are the non–group A streptococci. A growing (and still largely unpublished) experience indicates that the non–group A streptococci are isolated as frequently or more frequently than are the group A streptococci from adult patients with pharyngitis; furthermore, there is anecdotal evidence that the sickest of these patients seem to respond well to penicillin therapy. Thus, although the evidence is still inconclusive, it may be that we should not dismiss the presence of non–group A streptococci in a throat culture as a negative result, as we traditionally have been taught to do.

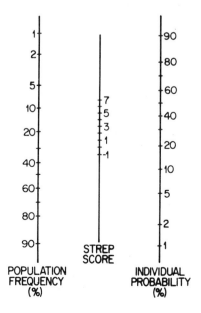

Figure 35–1. *Nomogram for predicting probability of group A streptococcal pharyngitis. To use the nomogram, determine the overall prevalence of positive cultures among adult patients presenting with sore throat at the site. Second, add the points based on the clinical findings to arrive at a strep score for an individual. Third, place a ruler on the figure so that it crosses the left line at the site prevalence and the center line at the strep score value. The point where the ruler crosses the right line is then the probability of a positive culture for that patient. As an example, if 20% of adult patients with sore throat at a site typically have positive cultures and a patient in this group has a strep score of 5, then a straight line connecting 20% on the left line with 5 points on the center line crosses the right line at a value of 55%, which indicates that this is the likelihood of a positive culture for this patient. From Komaroff AL, et al. J Gen Intern Med 1:1–7, 1986, with permission.*

Table 35–3. Treatment Regimens for Streptococcal Pharyngitis and Recommended Follow-Up

In Adults
1. Penicillin G, benzathine (Bicillin), 1.2 million U IM
2. Penicillin V, 250 mg q.i.d. × 10 days
3. Erythromycin, 250 mg q.i.d. × 10 days

In Children Below Age 12
1. Penicillin G, benzathine (Bicillin), 300,000–600,000 U IM
2. Penicillin V potassium, 25,000–90,000 U/kg per day in 3–6 divided doses × 10 days
3. Erythromycin, 30–50 mg/kg per day in 4 divided doses × 10 days

Follow-Up
1. Contacts who become symptomatic should have cultures performed.
2. Asymptomatic contacts who are at high risk from streptococcal pharyngitis (e.g., who have past history of acute rheumatic fever) should have cultures done.
3. Follow-up cultures to ensure streptococcal eradication should be obtained from patients with a past history of acute rheumatic fever.
4. In patients who do not respond to penicillin, the following causes should be considered:
   a. Poor compliance
   b. Coexisting infection with another organism (discussed later).

More intriguing, we have found serologic evidence of infection with chlamydial organisms in 21% and infection with *Mycoplasma pneumoniae* in 11% of adult patients with a sore throat. *M. pneumoniae* is an established pharyngeal pathogen, although it has not been isolated frequently from the throat. Chlamyd-ial organisms are respiratory tract pathogens: *Chlamydia trachomatis* is a common cause of pneumonia in neonates, and a newly recognized chlamydial organism called TWAR is a common cause of community-acquired pneumonia in adults. It remains to be proved whether they are common causes of pharyngitis.

Infectious Mononucleosis

Pharyngitis associated with heterophil antibody, which most often represents a recent new infection with Epstein-Barr virus, is seen in 2% of adult patients seeking primary care for a sore throat. Only a quarter of these patients have the full-blown infectious mononucleosis syndrome. On average, the patients do not have a prolonged illness compared with patients with other forms of viral pharyngitis. However, patients with the full-blown infectious mononucleosis syndrome do have a prolonged course of illness and may be susceptible to a number of potentially serious complications. Furthermore, some of the patients who do not have the full-blown syndrome when first seen may develop it.

Therefore, it may be valuable to identify a subset of patients with sore throat and without obvious infectious mononucleosis who should have hematologic and serologic tests for infectious mononucleosis. The clinical findings that

Table 35–4. Potentially Treatable Forms of Pharyngitis Other Than Group A Streptococcal Infection

Organism/Illness	Pursue Diagnosis If	Actions
Non–group A streptococci	Persistent pharyngitis	Repeat culture; treat with penicillin
Chlamydiae	Persistent pharyngitis and cough	Treat with erythromycin
Mycoplasma	Persistent pharyngitis	Treat with erythromycin
Haemophilus influenzae	Pharyngitis; otitis; positive culture results	Treat with amoxicillin, 500 mg q.i.d. × 10 days
Gonococci	Gay male; intercurrent urogenital infection; persistent pharyngitis	Treat with procaine penicillin G, 4.8 million U IM plus probenecid 1 g PO
Corynebacterium diphtheriae	Pseudomembrane; known epidemic	Culture on Löffler's medium; Rx antitoxin; isolation
Fusospirochetal infection (Vincent's angina)	Associated gingivitis	Rx penicillin
Mycobacterium tuberculosis	Single ulcer	Perform tuberculin test
Treponema pallidum	Single ulcer	Order serologic tests; dark-field microscopic examination
Peritonsillar abscess	Unilateral swelling/fluctuance	Incision and drainage; ? antibacterial drugs
Epiglottitis *(H. influenzae)*	Stridor; visible, red epiglottis	Rx amoxicillin/chloramphenicol; observe for respiratory obstruction
Neisseria meningitidis	Stiff neck; severe headache, motor deficits	Culture; consider lumbar puncture and blood culture
Yersinia enterocolitica	Persistent pharyngitis	Culture; treat with tetracycline
Corynebacterium haemolyticum	Pharyngitis and maculopapular rash of trunk and extremities	Culture; treat with penicillin

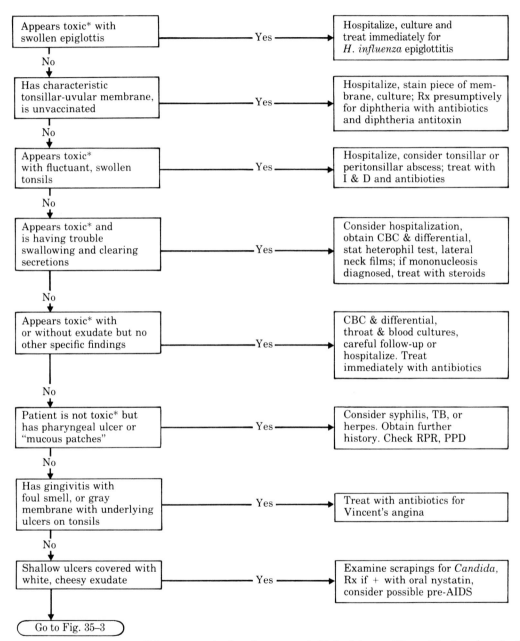

Figure 35–2. *Algorithm describing an evaluation for unusual, high risk conditions. *Toxic refers to the finding of high fever, prostration, tachycardia, thready pulse, and so on. From Branch WT Jr. Office Practice of Medicine, ed 2. Philadelphia, W. B. Saunders Co., 1987, p. 236.*

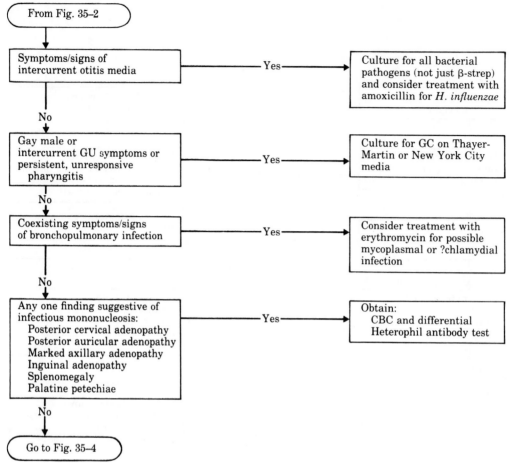

Figure 35–3. Algorithm describing an evaluation of more common nonstreptococcal causes of pharyngitis. From Branch WT Jr. Office Practice of Medicine, ed 2. Philadelphia, W. B. Saunders Co., 1987, p. 237.

are of value in this regard are summarized in Table 35–5.

Recently, a syndrome called chronic fatigue syndrome, chronic Epstein-Barr virus infection, or chronic mononucleosis has been described. Patients with this syndrome often present with recurrent pharyngitis and adenopathy in addition to chronic debilitating and sometimes disabling fatigue. This syndrome is related to a reactivation of latent Epstein-Barr virus infection in some patients, but other infectious agents also may produce the syndrome.

A Management Strategy

A reasonable strategy for suspecting various pathogens and therefore performing certain diagnostic or therapeutic maneuvers is summarized here and in Figures 35–2 to 35–4.

Streptococcal Pharyngitis. Because a throat culture or rapid antigen test can be false positive (i.e., can indicate a carrier state) and because penicillin treatment prescribed on the basis of a false-positive culture result can produce more suffering than it can be expected to eliminate, a good case can be made that patients who have a low probability of streptococcal pharyngitis based on clinical findings do not require a throat culture or rapid antigen test.

When the probability is below 3%, a throat culture can be avoided. As can be seen by Tables 35–1 and 35–2, clinical findings can be used to estimate such a low probability. (This recommendation does not apply to patients who have special risk factors for streptococcal disease: a past history of acute rheumatic fever, documented streptococcal exposure in the past week, residence in a community in which there is a current streptococcal epidemic, and

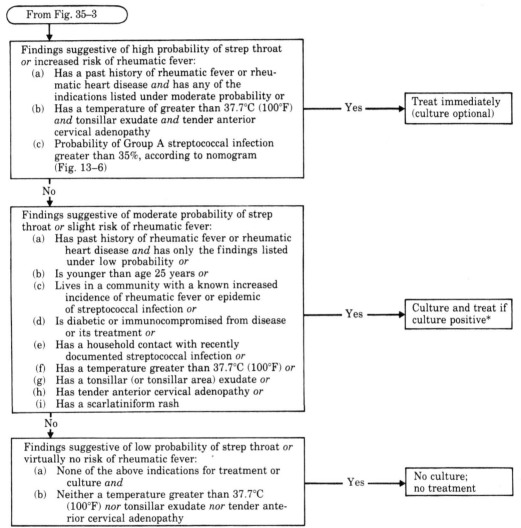

Figure 35–4. *Algorithm describing an evaluation of the probability of group A streptococcal pharyngitis and the risk of developing acute rheumatic fever. *Immediate treatment is preferred for those individuals whose throat culture results are not complete for 9 days into the illness (because treatment after that time has not been shown to be protective against rheumatic fever). From Branch WT Jr. Office Practice of Medicine, ed 2. Philadelphia, W. B. Saunders Co., 1987, p. 238.*

Table 35–5. Clinical Findings Suggesting a New Epstein-Barr Virus Infection

Finding	Predictive Value Positive*	Likelihood Ratio†
Palatine petechiae	0.11	5.8
Posterior auricular adenopathy	0.19	12.0
Marked axillary adenopathy	0.33	21.0
Inguinal adenopathy	0.06	2.9
Palatine petechiae, posterior auricular adenopathy, or marked axillary adenopathy	0.11	6.3

From Aronson MD, et al. Ann Intern Med 96:505–580, 1982, with permission.
*Predictive value positive is the fraction of all patients with a particular physical examination finding who have heterophil antibody.
†Likelihood ratio = true-positive rate/false-positive rate.

diabetes or other immunocompromising conditions.)

Conversely, because a throat culture or rapid antigen test can be false negative, we would advocate immediate antibacterial treatment for patients with a relatively high probability of streptococcal pharyngitis: greater than 40%. As can be seen in Tables 35–1 and 35–2, clinical findings can be used to identify patients with such a high probability.

Non–Group A Streptococcal Pharyngitis. When a non–group A streptococcus is repeatedly isolated from a patient with a sore throat persisting for more than 2 weeks, penicillin therapy probably should be prescribed.

New Epstein-Barr Virus Infection. A differential white blood count and heterophil test should be obtained for patients with any one of several findings that suggest a relatively high probability of a new Epstein-Barr virus infection (Table 35–5). Because both atypical lymphocytosis and heterophil antibody may not appear for 7 to 10 days after the onset of symptoms, each test can be false negative if obtained too early in the course of illness.

Haemophilus influenzae *Pharyngitis.* This entity should be suspected in an adult patient with concomitant symptoms or signs of otitis media or cough. It probably also should be suspected in patients with a sore throat persisting for more than 2 weeks.

Gonococcal Pharyngitis. Gonococcal pharyngitis should be suspected, and a culture on Thayer-Martin medium obtained, when the patient is a gay male, has associated symptoms of urogenital infection, or has a lingering sore throat.

Chlamydial and Mycoplasmal Pharyngitis. We know very little about these two possibly common forms of pharyngitis. It is our current recommendation that each should be considered when the patient has a sore throat persisting for more than 2 weeks—with a negative culture for group A streptococci or with a positive culture but failure to respond to penicillin treatment. The presence of a cough probably increases the likelihood of each of these entities.

Bibliography

Aronson MD, Komaroff AL, Pass TM, et al. Heterophil antibody in adults with sore throat: frequency and clinical presentation. Ann Intern Med 96:505–508, 1982.
Study of the typical and atypical presentations of primary Epstein-Barr virus infection in patients with sore throat.

Bridger RC. *Haemophilus influenzae*: the relationship to upper respiratory tract infection. N Z Med J 80:19–22, 1974.

Brock LL, Siegel AC. Studies on the prevention of rheumatic fever: the effect of time of initiation of treatment of streptococcal infections on the immune response of the host. J Clin Invest 32:630–632, 1953.
Evidence of the importance of early treatment in preventing nonsuppurative sequelae.

Centor RM, Witherspoon JM, Dalton HP. Non group A streptococci are associated with clinically significant sore throats. Clin Res 29:255, 1981.
Evidence that non–group A streptococci may occasionally be significant pharyngeal pathogens.

Centor RM, Witherspoon JM, Dalton HP, et al. The diagnosis of strep throat in adults in the emergency room. Med Decis Making 1:239–246, 1981.
Study of the clinical predictors of streptococcal pharyngitis.

Crawford G, Brancato F, Holmes KK. Streptococcal pharyngitis: diagnosis by gram stain. Ann Intern Med 90:293–297, 1979.
Demonstration that Gram's stain has predictive value in diagnosing streptococcal pharyngitis.

Denny FW, Perry WD, Wannamaker LW. Type-specific streptococcal antibody. J Clin Invest 36:1092–1100, 1957.
Demonstration that treatment can retard the increase of antistreptococcal antibodies.

DuBois RE, Seeley JK, Brus I, et al. Chronic mononucleosis syndrome. South Med J 77:1376–1382, 1984.
Clinical and laboratory findings for a new syndrome, now variably called chronic fatigue syndrome, chronic mononucleosis, or chronic Epstein-Barr virus infection syndrome.

Evans AS, Diete EC. Acute pharyngitis and tonsillitis in University of Wisconsin students. JAMA 190:699–708, 1964.
Description of the role of H. influenzae in producing pharyngitis.

Glezen WP, Clyde WA, Senior RJ. Group A streptococci, mycoplasmas, and viruses associated with acute pharyngitis. JAMA 202:455–460, 1967.
A survey of various etiologic agents in acute pharyngitis.

Grayston JT, Kuo C, Wang S, et al. A new *Chlamydia psittaci* strain, TWAR, isolated in acute respiratory tract infections. N Engl J Med 315:161–168, 1986.
Report of an important new respiratory tract pathogen.

Jones JF, Ray CG, Minnich LL, et al. Evidence for active Epstein-Barr virus infection in patients with persistent unexplained illnesses: elevated anti-early antigen antibodies. Ann Intern Med 102:1–7, 1985.
A report similar to that of DuBois and colleagues.

Kaplan EL, Top FH, Dudding BA. Diagnosis of streptococcal pharyngitis: differentiation of active infection from the carrier state in the symptomatic child. J Infect Dis 123:490–501, 1971.
Study of clinical and laboratory predictors of streptococcal pharyngitis in children.

Komaroff AL. The "chronic mononucleosis" syndromes. Hosp Pract 22:71–75, 1987.
A review of various syndromes producing chronic fatigue and, often, pharyngitis.

Komaroff AL, Aronson MD, Pass TM, et al. Serologic evidence of chlamydial and mycoplasmal pharyngitis in adults. Science 222:927–929, 1983.
Study of the possible chlamydial and mycoplasmal etiology of some cases of pharyngitis.

Komaroff AL, Pass TM, Aronson MD, et al. The prediction of streptococcal pharyngitis in adults. J Gen Intern Med 1:1–7, 1986.
Study of the clinical and laboratory predictors of streptococcal pharyngitis.

Siegel AC, Johnson EE, Stollerman GH. Controlled studies of streptococcal pharyngitis in a pediatric population: 2. Behavior of the type-specific immune response. N Engl J Med 265:566–571, 1961.
Detailed clinical and laboratory studies of streptococcal pharyngitis in children.

Straus SE, Tosato G, Armstrong G, et al. Persisting illness and fatigue in adults with evidence of Epstein-Barr virus infection. Ann Intern Med 102:7–16, 1985.
A report similar to those of DuBois and colleagues and Jones and colleagues with additional immunologic data.

Walsh BT, Bookheim WW, Johnson RC, et al. Recognition of streptococcal pharyngitis in adults. Arch Intern Med 135:1493–1497, 1975.
Study of the clinical predictors of streptococcal pharyngitis.

36

Diagnostic Evaluation of Lymphadenopathy

GRETCHEN KUNITZ, M.D.

Practicing internists and general practitioners are frequently faced with the task of evaluating an adult patient with peripheral lymphadenopathy. By definition, peripheral adenopathy is detectable by palpation. Lymph nodes in the mediastinum or retroperitoneum are central rather than peripheral and are not discussed in this chapter. Whether regional or generalized, adenopathy may be the presenting complaint of patients with a wide variety of underlying illnesses. Although many of these illnesses are self-limited or easily treated, the incidence of lymphatic malignancy increases steadily with age. Retrospective reviews of peripheral lymph node biopsies in patients younger than 25 years of age repeatedly have shown a less than 20% incidence of malignancy. In contrast, in the age group over 50, 55 to 80% of biopsies have shown a malignant process related to either primary lymphoma or metastatic carcinoma. In recent years, the emergence of human immunodeficiency virus (HIV) has made generalized lymphadenopathy common in urban primary care practice.

When a patient initially complains of localized or generalized swelling or when a practitioner first discovers presumptive adenopathy, the following questions must be asked: Is the swelling adenopathy? Is the adenopathy regional or generalized? If adenopathy is present, what is the likelihood that malignancy is present? What diagnostic tests are indicated? Is a biopsy necessary and if so, when should it be done? The answers to these questions vary considerably among patients. A thorough review of patient characteristics such as age and duration and severity of symptoms combined with an assessment of the character and location of the adenopathy aids practitioners in their evaluation and diagnostic plan. The in-

tent of this review is to provide a framework for diagnostic evaluation.

Is the Swelling Adenopathy?

During the initial evaluation, it is often difficult to distinguish actual adenopathy from swelling related to other causes. Neck cellulitis, periodontal abscess, lipoma, thyroglossal duct cyst, or parotitis may mimic cervical adenopathy. Similarly, an inguinal hernia or enlarged axillary sweat gland may be mistakenly identified as an enlarged node.

Adenopathy may present as lymphadenitis, an acute or chronic inflammation of lymph nodes associated with an adjacent infectious process. The pathologic appearance of the enlarged node depends on the infectious agent. In bacterial infections, the node may develop into a suppurative abscess, whereas a nonsuppurative or caseous inflammation is associated with nonpyogenic infections. Acute lymphangitis, in which the inflamed lymphatic channels result in visible red streaking, is most commonly associated with bacterial infection. However, a chronic lymphangitis may accompany sporotrichosis or the cutaneous infection associated with *Mycobacterium marinum*. Lymphedema caused by blockage of the lymphatic channels may follow radiotherapy, surgical node dissection, or fibrosis associated with chronic infection.

Determining the Likelihood of Malignancy

As a working definition, it is useful to consider the presence of one or more nodes larger than 1 cm or of multiple smaller nodes as grounds for further investigation. In addition to lymph node size, the character of the adenopathy must be evaluated. Although tender nodes often indicate an infectious process and rock-hard or rubbery nodes suggest malignancy, these axioms should serve as guidelines rather than as absolute rules. The location of the node is of diagnostic importance, as malignant tumors are most commonly found in cervical and supraclavicular sites. Isolated inguinal adenopathy is rarely associated with malignancy. Also important are the duration and rate of growth of the adenopathy. Steadily enlarging nodes over a period of months are more suspicious than newly discovered nodes that change little in size in the initial weeks of evaluation. Once the nodes have been evaluated, the characteristics of the patient need careful consideration. Bacterial infection accounts for 75 to 85% of adenopathy in the pediatric age group. Thus, a 10 year old with a tender, enlarged cervical node initially requires aspiration for a culture rather than excisional biopsy. In a recent retrospective study of 123 patients in the 9- to 25-year age group undergoing lymph node biopsy, lymph node size greater than 2 cm or an abnormal chest radiograph correlated with the finding of granuloma or tumor at the biopsy (or, in some cases, both). A history of ear, nose, or throat symptoms correlated with the absence of these biopsy findings. Discriminant analysis showed a wide range of other symptoms and signs to be unhelpful in predicting which biopsy specimens would show a granulomatous or malignant process. In an older adolescent or adult patient, an assessment based on patient and nodal characteristics is required. Reviewing the major causes of adenopathy by region aids in formulating a diagnostic plan.

Regional Adenopathy

Cervical Adenopathy

Of the hundreds of lymph nodes comprising the lymphatic system, the cervical nodes are most often noted by both the patient and practitioner to be enlarged. The most common cause of cervical adenopathy is a bacterial or viral infection of the face or oropharynx (Table 36–1). A careful examination of the throat and mouth may show the primary source of infection, thus mitigating the need for further evaluation.

With the recent influx of immigrants from Central and South America and Southeast Asia, the incidence of tuberculosis in the United States has increased. Eighty to 90% of persons with scrofula present with solitary enlargement of a cervical lymph node. Although patients usually have positive tuberculin results, tuberculous infection at other sites is rarely evident. Diagnosis rests on culture of the nodal aspirate, as the stain for acid-fast bacilli reveals tuberculous organisms only half the time.

The common house cat is the definitive host of the protozoan intracellular parasite causing toxoplasmosis. After contact with cat feces or after ingestion of undercooked pork or mutton, cervical or generalized adenopathy may develop. Although usually asymptomatic, this nontender adenopathy occasionally is associated with a low grade fever, malaise, and hepatosplenomegaly. The symptoms may persist for several months during which time the adenopathy may wax and wane. Abdominal pain may occur if retroperitoneal or mesenteric lymph nodes are involved. In immunocompromised hosts, toxoplasmosis may result in fulminant infection of the central nervous system. Treatment with pyrimethamine and sulfadiazine is warranted only for patients with severe symptoms or with underlying immunodeficiency. The diagnosis rests on detecting serum immunoglobulin antibodies. A titer of greater than 1:80 or a four-fold or greater rise in paired serum specimens establishes the diagnosis.

Infectious mononucleosis caused by the Epstein-Barr virus (EBV) is an acute self-limited illness of young adults. It is characterized by fever, pharyngitis (90%), splenomegaly (15%), palatal petechiae (25 to 50%), and symmetric posterior cervical adenopathy (90%). The pharyngitis is exudative in one third of infected patients and resembles streptococcal pharyngitis. The adenopathy may persist for many weeks, and typically the nodes are firm and tender to palpation. A physician who conducts a superficial examination of a patient with mononucleosis erroneously may prescribe antibiotic therapy for a presumptive bacterial pharyngitis. In as many as 90% of patients with mononucleosis, a maculopapular skin rash develops when they are treated with ampicillin. The diagnosis of mononucleosis rests on recording an absolute lymphocytosis (> 4000/mm^3) with 10% or more atypical lymphocytes in conjunction with a positive heterophil antibody or Monospot slide test. Of these two tests, the Monospot is both more sensitive

Table 36–1. *Cervical Adenopathy*

Disease	Clinical History and Presentation	Diagnostic Tests
Infectious		
Bacterial infection of face or oropharynx	Recent dental or facial exudative infection; acute pharyngitis	Leukocytosis; positive bacterial cultures (e.g., streptococcus)
Viral pharyngitis	Sore throat; constitutional symptoms	
Mononucleosis syndromes (EBV, cytomegalovirus)	Fever, pharyngitis; constitutional symptoms; nausea or anorexia	Leukocytosis; atypical lymphocytosis; elevated hepatic transaminase level; positive Monospot or heterophil test (EBV); rise in complement-fixing titers (cytomegalovirus)
Scrofula (*Mycobacterium tuberculosis*)	From tuberculosis-endemic area; known contact with infected person; constitutional symptoms	Positive tuberculin test; positive culture of nodal aspirate
Toxoplasmosis	Contact with cat feces; low grade constitutional symptoms	Positive immunoglobulin antibodies
Noninfectious		
Lymphoma	Constitutional symptoms; night sweats; pruritus	Anemia, elevated erythrocyte sedimentation rate, elevated hepatic transaminase levels; positive lymph node biopsy
Chronic lymphocytic leukemia	Older male patient; recurrent bacterial infections or low grade constitutional symptoms; 25% asymptomatic; splenomegaly	Lymphocytosis, anemia; abnormal bone marrow findings; hypogammaglobulinemia
Thyroid cancer	Prior radiation to neck; hoarseness; dysphagia; palpable thyroid nodule (familial endocrine abnormalities)	Cold nodule on radioactive iodine uptake scan; positive fine needle aspiration biopsy
Nasopharyngeal cancer	Facial pain or numbness; cranial nerve palsies	Mass on computed tomographic scan; positive biopsy of lymph node or tumor

and more specific, being positive in 90% of early infections. Determination of antibodies specific for EBV is rarely necessary.

Recently, a chronic form of an EBV-like infection has received attention in both lay and medical circles. Patients with this syndrome typically complain of severe fatigue associated with a low grade fever, myalgias, headaches, and recurrent pharyngitis. Gastrointestinal or neurologic symptoms may occur, and patients usually remember their symptoms beginning with a cold or flu-like illness. Fifty to 60% of patients report the presence of cervical adenopathy. Laboratory studies may reveal a mild leukopenia with increased numbers of monocytes or lymphocytes. Mild liver function abnormalities and high levels of EBV antibodies (viral capsid antigen: immunoglobulin G > 1:640; early antigen: antibody > 1:40) are associated with this syndrome. The exact cause remains unknown.

A clinical syndrome similar to mononucleosis is associated with cytomegalovirus. The adenopathy and pharyngitis seen with this illness are less pronounced than those associated with EBV. The diagnosis is confirmed by re-

cording a four-fold rise in complement-fixing titers or by cytologic examination of a tissue or urine specimen for cytomegalic cells with intranuclear inclusions. Patients with this syndrome are heterophil antibody negative.

Various malignant conditions may present with localized cervical adenopathy. Although this occurs most commonly with Hodgkin's disease, it may also occur with other lymphomas or leukemias or, rarely, with thyroid or nasopharyngeal carcinomas.

Preauricular and Postauricular Adenopathy

The differential diagnosis of isolated preauricular and postauricular adenopathy is limited to several common infections. Bacterial or viral conjunctivitis and infections of the eyelid may result in painful enlargement of the preauricular nodes (Parinaud's oculoglandular syndrome). Before the widespread use of rubella vaccine in the United States, postauricular adenopathy was common. The adenopathy may occur as early as a week before the appearance of the typical rash. The diagnosis is confirmed by recording a four-fold rise in serologic titers. The other major causes of postauricular adenopathy are infections of the scalp or ear and postauricular sinus tracts. Rarely, sarcoidosis may be associated with preauricular or postauricular adenopathy.

Supraclavicular Adenopathy

Most enlarged supraclavicular nodes are associated with malignancy. Rarely, scrofula is associated with supraclavicular adenopathy. The left supraclavicular node (Virchow's or sentinel node) drains the lymphatic system of the abdomen, kidney, and pelvis, whereas the right-sided node drains the mediastinum, lungs, and esophagus. Because they lie behind the clavicular head of the sternocleidomastoid muscle, these nodes often go undetected during routine physical examinations. Asking a patient to do Valsalva's maneuver may facilitate detection.

Axillary Adenopathy

Axillary adenopathy is most commonly associated with bacterial infections of the upper extremities and cancers of the breast. *Mycobacterium marinum* (fishtank granuloma) and sporotrichosis are uncommon causes of axillary adenopathy. Human infection with *M. marinum* usually follows minor trauma sustained in swimming pools or lakes. A small papule at the inoculation site enlarges with a characteristic bluish hue and may eventually suppurate. Sporotrichosis is a fungal disease affecting gardeners and florists in the United States. A single red or violaceous nodule most commonly on the hand is followed by the appearance of multiple nodules along regional lymphatics.

Another cause of axillary adenopathy is cat-scratch disease, a usually benign, self-limited illness thought to be caused by a pleomorphic gram-negative bacterium. Ninety per cent of persons thought to have this disease give a history of contact with cats. A primary inoculation site is obvious in 60 to 70% and tender adenopathy occurs in 80% of patients 1 to 2 weeks after contact. In one large study, 30% of patients reported a low grade fever and 25% reported fatigue. Rarely, encephalitis, purpura, and pneumonia are associated with this disease. Although a specific skin test has been developed, it is not readily available. A node biopsy may reveal typical organisms with a Warthin-Starry silver stain. Brucellosis, sporotrichosis, and, in rare instances, non-Hodgkin's lymphoma also may present with isolated axillary adenopathy.

Inguinal Adenopathy

It is useful to separate the causes of inguinal adenopathy into sexually and nonsexually transmitted cases (Table 36–2).

SEXUALLY TRANSMITTED DISEASES

In urban general medical practice, most cases of inguinal adenopathy are caused by the sexually transmitted diseases syphilis, herpes simplex infection, gonorrhea, chancroid, lymphogranuloma venereum, and granuloma inguinale.

The primary chancre of syphilis develops 3 to 4 weeks after exposure to *Treponema pallidum*. Bilateral inguinal adenopathy develops in 50 to 70% of patients about a week after appearance of the chancre. The nodes typically are nontender and firm; in women, adenopathy may be absent if only the deep inguinal system is affected. This regional adenopathy of primary syphilis must be distinguished from the generalized adenopathy of secondary lues, occurring 2 to 10 weeks postchancre. Diagnosis rests on dark-field microscopic examination of the primary lesion or on positive serologic tests. Of the several available serologic tests, the fluorescent antibody absorbed test is the most sensitive for primary syphilis.

The initial genital infection with herpes simplex virus type 2 invariably presents with vesicular eruptions and painful bilateral inguinal adenopathy 2 to 7 days after exposure. Low grade fever, malaise, and anorexia may also be present. In homosexual males, inguinal adenopathy is associated with primary herpes simplex virus type 2 perianal infection. Itching, tenesmus, discharge, and sacral paresthesias should alert the practitioner to this diagnosis.

The painful adenopathy seen in conjunction with chancroid infection is unilateral, occurring simultaneously with or shortly after the appearance of a genital ulcer. Ninety per cent of cases occur in males, and the disease often is associated with poor hygiene. The single ulcer is typically well demarcated and painful, and sometimes surrounded by an erythematous halo. Suppuration occurs in as many as 50%

Table 36–2. Inguinal Adenopathy

Disease	Clinical History and Presentation	Diagnostic Tests*
Sexually Transmitted		
Primary syphilis	Sexual contact with infected person; painless genital chancre; painless bilateral adenopathy	Positive dark-field microscopic examination of chancre; positive serologic test (positive VDRL 78% and FTA-abs 85%)
Herpes simplex virus infection	Sexual contact with infected person; painful vesicular eruption; painful bilateral adenopathy; low grade fever or malaise	Positive culture of vesicle
Gonorrhea	Sexual contact with infected person; urethral discharge; pelvic pain; painful bilateral adenopathy	Positive culture of cervical or urethral discharge
Chancroid	Male with poor hygiene; single painful ulcer; painful unilateral adenopathy	Evidence of gram-negative coccobacilli or culture of *Hemophilus ducreyi* from ulcer
Lymphogranuloma venereum	Chancre often unnoticed; painful unilateral adenopathy with bubo formation; proctitis, rectal abscess, or fistula; constitutional symptoms	Positive complement fixation titers; leukocytosis; elevated ESR in secondary stage
Granuloma inguinale	Chronic painless indolent ulcer	Donovan bodies on Wright's stain
Nonsexually Transmitted		
Lower extremity infection	Findings suggestive of infection	Leukocytosis; positive cultures
Cat-scratch disease	Prior cat scratch to lower extremity; mild constitutional symptoms	Diagnosis of exclusion; skin test not readily available
Bubonic plague	Flea bite 2–7 days before painful adenopathy; nausea, vomiting, diarrhea	Positive culture of blood and nodal aspirate
Tularemia	Contact with wild mammals or tics; painless ulcerated papule at inoculation site	Four-fold rise in agglutination titers
Lymphoma	Constitutional symptoms; night sweats; pruritus	Anemia; elevated ESR; elevated hepatic transaminase level; positive lymph node biopsy
Pelvic malignancy	Constitutional symptoms; vaginal bleeding; pelvic mass	Anemia; mass on pelvic ultrasound or computed tomographic scan

*VDRL, Venereal Disease Research Laboratory test; FTA-abs, fluorescent antibody absorbed test; ESR, erythrocyte sedimentation rate.

of infected patients. Diagnosis rests on finding gram-negative coccobacilli or by tissue culture of the organism *Haemophilus ducreyi*.

Lymphogranuloma venereum, caused by *Chlamydia trachomatis*, frequently presents with painful inguinal adenopathy 2 to 6 weeks after exposure. The genital chancre often goes unnoticed and the patient seeks medical attention because of the adenopathy. In 70% of cases, the adenopathy is unilateral. In men, a large, painful bubo grooved by the inguinal ligament (inguinal groove sign) may develop. This rarely occurs in women. Necrosis, suppuration, and draining fistulas mark the secondary stage of this infection, often associated with systemic symptoms, leukocytosis, and an elevated erythrocyte sedimentation rate. Con-

current proctitis, rectal abscess, or fistula may be seen, and in 5% of patients chronic adenopathy develops. Isolation of the organism from the nodal aspirate is possible in only 30% of cases. Diagnosis is made by documentation of a four-fold rise in complement fixation titers or a single titer of 1:64 or more.

The inguinal adenopathy seen in conjunction with granuloma inguinale is typically a chronic indolent enlargement caused by deposition of subcutaneous granulation tissue. The initial indurated nodule erodes into a granulomatous ulcer that is slow-growing and painless. Diagnosis rests on histologically documenting Donovan bodies with Wright's stain (clusters of blue or black organisms with a "safety pin" appearance).

Gonococcal urethritis may be associated with painful bilateral inguinal adenopathy, but, more commonly, no adenopathy is present.

NONSEXUALLY TRANSMITTED DISEASES

Infections of the lower extremities may cause inguinal adenopathy and should be carefully looked for during the physical examination. From 10 to 25% of patients with cat-scratch disease present with inguinal adenopathy, presumably related to a prior cat scratch on a lower extremity. Similarly, a bite to a lower extremity by a flea infected with *Yersinia pestis* results in bubonic plague, which is also associated with a unilateral inflammatory adenopathy. Although an uncommon disease affecting from 2 to 20 Americans yearly, mortality approaches 50 to 90% in the untreated patients. Two to 7 days after the flea bite, painful adenopathy develops in 60 to 70% of infected patients. Malaise, nausea, vomiting, diarrhea, and fever usually occur. Cultures of nodal aspirate and blood specimens are essential for an early diagnosis.

Tularemia caused by a small gram-negative coccobacillus infecting wild mammals and carried by tics is associated with an ulcerated, painless papule at the site of inoculation, followed by tender regional adenopathy in 60 to 70% of patients. The incidence of tularemia has increased steadily since 1975, with 200 to 300 cases reported yearly in the United States. As the organism is difficult to culture, diagnosis rests on documentation of a four-fold rise in agglutination titers.

In rare cases, lymphoma or pelvic malignancy may present with isolated inguinal adenopathy.

Generalized Adenopathy

Although a comprehensive discussion of generalized lymphadenopathy is beyond the scope of this chapter, the differential diagnosis is presented in Table 36–3 and is usefully divided into infectious causes, malignant tumors, collagen vascular diseases, dermopathies, and hypersensitivity reactions, which are commonly drug induced. Among gay men and intravenous drug users, generalized adenopathy may herald the onset of the acquired immunodeficiency syndrome (AIDS). In rare cases, sarcoidosis, hyperthyroidism, or the lipid storage diseases may result in generalized adenopathy.

For the purposes of this review, it is worthwhile discussing the causes of generalized adenopathy most commonly seen in primary care practice: secondary lues, lymphoma/leukemia, and infection associated with HIV.

Secondary syphilis is commonly associated with generalized firm, nontender adenopathy and constitutional symptoms. A maculopapular or pustular rash on the trunk and proximal extremities, condylomata lata in intertriginous areas (flat, grayish warts), and painless mucous patches may occur. As in a primary infection, the diagnosis is most readily accomplished by dark-field microscopic examination of skin or mucous membrane lesions. The VDRL has a 97% sensitivity rate in secondary infection but may be negative in the patient with AIDS. It is important to note that nonpathogenic treponemes from the mouth may give false-positive results.

Lymphomas and leukemias are varied in presentation. Although regional adenopathy (e.g., cervical) is the most common presenting complaint of patients with Hodgkin's disease, the adenopathy occasionally is generalized and symmetric. Non-Hodgkin's lymphoma when generalized tends to be asymmetric, whereas leukemia in its early stages may be associated with a symmetric multicentric adenopathy. Painless rubbery nodes associated with fever, night sweats, or weight loss should raise the question of malignancy.

As the prevalence of HIV infection increases, the primary practitioner must consider the diagnosis of AIDS or AIDS-related complex (ARC) in patients at risk who present with generalized adenopathy. This group includes homosexuals, bisexuals, intravenous drug users, persons who have had sexual contact with HIV-infected individuals, and recipients of blood products. The incidence of generalized adenopathy in this population is unknown, and it is unclear what percentage of patients with adenopathy progress to opportunistic infection or neoplasm. For an in-depth discussion of the HIV-related lymphadenopathy syndrome, refer to Chapter 37.

Use of Diagnostic Tests

A logical approach to a diagnostic evaluation must take into account the salient features of each patient's history combined with the clinical features of adenopathy. As it is neither cost efficient nor acceptable to patients to do an exhaustive evaluation at the first discovery

Table 36–3. Generalized Lymphadenopathy

Disease	Clinical History and Presentation	Diagnostic Tests
Infectious		
Bacteremia	Fever; evidence of localized infection; intravenous drug use; constitutional symptoms	Leukocytosis; positive blood cultures
Miliary tuberculosis	Exposure to infected person; pulmonary or constitutional symptoms	Positive tuberculin; abnormal chest x-ray; positive acid-fast bacilli on sputum smear
Brucellosis	Ingestion of contaminated milk products or infected meat; fever; sweats; myalgias; weight loss; splenomegaly	Positive agglutination test; culture positive in only 15–20%
Leptospirosis	Contact with infected animal or contaminated soil or water; headache; myalgias; fever; conjunctival suffusion; jaundice, meningitis	Positive agglutination test or culture; neutrophilia; proteinuria; urinary casts; hyperbilirubinemia
Secondary syphilis	History of genital chancre, papulosquamous rash involving palms and soles, condylomata lata, painless mucous patches	Positive serologic test (positive VDRL 97% and FTA 99%)
Histoplasmosis	Eastern and Midwestern United States; contact with infected soil; systemic symptoms; hepatosplenomegaly	Anemia; leukopenia; positive culture
Mononucleosis syndromes (EBV, cytomegalovirus)	Fever; pharyngitis; constitutional symptoms; nausea; anorexia	Leukocytosis, atypical lymphocytosis; elevated hepatic transaminase level; positive Monospot or heterophil test (EBV); rise in complement-fixing titers (cytomegalovirus)
Hepatitis B	Intravenous drug use; sexual contact with infected person; nausea; anorexia; malaise; jaundice	Elevated hepatic transaminase level; positive hepatitis B surface antigen
AIDS or AIDS-related complex	Intravenous drug use; sexual contact with infected person; recipient of blood products; constitutional signs and symptoms; seborrhea; oral thrush; herpes zoster	Anemia; neutropenia; elevated ESR; anergy; positive HIV antibody
Malignancy		
Leukemia (chronic lymphocytic)	See Table 36–1	
Lymphoma	See Table 36–1	
Inflammatory		
Systemic lupus erythematosus	Young woman; history of rash, arthritis, fever, malaise	Positive result for double-stranded DNA; anemia, positive antinuclear antibody or lupus erythematosus preparation, abnormal urinalysis
Rheumatoid arthritis	Woman with migratory asymmetric polyarthritis; pain and morning stiffness	Positive rheumatoid factor; mild anemia; increased ESR
Sarcoidosis	Pulmonary or constitutional; skin lesions; uveitis	Abnormal chest x-ray; anemia; hypercalcemia; elevated serum angiotensin-converting enzyme; anergy
Miscellaneous		
Hyperthyroidism	Weight loss; diarrhea; insomnia; tremor; exophthalmos	Elevated thyroid function tests
Eczema and chronic dermopathies	Chronic skin rash	—
Angioimmunoblastic reactions	Fever; constitutional symptoms; rash; hepatosplenomegaly	Hemolytic anemia; lymphopenia; hypergammaglobulinemia
Phenytoin (Dilantin) hypersensitivity	Dilantin exposure; constitutional symptoms may be present	Eosinophilia
Serum sickness	Drug exposure; fever; arthralgias; rash; edema	Leukocytosis; proteinuria; hypergammaglobulinemia

Table 36–4. Diagnostic Yield of Lymph
Node Biopsy

Biopsy Results	%
Diagnostic	50–63
Nondiagnostic	37–53
Children, excellent prognosis	—
Adults, disease will develop	25–50
Adults, lymphoma will develop	20
Problems in diagnosis include	
Poor choice of biopsy site	
Poor surgical technique	
Poor processing	
Poor interpretation	

of adenopathy, the practitioner must determine the extent and rapidity of diagnostic testing to use in each individual case.

If the adenopathy is regional, an initial search for an infectious process frequently leads to a diagnosis. Through a detailed history and physical examination, the practitioner can narrow the realm of diagnostic possibilities and avoid unnecessary laboratory or radiographic evaluations. The history should determine sexual preference, occupational and travel history, and use of drugs, together with a complete review of systems. The presence or absence of night sweats, weight loss, fever, or rash should be documented in the history.

The initial laboratory evaluation in most patients should include a complete blood count with differential leukocyte count. A leukocytosis is suggestive of bacterial infection, whereas a neutropenia or anemia may point toward malignancy or immunodeficiency. The presence of atypical lymphocytes suggests viral infection and a hypersensitivity reaction may be associated with eosinophilia. The sedimentation rate is often elevated in patients with malignancy, collagen vascular disease, or HIV infection, and abnormalities of liver function may also be present.

Serologic tests for specific infectious agents (e.g., *Treponema pallidum*, EBV, HIV) are useful to confirm a suspected diagnosis.

A chest radiograph is often useful in that 20% of patients with lymphomas show abnormalities as do patients with sarcoidosis, fungal disease, or other malignant processes. Mammography is recommended in a woman who presents with axillary adenopathy.

Pharyngeal cultures may help to diagnose a bacterial cervical adenitis, and cervical, urethral, or anal cultures often aid in the diagnosis of inguinal adenopathy.

When To Do a Biopsy

If an infectious work-up is nondiagnostic and the patient has a persistent or progressive adenopathy of unknown cause, a biopsy is indicated. Determining exactly when to proceed with a biopsy is often difficult. As cancers are most commonly found in cervical and supraclavicular nodes, it is reasonable to do a biopsy sooner in a patient with prominent cervical nodes. A woman with prominent axillary adenopathy also warrants an early biopsy, as does an older patient with diffuse, firm adenopathy. In general, the presence of significant localized adenopathy of longer than 2 to 3 weeks' duration without a documented infectious cause is grounds for a biopsy in *all* patients, regardless of age. An exception to this is the patient with AIDS-related complex who does not routinely require a biopsy. Although the adenopathy may be associated with both neoplastic and infectious conditions, the vast majority of patients with AIDS-related complex who have a lymph node biopsy show a nonspecific pattern of lymphoid hyperplasia. The presence of diffuse adenopathy in the absence of a known drug reaction, infection, or rheumatologic disease also warrants a biopsy.

A lymph node biopsy can be an extremely useful procedure. The internist, surgeon, and pathologist should work closely from the outset to ensure maximum yield. In several recent reviews, the diagnostic yield from peripheral lymph node biopsy in adults has been shown to be 37 to 63% (Table 36–4). For patients whose initial biopsies are nondiagnostic, a repeat biopsy is often useful. From 25 to 50% of these patients will show evidence of disease on repeat biopsy, and a substantial portion (20%) of this group will be diagnosed with lymphoma. The choice of the node for the biopsy and the proper biopsy technique are crucial. In general, it is best to choose the largest accessible node. Ideally, the entire node can be dissected for delivery to the pathologist. If pus or caseation is present, smears and cultures for bacteria and fungi are indicated. Frozen sections help in the diagnosis of nonlymphomatous malignancy, whereas specially stained slides are required for the diagnosis of lymphoma.

Bibliography

Abrams DI, Lewis BJ, et al. Persistent lymphadenopathy in homosexual men: end point or prodrome. Ann Intern Med 100:801–808, 1984.

A prospective study of 70 homosexual men with unexplained persistent adenopathy. Over a 1-year period, none of the patients developed more severe manifestations of AIDS.

Doberneck RC. The diagnostic yield of lymph node biopsy. Arch Surg 118:1203–1205, 1983.

A review of results of 169 patients undergoing lymph node biopsy. The overall diagnostic yield was 70.4% with an 80.6% yield if neoplasm was suspected. The yield from supraclavicular nodes was 90%, cervical nodes 76.4%, axillary nodes 62.5%, and inguinal nodes 38.5%.

Greenfield, Jordan MC. The clinical investigation of lymphadenopathy in primary care practice. JAMA 240:1388–1393, 1978.

A useful algorithm for the investigation of lymphadenopathy in ambulatory patients. Using principles of decision analysis, initial diagnostic steps are outlined and an approach is suggested for evaluation of patients with persistent enlarged nodes.

Libman, H. Generalized lymphadenopathy. J Gen Intern Med 2:48–58, 1987.

A comprehensive review of the clinical presentation and diagnosis of the major causes of generalized adenopathy.

Saltzstein SL. The fate of patients with non-diagnostic lymph node disorders. Surgery 58:659–662, 1965.

A retrospective analysis of the outcome of 177 lymph node biopsies. Of biopsies that initially were nondiagnostic, 17% developed lymphoma.

Sinclair S, Beckman E, Ellman L. Biopsy of enlarged superficial lymph nodes. JAMA 228:602–603, 1974.

A retrospective analysis of 135 patients undergoing lymph node biopsy in which 63% of biopsies were diagnostic. Fifty patients had lymphoma, 14 carcinoma, 6 tuberculosis, 1 histoplasmosis, 7 adenitis, and 1 phenytoin (Dilantin) hypersensitivity. Of the 50 patients with nondiagnostic biopsies, 9 eventually developed lymphoma. Biopsy yield was highest from cervical and supraclavicular sites.

Slap G, Brooks J, Schwartz S. When to perform biopsies of enlarged peripheral nodes in young patients. JAMA 252:1321–1326, 1984.

A retrospective review of pathologic diagnosis and clinical findings in 123 patients between the ages of 9 and 25 who underwent lymph node biopsy. Reactive hyperplasia, Hodgkin's disease, and granulomatous disease accounted for 68% of the diagnoses. By using discriminant analysis, a predictive model was developed to aid in the selection of young patients for biopsy.

37

Medical Evaluation of the Gay Male Patient

WILLIAM F. OWEN, JR., M.D.

Introduction

During the past decade there has been a growing awareness that gay men with multiple, anonymous sex partners are at increased risk of acquiring sexually transmitted diseases, which may be symptomatic or asymptomatic.[1] Because more than 70% of those with acquired immunodeficiency syndrome (AIDS) in the United States are gay men, much attention has been focused on the sexual practices and other lifestyle factors that might be linked to transmission of the etiologic agent of AIDS, human immunodeficiency virus (HIV), and on the expression of HIV-related illness in this risk group.[2]

Indeed, the American Medical Association, through its Council on Scientific Affairs,[3] has called on physicians to recognize the special health care needs of their gay and lesbian patients through "continuing medical education on the current state of research in and knowledge of homosexuality and in the taking of an adequate sexual history" and by "educating physicians to be attuned to recognize the physical and psychological needs of their homosexual patients."

A comprehensive discussion of the health concerns of lesbians is beyond the scope of this chapter. It should be noted, however, that lesbians have less risk of developing sexually transmitted diseases than either gay men or heterosexual men and women.[4] The clinician should keep in mind that some women currently in lesbian relationships may have been active heterosexually or may be bisexually active, which would increase their risk for acquisition of sexually transmitted diseases.

Medical and Sexual History

In the late 1940's, Kinsey published his report in which he estimated that 10% of white American men were predominantly homosexual and that 37% of men surveyed had at least one homosexual experience in their lifetimes. These statistics suggest that throughout their careers, most physicians treating adult patients see many gay patients and patients who engage from time to time in homosexual activity.

Because certain stereotypes of lesbians and gay men apply to only a small minority of gay patients, most physicians are probably unaware of these encounters unless they have specifically discussed sexual orientation with their patients. Even a person who is dating or married to an individual of the opposite sex is not necessarily heterosexual. Another study by the Kinsey Institute, for example, found that 20% of gay men and 35% of lesbians had been married at least once.

Physicians must become familiar not only with the clinical aspects of the viral, bacterial, fungal, protozoal, and traumatic conditions that particularly affect gay men, but also with how to elicit a complete sexual history. Emotional stresses arising from the traditional moral and social stigmas associated with homosexuality may lead gay patients to conceal their sexual orientation from their physicians.

Sexual Orientation Inquiry

Ideally, a discussion about sexual orientation should take place at the time of an initial comprehensive history and physical examination. In many situations, however, the physician may need to take the history when the patient comes with a problem that might be related to sexual intercourse.

Preface this question and "break the ice" by a brief comment such as, "Recently, we have become aware of certain medical conditions, such as AIDS, that may be related in part to a person's sexual practices." Then ask the question about sexual orientation using one of three methods.

Method 1. Ask directly. The question, "Are you heterosexual, bisexual, or homosexual?" is awkward because many gay patients feel uncomfortable with the clinical term homosexual. Phrasing the question, "Are you gay, bi, or straight?" may convey to the gay patient a sense of empathy and understanding.

Method 2. Ask about sexual partner choice: "Have you ever had sex with men, women, both, or neither?"

Method 3. Ask in the context of lifestyle: "Is there anything about your lifestyle, such as recent travel, sexual practices, diet, or use of drugs, that might help me to diagnose your medical problem?"[5]

Past History of Disorders Associated with Sexual Contact

Inquire about past sexually transmitted diseases and related conditions (Table 37–1). Ask specific questions about each of the sexually transmissible diseases and traumatic problems, and about HIV-related conditions, including lymphadenopathy, hairy leukoplakia, and thrush. Review previous medical records to determine results of any laboratory tests that may be correlated with HIV-related conditions, such as anemia, lymphopenia, thrombocytopenia, elevated sedimentation rate, cutaneous anergy by intradermal skin testing, decreased T helper (OKT4 or Leu 3[+]) cells, and decreased ratio of helper to suppressor (OKT8 or Leu 2[+]) T lymphocytes.

Review of Systems

Do a complete inventory of systems to determine if additional medical problems are present. Clinicians treating substantial numbers of gay men often find that making several concurrent diagnoses is the rule rather than the exception.

Table 37–2 provides examples of diagnoses that may be related to sexual intercourse.

Additional diagnoses should also be considered. The final diagnosis must, as always, be based on a synthesis by the clinician of several findings from the history, physical examination, and laboratory tests.

History of Sexual Partners

Does the patient currently have one regular partner or lover and, if so, are they in a closed (monogamous) or open relationship. Ask about the number of regular and nonsteady male and female sexual partners over the previous 24 months, and, to assess whether the pattern of sexual contacts has changed over time, the number of different male and female partners or contacts since 1978.

Whenever it is determined that a patient has had only one steady sexual partner since 1977, ask whether the sexual partner has also been monogamous before assuming that the patient is not at risk for HIV infection. Seroepidemiologic data from a sexually transmitted diseases clinic in San Francisco suggest that HIV antibodies were present in only 1% of gay men in 1978. Hence the year 1977 represents a period before most of the initial cases of HIV infection began to incubate.

History of Sexual Practices

An inventory of specific sexual practices can be of invaluable assistance in determining risk factors for sexually transmitted diseases and traumatic complications. Most gay men feel comfortable using the colloquial terms for these practices (Table 37–3), so use the common terminology or the anatomic descriptors rather than formal clinical terms. If you ask, "When having sex, does your partner's penis come in contact with your anus?" you are more likely to be understood than if you ask, "Do you participate in anogenital receptive sex?"

Does the patient participate in anal insertive or receptive sex or vaginal insertive sex? If so, then inquire about the use of a condom and the type of lubricant. Water-soluble lubricants are less likely to result in condom breaks than oil-based lubricants. Lubricants containing spermicidal substances, such as nonoxynol 9, have been shown to inactivate HIV in vitro. Discuss specific sexual practices in a frank and open manner. View this exchange as an op-

Table 37–1. *Diseases in the Gay Male Associated with Sexual Activity*

Etiologic Category	Specific Disease/Site
Traditional venereal diseases	Gonorrhea
	Urethral
	Anal
	Pharyngeal
	Chlamydial infections
	Nongonococcal urethritis
	Nongonococcal proctitis
	Lymphogranuloma venereum
	Bacterial prostatitis
	Syphilis
	Stage (primary, secondary, early latent, late latent, tertiary)
	Serologic titer (most recent and current)
Viral sexually transmitted diseases	Herpes
	Penile
	Anal
	Oropharyngeal
	Condylomata
	Anal (internal or external)
	Penile (external or urethral)
	Hepatitis A
	Hepatitis B
	Hepatitis B antigen and antibody titer
	Hepatitis B vaccine if negative serologic results
	Hepatitis, non A non B
	Cytomegalovirus infection
Enteric diseases	Shigellosis
	Campylobacter infection
	Amebiasis
	Giardiasis
Ectoparasitic diseases	Scabies
	Pubic lice (crabs)
Traumatic complications of sexual intercourse	Rectal injuries
	Hemorrhoids
	Anal fissures
	Fistulas
	Foreign bodies
	Genital injuries
	Penile bites and scrapes
	Penile edema
	Urethral instrumentation
	Scrotal trauma
	Nipple injuries
	Dermatologic conditions
	Allergic reactions to lubricants
	Inhaled nitrite burns
	Sexual assault of male victim
HIV-related conditions	Generalized lymphadenopathy
	Thrush
	Hairy leukoplakia
	Anemia, leukopenia, thrombocytopenia
AIDS	Kaposi's sarcoma and other neoplasms
	Opportunistic infections

From Owen WF Jr. Med Clin North Am 70:505, 1986, with permission.

portune time to educate the gay male patient nonjudgmentally about reduction of risk.

Location of Sexual Activity

Inquire about the location of sexual activity. Multiple, anonymous sexual contacts are probably more common at bathhouses. Anonymous encounters are also likely in parks and in back rooms of adult movie theaters, adult bookstores, health clubs, and bars but are less likely to be multiple in those locations.

Use of Drugs and Alcohol

Sharing needles for intravenous drug use has been said to be a risk factor for AIDS. Alco-

Table 37–2. Review of Systems of the Gay Male

System	Symptom	Diagnostic Considerations
General	Malaise	HIV-related condition, amebiasis, hepatitis
	Fatigue	HIV-related condition, amebiasis, hepatitis
	Unexplained weight loss	HIV-related condition, lymphoma
	Fever	Syphilis, opportunistic infection, lymphoma
	Night sweats	HIV-related condition, lymphoma
Dermatologic	Ulcer	Syphilis, lymphogranuloma venereum, chancroid, herpes
	Blister	Herpes, molluscum contagiosum, solitary lesion of disseminated gonococcal infection, staphylococcal folliculitis
	Wart	Condylomata acuminatum, condylomata latum of secondary syphilis, molluscum, cutaneous amebiasis
	Body rash	Secondary syphilis, hepatitis B, cytomegalovirus,
	Facial scaling	Seborrheic dermatitis of HIV-related conditions
	Local genital itching	*Candida* dermatitis, tinea cruris, streptococcal balanitis, staphylococcal folliculitis, herpes, lubricant contact dermatitis
	Bruise or scar	Trauma, Kaposi's sarcoma, idiopathic thrombocytopenic purpura
	Yellow skin	Hepatitis
Lymphatic	Generalized node enlargement	Lymphadenopathy syndrome, cytomegalovirus, secondary syphilis, lymphoma, Kaposi's sarcoma of lymph nodes, opportunistic infection involving lymph nodes
Visual	Loss of visual field	Cytomegalovirus retinitis, toxoplasma retinitis
	Red, painful, or itchy eye	Gonococcal conjunctivitis, herpes keratitis
Cardiopulmonary	Persistent cough	*P. carinii* pneumonia, pulmonary *Mycobacterium avium intracellulare,* cytomegalovirus pneumonia
	Shortness of breath	*P. carinii* pneumonia, pulmonary *M. avium intracellulare,* cytomegalovirus pneumonia
Oral	White spots	Thrush, mucous patches of secondary syphilis
	Ulcers	Herpes, canker sores, syphilitic chancre, inhaled nitrite burns, lubricant contact stomatitis
	Sore throat	Gonococcal pharyngitis, chlamydial pharyngitis, traumatic pharyngitis from fellatio
Gastrointestinal	Pain on swallowing	*Candida* esophagitis, herpetic esophagitis
	Nausea	Hepatitis
	Flatulence	Amebiasis, giardiasis
	Diarrhea	Shigellosis, *Campylobacter* enteritis, amebiasis, giardiasis, cryptosporidiosis
Proctologic	Anal itching	Fungal infection, gonorrhea, enterobiasis, condylomata acuminatum, lubricant contact proctitis
	Anal pain	Gonorrhea, lymphogranuloma venereum or non–lymphogranuloma venereum chlamydial proctitis, syphilis, herpetic proctitis, lubricant contact proctitis, traumatic proctitis, anal cancer
	Rectal bleeding	Gonorrhea, lymphogranuloma venereum or non–lymphogranuloma venereum chlamydial proctitis, syphilis, herpetic proctitis, amebic proctitis, trauma, foreign body, condylomata acuminatum, malignancy
	Lumps in anus	Condylomata acuminatum, hemorrhoids, Kaposi's sarcoma
Genitourinary	Genital ulcer	Syphilis, lymphogranuloma venereum, chancroid, herpes
	Urethral discharge	Gonorrhea, nongonococcal chlamydial urethritis, bacterial prostatitis
	Dark urine	Hepatitis, side effect of metronidazole used for amebiasis
	Urinary hesitancy	Bacterial prostatitis, traumatic prostatitis, urethral condylomata acuminatum, herpetic proctitis, traumatic urethritis from penile rings or urethral instrumentation
Neurologic	Persistent headache	Central nervous system toxoplasmosis, cryptococcal meningitis, herpetic meningoencephalitis, central nervous system lymphoma
	Confusion	Central nervous system toxoplasmosis, cryptococcal meningitis, progressive multifocal leukoencephalopathy, central nervous system lymphoma
	Loss of balance	Central nervous system toxoplasmosis, central nervous system lymphoma
	Localized nerve pain	Herpes zoster, HIV-associated neuropathy
	Tingling down thighs	Lumbosacral radiculitis of herpetic proctitis
Musculoskeletal	Joint pains	Tenosynovitis of disseminated gonococcal infection, arthritis of hepatitis B

From Owen WF Jr. Med Clin North Am 70:507–509, 1986, with permission.

Table 37–3. Gay Male Practices and Colloquial Terminology

Practice	Description	Colloquial Term	Comment
Mutual masturbation	Masturbation with partner	Jerking off; J/O; beating off	
Orogenital insertive	Insertion of penis into partner's mouth	Getting sucked	Does partner swallow semen ("cum")?
Orogenital receptive	Fellatio; insertion of partner's penis into patient's mouth	Sucking	Is partner's semen (cum) swallowed? Educate about risk of hepatitis B, cytomegalovirus, HIV transmission
Anogenital insertive	Insertion of penis into partner's rectum	Fucking	Coitus interruptus? Use of condom? Which lubricant?
Anogenital receptive	Insertion of partner's penis into patient's rectum	Getting fucked	Does partner use condom? Which lubricant? Use enema? Douche? Educate about risk of hepatitis B, cytomegalovirus, HIV transmission
Oroanal insertive	Anilinction; insertion of tongue into partner's anus	Rimming	Educate about transmission of enteric diseases, hepatitis A
Oroanal receptive	Insertion of partner's tongue into patient's anus	Getting rimmed	
Anodigital insertive	Insertion of finger into partner's rectum	Finger play; finger fucking	
Anodigital receptive	Insertion of partner's finger into patient's rectum	Partner lubricating rectum; getting finger fucked	Consider possibility of anorectal gonorrhea even if not anogenital receptive
Anomanual insertive	Insertion of hand or arm into partner's rectum	Fisting; fist fucking; handballing	Educate about possibility of trauma and transmission of HIV through contact of broken skin and rectal mucosa
Anomanual receptive	Insertion of partner's hand or arm into patient's rectum	Getting fisted	
Urination on/into partner	Urinating on partner or into partner's mouth or rectum	Giving water sports; golden showers	Educate about viral transmission via urine
Being urinated on/into	Patient being urinated on or receiving urine into mouth or rectum	Receiving water sports	
Erotic aids; erectile aids; dildoes	Using sexual appliances with masturbation or sex	Toys (tit or cock rings); dildoes	Caution against sharing; educate about trauma
Sadism; masochism; bondage; discipline	Using varying levels of sadomasochism or sadomasochistic fantasies	S/M (light or heavy); B&D	Determine type(s) and whether pain inflicted or received

From Owen WF Jr. Med Clin North Am 70:509, 1986, with permission.

hol, marijuana, sedatives, stimulants (e.g., cocaine and amphetamines, with street names such as MDA and crystal), and hallucinogens (e.g., LSD and phencyclidine, colloquially referred to as angel dust) may have a disinhibiting effect that might make some gay men more likely to engage in high risk sexual practices in which they otherwise would not. Inhaled amyl or isobutyl nitrites (colloquially, poppers) are also used by some gay men to cause a euphoric "rush" and facilitate anal sphincter relaxation during anal receptive intercourse. Anabolic steroids are used by some homosexual men to facilitate body building. Estrogens, however, do not appear to be abused by gay men. The effect of substance abuse on cellular immunity has not been adequately studied, but many clinicians working with HIV-infected patients are concerned that they might serve as cofactors in cellular immunosuppression. Advise your patients that it is best to avoid these substances.

Healthy Lifestyle Factors

Inquire about general measures, such as nutrition, exercise, rest, and stress reduction, that contribute to overall general health and are probably important in sustaining a healthy immune system. Ask about the duration and quality of sleep. Emphasize the importance of a regular exercise program, including aerobic exercise if indicated. Make a general assessment of the mood of the patient, with particular attention to any specific life stresses.

Sexual Identity and Sexual Dysfunction

Gay patients often consult their physicians because of concerns about sexual identity and sexual dysfunction. Reassure the gay patient who is just becoming aware of his or her identity ("coming out") that homosexuality is a normal variant rather than a medical illness. Refer the patient to the appropriate local service agencies and gay community organizations that have developed in recent years. These groups may be located through the National Gay and Lesbian Task Force Helpline at 1–800–221–7044. Refer patients with sexual dysfunctions to professional personnel who are as psychosexually objective with gay patients as they are with heterosexual patients with similar sexual dysfunctions.

Social Networks and Support Systems

Determine the support system of the gay patient. In times of crisis, patients may turn to parents, ex-wives and ex-husbands, children, lovers, former lovers, gay and non-gay friends, or, in certain metropolitan communities, volunteer organizations that have been established under the impetus of the AIDS crisis.

Encourage use of the Durable Power of Attorney for Health Care in those states that have enacted this law. If the patient is unable to make decisions regarding his health care, the Durable Power of Attorney grants this responsibility to an individual designated by the patient. The form also allows the patient to express his opinion about the use of life support equipment.

Confidentiality

Health care professionals have the responsibility to guarantee that knowledge of the sexual orientation of a patient remains inviolable. Homosexual intercourse is still illegal in many jurisdictions and is a cause for discharge from the U.S. military. Open or even presumed homosexuality has resulted in exclusion from certain fields of employment and in actual loss of jobs and housing.

Many gay patients are concerned about the issue of documentation of sexual orientation or of HIV antibody status. In certain medical practices, physicians have agreed informally on a coding system rather than writing homosexual or gay in the medical record. At the present time, it is best to keep HIV antibody status out of the medical record because many patients fear that such results could be used as conditions of employment or insurability or even as surrogate markers of homosexuality by governmental agencies charged with enforcing laws and regulations that relate to gay individuals. The physician might explain this position to the patient and ask him to remind the physician of his HIV antibody status whenever he returns for a visit. Alternatively, some practices keep a coded list of antibody test results that is separate from the medical record. The key for such a list should be kept in a separate locked site that is accessible only to physicians who have a need for this information.

Physical Examination

A number of diagnostic considerations may be suggested by physical findings (Table 37–4). Look for clues to HIV-related conditions such as persistent fevers, abnormal loss of weight, thrush, hairy leukoplakia, generalized lymphadenopathy, and violaceous macules or papules.

Anoscopy should be used for patients who have anorectal symptoms, who are anal receptive contacts of individuals with sexually transmitted diseases, who have abnormalities on digital rectal examination, or who are asymptomatic but have multiple, anonymous sexual contacts. Consider using a beveled, wide diameter operating anoscope that attaches to a fiberoptic light source. This instrument affords the best view of the lower rectum and anal canal. A disadvantage of the operating anoscope is that it must be sterilized, but disposable anoscopes that attach to a fiberoptic light source are now available.

Laboratory Screening of the Asymptomatic Gay Man

Many of the infectious diseases encountered by gay men may be present without associated

Table 37–4. Physical Examination of the Gay Male

Region	Sign	Diagnostic Considerations
Vital signs	Unexplained loss of weight	AIDS-related condition, lymphoma
	Fever	Syphilis, opportunistic infection, lymphoma
	Tachypnea	*P. carinii* pneumonia, pulmonary *Mycobacterium avium intracellulare*, cytomegalovirus pneumonia
Skin	Ulcer	Syphilis, lymphogranuloma venereum, chancroid, herpes
	Vesicle	Herpes simplex, herpes zoster, molluscum contagiosum, solitary lesion of disseminated gonococcal infection, staphylococcal folliculitis
	Wart	Condylomata acuminatum, condylomata latum of secondary syphilis, molluscum contagiosum, cutaneous amebiasis
	Generalized maculopapular rash	Secondary syphilis, hepatitis B, cytomegalovirus
	Localized genital rash	*Candida* dermatitis, tinea cruris, streptococcal balanitis, staphylococcal folliculitis, herpes simplex, lubricant contact dermatitis
	Purpura	Idiopathic thrombocytopenic purpura
	Violaceous papule, macule, or nodule	Ecchymosis or scar from trauma, Kaposi's sarcoma
	Jaundice	Hepatitis
Lymph nodes	Generalized lymphadenopathy	Lymphadenopathy syndrome, cytomegalovirus secondary syphillis, lymphoma, Kaposi's sarcoma of lymph nodes, opportunistic infection involving lymph nodes
	Regional inguinal lymphadenopathy	Primary syphilis, lymphogranuloma venereum, granuloma inguinale, fungal dermatitis, herpes simplex proctitis
Eyes	Cotton wool spots	Cytomegalovirus retinitis
	Keratitis	Herpes simplex
	Conjunctivitis	Gonococcal conjunctivitis
Chest	High pitched dry cough	*P. carinii* pneumonia
Mouth	White plaques	Thrush, mucous patches of secondary syphilis
	Ulcerations	Herpes simplex, canker sores, syphilitic chancre, inhaled nitrite burns, lubricant contact stomatitis
	Pharyngitis	Gonococcal pharyngitis, chlamydial pharyngitis, traumatic pharyngitis from fellatio
Abdomen	Hyperactive bowel sounds	Amebiasis, giardiasis, shigellosis, *Campylobacter* infections, cryptosporidiosis
	Hepatomegaly	Hepatitis
	Splenomegaly	Idiopathic thrombocytopenic purpura, HIV-related conditions, lymphoma
Anorectum	Perianal dermatitis	Fungal infections, herpes simplex, staphylococcal folliculitis, enterobiasis, lubricant contact dermatitis
	Perianal ulcerations	Herpes simplex, syphilitic chancre, lymphogranuloma venereum, anal fissures, anal fistulas
	Proctitis with mucus and friability	Gonorrhea, lymphogranuloma venereum or non–lymphogranuloma venereum chlamydial proctitis, syphilis, herpetic proctitis, amebic proctitis, trauma
	Warts	Condylomata acuminatum, condylomata lata
	Polypoid lesions	Condylomata acuminatum, polyps, hypertrophied papillae, neoplasia
	Violaceous anorectal macules	Trauma, Kaposi's sarcoma
	Prostate tenderness	Bacterial prostatitis, traumatic prostatitis
Genitalia	Genital ulcer	Syphilis, lymphogranuloma venereum, chancroid, herpes simplex, trauma
	Urethral discharge	Gonorrhea, nongonococcal chlamydial urethritis, bacterial prostatitis
	Urethral wart	Urethral condylomata acuminatum
	Penile edema	Edema from chronic use of penile rings

Table continued on following page

Table 37–4. Physical Examination of the Gay Male Continued

Region	Sign	Diagnostic Considerations
Neurologic system	Meningeal signs	Cryptococcal meningitis, herpetic meningoencephalitis, central nervous system toxoplasmosis, central nervous system lymphoma
	Disorientation	Central nervous system toxoplasmosis, cryptococcal meningitis, progressive multifocal leukoencephalopathy, central nervous system lymphoma
	Peripheral neuropathy	Herpes zoster, HIV-associated neuropathy, lumbosacral radiculitis of herpetic proctitis
	Ataxia	Central nervous system toxoplasmosis, central nervous system lymphoma
Extremities	Arthritis	Tenosynovitis of disseminated gonococcal infection, arthritis of hepatitis B

From Owen WF Jr. Med Clin North Am 70:514–515, 1986, with permission.

symptoms. The site of certain sexually transmitted diseases is determined by the occurrence of specific sexual practices (e.g., anal infection with *Chlamydia*). In addition, some infections (e.g., HIV infection) are often present for many years before symptoms develop, whereas others (e.g., urethral gonorrhea) have short incubation periods. To help decide which sexually transmitted diseases to screen for, obtain a careful history of sexual partners and practices.

Low Risk Group for HIV and for Recent Sexually Transmitted Disease

Gay men in this group have been celibate since 1977, monogamous since 1977 with one partner who is also known to have been monogamous since 1977, or have engaged only in no risk sexual activities (Table 37–5). Therefore, there is little risk of HIV infection in this category, but activities of the patient or of a partner prior to 1978 may have exposed the individual to syphilis or to hepatitis B. Screen for antibody to hepatitis B core antigen (anti-HB_c) to determine if the patient has been exposed to hepatitis B (Fig. 37–1). Review previous medical records to see if this screen for anti-HB_c has already been done and to avoid duplication of expensive tests. Because of the possibility that the patient's sexual practices might change in the future, consider recommending hepatitis B vaccine if anti-HB_c is negative. If anti-HB_c is positive, obtain hepatitis B surface antigen (HB_sAg) test to evaluate for the chronic hepatitis B carrier state. Also obtain a baseline syphilis serologic assay to detect late latent syphilis (Fig. 37–2).

High Risk for HIV but Low Risk for Recent Sexually Transmitted Disease

Gay men in this category have been following the no risk or low risk guidelines in recent years. Previous sexual activities of the patient

Table 37–5. Safer Sex Guidelines for HIV Risk Reduction

No Risk	Low Risk
Social dry kissing	Anal intercourse with latex condom*
Body massage	
Hugging	Vaginal intercourse with latex condom*
Body rubbing	
Using one's own sex toys	Orogenital contact before climax
Mutual masturbation	Orogenital contact with latex condom*
	Mouth-to-mouth kissing
	Oral vaginal contact with barrier
	Oral anal contact with barrier
	Anomanual contact with glove*
	Vaginal-manual contact with glove*

Moderate Risk	High Risk
Oral genital contact with climax	Anal receptive contact without condom
Oral anal contact	Anal insertive contact without condom
Oral vaginal contact	
Anomanual contact	Vaginal intercourse without condom
Sharing sex toys	
Ingestion of urine	

Modified from Scientific Affairs Committee of Bay Area Physicians for Human Rights. Safe sex guidelines for persons at risk for AIDS, in Campbell JM (ed). Medical Evaluation of Persons at Risk of Human Immunodeficiency Virus Infection. San Francisco, Bay Area Physicians for Human Rights, 1987, pp 15–17, with permission.
*Latex (not "natural" or intestinal) condom; condoms should always be used with a water-soluble lubricant containing nonoxynol 9, a spermicide.

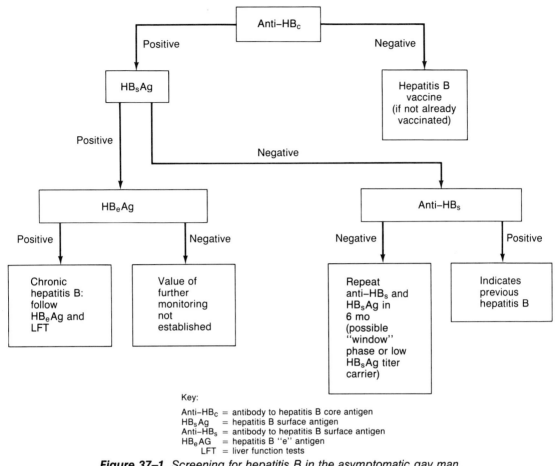

Key:

Anti–HB$_c$ = antibody to hepatitis B core antigen
HB$_s$Ag   = hepatitis B surface antigen
Anti–HB$_s$ = antibody to hepatitis B surface antigen
HB$_e$AG   = hepatitis B "e" antigen
     LFT   = liver function tests

Figure 37–1. *Screening for hepatitis B in the asymptomatic gay man.*

or of a partner, however, place men in this group at risk for HIV infection.

In addition to screening for hepatitis B (Fig. 37–1) and syphilis (Fig. 37–2), recommend that the patient obtain the enzyme-linked immunosorbent assay (ELISA) for HIV. In addition to concerns about confidentiality of medical records, many gay men are concerned about the anxiety associated with learning that their HIV antibody test is positive. Be prepared to counsel patients at length about the pros and cons of obtaining the HIV antibody test and about the meaning of a positive or negative test result. Suggest that the patient obtain the test results in the presence of a friend.

After confirming a positive HIV antibody test, do a careful physical examination, with particular attention paid to findings associated with AIDS-related complex in the skin (seborrheic dermatitis, perianal herpes simplex, dermatomal scars secondary to herpes zoster and onychomycosis), oral mucosa (thrush and hairy leukoplakia), and reticuloendothelial system (persistent generalized lymphadenopathy and

splenomegaly). Obtain a quantitative helper T lymphocyte (OKT4 or Leu 3$^+$) count along with a baseline complete blood count with differential count, platelet count, erythrocyte sedimentation rate (ESR), and chemistry panel (Fig. 37–3). Leukopenia, lymphopenia, an elevated ESR, elevated globulin level, very low total serum cholesterol level, and abnormal liver enzymes are frequently seen around or just before development of clinical manifestations of HIV infection. Analysis of T lymphocyte subsets (including OKT4) is now generally available from larger commercial laboratories and university medical centers and costs approximately $100 (US).

Some clinicians also recommend testing the HIV-positive patient for tuberculin skin test reactivity because patients with HIV infections have a higher incidence of tuberculosis, and treating tuberculin reactive patients with prophylactic isoniazid. Unfortunately, HIV-positive patients also have a high incidence of cutaneous anergy related to cellular immuno-

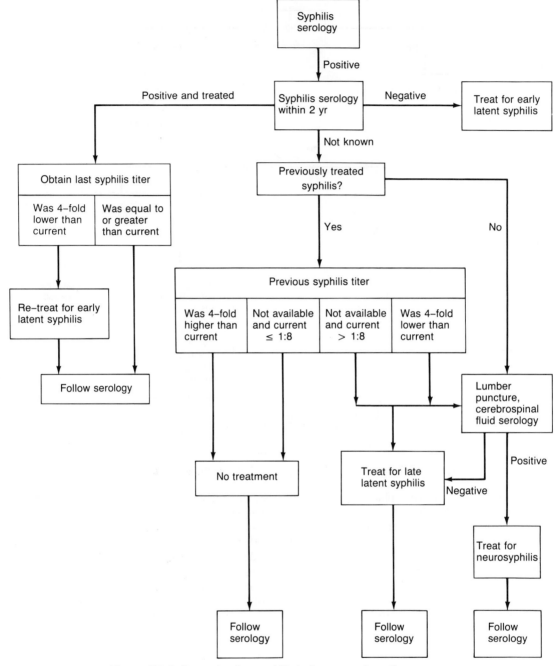

Figure 37–2. Screening for syphilis in the asymptomatic gay man.

deficiency, which results in many false-negative tuberculin skin tests.

Whatever the OKT4 level is, discuss implications of this result in the context of the symptoms, physical findings, and laboratory tests and emphasize the importance of risk reduction. If the OKT4 is less than 200 and signs of AIDS-related complex are present, recommend zidovudine (formerly called azidothymidine, AZT). The clinical manifestations of AIDS-related complex are frequently observed when the OKT4 is between 200 and 400. If the patient has between 200 and 300 helper T cells (low AIDS-related complex range), re-examine and repeat the OKT4 level in 3 months; between 300 and 500 helper T

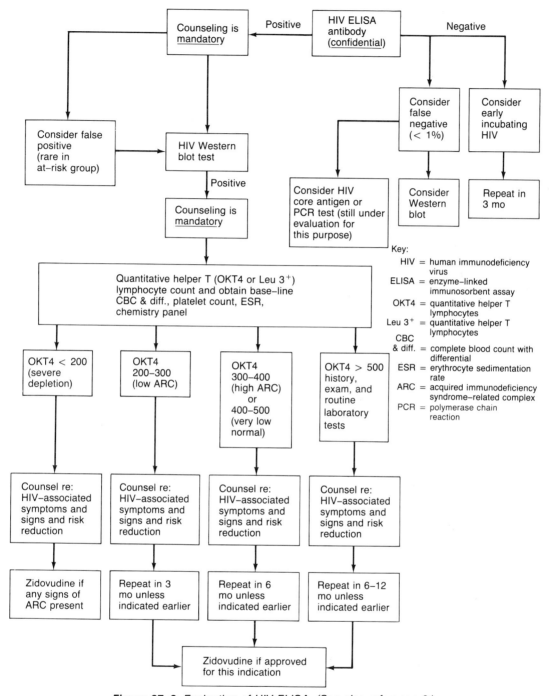

Figure 37–3. *Evaluation of HIV ELISA. (See also reference 6.)*

lymphocytes (high AIDS-related complex to low normal range), re-examine and repeat the OKT4 in 6 months; and above 500 helper T cells, repeat the examination and OKT4 in 6 to 12 months. Repeat the examination and assay for OKT4 level earlier if clinically indicated. The prognostic utility of the HIV core (p24) antigen and antibody tests and the beta₂-microglobulin level is currently under investigation. Preliminary reports indicate that individuals with high levels of p24 antigen and low levels of p24 antibody or with elevated levels of beta₂-microglobulin are at significantly higher risk for progression to full-blown AIDS compared with HIV-infected persons who are p24 antigen negative and have high levels of p24 antibody and low levels of beta$_2$-microglobulin.[7]

Studies are presently under way to determine if antiviral agents (e.g., zidovudine) are effective in slowing the progression of asymptomatic HIV antibody–positive patients to full blown AIDS. Therefore, new recommendations for evaluating and treating these patients are also likely to be made in the near future. Primary care physicians who infrequently care for HIV-positive patients should consult with colleagues who are familiar with zidovudine and its side effects before prescribing this drug. Zidovudine has been associated with significant hematologic side effects, including severe neutropenia and anemia, that frequently require red blood cell transfusions, reduction of the dosage, or even discontinuation of the medication. Patients receiving zidovudine should have a complete blood count with differential biweekly and a chemistry panel and platelet count monthly.

High Risk for HIV and for Recent Sexually Transmitted Disease

This group consists of asymptomatic gay men who have had one or more moderate risk or high risk contacts in recent months. In addition to screening for hepatitis B (Fig. 37–1), syphilis (Fig. 37–2), and HIV (Fig. 37–3), recommend a stool specimen for ova and parasites (with subsequent purged stool specimen if only nonpathogenic protozoa are present) and anal culture for gonorrhea (if it has been determined that the patient has engaged in anogenital, anomanual, or anodigital receptive activity since the patient's last anal culture for gonorrhea).

Safer Sex Guidelines

In counseling gay men, emphasize that reducing the risk of HIV infection may mean changing one's sexual practices, but it does not mean denying one's basic need for healthy sexual expression. Bay Area Physicians for Human Rights, founded in 1977 as the first organization of physicians in the United States dedicated to the health concerns of lesbians and gay men, has developed a set of guidelines that discuss the safety of various sexual practices based on our current knowledge of HIV transmissibility (Table 37–5).

Sexual transmission of HIV has been docu-

mented only from infected blood, semen, and vaginal secretions, which must then be introduced into the body. In the introduction to the current revision of the guidelines, the authors note that "our objective epidemiologic experience is still limited to relatively small numbers of people and short periods of time for observation, and these recommendations may require modification based on future experience."[8]

Prevention of HIV Transmission in Health Care Settings

Epidemiologic evidence has implicated only blood, semen, vaginal secretions, and possibly breast milk in transmission of HIV. The increasing prevalence of HIV increases the risk that health care personnel will be exposed to blood from HIV-infected patients, particularly if blood precautions are not adhered to. Health care personnel should consider *all* patients as potentially infected with HIV and should follow precautions to minimize risk of exposure to blood and other body fluids (Table 37–6).[9]

Clinical Syndromes

The infections encountered by gay men may be grouped conveniently into several syndromes based on the organ system involved and on clinical manifestations. The syndromes may be clustered into two groups based on association with HIV. Some causative agents are found in both groups (e.g., herpes simplex virus infections).

Syndromes Related to HIV

FEBRILE SYNDROME (Table 37–7 and Fig. 37–4)

It is important to look first for potentially life-threatening infections, such as *Pneumocystis carinii* pneumonia, infections causing acute appendicitis, and bacterial septicemia. In my experience, certain bacterial infections, such as those causing acute appendicitis or related to anorectal fistulas, and bacterial sepsis, are encountered more commonly in HIV-positive patients than in the rest of the population. The first diagnosis to be considered in the patient who is at risk for AIDS, however, is *P. carinii* pneumonia, the most common of the oppor-

Table 37–6. Prevention of HIV Transmission in Health Care Settings

Category	Preventive Practice
Barrier precautions	1. Wear gloves when touching blood or body fluids or items soiled with blood or body fluids for *all* patients. 2. Wear gloves for venipuncture, vascular access, and all invasive procedures including vaginal and cesarean deliveries. 3. Change gloves between examining patients and when a glove is torn or a sharp injury occurs. 4. Wear masks, goggles, or face shields during procedures that generate droplet particles. 5. Wear gowns or aprons during procedures that generate splashes of blood or other secretions, including vaginal and cesarean deliveries.
Hand washing	1. Wash immediately if contaminated with blood and other body fluids. 2. Wash immediately after gloves are removed. 3. Always wash hands between examining patients.
Prevention of injury by sharp implements	1. Do not recap, bend, or break needles by hand. 2. Do not remove needles from disposable syringes. 3. Place the syringe-needle unit and scalpel blades in puncture-resistant containers located close to the use area.
Handling of laboratory specimens	1. Place specimen in a well-constructed container with a secure lid. 2. Wear gloves when processing all specimens and change gloves and wash hands after completion. 3. Wear masks and goggles if mucous membrane contact is anticipated. 4. If a spill of blood or other body secretions occurs, decontaminate surfaces with a tuberculocidal germicide or household bleach (1:10 dilution). 5. Consider blood and body fluids of *all* patients to be infective. (This eliminates the need for warning labels.)
Resuscitation devices	1. Place resuscitation mouthpieces, bags, and other ventilation devices in areas where need for their use is predictable.
Health care personnel	1. If exudative lesions or weeping dermatitis is present, refrain from all direct patient care and handling patient care equipment until the condition resolves. 2. Pregnant personnel are not at increased risk, but because an HIV-infected person can transmit HIV perinatally, pregnant health care personnel must also strictly adhere to these precautions.

tunistic infections. Ask the patient whether he has a cough or shortness of breath. Rarely, this pneumonia presents with fever only and without respiratory manifestations. In this circumstance, pulmonary uptake seen on a gallium radionuclide scan may lead the clinician to consider *P. carinii* pneumonia.

The history and physical examination may also provide clues to the origin of the fever. Ask about medications frequently used for AIDS-related infections (e.g., trimethoprim-

sulfamethoxazole, penicillins, rifampin, and ansamycin), which are often associated with fever. During the physical examination, check for local sites of infection (e.g., rectal abscesses) or neoplasm (e.g., change in size or texture of a previously stable lymph node).

Do blood cultures to look for bacterial or atypical mycobacterial sepsis, as well as for clues to viral and deep mycotic infections. Do a gallium scan to look for occult sources of fever (e.g., *P. carinii* pneumonia or non-Hodg-

Table 37–7. Febrile Syndrome Related to HIV

> *P. carinii* pneumonia
> Atypical mycobacterial infections
> Cytomegalovirus infections
> Deep mycoses
> Non-Hodgkin's lymphoma
> Toxoplasmosis
> Nonopportunistic bacterial infections
>   Acute appendicitis
>   Catheter-associated septicemia
> HIV-associated fever
> Drug fevers

Table 37–8. Respiratory Syndrome Related to HIV

> *P. carinii* pneumonia
> Common nonopportunistic bacterial pathogens
> *Hemophilus influenzae* pneumonia
> Pneumococcal pneumonia
> Mycoplasma pneumonia
> Legionella pneumonia
> Mycobacterial pneumonias
> Cytomegaloviral pneumonia
> Fungal pneumonias
> Pulmonary cryptococcosis
> Pulmonary histoplasmosis
> Pulmonary coccidioidomycosis
> Pulmonary non-Hodgkin's lymphoma
> Lymphocytic interstitial pneumonitis

kin's lymphoma). Do a cryptococcal antigen test to check for the presence of cryptococcal disease that requires further diagnostic evaluation.

If the fever persists, consider a magnetic resonance imaging scan of the brain. This imaging technique is far superior to the computerized tomographic scan of the brain for detecting central nervous system toxoplasmosis, lymphoma, progressive multifocal leukoencephalopathy, and HIV-associated encephalopathy.

Fever may be seen in association with HIV itself, but do not assume that HIV is the cause of the fever unless you are certain that you have excluded other sources. If further evaluation by an infectious disease consultant does not reveal a specific source of the fever, consider empiric treatment of HIV with an antiretroviral agent (e.g., zidovudine), if the patient meets other indications for use of such an agent. If the fever is causing significant discomfort to the patient, also consider use of a nonsteroidal anti-inflammatory agent such as ibuprofen 600 mg orally every 8 hours or sustained-release indomethacin 75 mg orally every 12 hours.

RESPIRATORY SYNDROME (Table 37–8 and Fig. 37–5)

Dyspnea on exertion is a frequent symptom of *P. carinii* pneumonia. Ask the patient whether he notices slight shortness of breath on walking a flight of stairs or after walking from his car to your office. A cough that occurs after deep inspiration is another suggestive finding. Obtain a chest film, serum lactate dehydrogenase (LDH) test, ESR, and arterial blood gas or oxygen saturation assay by pulse oximetry, $A-a$ O_2 gradient, or diffusing capacity (DL_{CO}). Assuming that one has baseline measures, a rise in lactate dehydrogenase level and ESR is typically observed in patients developing this pneumonia. The magnitude of

rise of the lactate dehydrogenase is directly proportional to the extent of *P. carinii* pneumonia.

If these tests are abnormal or if the patient has persistent cough, dyspnea, or fever, induce a sputum sample for Toluidine Blue stain, Giemsa's stain, or a monoclonal antibody stain for *P. carinii*. To obtain a sputum specimen that is more likely to be of diagnostic value, request that a respiratory therapist treat the patient with intermittent positive pressure breathing using a bronchodilator such as albuterol. The therapist should follow the bronchodilator treatment with a nebulized saline mist treatment, while encouraging the patient to cough.

If the induced sputum does not reveal *P. carinii* or other causative organisms, request that a chest disease consultant do an endobronchial lavage. (Note: some clinicians would do a gallium radionuclide scan first, although this procedure adds 24 to 72 hours and several hundred dollars to the evaluation.) If the lavage does not reveal *P. carinii* and cough and dyspnea persist, proceed to bronchoscopy with biopsy and, if necessary, to open lung biopsy. It is important to confirm the diagnosis of *P. carinii* pneumonia, at least at the first such episode, because the microscopic diagnosis confirms the presence of AIDS and is often required for therapeutic drug trials.

Although cytomegalovirus is frequently isolated from endobronchial lavage cultures, the diagnosis of this type of pneumonia may be made only on the basis of histopathologic examination for the typical inclusion bodies. Lymphocytic interstitial pneumonitis (also referred to as nonspecific interstitial pneumonitis) is a diagnosis generally made on the basis of open lung biopsy and is thought to be caused directly by HIV.

If there is any question about the patient's

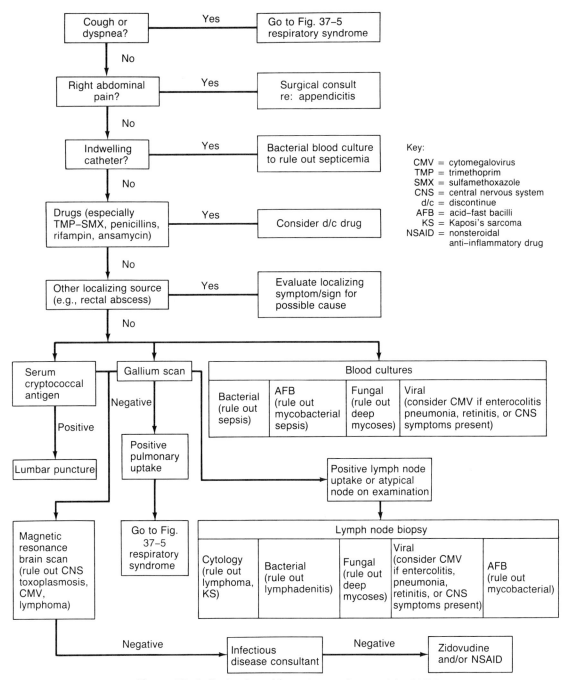

Figure 37–4. Evaluation of fever in a patient at risk of HIV.

respiratory status (e.g., Po$_2$ < 70 in a non-smoker at sea level), then admit him to the hospital at least for the first week of treatment. Some clinicians believe that the cure rate for pentamidine against *P. carinii* pneumonia is greater than that for trimethoprim-sulfamethoxazole and is not associated with the drug rash and fever that frequently occur in the second or third week of the oral therapy. The oral treatment, however, is easier to use on an outpatient basis and is less expensive.

DIARRHEAL SYNDROME (Table 37–9 and Fig. 37–6)

Diarrhea is a frequent complaint of many patients with AIDS. Diarrhea may herald the

Table 37-9. *Diarrheal Syndrome Related to HIV*

Cytomegaloviral enterocolitis
Mycobacterial enterocolitis
Nonopportunistic bacterial enteritis
    Shigellosis
    Campylobacter infections
    Clostridium difficile enterotoxin
Nonopportunistic protozoal infections
    Amebiasis
    Giardiasis
    Blastocystis hominis enterocolitis
Cryptosporidiosis
Gastrointestinal non-Hodgkin's lymphoma

onset of a new opportunistic infection or enteric pathogen, or it may be chronic, requiring management as a symptom after careful evaluation for and treatment of any causative agents. Diarrhea not associated with any specific pathogen is sometimes present for several days before development of the cough and dyspnea that are characteristic of *P. carinii* pneumonia.

Do a stool culture and up to three stool analyses for ova and parasites. Be sure to culture for *Campylobacter jejuni* and request an analysis for *Cryptosporidium* on the stool ova and parasite examination. If the patient has been taking antibiotics, request a stool analysis for the toxin produced by *Clostridium difficile*.

If the stool culture and ova and parasite test are negative and diarrhea persists, use sigmoidoscopy to determine if proctitis (inflammation of the anus and rectum) or proctocolitis (inflammation of the bowel beyond 15 cm) is present. Perform a biopsy of the inflamed area and send for a bacterial culture, *Chlamydia* culture or immunofluorescent smear, acid-fast bacterial smear and culture, fungal culture, and viral culture. Ask the pathologist to look specifically for protozoa (particularly *Cryptosporidium*), cytomegalovirus inclusion bodies, and neoplasms (particularly Kaposi's sarcoma and non-Hodgkin's lymphoma).

If sigmoidoscopic results are normal or rectal biopsy does not reveal a causative organism and diarrhea persists, request gastroduodenoscopy with biopsy. Send the biopsy material for bacterial culture, acid-fast smear and culture, fungal culture, and viral culture. Ask the pathologist to look for cytomegalovirus inclusion bodies, *Cryptosporidium*, and neoplasms (particularly Kaposi's sarcoma and non-Hodgkin's lymphoma).

When diarrhea persists, either because a cause cannot be found, or because of a lack of response to specific antimicrobial therapy, empiric treatment with a nonsteroid anti-inflammatory drug is sometimes useful, particularly if there is no response to opiate antidiarrheal agents. Sustained-release indomethacin 75 mg orally every 12 hours is a regimen that appears to decrease diarrhea by its prostaglandin-inhibiting mechanism.

ORAL MUCOSAL SYNDROMES

Oral Candidiasis (Thrush). Oral candidiasis is one of the most common fungal infections seen in patients with AIDS and AIDS-related complex. Look for white cottage cheese–like plaques on the palate, buccal mucosa, pharynx, gingiva, or tongue. Treat with clotrimazole oral troches one five times daily for 2 weeks. If thrush recurs, repeat treatment and consider maintenance clotrimazole, one to three oral troches daily.

Hairy Leukoplakia. Hairy leukoplakia is sometimes confused with thrush. Look for white vertical streaks or plaques along the lateral aspects of the tongue. Hairy leukoplakia has been described only in patients who have been infected with HIV, and its presence is considered to be highly associated with eventual progression to full-blown AIDS. Both Epstein-Barr virus and human papillomavirus have been isolated from hairy leukoplakia lesions. Very high dose acyclovir 800 mg orally every 4 hours around the clock for 2 weeks appears to have some activity against Epstein-Barr virus, which is a member of the herpesvirus family. Although this treatment may result in disappearance of the hairy leukoplakia, it is not known whether this effect is substantive or merely cosmetic.

Necrotizing Gingivitis. Necrotizing gingivitis can be very severe, particularly in advanced AIDS. Penicillin does not appear to be very effective. Rinsing with dilute hydrogen peroxide or povidone-iodine solutions may be of some value.

Oral Kaposi's Sarcoma. Oral Kaposi's sarcoma generally has the same purple bruise-like appearance as Kaposi's sarcoma of the skin. Radiation therapy is sometimes useful when the lesions are growing or painful.

ESOPHAGEAL SYNDROMES

Esophageal Candidiasis. Patients usually complain of dysphagia in this syndrome. Ask the gastroenterologist to look for the white plaques characteristic of esophageal candidi-

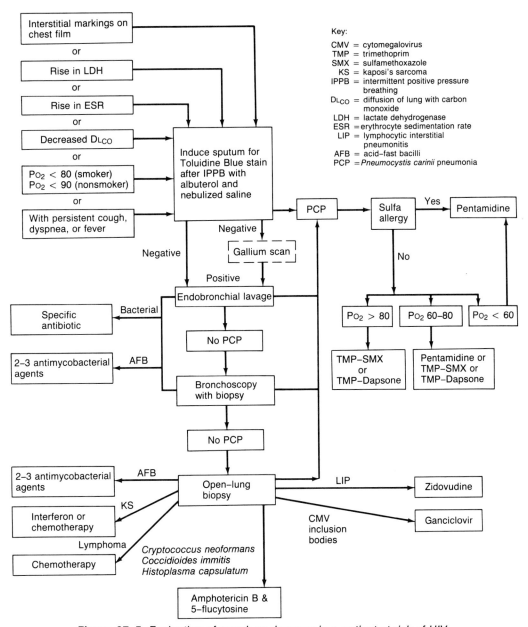

Figure 37–5. *Evaluation of cough or dyspnea in a patient at risk of HIV.*

asis during esophagogastroscopy. If these are not present, the gastroenterologist should perform a biopsy and send cultures for herpes simplex virus infection and cytomegalovirus infection.

Treat esophageal candidiasis with a 2-week course of ketoconazole 200 mg orally twice daily, followed by a maintenance regimen of clotrimazole oral troches five times daily. If odynophagia recurs, repeat treatment with ketoconazole and consider a maintenance program of ketoconazole 200 mg orally daily.

Esophageal Herpes Simplex Virus Infection.

Treat with high dose acyclovir 400 mg orally every 4 hours for 10 days. If symptoms recur, repeat the treatment and consider maintenance acyclovir 200 mg or 400 mg three times daily.

Esophageal Cytomegalovirus Infection.
Treat only if characteristic inclusion bodies are present and if the patient is having severe odynophagia. Ganciclovir (9-[2-hydroxy-1-(hydroxymethyl)ethoxymethyl] guanine, formerly known as dihydroxymethylpropoxymethylguanine or DHPG) may be obtained on an investigational basis from the manufacturer, Syntex Corporation, Palo Alto, CA.

NEUROLOGIC SYNDROME
(Table 37–10 and Fig. 37–7)

Inquire whether one or more of the following symptoms are present: headaches, personality changes or depression, a decreased level of consciousness or dementia, seizures, other focal neurolgic findings, and fever.

Fever and headache are seen in cryptococcal meningitis, herpes simplex virus meningoencephalitis, and toxoplasmosis. Seizures and other focal (e.g., hemiparesis) and general (e.g., hiccups) neurologic findings are characteristic of toxoplasmosis. Changes in mental status occur in HIV encephalopathy and in progressive multifocal leukoencephalopathy but may occur in any of the other neurologic conditions associated with AIDS. Pain or paresthesias in the lower extremities generally occur in the HIV-related peripheral neuropathy. Unilateral or bilateral flaccid paralysis and neurogenic bladder have been described in HIV-associated myelopathy.

Clinicians must be aware that in HIV-infected patients, syphilis may be difficult to diagnose and may have unusual presentations. The serologic response to syphilis may be altered, requiring the use of sequential tests or other diagnostic modalities including biopsy of skin lesions and evaluation of the cerebrospinal fluid. Neurosyphilis may be an early infectious complication of HIV infection or may even be the presenting manifestation. Patients may be asymptomatic or may present with various neurologic findings including hemiparesis and cranial nerve palsies. Standard regimens for treatment of primary, secondary, and latent syphilis do not result in treponemicidal antibiotic levels in the cerebrospinal fluid.

Unless otherwise contraindicated, do a lumbar puncture. In addition to standard tests of cerebrospinal fluid, send for analysis of cryptococcal antigen (or for India ink stain if the cryptococcal antigen test is not available). Order an immunofluorescent assay for immuno-

Table 37–10. Neurologic Syndrome Related to HIV

HIV encephalopathy
HIV neuropathy
Cryptococcal meningitis
Toxoplasmosis
Progressive multifocal leukoencephalopathy
Herpes simplex virus meningoencephalitis
Cytomegaloviral meningoencephalitis
Central nervous system mycobacterial infections
Central nervous system lymphoma
Central nervous system Kaposi's sarcoma
HIV myelopathy

globulin M toxoplasma antibody (available through Jack Remington, M.D., Director, Palo Alto Research Laboratory, Palo Alto, CA) and quantitative Venereal Disease Research Laboratory (VDRL) test. Obtain a Gram's stain and bacterial culture, acid-fast bacterial smear and culture, fungal culture, viral culture (including herpes and cytomegalovirus), and cytologic tests.

If the cerebrospinal fluid does not reveal the cause of the neurologic symptoms, obtain a magnetic resonance imaging scan of the brain. HIV encephalopathy on this brain scan appears as patchy white matter disease with widened sulci often extending into the cerebellum. Toxoplasmosis appears as lesions in the basal ganglia or as abscesses elsewhere in the brain.

Because findings of HIV encephalopathy can sometimes overlap with those of progressive multifocal leukoencephalopathy, a trial of zidovudine, an antiviral agent with demonstrated in vitro and in vivo activity against HIV, is useful diagnostically. A dramatic improvement in dementia has been observed in patients with HIV encephalopathy.

Single or multiple discrete lesions seen on the magnetic resonance imaging brain scan may be caused by toxoplasmosis, lymphoma, or tuberculous abscesses. To distinguish toxoplasmosis from the other causes of brain lesions and to avoid the cost and trauma of a diagnostic brain biopsy, an empiric course of pyrimethamine and sulfadiazine, followed by a repeat brain scan in 3 to 4 weeks, can be useful. If no response is noted to therapy, then proceed with a diagnostic brain biopsy if the lesion is easily accessible.

The neuropathy associated with HIV has shown only limited response to zidovudine. Pain and paresthesias caused by HIV-related neuropathy may respond to amitriptyline 50 to 100 mg at bedtime.

OCULAR SYNDROMES

Retinal Cotton Wool Spots. Cotton wool spots are frequently observed on routine funduscopic examination of immunocompromised patients. Their etiology and prognostic value have not been adequately studied.

Cytomegalovirus Retinitis. Cytomegalovirus causes retinitis in many patients with AIDS, which has progressed in most untreated cases to blindness. Ask the patient whether he has noted spots, loss of part of the visual field, or blurring of vision. Request ophthalmologic consultation immediately. Treatment with ganciclovir has resulted in reduction or remission of retinal lesions in over 80% of patients.

Cryptococcal Ophthalmoplegias. Patients with cryptococcal meningitis frequently have cranial nerve palsies early in the disease process, usually involving the third and sixth cranial nerves. Ask the patient about double vision. The ophthalmoplegias usually resolve with amphotericin B and flucytosine treatment.

DERMATOLOGIC SYNDROMES

Seborrheic Dermatitis. Seborrheic dermatitis and fungal infections of the skin are the most common dermatologic manifestations in individuals infected with HIV. Some clinicians believe that seborrheic dermatitis is caused by a fungus, whereas others maintain that it results from a direct effect of HIV. Look for scaling and erythema in a malar distribution or in a more generalized pattern over the anterior chest, abdominal skin, and, less commonly, on the extremities. Treatment is with topical ketoconazole cream or with a low potency, nonfluorinated topical corticosteroid cream. Spontaneous improvement in seborrheic dermatitis has been observed in some patients receiving zidovudine.

Nonopportunistic Fungal Dermatoses. Superficial mycoses, such as tinea pedis and tinea cruris, are easily treated with topical ketoconazole, clotrimazole, or miconazole cream. Look for scaling on the plantar surface and interdigital spaces or erythema on the lateral aspects of the feet in tinea pedis. Look for well-marginated erythematous rashes in the groin and perianal areas in tinea cruris. Onychomycosis is usually asymptomatic but appears as a ragged or thickened growth pattern of the nails. Treatment may be attempted with oral griseofulvin or ketoconazole, but the need to monitor systemic side effects of these medications and the slow response to treatment make the use of these drugs generally unrewarding. Spontaneous improvement in onychomycosis has been observed in some patients receiving zidovudine.

Herpes Simplex Virus Infections. Herpes simplex virus infections in patients infected with HIV may be severe and persistent. The most common area of involvement is the perianal area and rectum, but the perioral and intraoral regions, genitalia, and other areas of the skin may also be involved.

Herpes Zoster Infections. Herpes zoster infections (shingles) are also seen frequently in patients infected with HIV. Look for vesicles in various stages of development after the course of a dermatome.

Kaposi's Sarcoma. After *P. carinii* pneumonia, Kaposi's sarcoma is the most prevalent opportunistic disorder in gay men with AIDS. It may be indolent or aggressive, involving multiple sites on the skin and viscera. Look for indurated lesions, varying in size from a few millimeters to several centimeters and in color from red to purple to black, which are located anywhere on the skin, conjunctivae, and oral and rectal mucosa. Treatment does not favorably influence survival and may result in further immunosuppression and myelosuppression. Therefore, the goal of therapy should be directed at lesions that are either disfiguring or are causing lymphatic obstruction, gastrointestinal hemorrhage, or respiratory compromise.

Radiation therapy has been used most effectively in small lesions on the face and in the oropharynx. Vincristine and vinblastine may be employed where lesions are causing lymphatic obstruction or respiratory distress. Alpha interferon, an immune modulator given subcutaneously or intramuscularly in doses up to 36 million units daily, with or without zidovudine, has resulted in objective response in up to 40% of patients receiving the agent in uncontrolled studies. Patients showing an objective response with alpha interferon usually have higher OKT4 levels than patients not demonstrating a response.

Drug Rash. Many of the drugs used to treat AIDS-related opportunistic infections may be associated with a rash. The most common is the reaction that occurs between 10 and 15 days after starting treatment with trimethoprim-sulfamethoxazole or trimethoprim and Dapsone. More than 80% of HIV-positive people are said to develop this maculopapular morbilliform rash, which begins on the trunk and upper extremities, spreads to the face and sometimes to the lower extremities, and becomes confluent and produces a sunburned appearance. The rash is frequently associated with a fever. The rash and fever subside after 4 or 5 days despite continuing treatment with the medication.

Rashes have also been associated with a medication used to treat mycobacterial infection, rifampin, and with an investigational antimycobacterial agent, ansamycin. These exanthems may be accompanied by severe fevers, and discontinuation of the medication may be required.

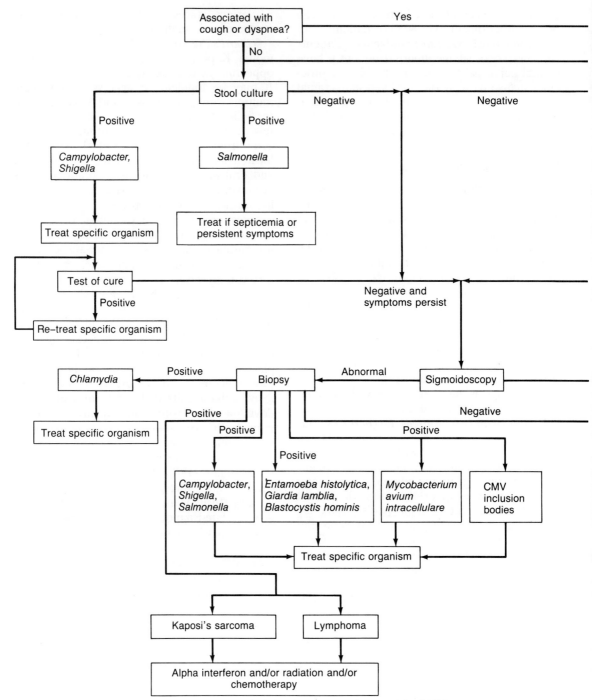

Figure 37–6. *Evaluation of diarrhea in a patient at risk of HIV.*

LYMPHADENOPATHIC SYNDROMES

Persistent Generalized Lymphadenopathy.
Shortly after 1979, physicians began to encounter substantial numbers of gay men with generalized lymphadenopathy, with or without constitutional symptoms.[10] The nodes were at least 1 cm in diameter, located in at least two noncontiguous, extrainguinal sites, and present for at least 6 months. A lymph node biopsy usually revealed benign reactive hyperplasia. Analysis of a cohort of such men after 6 years indicated that up to 40% developed full-blown AIDS. As HIV infection progresses and lym-

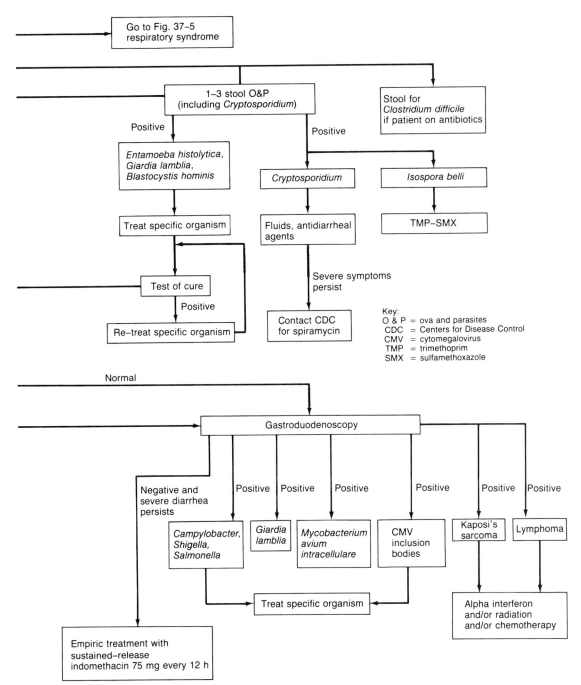

Figure 37–6 Continued

phocytic depletion occurs, lymph nodes frequently decrease substantially in size or disappear. This sometimes occurs within several weeks before development of an AIDS-defining opportunistic infection.

Because lymph node biopsy in this group of patients has been of little value, certain criteria

have been suggested to help determine when a biopsy is indicated.[11] Look for severe constitutional symptoms (e.g., persisting fevers, severe malaise and fatigue, or weight loss of more than 10% of body weight); new or increasing lymph node enlargement; and laboratory abnormalities (e.g., ESR greater than

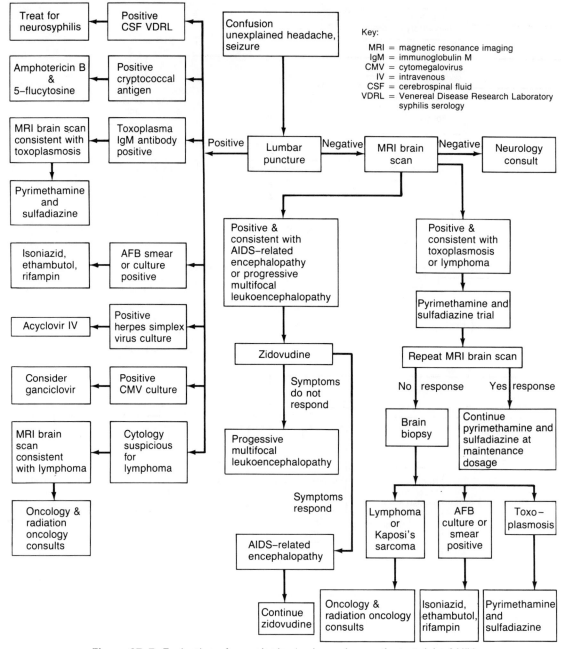

Figure 37–7. Evaluation of neurologic syndrome in a patient at risk of HIV.

50 or intrathoracic lymphadenopathy demonstrated by chest film).

When a lymph node biopsy is performed, send the specimen to the pathologist to examine for Kaposi's sarcoma, non-Hodgkin's lymphoma, and toxoplasmosis. Also send part of the specimen for a Gram's stain and bacterial culture, acid-fast bacterial smear and culture, fungal culture, and viral culture (including cytomegalovirus).

Lymphadenopathic Kaposi's Sarcoma. Kaposi's sarcoma lesions of the skin usually precede Kaposi's sarcoma lesions of nodes. Note that lymph nodes containing Kaposi's sarcoma feel firm to hard on examination compared with nodes resulting from benign reactive hyperplasia. Lymphadenopathic Kaposi's sarcoma is frequently associated with obstruction of local lymphatic vessels. Check for local edema surrounding the node or for asymmetric enlargement or asymmetric peripheral edema of the lower extremities.

Non-Hodgkin's Lymphoma. Non-Hodgkin's lymphoma is considered to be an opportunistic neoplasm defining AIDS in individuals infected with HIV. Results of treatment of AIDS-associated non-Hodgkin's lymphoma have been discouraging, and multiagent chemotherapy has been complicated by a high incidence of opportunistic infections and by pancytopenia.[12] Treatment has been associated with a low complete response rate (33 to 50% a high relapse rate, and a high mortality rate.

Syndromes Not Necessarily Related to HIV

URETHRAL SYNDROME (Fig. 37–8)

Obtain a Gram's stain of urethral material. If gram-negative diplococci are seen within polymorphonuclear leukocytes, treat for gonorrhea. Penicillinase-producing strains of *Neisseria gonorrhoeae* are endemic (as of early 1987) in many major metropolitan areas of the United States, including New York City, Los Angeles, Philadelphia, Detroit, San Diego, and San Francisco. In these areas, treat with ceftriaxone 125 mg intramuscularly. Add doxycycline 100 mg orally twice daily for 7 days to treat possibly coexisting *Chlamydia*. Spectinomycin 2.0 g intramuscularly may be used in place of ceftriaxone, but it is more expensive and does not treat pharyngeal gonorrhea adequately. In areas of the United States not endemic for these strains, aqueous procaine penicillin G 4.8 million units intramuscularly may be used in conjunction with probenecid 1.0 g. Add doxycycline to treat possibly coexisting *Chlamydia*. Be sure that any known partners are treated and obtain a test culture for *N. gonorrhoeae* 3 to 7 days after treatment has been completed.

If gram-negative intracellular diplococci are not seen within polymorphonuclear leukocytes, obtain a culture for *N. gonorrhoeae* and treat for nongonococcal urethritis with doxycycline 100 mg orally twice daily for 7 days. If symptoms persist, obtain a monoclonal immunofluorescent antibody smear for *Chlamydia*, re-treat for nongonococcal urethritis (possibly caused by the 6 to 10% of ureaplasmas that are resistant to tetracyclines) with erythromycin 250 mg orally four times daily for 7 days, and consider whether the patient has been reinfected from an asymptomatic untreated partner. Also consider other diagnoses, such as herpes simplex virus infection (look for vesicles around the urethral meatus) and chronic prostatitis (do a rectal examination and send expressed prostate secretions for a Gram's stain and culture).

MUCOCUTANEOUS LESIONS

Syphilis. In primary syphilis, look for a painless ulceration on or around the genitalia, mouth, pharynx, or anorectum. Chancres in the anal region may be asymptomatic, like classic penile chancres, or painful. Anoscopy may be required to visualize an anorectal chancre.

In secondary syphilis, look for the classic maculopapular rash with or without fever. Secondary syphilis may also appear as a hepatitis-like syndrome with malaise, fatigue, right upper quadrant abdominal tenderness, and low grade elevations in liver enzyme levels. In HIV-positive patients, the serologic response may be altered, requiring sequential VDRL tests or a biopsy of suspected syphilitic lesions.

Latent syphilis is diagnosed on the basis of a positive serologic test for syphilis in the absence of recent treatment for syphilis. Obtain results of previous syphilis serologic tests to determine whether early latent or late latent syphilis is present. As noted in the discussion on the neurologic syndrome associated with HIV infection, the incubation period for neurosyphilis may be unusually short, and the antibody response may be impaired, thus obscuring the diagnosis.

Herpes Simplex Virus Infection. Look for the characteristic cluster of painful or pruritic blisters on or around the genitalia, on the mouth, in the oropharynx, around the anus, or in the anal canal. Anoscopy for anorectal herpes reveals congestion and sometimes pus and ulcerations. Complications include lumbosacral radiculomyelopathy or sacral meningomyelitis manifested by sciatica, paresthesias in the lower extremities, and urinary dysfunction.

Venereal Warts. The genital wart virus may cause cauliflower-like lesions on or around the genitals, in the perianal area, or within the anal canal. On male genitals, warts are most frequently seen on the corona or shaft, but they may also occur within the urethra or on the skin of the groin.

In the perianal region and in the anal canal, condylomata acuminata may be small or extensive. They should be distinguished from the

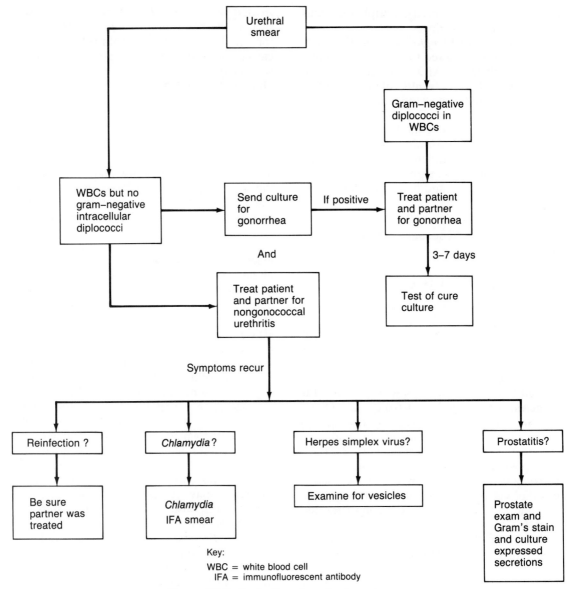

Figure 37–8. Evaluation of urethral syndrome.

condylomata lata of secondary syphilis, which are generally flatter and smoother.

Treat small genital or perianal warts with podophyllin 25% solution applied to the lesions. Instruct the patient to wash the podophyllin off in 4 to 6 hours. A reapplication of podophyllin in 1 or 2 weeks is often necessary. Minor lesions may also be treated with cryotherapy or bichloroacetic acid. For more extensive condylomata, anorectal condylomata, or lesions not responding to podophyllin, electrocautery, surgical excision, and intralesional or systemic alpha interferon are alternative treatments.

Pubic Lice and Scabies. Pubic lice and their egg sacs are visible. Scabies (mites) may be seen on microscopic examination of a scraping from an unroofed burrow. Both ectoparasites cause intense itching. Treat pubic lice with topical overnight application of pyrethins with piperonyl butoxide or with lindane 1% lotion. Recommend reapplication in four nights to kill lice that have not yet hatched from nits at the time of the first treatment. Treat scabies with topical application of lindane 1% lotion or crotamiton 10%.

PROCTITIS SYNDROME (Fig. 37–9)

Inquire about tenesmus, a sensation of urgency to defecate frequently with production

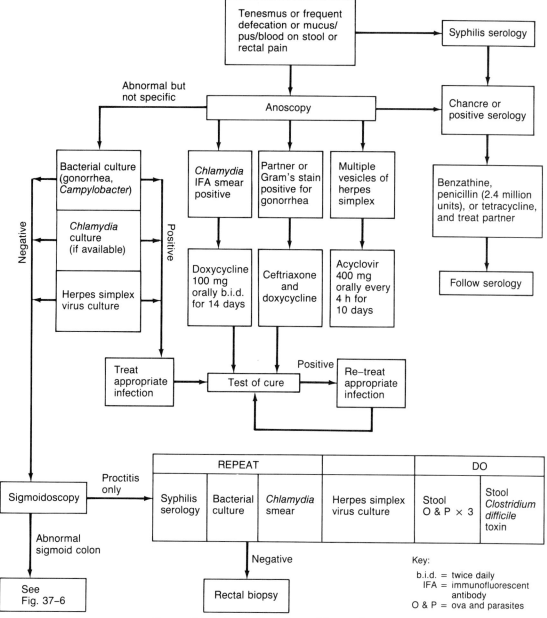

Figure 37–9. *Evaluation of proctitis syndrome.*

of only scant stool, usually associated with pain and sometimes accompanied by mucus and blood. Do an anoscopic examination and obtain a serologic test for syphilis. If a chancre is seen or the serologic result is consistent with primary syphilis, treat with benzathine penicillin or tetracycline. Because syphilis serologic results may be positive in only 50% of cases of primary syphilis, however, advise a follow-up serologic test in 1 month if syphilis is suspected, even if the initial serologic test for syphilis is negative.

Obtain a Gram's stain of the anal mucosa smear to look for gram-negative intracellular diplococci characteristic of *N. gonorrhoeae*, an immunofluorescent antibody smear for *Chlamydia*, and a scraping of anal ulcerations, abrasions, or fissures for herpes simplex virus culture. Also do a bacterial culture of the anal mucosa; specify both *N. gonorrhoeae* and *Campylobacter* species. Treat any of these infections according to the regimens outlined in Table 37–11.

If the initial evaluation of proctitis is nega-

Table 37–11. Treatment Regimens for Sexually Transmitted
Infections and Opportunistic Diseases in Gay Men*

Infection	Treatment	Alternative	Comment
Therapy for Infections Not Necessarily Associated with HIV			
N. gonorrhoeae in PPNG areas	Ceftriaxone 125 mg IM	Spectinomycin 2–4 g IM	Spectinomycin not adequate for pharyngeal gonorrhea
N. gonorrhoeae in non-PPNG areas	Aqueous procaine penicillin G 4.8 million U IM *with* probenecid 1 g PO	Spectinomycin 2–4 g IM *or* doxycycline 100 mg PO b.i.d. × 7 days	Spectinomycin alternative for urethral or anorectal infection Doxycycline alternative for pharyngeal infection
Chlamydia trachomatis non-LGV strain	Doxycycline 100 mg PO b.i.d. × 7 days	Erythromycin 500 mg PO q.i.d. × 7 days	
C. trachomatis LGV strain	Doxycycline 100 mg PO b.i.d. × 21 days	Erythromycin 500 mg PO q.i.d. × 21 days	
Syphilis (HIV negative) (primary, secondary, or early latent)	Benzathine penicillin G 2.4 million U IM	Doxycycline 100 mg PO t.i.d. × 15 days	
Syphilis (HIV positive) (primary, secondary, or latent)	Aqueous penicillin 2.4 million U IV every day × 14 days *or* procaine penicillin 2.4 million U IV every day × 14 days *with* probenecid 1.5 g PO every day × 14 days *or* amoxicillin 3 g PO b.i.d. × 14 days *with* probenecid 1 g PO every day × 14 days	Doxycycline 100 mg PO b.i.d × 21 days	
Shigella spp	Trimethoprim-sulfamethoxazole 160 mg/ 800 mg PO b.i.d. × 7 days	Ampicillin 500 mg PO b.i.d. × 7 days or ciprofloxacin 500 mg PO b.i.d. × 7 days	
Salmonella spp	Antibiotics recommended only in severe cases	Ceftriaxone 2 g IM or IV every day × 10 days *or* ciprofloxacin 500 mg PO b.i.d. × 10 days *or* chloramphenicol 500 mg IV every 6 h × 10 days	Norfloxacin investigational for this indication
Campylobacter spp	Erythromycin 500 mg PO q.i.d. × 7 days	Ciprofloxacin 500 mg PO b.i.d. × 7 days	
Clostridium difficile	Metronidazole 15 mg/kg IV loading then 7.5 mg/kg every 6 h	Vancomycin 1.0 g IV every 12 h	
Entamoeba histolytica	Metronidazole 750 mg PO t.i.d. × 10 days *with* iodoquinol 650 mg PO t.i.d. × 20 days	Paramomycin 25–30 mg/kg per day in 3 doses × 7 days	Paramomycin may eradicate luminal but not tissue phase *E. histolytica* infections
Dientamoeba fragilis	Iodoquinol 650 mg PO t.i.d. × 20 days	Paramomycin 25–30 mg/kg per day in 3 doses × 7 days	
Giardia lamblia	Quinacrine HCl PC 100 mg PO t.i.d. × 21 days	Metronidazole 250 mg PO t.i.d. × 5 days	Metronidazole investigational for this indication
Blastocystis hominis	Value of treatment not established	Iodoquinol 650 mg PO t.i.d. × 20 days	
Herpes simplex virus infections (oral or genital)	Acyclovir 200 mg PO 5 times daily × 5 days	Supportive therapy	
Hepatitis B	Supportive therapy		Advise unvaccinated sexual contacts to obtain anti-HB$_c$. If anti-HB$_c$ is negative, give hepatitis B immune globulin and hepatitis B vaccine.

Table 37–11. *Treatment Regimens for Sexually Transmitted Infections and Opportunistic Diseases in Gay Men** Continued

Infection	Treatment	Alternative	Comment
Therapy for Infections Not Necessarily Associated with HIV Continued			
Condyloma acuminatum (genital or perianal)	Podophyllin 25% to lesion every 1–2 wk	Electrocautery *or* cryotherapy	Instruct to remove podophyllin in 4–6 h
Condyloma acuminatum (intra-anal)	Electrocautery	Bichloroacetic acid *or* surgery *or* intralesional alpha interferon	
Pubic lice	Pyrethrins with piperonyl butoxide	Lindane 1% lotion	Apply overnight repeat in 4 days, wash clothes and linens
Mites (scabies)	Lindane 1% lotion	Crotamiton 10%	Apply topically
Therapy for Diseases Associated with HIV			
HIV	Zidovudine (formerly called azidothymidine or AZT) 100–200 mg PO every 4 h		Currently indicated if history of *P. carinii* pneumonia or if OKT4 < 200; reduce dose to 100 mg PO every 4 h if Hgb < 9–10 or if neutrophils < 750; suspend if Hgb < 8 or if neutrophils < 500
P. carinii pneumonia	Trimethoprim-sulfamethoxazole (given PO or IV as 15–20 mg/kg per day of trimethoprim divided in 3–4 doses) × 14–21 days *or* pentamidine isethionate 4 mg/kg per day IV × 14–21 days	Dapsone 100 mg PO daily × 14–21 days *with* trimethoprim 15–20 mg/kg per day PO divided in 3–4 doses × 14–21 days	Continue therapy through rash and fever if otherwise tolerated; Dapsone investigational for this indication; reduce pentamidine to 3 mg/kg per day if significant adverse effects
Toxoplasmosis	Sulfadiazine 1 g PO q.i.d. × 6 wk *with* pyrimethamine 25 mg PO b.i.d. *and* leucovorin 5 mg PO b.i.d.	Clindamycin 900 mg IV or PO every 6 h *with* pyrimethamine 25 mg PO b.i.d. *and* leucovorin 5 mg PO b.i.d.	Maintain using sulfadiazine 1 g PO b.i.d. *with* pyrimethamine 25 mg PO daily *and* leucovorin 5 mg PO b.i.d.; clindamycin use for this indication investigational
Cryptosporidiosis	Supportive therapy	Spiramycin 1.0 g PO q.i.d.	Investigational agent available in the United States only from the FDA 1-301-443-4310
Isosporiasis	Trimethoprim-sulfamethoxazole 160 mg/800 mg q.i.d. × 10 days then b.i.d. × 3 wk		Trimethoprim-sulfamethoxzole investigational for this indication
Candidiasis (oral thrush)	Clotrimazole one oral troche 5 × per day *or* nystatin gargle 500,000 U q.i.d.	Clotrimazole one vaginal troche PO q.i.d.	Suppress with one troche daily
Candidiasis (esophageal)	Ketoconazole 200 mg PO b.i.d. × 10 days		May need to suppress with ketoconazole 200 mg PO daily
Cryptococcosis (including meningitis)	Amphotericin B 0.4–0.6 mg/kg per day IV × 3 wk *with* flucytosine 100 mg/kg per day PO in 4 divided doses		Escalate amphotericin in 5-mg increments IV daily from 5 mg to full dose; maintain using amphotericin B 50 mg IV twice weekly after 3 wk *with* flucytosine

Table continued on following page

Table 37–11. Treatment Regimens for Sexually Transmitted
Infections and Opportunistic Diseases in Gay Men* Continued

Infection	Treatment	Alternative	Comment
Therapy for Diseases Associated with HIV Continued			
Mycobacterium avium intracellulare infections of blood, bone marrow, lymph nodes, and gastrointestinal tract	Ethambutol 15 mg/kg per day PO *with* rifampin 600 mg PO daily *or with* ansamycin 300 mg PO daily *and with* ciprofloxacin 500 mg PO b.i.d. *and with* isoniazid 300 mg PO daily *and with* clofazimine 100 mg PO daily	No therapy (because value of therapy has not yet been shown)	Ansamycin, clofazimine, and ciprofloxacin are investigational agents; other investigational drugs include trimetrexate and amikacin
Mycobacterium tuberculosis	Ethambutol 15 mg/kg per day PO *with* rifampin 600 mg PO daily *and with* isoniazid 300 mg PO daily		Pyridoxine (vitamin B₆) should also be given with isonizid to prevent peripheral neuropathy
Anorectal herpes simplex (especially in immunocompromised patient)	Acyclovir 400 mg PO 5 times daily × 10 days	Supportive therapy if mild or foscarnet if severe	Foscarnet is investigational agent available from Astra Pharmaceutical Co., Westboro, MA
Herpes zoster (shingles)	Acyclovir 800 mg PO every 4 h × 10 days	Supportive therapy	Acyclovir investigational for this indication
Hairy leukoplakia	Acyclovir 800 mg PO every 4 h × 10 days *or* Peridex mouthwash	No treatment (consequences of untreated hairy leukoplakia have not been shown)	Acyclovir investigational for this indication; maintenance dose not established
Cytomegalovirus infections of retina, brain, gastrointestinal tract, lungs	Ganciclovir		Investigational drug available from Syntex Inc., Palo Alto, CA
Progressive multifocal leukoencephalopathy	Supportive therapy		
Kaposi's sarcoma	Supportive therapy *or* alpha interferon 3 million–30 million U daily for 4–6 wk with or without zidovudine	Radiation therapy *or* vincristine 2 mg IV biweekly *alternating with* vinblastine 0.1 mg/kg IV biweekly	Interferon use for KS investigational and has not been approved by the FDA; if KS responds to interferon, maintain with 3 million–36 million U SC 3 times weekly; radiation used for palliation of cosmetically undesirable KS; vincristine and vinblastine are used to treat extensive KS with morbidity
Non-Hodgkin's lymphoma	Radiation therapy for localized tumors	Multiagent chemotherapy *or* alpha interferon	Chemotherapy in AIDS-related NHL associated with severe pancytopenia and opportunistic infections; interferon use in NHL still investigational

*Key to abbreviations: AIDS, acquired immunodeficiency syndrome; anti-HBc, antibody to hepatitis B core antigen; b.i.d., twice daily; d, day(s); FDA, U.S. Food and Drug Administration; HCl, hydrochloride; Hgb, hemoglobin (in g/dl); IM, intramuscularly; IV, intravenously; KS, Kaposi's sarcoma; LGV, lymphogranuloma venereum; NHL, non-Hodgkin's lymphoma; OKT4, total number of T helper lymphocytes; PC, after meals; PO, orally; PPNG, penicillinase-producing *N. gonorrhoeae*; q.i.d., four times daily; SC, subcutaneously; t.i.d., three times daily.

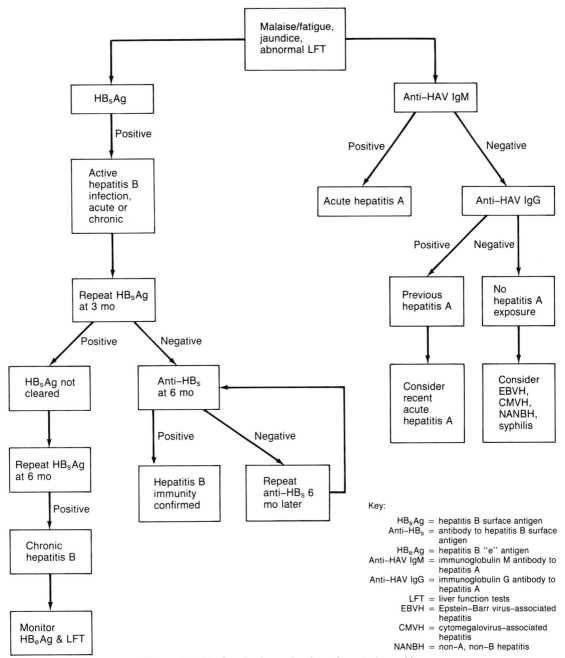

Figure 37–10. *Serologic evaluation of acute hepatitis.*

tive, do a proctosigmoidoscopic examination. If involvement of only the anorectum is noted, re-evaluate for syphilis, gonorrhea, *Campylobacter* species, *Chlamydia*, and herpes simplex virus. Also do stool tests for ova and parasites. If the sigmoid colon is involved, then continue the evaluation according to the algorithm outlined for the enterocolitis syndrome (see next chapter).

For all of the bacterial and protozoal infec-

tions, do cultures or stool analyses to determine whether treatment has been efficacious. These tests should be done several days after the course of antimicrobial therapy has been completed.

ENTEROCOLITIS SYNDROME (see Table 37–9 and Fig. 37–6)

The initial diagnostic evaluation for diarrhea in gay men not at risk for HIV infection is similar to the evaluation of patients infected with HIV, but an intensive search for opportunistic infections and neoplasms is not as important. Obtain a stool culture and a stool examination for ova and parasites. If nonpathogenic amebae are seen (which can serve as surrogate markers for the possible presence of pathogenic amebae) and symptoms persist, obtain one or two additional specimens after a bisacodyl suppository or magnesium citrate purge. If these are negative and symptoms still persist, do a sigmoidoscopic examination and obtain a biopsy if the former shows abnormal mucosa.

Treat infections associated with the enterocolitis syndrome according to the recommendations in Table 37–11. For any of the enteric infections, obtain a stool specimen to determine that the therapy has been efficacious.

HEPATITIS (Fig. 37–10)

Classic symptoms of both hepatitis A and B include malaise, fatigue, anorexia, dark urine, light stools, and jaundice. Most cases of hepatitis B occurring in gay men, however, are clinically inapparent. Obtain assays for hepatitis B surface antigen (HB_sAg) and the immunoglobulin M antibody to hepatitis A virus (anti-HAV IgM). Other viral etiologies of hepatitis include Epstein-Barr virus (infectious mononucleosis), cytomegalovirus, and non-A, non-B hepatitis. Secondary syphilis with syphilitic hepatitis can also mimic acute viral hepatitis.

Treatment Regimens

Recommendations for treatment of the sexually transmitted diseases and AIDS-related opportunistic infections and neoplasms discussed in this chapter are given in Table 37–11. Some of the therapies are still investigational and have not been approved by the U.S. Food and Drug Administration. As with any treatment regimen, caution should be exercised in the use of investigational drugs and, if the treating physician is not familiar with these agents, specialty consultation or a review of the current literature is suggested.

Summary

During the past decade, clinicians have become increasingly aware of the special health care needs of gay men. A substantial minority of men are at some time in their lives homosexually active, but the vast majority of gay men are not readily visible to their physicians. Because gay men who engage in certain sexual practices may be at increased risk for a variety of sexually transmitted diseases and HIV-associated conditions, it is important for physicians to inquire about the sexual orientation of all patients and to take a history of sexual practices. Physical findings may also provide clues to sexually transmitted diseases and to illnesses associated with HIV. Because homosexual activity is still illegal in some jurisdictions and is attached to cultural and religious stigmas even in areas where it has been legalized, physicians need to be keenly aware of the issue of confidentiality as it applies to documentation in medical records and in research.

Laboratory screening tests are frequently useful in detecting sexually transmitted diseases in the asymptomatic gay man or in helping the clinician, in conjunction with findings from the history and physical examination, identify patients who are at risk for HIV-associated conditions. Decisions about whether to use laboratory screening tests should take into account the incubation period for infections and specific sexual practices. The HIV antibody test should be ordered and recorded in a confidential manner only after the patient understands the potential implications and limitations of this test, and ideally it should be done at an anonymous testing site. The physician ordering or recommending the HIV antibody test should be prepared to counsel the patient after a discussion of the results, particularly if this service is not provided at the testing site.

Physicians have a responsibility to advise gay men about sexual practices that may be associated with a high risk of infection or trauma and to provide counsel about sexual practices that are considered to be safe. It should be emphasized at the same time that emotional intimacy is still an important component of a healthy lifestyle. Physicians should also become familiar with the sources of emotional support used by the gay patient, whether traditional sources, such as members of the patient's nuclear family, or nontraditional sources, such as lovers, close friends, or community organizations.

References

1. Owen WF Jr. Sexually transmitted diseases and traumatic problems in homosexual men. Ann Intern Med 92:805–808, 1980.

An early review of sexually transmitted diseases affecting gay men published 1 year before the first reports of AIDS.

2. Castro KG, Hardy AM, Curran JW. The acquired immunodeficiency syndrome: epidemiology and risk factors for transmission. Med Clin North Am 70:635–649, 1986.

    A succinct review of the epidemiology of AIDS, including case definition and risk factors.

3. Council on Scientific Affairs of the American Medical Association. Health care needs of a homosexual population. JAMA 248:736–739, 1982.

    An authoritative statement that physicians at all levels of training need to recognize the special health needs of their lesbian and gay patients.

4. Robertson P, Schachter J. Failure to identify venereal disease in a lesbian population. Sex Transm Dis 8:75–126, 1981.

    Landmark study showing that lesbians have sexually transmitted diseases only rarely but do have other health care needs.

5. Owen WF Jr. The clinical approach to the homosexual patient. Ann Intern Med 93:90–92, 1980.

    An early discussion of the importance of obtaining a complete sexual history, including a history of sexual practices.

6. Farzadegan H, Polis MA, Wolinsky SM, et al. Loss of human immunodeficiency virus type 1 (HIV-1) antibodies with evidence of viral infection in asymptomatic homosexual men: a report from the muticenter AIDS cohort study. Ann Intern Med 108:785–790, 1988.

    Four asymptomatic men of 1000 HIV seropositive individuals were found to have lost antibodies to HIV p24, gp160, and gp155 on the Western blot test. By using the polymerase chain reaction (PCR), which amplifies specific genetic elements, two of the four patients were shown to have HIV DNA sequences in circulating peripheral blood mononuclear cells throughout the study.

7. Moss AR, Bacchetti P, Osmond D, et al. Seropositivity for HIV and the development of AIDS or AIDS related condition: three year follow up of the San Francisco General Hospital cohort. Br Med J 296:745–750, 1988.

    Five percent of 462 initially asymptomatic homosexual men progressed to AIDS at 1 year, 11% at 2 years, and 22% at 3 years; 50% were predicted to progress to AIDS by 6 years. Five independent predictors of progression were elevated (> 5) beta$_2$-microglobulin levels, HIV p24 antigenemia, decreased (< 200) CD4 lymphocytes, decreased hematocrit, and decreased (< 3000) white blood cells.

8. Scientific Affairs Committee of Bay Area Physicians for Human Rights. Safe sex guidelines for persons at risk for AIDS, in Campbell JM (ed). Medical Evaluation of Persons at Risk of Human Immunodeficiency Virus Infection. San Francisco, Bay Area Physicians for Human Rights, 1987, pp 15–17.

    Latest issue of the first "safer sex" guidelines to be published based originally on epidemiologic data about AIDS before identification of HIV. This highly recommended publication also contains chapters on evaluation of the worried well patient and AIDS-related clinical syndromes. (Reprint information: BAPHR, P.O. Box 14546, San Francisco, CA 94114.)

9. Centers for Disease Control. Recommendations for prevention of HIV transmission in health-care settings. MMWR 36(Suppl 25):15–185, 1987.

    Good review of risk to health care personnel of acquiring HIV in health care settings and of recommended precautions to prevent transmission.

10. Abrams DI. Lymphadenopathy related to the acquired immunodeficiency syndrome in homosexual men. Med Clin North Am 70:693–706, 1986.

    Thorough discussion of one early clinical manifestation of infection with HIV.

11. Hollander H. Practical management of common AIDS-related medical problems. West J Med 146:237–240, 1987.

    Discussion of several clinical syndromes associated with HIV highlighted by succinct text and clear tables.

12. Kaplan LD, Wofsy CB, Volberding PA. Treatment of patients with acquired immunodeficiency syndrome and associated manifestations. JAMA 257:1367–1374, 1987.

    Excellent presentation of therapeutic options in and investigational approaches to management of opportunistic infections and neoplasms.

38

Infectious Diseases and Travel: Risk, Recognition, Remedies, and Prevention

JAY A. JACOBSON, M.D., F.A.C.P.

Introduction

Travel for business and for pleasure has grown increasingly popular during the past decade. Jet aircraft have made international destinations seem closer and more convenient, with trips measured in hours rather than days or weeks. The need for exploration to discover additional natural resources and the desire for adventure and new and different experiences have drawn many Americans to previously unvisited or unaccessible places. Travel clearly has its financial, emotional, and intellectual rewards, but it is usually stressful and occasionally hazardous. Between 20 and 25% of travelers to developing nations become ill during their trips.

Accidents and acute illness can, of course, occur anywhere, but their outcome may be influenced by the accessibility and quality of medical care. Exacerbations of chronic diseases such as arthritis, coronary artery disease, and chronic lung disease are not unusual during an extended trip. Detailed discussion of the prevention and management of these problems is beyond the scope of this chapter, but some basic principles are worth restating. Table 38–1 provides a checklist whose relevant points should be reviewed with individual patients planning trips. Patients should be cautioned about behavior such as exposing oneself for unduly long periods to the sun; driving in areas where practices, regulations, and vehicles may be unfamiliar; and participating in activities for which there has been inadequate physical or mental preparation. Patients with chronic illnesses or who are at risk of acute disease should be knowledgeable about their

circumstances and should carry an ample supply of appropriate medicines. It would be desirable for them to have a medical description of their illness and therapy available for another physician if they must see one. Finally, all travelers, but especially those likeliest to become ill, should know how to obtain medical care while traveling. A mechanism for paying for the care should also be established because many medical insurance plans may not be applicable or acceptable in some locations. In this chapter I will address the infectious diseases that are associated with travel; how they are acquired; how they are recognized and managed; and how they may be prevented.

Risk Factors for Infections in Travelers

The risk of travel-associated infection varies substantially for particular itineraries and for individual travelers. Circumstances most com-

Table 38–1. *Basic Principles for Safe Travel*

Contact physician 6 wk before foreign travel for medical summary of health problems and adequate supplies of prescription medicines for existing and potential travel-related illnesses.

Obtain names of available physicians from International Association for Medical Assistance to Travelers, 736 Center Street, Lewiston, NY 14092; 1–716–754–4883.

Arrange for necessary immunizations.

Review health and automobile insurance coverage.

Be aware and prepared for anticipated extremes of temperature and exposure to sun.

Be aware of potential hazards associated with swimming or drinking water.

Be aware of foods most likely to transmit infection and be prepared to prevent or treat gastroenteritis.

monly linked with infections are noted in Table 38–2. Infectious agents that have humans as their reservoir and depend on person-to-person transmission are not uniformly distributed around the world. Tuberculosis and hepatitis B virus infections are more prevalent in lesser developed countries than in the United States. Travel in such countries is likely to increase one's risk of tuberculosis because it is transmitted by droplet nuclei through the air. On the other hand, more intimate exposure, usually sexual, is required before the increased prevalence of hepatitis B constitutes a risk to the traveler. Where personal hygiene and culinary hygiene are not rigorously maintained and water quality is not regularly evaluated or ensured, food-borne and water-borne infections are of course more likely. Even differences in the prevalent gastrointestinal flora, which inevitably make their way to some foods, may account for the frequency of infectious gastroenteritis in travelers to and from many countries. The environment itself may pose some risk of infection to the newly arrived visitor. Some parts of the American Southwest and Mexico harbor the arthrospores of *Coccidioides immitis* in soil and dust. Even travelers simply passing through this region are at some risk of valley fever, whereas some individuals, such as pregnant women, immunocompromised patients, and black visitors, may be at increased risk of more severe coccidiodomycoses. An increased prevalence of an infectious agent in humans or animals and an appropriate vector for transmission may together increase the risk of infection to visitors and residents. Such is the case with insect- or arthropod-borne infections such as malaria in Asia, Africa, and South America and tularemia, Rocky Mountain spotted fever, and Lyme disease in the United States.

Infections acquired while traveling, although

Table 38–2. *Circumstances Increasing the Risk of Travel-Associated Infections*

Travel to developing nations
Prolonged exposure
Visiting areas with high endemic rates of particular
  diseases
Lodging and eating at unregulated or uninspected
  facilities
Travel to rural areas
Failure to adhere to recommendations regarding
  immunization, food, water, and antimicrobial
  prophylaxis
Personal health factors such as immunosuppression,
  achlorhydria, use of H_2 blockers, or prior gastric
  resection

perhaps more common than those acquired while remaining at home, are still the exception rather than the rule. Most travelers escape even the milder infections such as traveler's diarrhea, although in very high risk areas up to 40% of visitors may be affected. Fortunately, it is quite rare for travelers to develop a more serious infection such as typhoid fever or malaria. The likelihood of developing a travel-associated infectious disease is dependent on a number of factors. First is the endemicity of a particular infection. Gastroenteritis can be acquired virtually anywhere, but Colorado tick fever is not likely to be acquired anywhere except the mountainous West of the United States. Second, and perhaps most obvious, is the duration of the trip. Most exposure risk is time-dependent, so that trips of several days have predictably less risk than visits of weeks to months. Third, the nature of the travel influences the risk of infection. Tourists who do their traveling in air-conditioned buses, who stay in only first-class hotels, and who congregate only with each other have minimal risk of exposure to infections dependent on poor hygiene, personal exposure, or contact with the animate or inanimate environment. Conversely, extensive rural travel, adoption of the native style of eating and food preparation, and activities that result in sustained exposure to insects and arthropods constitute an increased risk.

The degree to which travelers adhere to medical recommendations for risk reduction also affects development of infectious diseases. Traveler's diarrhea, for example, is less common in those who consume only cooked food and avoid untreated water, and malaria is rare in individuals who scrupulously follow their schedule for prophylaxis. Unfortunately, less than half of the visitors to areas in which malaria is endemic report using chemoprophylaxis.

The vast majority of travel-associated infections involve the gastrointestinal tract. Toxigenic and enteropathogenic *Escherichia coli* infections are most common, but the bacterial and protozoal agents of diarrhea are also encountered with regularity as is hepatitis A virus. Fortunately, diseases such as yellow fever, schistosomiasis, trypanosomiasis, and filariasis, although thought of as virtually synonymous with travel-related infections and associated with visits to unusual or exotic places, are rarely seen in Americans returning from short visits to endemic areas. With this being the case, it is highly likely that returning travelers with symptoms other than diarrhea actually have an illness that is coincidental with their travel rather than caused by it.

Syndromes Caused by or Confused with Travel-Associated Infections

Diarrhea

The differential diagnosis and management of acute diarrhea are discussed in Chapter 21.

In travelers with chronic diarrhea who have had protracted visits or temporary residence in Southeast Asia or the Caribbean, some consideration should be given to tropical sprue, an entity usually manifested as a malabsorption syndrome. The diagnosis is established by seeing blunting of intestinal microvilli by small bowel biopsy. Treatment includes tetracycline and vitamin B_{12} and folate supplements.

Rash

Rashes are, of course, common, and when they occur in travelers may raise suspicions about exotic infections such as typhoid fever, filariasis, or schistosomiasis. In most cases, however, they are not infectious but rather related to a hypersensitivity, contact, or adverse drug reaction. Common noninfectious examples include photosensitivity dermatitis associated with tetracycline, rhus dermatitis caused by poison ivy or similar plants, and contact dermatitis related to new clothing or products acquired for or during travel. Particularly severe rashes and the Stevens-Johnson syndrome have been linked with the use of sulfonamides and the antimalarial drug Fansidar (pyrimethamine-sulfadoxine).

Most infectious diseases characterized by a rash also include a fever, which may prove helpful in distinguishing between the many potential causes of a rash. The character and appearance of the rash are useful in narrowing a differential diagnosis. A petechial rash suggests meningococcal infection, rickettsial infection such as Rocky Mountain spotted fever, and dengue. A morbilliform rash is typical of measles, and it should be recognized that measles remains common in most developing countries. Susceptible travelers may develop classic measles, whereas partially immune individuals such as those who received a less

effective vaccine or who were vaccinated before 12 to 15 months of age may develop an illness with an atypical rash and prominent joint pains. Rose spots, although said to be characteristic of typhoid fever, are rarely seen, and the rash is usually not prominent in that infection. Jaundice suggests hepatic involvement or hemolysis and can be an important clue to viral hepatitis, yellow fever, leptospirosis, or some forms of malaria. In most returning travelers, more common conditions such as gallbladder disease and alcoholic liver disease often prove to be the explanation of an elevated bilirubin level.

Fever

Fever, like rash, is a common complaint. Most fevers in travelers, as in other patients, prove to be of viral origin and are generally due to self-limited upper respiratory infections. Influenza can produce a more severe and protracted febrile illness, which is readily suspected and diagnosed during our flu season. It should be recalled, however, that during our summer, influenza is occurring in the Southern hemisphere and so returning travelers from South America may be manifesting or incubating an influenza virus infection.

More serious causes of fever that can have major consequences if unrecognized and untreated are Salmonella typhi infections, malaria, tuberculosis, amebiasis, brucellosis, and schistosomiasis. Each should be suspected under appropriate clinical circumstances. Typhoid fever is an illness that may persist for weeks with symptoms that include malaise, weight loss, constipation, abdominal pain, and cough. The pulse rate may be paradoxically slow for the temperature. Laboratory results including serologic tests for antibody to Salmonella antigens may be nonspecific and unreliable. The diagnosis is best established by a blood culture and occasionally by a stool culture. Therapy is with ampicillin or chloramphenicol.

Malaria should be suspected in anyone who has traveled in an endemic area. The onset of a malarial paroxysm may follow return from the site of exposure by several months to several years. Early in the course malaria may seem much like the flu with erratic chills, fever, and myalgias. If untreated, a more regular periodic pattern of fevers is established. Most patients feel relatively well between febrile episodes. A more persistent and progressive illness accompanied by jaundice, dark urine, and central nervous system abnormalities suggests falciparum malaria and constitutes a medical emergency. In all cases, a rapid diagnosis is desirable and generally possible by examining thick and thin blood smears for malarial organisms. Specimens obtained just before or at the beginning of a rigor are most useful. If smears are positive or if the patient is strongly suspected to have malaria, especially falciparum, empiric therapy with quinine should be started. If infection with a relapsing strain that has extraerythrocytic forms is diagnosed or suspected, concomitant treatment with primaquine should be administered. Primaquine should be used with caution in patients with glucose-6-phosphate dehydrogenase deficiency because of hemolysis, and it should not be given with other potentially hemolytic agents or quinacrine.

Fever of unknown origin is often the only clue to an abscess. In travelers with a history of diarrhea, with right upper quadrant tenderness, or with abnormal liver function studies, an amebic liver abscess should be suspected and investigated. Serologic tests and ultrasound or computed tomography examination of the liver generally establishs or excludes this diagnosis. Amebic abscesses can be treated with metronidazole.

Brucellosis should be considered in febrile patients who had occupational exposure to cattle, swine, or goats while traveling or in those who consumed dairy products from potentially infected animals. The diagnosis can be sought by serologic tests and blood culture on brucella agar. The treatment is tetracycline and gentamicin or high dose trimethoprim-sulfamethoxazole.

Travel to certain parts of the United States enhances the risk of several febrile diseases. Travelers to the Southwest and especially the San Joaquin Valley may develop valley fever or coccidioidomycosis, an acute respiratory illness characterized by cough, fever, and pulmonary infiltrate seen on a chest radiograph. Visitors to the Mississippi River valley, especially if they visit caves or have substantial exposure to soil, may develop a similar illness, histoplasmosis. In both cases, infection is generally self-limited and requires no treatment, although in some high risk individuals the disease may become progressive or disseminated, in which case therapy with amphotericin may be necessary. Diagnosis is established by a sputum stain and culture for fungi. Additional helpful information is provided by skin tests and relevant antibody measurement.

Travel to the western United States entails possible exposure to Colorado tick fever, a viral infection; relapsing fever related to a spirochete; or Rocky Mountain spotted fever, which is caused by rickettsia. All are transmitted by ticks, and a history of outdoor activity is usually present, but even spending a night in a cabin where the interior or the firewood harbors ticks may be sufficient. An actual history of a tick bite or seeing a tick is often absent. Relapsing fever is, as the name suggests, a series of febrile episodes separated by several days during which the patient feels well (similar to malaria). The diagnosis is made by seeing the *Borrelia* spirochetes in a peripheral blood smear obtained during a bout of illness. Tetracycline and chloramphenicol are the treatments of choice. Colorado tick fever is also characterized by a period of remission between several febrile days, giving rise to a "saddle-back" fever pattern. The most striking laboratory abnormality is usually leukopenia, but the diagnosis rests on a rising antibody titer or recovery of virus from blood. There is no specific treatment, and the illness generally resolves without sequelae in 7 to 10 days. Rocky Mountain spotted fever should be suspected in patients with outdoor exposure in the mountainous west but even more so in other endemic areas such as those along the eastern seaboard. In its early stages, this infection may be difficult to separate from other acute febrile illnesses. As it progresses, however, multiorgan involvement and evidence of vasculitis and the characteristic petechial rash may make the diagnosis more obvious. Diagnosis may be made rapidly by fluorescent antibody staining of a biopsy of involved skin. Serology can establish the diagnosis also, but usually only in retrospect. Prompt treatment of this serious disease can be life-saving, and waiting for confirmation of the diagnosis may imperil the patient. Thus, early and often empiric therapy for a highly suspected case with tetracycline or chloramphenicol is appropriate.

Most patients with active tuberculosis have at least a low grade fever. The presentation of tuberculosis in travelers, however, may be different from that seen in other patients because the latter generally have reactivation disease, whereas travelers are more likely to have primary infection. Both groups of patients are likely to have a cough. In travelers, one is more likely to see lower lobe infiltrate and possibly adenopathy on a chest radiograph rather than upper lobe cavitation. The diagnosis, however, proceeds in similar fashion. A positive tuberculin test, especially in a previously negative individual, substantially raises the probability of tuberculosis, but the diagnosis is confirmed, of course, by seeing acid-fast bacteria in the sputum and growing *Mycobacterium tuberculosis* from the specimen. Isoniazid and rifampin constitute the most commonly used therapy. Family contacts and traveling companions should also be evaluated with skin tests if this diagnosis is made.

Prevention of Travel-Associated Infections

Many of the minor and most of the major travel-associated infections are preventable. Effective strategies range from measures designed to reduce contact with infectious material such as avoiding raw foods or using insect repellant to augmenting the traveler's defenses through passive or active immunization or chemoprophylaxis.

Because diarrhea is the most common affliction of vacationers and business travelers, advice about its prevention should be a regular part of pretrip counseling. Table 38–3 summarizes recommendations for prevention of gastrointestinal infections. For visitors to tropical countries where sanitation practices are not like Western standards, untreated water should be avoided. Water can be rendered safe by boiling for 10 minutes or adding one iodine tablet per quart or five drops of tincture of iodine per quart and waiting 30 minutes. Sealed bottled water, carbonated soft drinks, beer, hot coffee, hot tea, undiluted fruit juice, and pasteurized milk are generally safe. Ice added to drinks reintroduces the risk of contaminated water and should be omitted. Fresh

Table 38–3. *Recommendations for Prevention of Travel-Associated Gastrointestinal Infections*

Avoid untreated water including ice.
Water can be made safe by
   Boiling for 10 min.
   Adding iodine tablets, one per quart, and waiting 30 min.
   Adding tincture of iodine, 5 drops per quart, and waiting 30 min.
Carbonated drinks, beer, coffee, tea, undiluted fruit juice, and pasteurized milk are generally safe.
Avoid fresh leafy and raw vegetables. Eat only fruits you can peel or slice yourself.
Avoid uncooked or buffet-style meats, fish, and shellfish. Eat well-cooked food served hot.
Avoid nonpasteurized dairy products in rural areas.

leafy vegetables and raw vegetables are likely to be intrinsically contaminated or are likely to become so during handling or rinsing with water. Therefore, such items and salads made from them should be eschewed. Fruits that can be peeled and sliced personally are safe. Food that is thoroughly cooked and served hot is not likely to be a source of any infection. Avoiding dairy products that are not pasteurized reduces the risk of gastroenteritis, brucellosis, and tuberculosis.

Expert opinion varies substantially regarding the choice and use of prophylactic or therapeutic medicines for traveler's diarrhea. A universal recommendation for antimicrobial prophylaxis seems a bit excessive in view of variable but often low rates of infection, mildness and brevity of the usual illness, and the expense and possible side effects of the drugs. Selected individuals such as those whose visit is of a critical nature or those who are at increased risk because of constitutional, surgical, or medically induced low gastric acidity may be appropriate candidates for prophylaxis, if their visit is for less than 2 weeks. In such persons, prophylaxis should commence on arrival in the high risk area and continue for 2 days after leaving. Several prophylactic regimens have demonstrated efficacy. Doxycycline 100 mg daily, trimethoprim-sulfamethoxazole one double-strength tablet daily, and Pepto-Bismol 2 oz or two tablets orally four times a day have all reduced the incidence of "turista" in short-term visitors to tropical countries. Each has some disadvantages. The tetracyclines can cause a photosensitivity dermatitis and are contraindicated in children and pregnant women because of their effect on teeth and developing bone. Sulfonamides may produce a variety of adverse effects but most commonly are associated with a skin rash that can be quite severe. Trimethoprim alone 200 mg daily and norfloxacin 400 mg daily are also effective and may be less likely to induce allergic or other adverse reactions. All of the effective prophylactic antimicrobials add to the cost of traveling and may predispose to more severe and resistant infections. Pepto-Bismol is a more innocuous agent that interferes with the effect of toxigenic *E. coli* in the intestine. It is a bit cumbersome to carry and to take the required amount each day, but tablets of this over-the-counter preparation are also effective and more convenient. Patients should be told that the bismuth in this product may color their tongue and their stool black. This should not be confused with melena. It may also cause mild tinnitus.

If traveler's diarrhea does occur, it is usually self-limited, but symptomatic improvement or cure can be achieved more rapidly if some of the medicines cited earlier are used in a therapeutic mode. The decision to treat and with what agent should be based on severity of illness and the probability of particular pathogens being present. Table 38–4 summarizes some suggestions regarding this. Effective regimens include bismuth subsalicylate 1 oz every 0.5 hour up to eight doses/day or trimethoprim/sulfamethoxazole one double-strength tablet twice daily for 5 days, trimethoprim 200 mg twice daily for 5 days, or ciprofloxacin 500 mg orally twice daily for 5 days. Loperamide 4 mg then 2 mg after each loose movement up to eight capsules per day or diphenoxylate up to two tables four times a day may provide exclusively symptomatic relief. The latter drugs should not be used in patients with fever and the dysentery syndrome.

If symptoms do not improve spontaneously or after treatment for a week the patient should consult a physician. Other conditions that make medical consultation desirable are the presence of fever, severe abdominal pain, or blood and pus in the stool. Patients with these complaints are more likely to have salmonella, shigella, or campylobacter gastroenteritis. Ampicillin can be used for severe cases of salmonella or shigella infection, whereas erythromycin is the appropriate therapy for cases caused by campylobacter. In endemic cholera areas, if profound watery diarrhea develops, balanced fluid replacement, treatment with tetracycline, and medical evaluation are imperative. Recipes for fluid replacement can be readily prepared with the following ingredients: one fluid has 8 oz of orange, apple, or fruit juice for potassium, ½ teaspoon of honey or corn syrup for glucose, and a pinch of table salt; the other fluid has 8 oz of carbonated or boiled water and ¼ teaspoon of baking soda for sodium bicarbonate. The patient consumes glasses of each fluid alternately until thirst is quenched. Other safe fluids can also be added.

Although less common than diarrhea, malaria can be much more serious. Several types of malaria are found in tropical countries, the most serious of which is caused by *Plasmodium falciparum*. Unfortunately, chloroquine-resistant falciparum strains have become widely established around the world. This has made prophylactic recommendations a bit more complex. Chloroquine continues to be recommended for all travelers to endemic areas because chloroquine-sensitive strains are ubiquitous. Chloroquine should be given as 500 mg orally weekly for 1 week before entering the endemic region, continued once weekly throughout the stay, and once weekly for 6 weeks after departure. Side effects such as rash and telogen effluvium (falling out of the hair) are rare, and retinopathy does not occur with prophylaxis given for less than 5 years.

Fansidar (pyrimethamine-sulfadoxine) is effective prophylaxis for chloroquine-resistant falciparum strains when taken once per week. However, its side effects, such as Stevens-Johnson syndrome and toxic epidermal necrolysis, and its contraindication in pregnant patients and those allergic to sulfonamides make its routine use inappropriate. It probably should be given to individuals with prolonged (>3 weeks), sustained, high risk exposure to places such as East and Central Africa. For short-term visitors, the risks seem to outweigh the benefits. For them, provision of at least one treatment dose (three tablets) with instructions to take them and seek medical advice for a fever of 102°F or more is a reasonable compromise.

Other reasonable precautions against malaria include avoiding mosquito-infested areas when possible, wearing protective clothing, and using diethyltoluamide insect repellent where mosquito exposure is likely.

Table 38–4. Indications for Empiric Therapy of Traveler's Diarrhea

Symptoms	Treatment
Mild illness (≤ 3 unformed stools/day) with few or no associated symptoms	Fluids only
Moderate illness (3–5 unformed stools/day) without fever, bloody stools, or disabling associated symptoms	Symptomatic treatment with loperamide or bismuth subsalicylate (Pepto-Bismol)
Severe illness (≥ 6 unformed stools/day) or diarrhea with fever, bloody stools, or disabling associated symptoms	Antimicrobial therapy with or without symptomatic treatment trimethoprim/ sulfamethoxazole, trimethoprim, or ciprofloxacin

Schistosomiasis is an uncommon disease of visitors to endemic areas in North Africa and Asia. It can be avoided simply by not bathing or swimming in potentially infected lakes, rivers, or streams.

Acquired Immunodeficiency Syndrome and Human Immunodeficiency Virus

Many travelers now express concern about their risk of this syndrome when visiting other lands, especially Africa, because they are aware that the disease is highly prevalent there. Their questions often focus on the risk of transmission by casual contact, food, and mosquitos. There is no evidence that these routes are implicated in the transmission of human immunodeficiency virus infection. The manner in which the infection is acquired is known: it involves percutaneous exposure to blood or blood products or intimate sexual contact. Travelers who avoid sexual relations with persons conceivably at risk and who have no contact with blood should not be at increased risk of acquiring the virus. If during the course of treatment for an accident or illness, it becomes necessary to receive blood or blood products, it would be reasonable and prudent to inquire about its origin and testing. Blood and blood products manufactured in North America, Japan, and Western Europe are tested and/or treated in such a way that they are quite safe with respect to this virus.

Immunizations

Preparing for a trip provides a good opportunity to assess the routine immunization status of children and adults. A consultation should be scheduled at least 6 weeks before departure so that necessary boosters and new immunizations can be given and an antibody response can develop. Table 38–5 summarizes recommended immunizations. Everyone should be fully immunized against diphtheria and tetanus. This requires an initial series and boosters every 10 years. Measles vaccination should be provided for individuals without a history of measles who have not been vaccinated with live measles vaccine (birth date before 1956). If the individual has not had rubella, mumps, or both, the combined measles-mumps-rubella vaccine is recommended. Although not routinely required within the United States, travelers to developing countries should have polio

Table 38–5. *Immunizations for the Traveler*

Routine (these vaccinations should be up to date or unnecessary because of history of illness):
  Diphtheria-tetanus (booster every 10 yr)
  Measles*
  Mumps*
  Rubella*
  Poliomyelitis (booster every 5 yr for those traveling to rural areas of developing countries)
Sometimes required for international travel:
  Cholera (valid for 6 mo)
  Yellow fever* (valid for 10 yr)
  Typhoid (booster every 3 yr)
  Immune globulin for hepatitis A prophylaxis (repeat every 3–6 mo)
Vaccines for special circumstances:
  Rabies (human diploid cell vaccine booster every 2 yr)
  Meningococcus
  Plague
  Hepatitis B

*Live attenuated viral vaccine.

boosters with the inactivated vaccine. The boosters need not be repeated more often than at 5-year intervals.

Certain areas of the world are endemic for specific diseases not encountered elsewhere, such as yellow fever in South America, and some countries require evidence of vaccination for particular diseases to avoid their importation. For this reason, it is necessary to discuss a traveler's itinerary, consult the sources mentioned later in this chapter, and determine which vaccines are medically appropriate and which are legislatively required. For visitors to yellow fever endemic areas of South America, Africa, and Trinidad, yellow fever vaccine is recommended. It must be repeated at 10-year intervals. It is generally available at large urban public health departments and a limited number of other officially designated centers.

Cholera vaccine is neither particularly effective nor long-lasting, but many countries require evidence of cholera vaccination within 1 year for travelers passing through endemic areas.

Typhoid vaccine should be considered for all travelers whose risk to contaminated food and water is unavoidably high and prolonged because of the nature of their visit. Most cases are seen in individuals traveling in Mexico or India. The vaccine is given in two doses, 1 month apart, and provides protection for 3 years.

Special circumstances may suggest the use of vaccines that are not routinely recommended either for U.S. residents or travelers. Individuals likely to have accidental or occupational exposure to rabid animals in Africa, Latin America, and the Indian subcontinent should receive the human diploid cell rabies vaccine in three doses. Plague is endemic in animals in some areas of rural Africa, Asia, and South America, as it is in parts of the western and southwestern United States. Only exceptional travelers—those contemplating occupational exposure to rodents and their fleas—are candidates for plague vaccine. Hepatitis B, like human immunodeficiency virus, is transmitted by exposure to blood and sexual contact. Some travelers, such as those engaged in health care or those who are likely to be sexually active with individuals at risk, should be vaccinated with three doses of hepatitis B vaccine. It should be administered in the deltoid area rather than the buttock for a better immune response.

Meningococcal disease is endemic in sub-Saharan Africa in the dry season, and in the last decade has been epidemic in diverse areas around the globe including Brazil, Finland, India, and Nepal. Travelers to endemic areas are potential candidates for the vaccine, although unless they have exceptionally intimate contact with the residents the risk is quite small.

Hepatitis A is spread by the fecal-oral route, and contaminated food can serve as a vehicle. Precautions aimed at lowering the risk of other food-borne infections should also reduce the likelihood of hepatitis A. However, travelers who by necessity or choice adopt a native lifestyle in the developing world and along the Mediterranean coast may benefit from the passive protection afforded by immune globulin. Administration of the globulin would need to be repeated at approximately 3-month intervals for the duration of exposure to provide optimal protection. Visitors who stay for a short time at Western-style hotels and resorts are at such low risk that vaccination is unnecessary.

Sources of Information

Because epidemics are often unpredictable, because recommendations regarding vaccination and prophylaxis are constantly changing, and because governmental requirements for travelers are sometimes complex and obscure, it is important that physicians have reliable and up-to-date sources of accurate information for their traveling patients.

State and large city health departments receive regular communications from the Centers for Disease Control (CDC) regarding rec-

ommendations for travelers. The CDC also regularly issues an almost indispensable paperback handbook called Health Information for International Travel, available from the Superintendent of Documents, U.S. Government Printing Office, Washington, DC 20402. The CDC's weekly publication Morbidity and Mortality Weekly Report is also an extremely valuable and unrivaled source of current information on travel-associated infections. For additional up-to-date information, the CDC's Center for Prevention Services, Atlanta, GA 30333 can be contacted directly (telephone 1–404–329–1800). Advice about physicians and medical facilities available abroad can be obtained from International Association for Medical Assistance to Travelers, 736 Center Street, Lewiston, NY 14092 (telephone 1–716–754–4883).

Good information, good advice, and good judgement should prevent most infections in travelers.

Bibliography

Advice for travelers. Med Lett 29:53–56, 1987.
> *The virtue of this reference is brevity. Most common infectious disease and immunization concerns are addressed concisely.*

Committee on Immunization, Council of Medical Societies. Guide for Adult Immunization. Philadelphia, American College of Physicians, 1985.
> *This is a useful pamphlet that provides recommendations on routine immunizations, prophylaxis for a variety of conditions, and a short section on travel-related conditions and immunization. The material on specific vaccines such as duration of immunity, adverse reactions, and precautions and contraindications is quite useful.*

Division of Quarantine, Center for Prevention Services, Centers for Disease Control. Health Information for International Travel. Washington, DC, U.S. Department of Health and Human Services, 1987.
> *This is the most complete and detailed source of information on recommended and required immunizations and prophylaxis. It also includes an excellent section on other travel-related issues called Helpful Hints for the Traveler. A new edition is issued each year and is available from the U.S. Government Printing Office.*

Dupont HL. Infectious diarrhea: a patient outside the United States, in Bayless TM, Brain MC, Cherniack RM (eds). Current Therapy in Internal Medicine—2. Toronto, BC Decker, 1987, pp 213–214.
> *This chapter provides a short tabular summary of risk factors for traveler's diarrhea, medical and practical ways to reduce risk, and indications for empiric therapy.*

Gorbach SL, Edelman R (eds). Travelers' diarrhea. National Institutes of Health Consensus Development Conference. Rev Infect Dis 8(Suppl 2):S109, 1986.
> *The risks and benefits of various prophylactic and therapeutic strategies are discussed.*

Hill DR, Pearson RD. Health advice for international travel. Ann Intern Med 108:839–852, 1988.

This is a thorough review, with especially helpful sections on immunizations and malaria prophylaxis.

Lange WR. Travel medicine resources for the primary care physician. Postgrad Med 81:293–300, 1987.

This article is a valuable guide to books, journals, and organizations concerned with illness in travelers. It lists references suitable for both the physician and his or her patient.

Mann JM. Emporiatric policy and practice: protecting the health of Americans abroad. JAMA 249:3323–3325, 1983.

This concise commentary with useful facts pertaining to the number of travelers and their destinations mentions two major problems related to emporiatrics, the science of the health of travelers: lack of expertise in this area by private physicians and a paucity of data about the epidemiology of diseases in travelers and the cost-effectiveness of various methods of prevention.

Sears SI, Sach RB. Medical advice for the international travelers, in Barker LR, Burton JR, Zieve PD (eds). *Principles of Ambulatory Medicine*, ed 2. Baltimore, Williams & Wilkins, 1986, pp 400–414.

This chapter takes a disease- and vaccine-specific approach to the problems of international travel. It contains some interesting material on noninfectious travel-associated problems such as high altitude exposure, snake bite, and special problems of women and children.

Smith RP Jr. Health advice for travelers, in Branch WT (ed). Office Practice of Medicine, ed 2. Philadelphia, WB Saunders, 1987, pp 1264–1276.

This chapter also takes a disease- and vaccine-specific approach to the problems of international travel. It includes a useful section on the evaluation of the returning traveler.

Wolfe MS. Diseases of travelers. CIBA Clin Symp 36(2):1–32, 1984.

This valuable reference is particularly strong with respect to protozoan and parasitic infections and is distinguished by its excellent illustrations of both pathogens and their clinical manifestations.

39

Herpes Simplex and Varicella-Zoster Virus Infections

DAVID C. CLASSEN, M.D.
CHARLES B. SMITH, M.D.

Herpes Simplex Virus

Introduction

Herpes is derived from the Greek word *herpe*, which means to creep. A documented problem in prebiblical times, herpes simplex virus (HSV) infections continue to creep into everyday modern life and remain among the most common infections of humans. For most patients, these infections are more of an annoyance than a significant clinical problem. However, for the immunocompromised patient or the neonate, HSV infections can be life-threatening. During the last two decades, we have dramatically increased the understanding of HSV infections as well as the availability of new and promising methods of treatment, including the use of antiviral drugs and vaccines. The internal medicine practitioner is now faced with issues raised by these common infections, including diagnostic considerations, therapeutic alternatives, public health implications, and the sexual and emotional impacts on patients.

Epidemiology

HSV is a member of the large group of herpesviruses, which also includes cytomegalovirus, Epstein-Barr virus, and varicella-zoster virus (VZV). Human HSV infections are caused by two biologically related but antigenically distinct viruses, HSV type 1 (HSV 1) and HSV type 2 (HSV 2). Both strains cause mucocutaneous disease and can infect any part of the body. However, HSV 1 typically causes infections in the orofacial area and HSV 2, in the genital area. Like all herpesviruses, HSV can cause acute, chronic, latent, or reactivated infections. Although some animals can be experimentally infected with HSV, humans are the only known natural reservoir.

HSV infections occur worldwide and affect all age groups and socioeconomic classes. Approximately a half million episodes of primary herpes labialis infections and 100 million episodes of recurrent herpes labialis infections occur each year, and there are 100,000 to 500,000 cases of primary herpes genitalis and 2 to 20 million recurrences of herpes genitalis infections each year in the United States.

Surveys of the prevalence of antibodies to HSV indicate that primary HSV 1 infection occurs during childhood and that 40 to 60% of young adults show serologic evidence of previous infection, although in lower socioeconomic groups most young adults are seropositive. In contrast, antibodies to HSV 2 do not appear until young adulthood, which reflects the primary role of sexual transmission of HSV 2. The prevalence of antibodies to HSV 2 is related to sexual activity and socioeconomic factors and ranges from 3% for nuns to 25% for middle class patients to more than 80% for prostitutes.

The majority of patients with antibody to HSV 1 or 2 are asymptomatic. Some asymptomatic patients may periodically excrete HSV 1 or 2 in their pharyngeal or genital secretions and may be a source for infecting others. The titer of HSV in cultures from symptomatic lesions is 100 to 1000 times higher than that from cultures of the oral or genital tracts of asymptomatic excreters; thus, transmission of HSV infections is more likely to occur from patients with symptomatic lesions. Transmission occurs by direct physical contact and involves direct inoculation of virus into mucocutaneous sites or abraded skin.

Recurrent Infections

After replication of HSV in epithelial cells of mucous membranes or the skin, the virus spreads to the sensory nerves and is transported intraxonally to proximal ganglia. HSV can remain in the ganglion in a latent state for the life of the patient; recurrent infections are due to reactivation of HSV from its latent state. Factors that have been documented to stimulate reactivation include fever, exposure of the skin (particularly of the lips) to ultraviolet light, surgical trauma to the trigeminal nerve roots, and immunosuppression (as seen with cancer chemotherapy or acquired immunodeficiency syndrome [AIDS]). Other suggested causes of reactivation include hormonal changes associated with menses and emotional and physical stresses. Recurrences generally occur in the same areas as the initial infection and are clinically less severe than the initial infection. Reinfections also occur with both HSV 1 and 2 as a result of new contacts with infected individuals. These can occur at any site and are less severe than the primary infections, presumably because of pre-existing immunity.

Clinical Features

HERPES LABIALIS

Primary infection with HSV 1 usually occurs in childhood and is most often asymptomatic. Infection is acquired by contact with infected oral secretions. Symptomatic primary infections present as gingivostomatitis or pharyngitis, both of which can be quite severe. HSV 1 has a 2- to 12-day incubation period followed by fever and sore throat with the development of pharyngeal edema and erythema. Vesicular lesions then appear on the pharynx, buccal mucosa, tongue, soft palate, and floor of the mouth. Lesions on the mucous membrane quickly ulcerate, so that the vesicular phase can be missed. Breath is usually fetid and cervical adenopathy is often present. Mouth pain can be so severe that some children become significantly dehydrated. Systemic symptoms can persist for as long as 7 to 10 days. In college-age students, primary infection can present as a posterior pharyngitis alone. In one

study, HSV was isolated from the pharynx of 11% of college students admitted to an infirmary with pharyngitis. In this population, ulcerative or exudative lesions could be seen on the tonsils or posterior pharynx. The total duration of the illness is about 10 to 14 days for both children and adults.

Recurrent infection occurs in 20 to 40% of individuals with herpes labialis. Serial cultures of oral and pharyngeal secretions indicate that recurrent infection is frequently asymptomatic. However, when symptomatic, it is manifested clinically as blistering lesions on the lips (cold sores), gums, or anterior hard palate. Often a prodrome of pain, burning, or itching for 6 to 48 hours precedes the appearance of vesicular lesions on the vermilion border of the lips. The lesions ulcerate over the next day or two and then form a crust. Cervical adenopathy may occur but fever is unusual. Resolution occurs within 8 to 10 days. The nose, chin, and cheek can also be involved, as can the eye in the form of keratitis, conjunctivitis, and blepharitis. In immunosuppressed patients, burn patients, and patients with severe atopic eczema, severe recurrent infections of the skin and mucous membranes can occur. The mucositis of HSV 1 can mimic mucositis from other etiologies such as radiation, cytotoxic therapy, or fungal infection.

HERPES GENITALIS

The first clinically apparent genital infection with HSV 1 or 2 is called primary if there has been no prior infection with HSV 1 or 2 by history or serology; it is called initial if there is evidence of a prior HSV infection. It appears that initial HSV 2 disease can first manifest years after an unrecognized HSV 1 primary infection and that prior infection with HSV 1 limits the severity of the initial infection with HSV 2. Approximately 80% of herpes genitalis is due to HSV 2; however, initial episodes of genital HSV 1 or 2 are clinically indistinguishable. The primary or initial episode of herpes genitalis usually occurs during young adulthood and correlates with sexual activity. The high degree of infectivity of HSV 2 is documented by reports that 85 to 90% of women get herpes genitalis if sexually exposed to a male with active lesions. The incubation period is from 2 to 7 days, and lesions are often preceded by a prodrome including fever, anorexia, malaise, headache, and lassitude. Local symptoms include pain, itching, dysuria, vaginal and urethral discharge, and bilateral tender inguinal adenopathy. Then, widely scattered papules develop in the genital area, usually on the penile shaft or glans in men and on the vulva, perineum, buttocks, vagina, and cervix in women. The papules quickly become vesicles on an erythematous base that can persist for several days on the skin. However, lesions on mucosal surfaces quickly ulcerate and are covered by a grayish-white exudate, and thus the vesicular phase can be missed, especially in women. Skin and mucous membrane lesions are often exceedingly painful. Lesions usually form a crust by 5 days and heal by 10 to 14 days. The total duration of illness can be 3 weeks, although systemic symptoms usually resolve by 1 week. The most significant complication is local neurologic involvement, which can lead to sacral neuralgia characterized by urinary retention, constipation, and loss of anal tone. In 20 to 30% of primary cases, transient aseptic meningitis can develop, which usually is self-limited and benign and manifested only by inflammatory cells in the spinal fluid.

RECURRENT HERPES GENITALIS

Although recurrences are often less severe than the initial infection, they can still be quite disturbing and emotionally disruptive. The frequency of recurrences can vary from monthly to yearly or every few years. Recurrence rates tend to decrease over time after the initial infection. In contrast to initial infections, recurrent infections generally do not produce systemic symptoms. Prodromes occur in half of all recurrences and include hyperesthesia/dysesthesia, tenderness, itching, and burning, which occur 3 to 24 hours before the lesions appear. Vesicles rapidly progress to ulcers on mucous membranes or they form a crust on the skin as in the initial infection. All lesions are usually healed by 10 days, although in 10% of patients, new lesions may continue to form during the first week. Symptoms that also may complicate recurrences include dysuria, vaginal discharge, and persistent neuralgia.

OTHER INFECTION SITES

HSV can cause infection in many other sites. Herpetic whitlow is HSV infection of fingers and hands that most often occurs in medical and dental personnel after virus from infected mucosal surfaces of patients is introduced through abraded skin. Infection is characterized by pustular or vesicular lesions at the site of inoculation and is associated with fever, malaise, and regional adenopathy, which often leads to a mistaken diagnosis of bacterial infection. The course is usually self-limited unless surgical drainage is attempted, which can spread and prolong the viral infection.

Homosexual men or heterosexual women who participate in anal intercourse can develop HSV infections of the perianal area, rectum, or colon. Proctitis can present with pain, discharge, tenesmus, and sacral neuralgia. Systemic symptoms and inguinal adenopathy are very common. The disease is usually self-limited, and healing occurs by 2 to 3 weeks unless the patient has an underlying immunodeficiency, in which case the disease can have a prolonged and progressive course.

HSV infections of the eye can present as conjunctivitis, blepharitis, and keratitis. Because untreated infections can lead to permanent blindness, patients suspected of having HSV infections of the eye should be promptly referred to an ophthalmologist. The primary infection presents as a conjunctivitis and blepharitis, and the presence of vesicles on the conjunctiva or satellite lesions should suggest the diagnosis. Recurrent infections usually present with a typical dendritic keratitis, which is easily identified by an examination of the cornea with the aid of fluorescein dye and a slit lamp. Several antiviral drugs including trifluridine and idoxuridine are effective in controlling this infection. Topical corticosteroids are contraindicated in the early stages of infection, a proscription that needs emphasis because some physicians inappropriately use such agents in empirically treating pinkeye.

Neonatal HSV infections usually occur within a few days of delivery and are often systemic, rapidly progressive, and associated with a significant mortality even with treatment. Infections are transmitted during vaginal delivery of an infant to a mother with herpes genitalis. The risk of neonatal infection is high when delivery occurs in conjunction with an episode of primary herpes genitalis, and elective cesarean section is recommended. However, the risk of transmission is much lower with symptomatic recurrences, and recommendations for a cesarean section are much less clear in this setting. The risk of serious neonatal infection is much lower if mothers are asymptomatic shedders of HSV or if their primary infection occurs in the first or second trimester. A cesarean section is not usually recommended for either group. These mothers do not need to be screened for HSV infection, nor do they need acyclovir prophylaxis. However, primary herpes infection during the first 20 weeks of pregnancy has been associated with an increased risk of spontaneous abortion, congenital abnormalities, and premature birth. Pregnant women who are the sexual partners of persons with active HSV lesions should abstain from sex during the third trimester and should use barrier protection during the first two trimesters. Women can be advised that the presence of recurrent herpes genitalis is not a valid reason to avoid a wanted pregnancy and that the risk of severe neonatal herpes can be made quite small with proper medical care and advice.

Herpes encephalitis is a life-threatening disease and commonly presents in otherwise healthy patients with the rapid onset of fever, confusion, and seizures; there is usually no evidence of skin lesions. Spinal fluid analysis reveals pleocytosis with mononuclear cells; however, the cerebrospinal fluid findings are variable, and normal findings do not rule out the diagnosis. Diagnosis is aided by computed axial tomographic scan, magnetic resonance imaging, brain scan, or arteriographic evidence of focal lesions in the temporal lobe and an electroencephalogram showing focality in the temporal lobe. A definitive diagnosis is made by brain biopsy. Current therapy is intravenous acyclovir for 2 to 3 weeks. The mortality rate is quite high and the survivors are often significantly disabled even with appropriate therapy.

HSV infections have also been associated with erythema multiforme, Stevens-Johnson syndrome, Bell's palsy, trigeminal neuralgia, and temporal lobe epilepsy, but further work is needed to confirm and explain these observations. The epidemiologic association of HSV infections with cancer of the cervix has been complicated by evidence that the human papilloma virus can also cause cervical cancer. Therefore, all women with a history of genital herpes infections should be advised that yearly pelvic examinations with Pap smears are appropriate.

Psychologic Implications

Although the clinical illness associated with recurrent herpes is usually quite mild, the stigma of this sexually transmitted disease, which may affect newborn children, has understandably generated strong emotional feelings among the affected patients. The goal of counseling patients with genital herpes is to alleviate unnecessary and inappropriate anxieties while instructing the patient regarding the prevention of transmission of the disease and the availability of therapy. The physician should attempt to provide truthful and accurate information and to address each issue of concern in a direct nonjudgmental and compassionate manner. It is reasonable to present all information in as positive a light as possible and to point out that the disease is not as severe as the lay community has been led to believe. Emphasis should be placed on the usual lack of serious medical complications and on the effective therapies available. Other issues that need to be addressed include methods for prevention of transmission, how and when to tell present or future partners, concerns about childbirth, and cervical cancer.

Diagnosis

The initial clinical diagnosis must rely on symptoms and typical lesions in a patient with a history of prior infection or recent exposure to someone with HSV infections. In the case of typical herpes labialis, the clinical diagnosis is usually sufficient. Herpes genitalis, in contrast, should be confirmed by laboratory testing because of the significant implications of the diagnosis and because other conditions can mimic the genital ulcers seen with HSV.

Viral isolation is the best method for confirmation of diagnosis (Table 39–1). It is highly specific (100%) and sensitive (80 to 90%) if the sample for culture is taken during the vesicular stage and plated within 6 hours. False-negative results may be due to improper collection techniques, improper sample transport, or prior use of topical or oral antiviral medications. A more rapid alternative is the abbreviated cell culture method followed by fluorescent antibody staining (shell-vial technique). It has specificity and sensitivity comparable to those of viral culture and offers savings of time (< 24 hours) and cost.

Cytologic examination of cells scraped from the bottom of lesions (Tzanck's smear) may show multinucleated giant cells and inclusions suggestive of HSV infection; however, this technique is not very sensitive (40 to 57%) and not very specific (60%).

Detection of HSV viral antigens in cells scraped from active lesions by using monoclonal antibodies and the indirect fluorescent technique has the advantage of rapidity (< 24

Table 39–1. Diagnosis of HSV Infections

Test	Sensitivity (%)	Specificity (%)	Time	Cost ($)
Viral isolation (cell culture)	80–90	100	1–7 days	25
Nonspecific stain (Tzanck)	40–57	60	1–2 h	15
Specific stain (immunofluorescent monoclonal antibodies)	48–100	80–98	2–5 h	75
Abbreviated cell culture with specific stain	65–100	88–100	1–2 days	100
Electron microscopy	10–88	50–80	2 h	125
Enzyme immunoassay	40–96	62–95	4–6 h	35
Serologic tests				
Immunoglobulin G	Unknown	60–95	2–24 h	35
Immunoglobulin M	Unknown	90–100		35

Adapted, with permission, from Straus SE. Herpes simplex virus infections: biology, treatment, and prevention. Ann Intern Med 1985; 103:404.

hours), but this method is also less sensitive and specific than viral culture and is not available at most centers. A new technique that holds much promise is the use of DNA probes for the detection of specific viral DNA or RNA in clinical specimens. It is quick, sensitive, and specific; however, it is not yet generally available.

Serologic studies are not helpful for the reliable diagnosis of HSV infections in individual patients. When an initial suspicion of herpes genitalis is not confirmed by laboratory testing, further evaluation should be done for veneral diseases such as syphilis and chancroid, which can present as genital ulcers.

Management

The major goals of treatment of HSV infections are to decrease the severity of acute symptoms, prevent local spread of lesions, prevent recurrences, and reduce the transmission to others. The emergence of antiviral drugs has offered hope for meeting some of these goals. Multiple antiviral agents are now under study; however, currently only acyclovir appears efficacious and relatively nontoxic for treatment of some oral and genital HSV infections. Acyclovir is a nucleoside analogue that is phosphorylated to its active form by a viral-coded thymidine kinase and consequently is activated only in HSV-infected cells. This activated form works by inhibiting viral replication. Acyclovir is available in topical, oral, and intravenous formulations. Only 15 to 30% of the oral dose is absorbed and the half-life is short; thus, high doses are needed (200 mg orally five times a day). Oral acyclovir is generally well tolerated. Elevated blood levels occur rapidly in patients with renal impairment, leading to confusion, somnolence, and other central nervous system aberrations; ad-

justment of dose in this setting is necessary. Other side effects have been reported with long-term therapy, including diarrhea (8%), headache (13%), arthralgias (3.6%), and slight elevations in bilirubin (14%). There have been some reports of leukopenia and thrombocytopenia.

IMMUNOCOMPROMISED PATIENTS

Immunocompromised patients may develop prolonged local disease or may face local progression and dissemination. Those particularly at risk include patients with hematologic or lymphoreticular malignancies, inherited athymic disorders, organ transplants (particularly bone marrow), AIDS, and significant burns. In such patients, multiple studies have shown that acyclovir in oral or intravenous form decreases the formation of new lesions, decreases the time to healing, decreases the time of viral shedding, and prevents local progression or dissemination. Acyclovir therapy is clearly indicated for all immunocompromised patients with local or disseminated disease (Fig. 39–1). Oral therapy is usually adequate for mild disease, although intravenous therapy should be used in the seriously ill patient. The usual intravenous dose is 5 mg/kg every 8 hours.

Antiviral prophylaxis can prevent HSV reactivation in immunosuppressed patients. Acyclovir prophylaxis has been advocated for bone marrow and heart transplant patients as well as during periods of immunosuppression in other patients (chemotherapy and radiotherapy). Reports of success without serious toxicity have appeared.

IMMUNOCOMPETENT PATIENTS

OROFACIAL HERPES

For primary herpes infection of the oral cavity, no oral or topical agent has been shown

Mucocutaneous HSV Infection

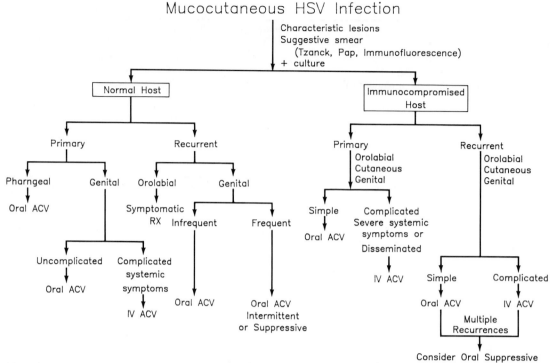

Figure 39–1. Decision tree for choice of therapy for HSV infections. Doses for oral and intravenous (IV) acyclovir (ACV) therapy are discussed in the text. Adapted from Whitley RJ and Barnes DW. Herpes simplex virus infection, in Kass E and Platt R (eds). Current Therapy in Infectious Diseases–2. Toronto, B. C. Decker, 1986: 380.

to be clearly efficacious in treating the acute infection or preventing recurrent infection. However, oral acyclovir has been shown to reduce the severity of primary genital infection and by extrapolation, we believe that it is appropriate to treat primary HSV gingivostomatitis and pharyngitis with oral acyclovir (200 mg five times a day for 10 days). We do not recommend treatment of recurrent orofacial herpes labialis because it is usually a benign and self-limited disease and all available agents have at best shown limited benefit in treatment studies. However, prophylaxis may be appropriate for patients who have particularly severe recurrences, for patients who have severe atopic eczema, or for patients whose recurrences are complicated by erythema multiforme. These patients may receive prophylactic oral acyclovir at a dose of 200 mg three times a day for up to 1 year. However, prophylaxis is not recommended for pregnant or breast-feeding patients.

HERPES GENITALIS

Multiple studies have shown the efficacy of oral and intravenous acyclovir in acute primary or initial herpes genitalis. Decreases in duration of pain, viral shedding, and time to healing have all been noted. However, no trial has shown prevention of latent infection or a decrease in the frequency of recurrences with short-term treatment of primary or initial genital infection. Topical preparations have been shown to be clearly inferior to systemic therapy. Thus, for the treatment of initial or primary herpes genitalis, oral acyclovir 200 mg five times a day for 10 days is recommended. Intravenous therapy may be indicated for severe cases and for patients with neurologic complications.

Treatment of symptomatic recurrences is more controversial. No topical agent has been found to be clearly efficacious in moderating symptomatic recurrences. Oral acyclovir has been shown to decrease the frequency of appearance of new lesions, to reduce the time to healing, and to decrease viral shedding if used within 3 days of the onset of symptoms. Thus, for sporadic severe recurrences of herpes genitalis, oral acyclovir 200 mg five times a day for 5 days is recommended.

Prevention of recurrences has been studied in patients who experience at least six recurrences a year. Trials have been done with daily doses of 400, 600, and 1000 mg of acyclovir; all were shown to be more effective than a placebo in decreasing, but not eliminating, the frequency of recurrences. All trials have found that recurrence rates return to pretreatment levels after therapy stops. The use of acyclovir for longer than 1 year has not been evaluated in any trial to date; thus, the risks of long-term use have not been elucidated. At this time, we recommend prophylaxis only for patients who have a history of more than six recurrences of herpes genitalis per year and who are severely distressed by their illness. The dose is 200 mg of acyclovir orally three times a day for a maximum of 6 months.

Because chances of transmission of HSV are greatest when lesions are active, abstinence from sexual intercourse is the recommended method of prevention during recurrences. There is no evidence that the use of acyclovir prevents transmission during episodes of recurrences. Condoms are believed to reduce the transmission of HSV significantly, and their use should be encouraged. However, during the last trimester of pregnancy, women should abstain from intercourse with infected male partners regardless of the use of acyclovir or condoms.

Varicella-Zoster Virus

Introduction

VZV is a herpesvirus that causes the common childhood illness varicella (chicken pox) and that can reactivate in later life to cause herpes zoster (shingles). In most children, varicella is a relatively minor and self-limited illness, whereas zoster, which occurs in 50% of adults, is associated with significant morbidity in the form of postherpetic neuralgia (PHN) and mortality associated with dissemination. PHN is primarily a problem in elderly patients, whereas disseminated zoster is a significant problem in immunocompromised patients.

Epidemiology

Initial infection with VZV usually occurs during childhood, and few escape infection with the virus before reaching adulthood. Reactivation of VZV infection in the form of zoster occurs at an increasing rate with age. It is estimated that in a population of 1000 pa-

tients who live until they are 85 years old, 500 have had at least one episode and 10 have had two episodes of VZV infection. In addition to increased risk with increasing age, this infection is also more common in patients with malignancy or immunosuppression than in immunocompetent patients. Zoster has been estimated to occur in 50% of bone marrow transplant patients, in 40% of AIDS patients, and in 15 to 30% of patients with Hodgkin's disease, especially those undergoing radiation therapy and/or chemotherapy. Unlike chicken pox, which has a seasonal predominance, zoster occurs throughout the year. Although there have been reports that the incidence of zoster is related to exposure to acute varicella, there are no accepted data linking the two. Conversely, the lesions of zoster patients are infectious and can be the source of chicken pox, a problem of particular concern in hospitals.

Pathogenesis

Transmission of VZV usually occurs by respiratory spread of the virus in aerosols. The virus is rapidly disseminated from the respiratory tract through the bloodstream to the skin and other organs. VZV has a predilection for damaging epithelial cells of the lung and skin, and it is unusual to see direct damage to other organs. Although initial infection is brief and self-limited, epidemiologic data on the incidence of VZV indicate that latent infection develops in a least 50% of individuals. Latent infection is presumed to occur in sensory ganglia because at reactivation zoster follows dermatomal patterns of involvement and because autopsy studies done during early reactivation show destruction of dorsal root ganglia from which VZV has been cultured.

Clinical Features of Acute Zoster

Zoster begins with a prodrome of fever, malaise, chills, neuritic pain, and occasionally gastrointestinal symptoms that can last for as long as 4 to 6 days before appearance of the rash. The rash erupts as erythematous papules that progress in 24 hours to vesicular lesions on an erythematous base. New lesions commonly develop over 2 to 3 days but are quite unusual after 5 days. The rash is usually confined to one or more sensory dermatomes and rarely crosses the midline (less than 1% of cases occur bilaterally). Thoracic dermatomes are most commonly involved followed by trigeminal, cervical, and lumbar dermatomes. It is not uncommon to find a few lesions adjacent to the primary dermatomes, and this finding does not represent dissemination. Vesicular lesions commonly form a crust by 5 to 7 days and resolve by 2 weeks, except in patients who develop secondary bacterial infections or in immunocompromised patients in whom the rash can progress over many weeks or months if untreated.

Neuritic pain in the same distribution as the rash usually occurs before the onset of the rash and at this stage may be a difficult diagnostic problem. The pain of acute zoster varies from an annoying itching to a dull aching or burning pain in the area of the rash. The skin in the area of the rash is typically hyperesthetic, and irritation or motion of the affected area may induce severe lancinating and sharp radiating pains. The pain usually resolves when the cutaneous lesions disappear.

In most patients, the clinical course of zoster is benign and self-limited. Cutaneous lesions heal completely within 3 weeks and neuritic pain resolves in about the same time. Most patients suffer no long-lasting complications from their illness.

Complications

PHN is the most common complication of herpes zoster and can be defined as prolonged neuritic pain after resolution of the cutaneous lesions of zoster. PHN persists for 2 to 12 months and gradually resolves, although it can persist for up to 2 years and can produce such severe symptoms that it can totally incapacitate patients. Although PHN is quite unusual in young patients, it occurs in 50 to 75% of patients over age 60.

The pain of PHN is similar to that seen in acute zoster and varies in severity from an annoying itching sensation to a constant, severe burning pain with intermittent attacks of stabbing radicular pain. The pain of PHN can be especially distressing because of its chronic and unrelenting nature. Many patients suffer from associated depression, which can severely alter lifestyle and ability to function normally.

Dissemination of zoster appears as cutaneous spread to other dermatomes. The spread of the rash occurs from 4 to 11 days after its initial appearance and indicates that the host is no longer able to control the viral infection. Visceral dissemination to the lungs, liver, and central nervous system also can occur at the same time. Although dissemination can occasionally occur in immunocompetent patients, it is more common in immunocompromised patients with an incidence of 5 to 15%. Even in hospitalized immunocompromised patients, the mortality with dissemination is less than 10%.

Central nervous system complications of zoster are diverse but infrequent. Ramsay Hunt syndrome is characterized by tympanic membrane involvement and unilateral 12th nerve paralysis. Bell's palsy of the facial nerve has also been observed. Sacral nerve dysfunction is manifested by incontinence, impotence, and constipation. Transverse myelitis, Guillain-Barré syndrome, aseptic meningitis, and encephalitis have been seen. Neurologic complications are usually self-limited except in the severely compromised patient.

Reactivation in the ophthalmic division of the trigeminal nerve can lead to a spectrum of involvement that includes conjunctivitis, keratitis, glaucoma, and optic neuritis. Herpes simplex can mimic herpes zoster, especially in the trigeminal distribution, and this possibility should prompt concern and evaluation to separate the two.

Diagnosis

Diagnosis of zoster is most frequently made on clinical observation of the typical vesicular rash in a dermatomal pattern that respects midline definition. Although this is a reasonably accurate method for diagnosis, a note of caution is appropriate because herpes simplex can mimic herpes zoster in appearance, especially in the trigeminal distribution and in the genital area. One study revealed that up to 13% of cases of presumed zoster were found to be HSV on culture. Therefore, in clinically vague presentations or in trigeminal involvement, supporting evidence should be collected. Staining of lesion scrapings (Tzanck's smear) when positive shows the presence of multinucleated cells with inclusions but does not help separate VZV from HSV. Acute serologic titers have not been found to be a reliable indicator in diagnosis. The most reliable method of diagnosis is culture of HSV from vesicular fluid within 3 days of onset of lesions. The sensitivity of viral culture of vesicular lesions is much higher for HSV than for VZV, and HSV tends to grow out within 5 days. Therefore, a negative culture at 1 week suggests the diagnosis of VZV rather than HSV.

Zoster occurs in many patients with untreated malignancy, especially those with leukemia and lymphomas. This association has raised the question of whether all patients with zoster without evidence of malignancy should undergo an exhaustive evaluation to rule out any underlying malignancy. In most patients, malignancy has been diagnosed before zoster appears. Most authorities do not believe that an extensive work-up for malignancy is fruitful or appropriate in patients with zoster who are otherwise healthy and have no obvious underlying malignancy after a routine history, physical examination, and screening laboratory tests.

Zoster has recently been noted with increasing frequency in young patients who later develop AIDS. Zoster patients who are also in a high risk group for AIDS should have their HIV status clarified, and clinicians should be aware that zoster may present as the first infectious complication of AIDS or AIDS-related complex.

Treatment

ACUTE ZOSTER

IMMUNOCOMPROMISED PATIENTS

For treatment of zoster infections in immunocompromised patients with localized or disseminated disease, intravenous vidarabine, interferon, and acyclovir have all been shown to be effective in decreasing length of viral shedding, decreasing time of formation of new lesions, and preventing dissemination. Acyclovir currently appears to be the best-tolerated and most effective regimen for the treatment of zoster in immunocompromised patients (Fig. 39–2). A few studies suggest that oral therapy with acyclovir may also be effective in immunocompromised patients, and this route might be tried in patients with mild illness and limited dissemination; however, the intravenous route is most appropriate in the setting of severe systemic illness. The oral dose of acyclovir is 800 mg five times daily, and the intravenous dose is 5 mg/kg given every 8 hours.

IMMUNOCOMPETENT PATIENTS

The treatment of zoster infections in immunocompetent patients is more controversial. Zoster is usually a self-limited process, and appropriate therapy for young, health patients is reassurance and local care to prevent bacterial suprainfection of vesicular lesions. Although intravenous and possibly oral treatment with acyclovir may accelerate clinical improvement, we do not believe that the benefits justify the costs and potential risks of antiviral therapy in this group. An exception to this recommendation is for immunocompetent patients with involvement of the ophthalmic branch of the trigeminal nerve, who should be aggressively treated with intravenous acyclovir because of the potential for blindness.

Most controversy now focuses on the treatment of zoster in elderly patients who suffer from the acute effects of zoster and particularly from PHN. Oral acyclovir at dosages used for HSV infections has not been effective in controlling any of the acute symptoms of zoster. However, a recent British study evaluating the efficacy of acyclovir in high doses (4 g/day for 5 days) for the treatment of acute zoster in immunocompetent patients over age 60 revealed a significant efficacy in reducing the symptoms of acute zoster. Based on this study, we believe that it is appropriate to use high doses of oral acyclovir (800 mg orally five times a day) for the acute symptoms of zoster in all patients over age 60.

The complication of PHN is a common and disabling problem in the elderly population, and effective preventive therapy is needed for this group. Unfortunately, studies to date indicate that the occurrence of PHN does not appear to be influenced by intravenous or oral antiviral therapy of acute zoster. Corticosteroids are used by some physicians to prevent PHN in elderly persons, but this practice remains very controversial. Reports suggesting the efficacy of corticosteroids in preventing PHN have, for the most part, been anecdotal and inconclusive. The most recent and best controlled study failed to show that a 3-week course of oral prednisone affected the development of PHN, and at this time we cannot recommend corticosteroids for prevention or therapy of PHN.

SYMPTOMATIC THERAPY FOR PAIN IN ACUTE ZOSTER AND PHN

The neuritic pain associated with acute zoster and PHN is often of sufficient intensity to require symptomatic treatment. Failure to adequately control the pain in patients with the prolonged symptoms of PHN is often associated with clinical depression and significant loss of function, particularly in elderly patients.

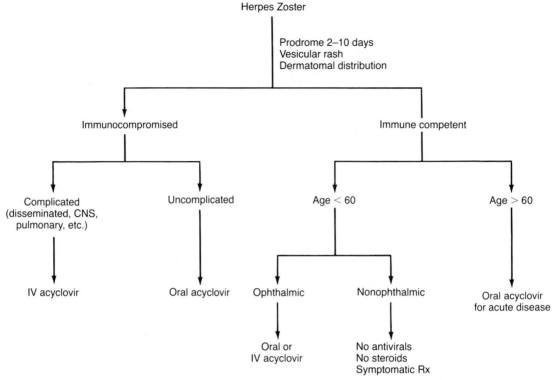

Figure 39–2. *Decision tree for choice of therapy for herpes zoster virus infections. Doses are discussed in the text.*

In the acute phase of the illness, it is reasonable to begin therapy with nonaddicting analgesics such as aspirin or nonsteroid drugs combined with topical agents such as Zostrix (capsaicin 0.025% cream [nonprescription]).

When the pain of acute zoster progresses and is not controlled by initial measures, antidepressants (tricyclics) and anticonvulsants (carbamazepine) should be tried. Some experts believe that neuroaugmentive techniques (acupuncture and counterirritation) can dull the pain by way of overstimulation of the afferent pathway. Occasionally, patients fail to respond to these measures and need more aggressive therapy with either narcotic agents or aggressive surgical intervention (nerve interruption); however, success at this point is often limited.

Bibliography

Balfour HM, Bean B, Laskin OL, et al. Acyclovir halts progression of herpes zoster in immunocompromised patients. N Engl J Med 308:1448–1453, 1983.
Ninety-four immunocompromised patients with zoster were entered in a randomized double-blind trial of intravenous acyclovir versus placebo for 1 week. Treated patients had a quicker resolution of symptoms and lack of progression of the infection.

Brunell PA. Varicella-zoster virus, in Mandel J, Douglas RG, Bennett JE (eds). Principles and Practice of Infectious Diseases. New York, Wiley Medical Publications, 1985, pp 952–960.
This is an excellent review of herpes simplex and herpes zoster.

Bryson YJ, Dillon M, Lovett M, et al. Treatment of first episodes of genital herpes simplex infection with oral acyclovir. A randomized double-blind controlled trial in normal subjects. N Engl J Med 308:916–921, 1983.
This excellent trial shows acyclovir's ability to decrease viral shedding time and new lesion formation as well as to shorten lesion duration.

Corey L, Spear PG. Infections with herpes simplex viruses. N Engl J Med 314:686–690, 749–757, 1986.
This reference is an excellent review of herpes simplex and herpes zoster.

Douglas JM, Critchlow C, Benedetti J, et al. A double-blind study of oral acyclovir for suppression of recurrences of genital herpes simplex virus infection. N Engl J Med 310:1551–1556, 1984.
Oral acyclovir in two dosage regimens was compared in a randomized double-blind trial. Both 1000- and 400-mg regimens were shown to markedly reduce but not eliminate recurrences of genital herpes. After treatment stopped, the recurrence rate returned to pretreatment levels.

Esmann V, Geil JP, Kroon S, et al. Prednisolone does not prevent post-herpetic neuralgia. Lancet 126–129, 1987.
A placebo controlled double-blind trial evaluating the efficacy of prednisolone in the prevention of PHN in elderly patients. The trial failed to show a benefit in the corticosteroid-treated group.

Hirsh MS. Herpes simplex virus, in Mandel J, Douglas

RG, Bennett JE (eds). Principles and Practice of Infectious Diseases. New York, Wiley Medical Publications, 1985, pp 945–952.

This chapter is an excellent review of herpes simplex and herpes zoster.

Kalman CM, Laskin OL. Herpes zoster and zosteriform herpes simplex infections in immunocompetent adults. Am J Med 81:775–778, 1986.

In this review of zoster in immunocompetent adults without underlying illness or malignancy, 13% of patients thought to have zoster infection who were cultured were found to have simplex infection.

Mazur MH, Dolin R. Herpes zoster at the NIH: a 20 year experience. Am J Med 65:738–744, 1978.

A review of 107 cases of zoster at the National Institutes of Health mainly among immunosuppressed patients detailed associated morbidity but a low rate of mortality.

McKendrick MW, McGill JI, White JE, et al. Oral acyclovir in acute herpes zoster. Br Med J 293:1529–1532, 1986.

Oral acyclovir at 4 g/day was compared with placebo in 205 immunocompetent patients with zoster. Acyclovir significantly reduced time to arrest of new lesions, loss of vesicles, and new lesion formation. Also, treated patients had less pain. No significant toxicity was noted at this dose.

Pazin GJ, Harger JH. Management of oral and genital herpes simplex virus infections: diagnosis and treatment. DM 32:725–824, 1986.

This complete review of the approach to diagnosis and treatment of herpes simplex infections has an emphasis on psychologic factors and guide for counseling.

Portenoy RK, Duma C, Foley KM. Acute herpetic and post-herpetic neuralgia: clinical review and current management. Ann Neurol 20:651–664, 1985.

Current understanding of PHN is reviewed, with emphasis on multiple therapeutic approaches.

Shepp DH, Dandliker PS, Meyers JD. Treatment of varicella-zoster infections in severely immunocompromised patients. N Engl J Med 314:208–212, 1986.

Comparison of intravenous acyclovir and intravenous vidarabine in the treatment of VZV infections in immunocompromised patients showed that acyclovir was more effective in preventing progression, preventing complications, shortening the lesion time, and shortening the viral shedding period.

Straus SE. Herpes simplex virus infections: biology, treatment, and prevention. Ann Intern Med 103:404–413, 1985.

An excellent review of herpes simplex and herpes zoster is provided.

Straus SE, Takiff HE, Seidlin M, et al. Suppression of frequently recurring genital herpes. N Engl J Med 310:1545–1550, 1984.

Oral acyclovir 200 mg t.i.d. markedly reduced but did not eliminate recurrences in this randomized trial. Recurrences returned after therapy was stopped.

Straus SE, Ostrove JM, Inchanspé G, et al. Varicella-zoster virus infections. Ann Intern Med 108:221–237, 1988.

This is a well-written, thorough review of the subject. In immunocompetent hosts with herpes zoster infection, the authors recommend limiting oral acyclovir to those patients with ophthalmic zoster (132 references).

Weller TH. Varicella and herpes zoster. N Engl J Med 309:1362–1368, 1434–1440, 1983.

This article is an excellent review of herpes simplex and herpes zoster.

PART NINE

Neurology

40

Diagnosis and Treatment of Headaches

ROBERT V. STEINMETZER, M.D.

Introduction

Headaches are one of the most common symptoms seen by primary care physicians. A typical general medicine practice includes 25 to 30% of patients who have headaches as one of their primary complaints. The economic impact of this condition is demonstrated by the fact that more than 150 million workdays are lost annually because of headaches and that analgesic consumption costs billions of dollars. Most patients have one of the common, generally benign forms of headaches. However, the physician must be careful not to overlook a rare but potentially life-threatening condition that can masquerade as simple headache. The physician should establish good patient rapport, clearly state the objectives of therapy, and stress that symptoms may take time and patience to control.

Clinical Approach to the Headache Patient

In more than 90% of the cases, a detailed and well-organized history gives the correct diagnosis. Characteristics of the most common headaches are noted in Table 40–1. Important characteristics of the headache include type (e.g., dull, sharp), location and radiation, intensity, and duration. Certain factors (foods, medications, menses, stress, physical exercise) that precipitate or worsen headaches should be noted (Table 40–2). Past head or neck injury can lead to post-traumatic or muscle contraction headaches. Associated symptoms frequently suggest certain diagnoses. For example, an aura may precede migraine headaches, and altered sleep patterns are commonly seen with muscle contraction headaches. A recent onset or change in a headache raises the suspicion of a structural lesion, such as an intracranial mass or vascular lesion. In contrast, a long duration of headache helps to exclude serious occult disorders. The physician must always determine whether the patient has more than one type of headache to avoid incomplete diagnosis and partial treatment.

A detailed physical examination with emphasis on the head and neck and the neurologic system is essential. Although major intracranial lesions are frequently obvious, they may also present with the loss of function of a single cranial nerve or a minor gait disturbance. The eye examination should note pupillary responses, extraocular movements, fundoscopic changes, visual field disturbances, and ocular bruits. An ear, nose, and throat examination helps exclude inflammatory and neoplastic processes that can lead to head pain. Temporomandibular joint disturbances cause local tenderness and limit the range of motion. The temporal arteries may be raised and tender in temporal arteritis. Scalp tenderness, especially over the occipital ridge, is common. Cervical and trapezius muscles are commonly painful to palpation in muscle contraction and mixed headaches. Measuring blood pressure is an important part of the physical examination. However, hypertension alone is an unlikely cause of headache unless the readings exceed 210/120 mm Hg.

Laboratory tests are generally not helpful in diagnosis. Serum chemistry analyses and complete blood counts are not necessary unless the history or physical examination suggests an abnormality. An older patient with a new onset of headache suggesting temporal arteritis requires an erythrocyte sedimentation rate.

The most important radiologic procedures

Table 40–1. Characteristics of Certain Headache Types

Type of Headache	Characteristics
Migraine	Quality: pressure, pounding, throbbing Duration: hours to several days Frequency: intermittent, with pain-free intervals Location: unilateral but sometimes global Prodrome: aura in classic migraine Associated symptoms: nausea, vomiting, diarrhea, visual abnormalities Other: positive family history in 60% of cases
Cluster	Quality: steady pressure, extreme severity Duration: 0.5 to 4 h Frequency: intermittent; headaches grouped over weeks or months, one to several per day; nocturnal attacks common Location: strictly unilateral, often involving the orbit Prodrome: none Associated symptoms: lacrimation, rhinorrhea; Horner's syndrome may be present during an attack Other: negative family history, male predominance
Muscle contraction headaches	Quality: dull, band-like pressure Duration: may be continuous Frequency: daily or almost daily Location: fronto-occipital or global Prodrome: none Associated symptoms: neck pain, depression
Mixed headaches	Quality: pressure and/or pounding; variable intensity Duration: may be continuous Frequency: daily Location: fronto-occipital or global Prodrome: none Associated symptoms: occasional photophobia, nausea Other: may have previous history of migraines; frequent medication abuse

Table 40–2. Medications and Foods Commonly Causing Headaches

Medications	Foods
Caffeine-containing analgesics	Alcohol
Reserpine	Chocolate
Indomethacin	Caffeine
Beta blockers	Aged cheese
Diuretics, especially loperamide and triamterene	Cured meats Nuts Citrus fruits
Ergotamine	Pods of broad beans
Nitrates	Monosodium glutamate, sulfites, nitrites, and other preservatives
Nifedipine	
Oral contraceptives	

are computed tomographic (CT) scanning and magnetic resonance imaging (MRI). The head CT scan with contrast is the single most helpful and available procedure. The high initial cost is rapidly offset by elimination of the need for less sensitive tests. If it leads to a faster diagnosis and recovery, a CT scan may help save money for the patient and the third-party payer. Any patient with an otherwise unexplained new onset headache or a definite change in symptoms should undergo a scan, even though the probability of uncovering an organic lesion is less than 5%. Additional sector scans of the sella turcica and the cerebellopontine angle may be needed if more details of these poorly visualized areas are required. Posterior fossa views are especially important in the presence of cranial nerve involvement, cerebellar signs, or highly localized occipital headaches.

In some medical centers, MRI is the procedure of choice to evaluate headache. By allowing high resolution imaging without the use of contrast material, MRI is particularly advantageous in elderly patients or those with compromised renal function. It is more sensitive than CT for detecting early infiltrating tumors and multiple sclerosis plaques and can clearly show the posterior fossa, brain stem, and congenital abnormalities. The major limitations of MRI are cost and availability. If symptoms are absolutely typical such as in the young patient with migraine or cluster headaches and if the subject is quickly responsive to therapy, one can forego the CT or MRI scan.

Other radiologic tests are less useful in diagnosing the cause of headache. Skull films may reveal evidence of fracture, multiple myeloma, or Paget's disease but are too insensitive to detect other intracranial abnormalities. Cervical spine films are mandatory in head and neck trauma and are also helpful to assess the presence of spondylosis or foraminal encroachment in patients with occipital headache. Sinus films are greatly overused and lack both sensitivity and specificity. If lesions are suspected in either the sinuses or the orbits, sector CT scanning is necessary if plain films are normal. Angiography is the best examination to detect arteriovenous malformations, aneurysms, and cerebral vasculitis but should not be used in the routine evaluation of headache patients.

Some other diagnostic test may be useful in

carefully selected patients. Electroencephalography is useful only for patients with suspected seizure disorders. Lumbar puncture should be limited to patients with suspected central nervous system infections or subarachnoid hemorrhage. In most instances, it should be preceded by either CT scanning or MRI to rule out an intracranial mass lesion. Psychologic testing using personality profiles such as the Minnesota Multiphasic Personality Inventory are helpful in assessing underlying traits or affective disorders. The knowledge gained from testing may be helpful if relaxation or biofeedback techniques are used.

Migraine Headaches

The incidence of migraine varies from 5 to 20% in the population, and has a female/male ratio of about 3:1. The age of onset is most frequently in the second and third decade but may range from childhood to late adulthood. New onset of migraines after age 50 is unusual and should alert the physician to look for a structural lesion. Although the term migraine suggests a hemicranial headache, about 40% of patients describe a bilateral or global headache. The pain may be either pulsating or steady and pressure-like. Associated symptoms may include visual disturbances (photophobia, scotomas, distortions), gastrointestinal dysfunction (nausea, vomiting, diarrhea), and occasionally neurologic deficits (hemiparesis, dysesthesias, dysarthria, vertigo, altered mental status). Migraines are generally intermittent, and patients should have symptom-free intervals. Exceptions are patients who have either another underlying disease or have evolved into a pattern of daily mixed vascular-tension headaches. Common precipitants of migraines include certain foods and food additives (Table 40–2), menses, insomnia or excessive sleep, stress, and barometric changes.

Most experts consider migraines to be vascular headaches, although neurogenic mechanisms are also postulated. The prodromal phase seen in some patients may be due to vasoconstriction, whereas vasodilatation is seen during the headache phase. Biochemical substances including serotonin, bradykinins, and prostaglandins are putative mediators in the attack. The headache itself represents just one facet of an intermittent autonomic dysregulation that is responsible for such symptoms as nausea, vomiting, diarrhea, vertigo, sweating, and vasomotor instability.

Common and classic migraines are the two most common types. Classic migraine, which represents less than 20% of cases, is preceded by transient visual or neurologic symptoms (aura); an aura does not precede common migraine. There are several uncommon types of migraine worth noting. Basilar artery migraine is characterized by a severe occipital headache accompanied by bilateral visual field defects, ataxia, and impaired or sudden loss of consciousness. In ophthalmoplegic migraine, the headache is located on the same side as the oculomotor paralysis, which may outlast the headache by several days. Hemiplegic migraine occurs in both familial and nonfamilial forms. The hemiplegia persists for more than 24 hours than the actual headache.

The treatment of migraines depends on their severity and frequency. All patients should establish regular sleep habits and, if possible, identify and eliminate any precipitating factors. Patients with occasional, mild attacks may obtain relief from simple analgesics, such as aspirin or acetaminophen, and from resting in a dark room. A small amount of caffeine may be useful adjunctive therapy for some patients. Patients unresponsive to these measures generally respond to one of several agents: other nonsteroidal anti-inflammatory drugs (NSAIDs) such as naproxen or meclofenamate, Midrin (isometheptene mucate, dichloralphenazone, acetaminophen), or ergot derivatives. These medications are most effective when taken early during the attack. Nausea and vomiting are frequently more disabling than the headache. Antiemetics such as metoclopramide or phenothiazines are usually effective.

Ergot derivatives are presently the most widely used and effective drugs for the acute migraine attack (Table 40–3). Sublingual and inhaler preparations work the fastest, but their unpleasant tastes frequently deter use. The utility of oral tablets is sometimes limited by slow absorption in the presence of gastroparesis and nausea. In such cases metoclopramide, 20 mg orally at the onset of the migraine, is a useful adjunct that allows for improved efficacy of an oral ergotamine or analgesic. Patients with uncontrolled vomiting respond well to suppositories. Resistant cases or those requiring emergency room care may respond to subcutaneous or intramuscular dihydroergotamine (D.H.E. 45). The maximal weekly dose of ergots is 10 mg. Exceeding this dose increases the risk of adverse side effects including ergotism and rebound headaches.

Table 40–3. Ergotamine Preparations and Use

Preparation	Dosage
Ergotamine tablets (Cafergot)	Two tablets at headache onset, 1 tablet every 0.5 h until relief is obtained; maximum dose: 6 tablets per day, 10 tablets per week
Ergotamine aerosol (Medihaler Ergotamine)	One inhalation at onset, 1 inhalation every 5 min until relief; maximum dose: 6 inhalations per day and 15 per week
Ergotamine sublingual tablets (Ergomar or Ergostat)	One tablet under the tongue at onset, 1 every 0.5 h until relief is obtained; maximum dose: 3 tablets per day and 5 per week
Ergotamine suppositories (Cafergot suppositories)	One suppository rectally at onset, may repeat in 1 h if needed; maximum dose: 2 suppositories per attack and 5 per week
Dihydroergotamine mesylate (D.H.E.)	One milliliter subcutaneously or intramuscularly at onset, repeat in 1 h if needed; maximum dose: 3 ml/day and 6 ml/wk

Contraindications to ergotamine use include coronary artery disease, peripheral vascular disease, and noncompliant patients who may overuse the medication.

Migraine prophylaxis is indicated in patients who have frequent attacks (three to four per month), severe attacks that respond poorly to abortive therapy, medical contraindications for symptomatic therapies, or attacks that occur predictably (e.g., during menstrual periods). A variety of agents have been used for prophylaxis (Table 40–4). Beta blockers are the initial drug of choice for most patients. Either selective or nonselective beta blockers are effective; however, agents with intrinsic symphathomimetic activity (e.g., pindolol and acebutolol) appear to be less useful. Most therapeutic failures are due to insufficient doses rather than true resistance. Failure to respond to one agent does not exclude other beta blockers from being effective. Patients who fail beta-blocker therapy or have contraindications to their use should have a trial of calcium blockers. Verapamil and diltiazem appear to be the most useful agents. In our experience, nifedipine is less effective and causes side effects such as flushing, edema, or an increase in headaches. Tricyclic antidepressants with reduced anticholinergic activity, such as nortriptyline, are useful in some patients and generally well tolerated. Starting with a small dose at bedtime lessens side effects and improves compliance. If sedation is a troublesome side effect, protriptyline may be used instead.

Methysergide, at a daily dose of 6 to 8 mg, is frequently effective when other agents have failed. It should never be used for more than 4 to 6 consecutive months because of the risk of serious toxicity. Several small trials suggest that NSAIDs such as naproxen, tolfenamic acid, and fenoprofen are effective in prevention. Until more data are available, NSAIDs should be used mainly in prophylaxis of menstrual migraines. Cyproheptadine, clonidine, guanabenz, and lithium are less effective and limited by troubling side effects. Monoamine oxidase inhibitors should be reserved for resistant cases.

Cluster Headaches

Cluster headaches (Horton's or histamine cephalgia) are a type of vascular headache that occurs predominantly in males. The pain is severe, boring, unilateral, steady, and frequently centered around the eye or the temporal region. A typical attack lasts from 30 to 90 minutes and is frequently associated with ipsilateral lacrimation, rhinorrhea, nasal stuffiness, and/or salivation. A bilateral cluster headache is unusual. The headache frequently awakens the patient from sleep. As opposed to the migraine sufferer, the cluster patient does not lie down but rather paces the room or engages in some restless activity. The term cluster refers to the unique rate and periodicity of the headache attacks. It may occur once a day or repeat itself several times each day. After a few weeks or months, the attacks decrease in frequency and the patient becomes asymptomatic for months or years. In a small number of patients, headaches do not completely remit, and the patients develop chronic cluster headaches.

Abortive therapy is generally less successful for cluster headaches than for migraine. Ergot derivatives may be tried. Some patients get relief with inhalation of high flow oxygen.

Table 40–4. *Migraine Prophylaxis*

Preparation	Daily Dose (mg)	Comments
Beta blockers		Avoid in pregnancy, asthma, Raynaud's
Propranolol	80–320	disease, congestive heart failure,
Nadolol	40–160	bundle branch blocks
Atenolol	50–100	
Timolol	20–40	
Metoprolol	100–200	
Calcium channel blockers		Nimodipine may soon be drug of
Verapamil	240–480	choice; U.S. Food and Drug
Diltiazem	180–360	Administration approval pending
Tricyclic antidepressants		
Amitriptyline	25–150	Sedation and anticholinergic effects vary
Doxepin	25–150	among the agents
Nortriptyline	25–150	
Protriptyline	15–40	
Methysergide	6–8	Fibroproliferative syndromes limit use to 4–6 consecutive mo
Lithium	900–1500	Monitor blood levels, renal and thyroid function
Nonsteroidal anti-inflammatory drugs		Avoid in volume-contracted states, renal dysfunction
Ibuprofen	1600–2400	
Indomethacin	75–200	
Naproxen	500–1000	
Alpha receptor stimulants		
Clonidine	0.2–0.4	
Guanabenz	8–24	
Cyproheptadine	4–16	Sedation and weight gain may limit effectiveness
Monoamine oxidase inhibitor		
Phenelzine	45–90	Avoid tyramine-containing foods and sympathomimetics

Another interesting alternative is the intranasal instillation of 1 ml of 4% lidocaine (Xylocaine) into the area of the sphenopalatine fossa. The patient is instructed to lie supine, hyperextend the neck, and turn toward the side of the pain.

The main goal in the treatment of cluster patients is prophylaxis. In the absence of contraindications, methysergide is the drug of choice. There is less concern for long-term side effects of methysergide in cluster patients. A clinical response is generally seen within a few days, but the patient should remain on the drug for another few weeks. Cluster patients who are not improved within 1 week to 10 days should either have the medication discontinued or have steroids (prednisone 30 to 60 mg/day or methylprednisolone 24 to 48 mg/day) added. If this combination is successful and the patient is free from headaches for several days, the medications can be tapered over 2 to 3 weeks. Other agents should be tried for patients who do not respond to combination therapy within a week. These include calcium blockers, indomethacin, tricyclic antidepressants, lithium, cyproheptadine, or a small daily dose of ergotamine in the form of Bellergal-S (phenobarbital 20 mg, ergotamine 0.3 mg, and belladonna 0.1 mg). The calcium blockers verapamil and diltiazem are most effective for chronic cluster headaches. In addition, alcohol and food containing vasoactive substances should be avoided during the active headache phase. In some cases, the cluster headaches occur at a predictable time, such as 1 hour after going to sleep. In these situations, using an ergot derivative at bedtime may be beneficial.

Muscle Contraction Headaches

Eighty percent of headaches seen by primary care practitioners are muscle contraction headaches. The age of onset is typically 20 to 40, and there is a female predominance. Most patients have an acute, self-limited form that is generally responsive to over-the-counter analgesics. However, about 20% of patients develop chronic headaches with persistent pain at least four times per week.

The headache pain is frequently described as pressure, band-like, or a steady ache. The areas of headache pain vary; they may be distributed in a fronto-occipital pattern or localized to the forehead, temporal areas, or the occiput and neck. The pain may be either unilateral or bilateral. Trigger points similar to those seen in fibromyalgia are common and often include the neck and shoulder muscles. Pain may be alleviated by limiting the movement of the head, neck, and jaws, or by producing muscle relaxation with gentle massage or the use of heat.

Depression frequently precipitates chronic muscle contraction headaches. Common clinical features of depression that accompany these headaches include sleep disturbances (e.g., insomnia, hypersomnia, early awakening), weight loss, and decreased libido. The headaches are often most severe in the early morning and evening; this diurnal variation is considered by some to be a distinctive characteristic of depression-associated headaches. These headaches are unremitting and often poorly responsive to analgesic preparations. Preventive therapy should be considered in most of these patients. The most helpful agents are the tricyclic antidepressants. Besides acting on the central pain control mechanisms, they improve sleep patterns and have muscle relaxant and antidepressant properties. Amitriptyline and doxepin given at bedtime are the most commonly used agents. In the older population sensitive to anticholinergic side effects, use of nortriptyline or desipramine is advisable. If excessive sedation is a problem, protriptyline may be substituted for the other agents.

In some patients, cervical spine disease may precipitate chronic muscle contraction headaches. Common clinical features include constant occipital aching that starts in the morning and lasts all day, muscle spasm, suboccipital tenderness, and limited range of neck motion. NSAIDs and in some patients a soft cervical collar are useful therapies.

Mixed Headaches

Mixed headaches have features of both vascular and muscle contraction headaches. They may develop de novo or in a patient with a past history of typical migraines. The pain has characteristics of muscle contraction headaches with superimposed vascular features, such as visual symptoms, nausea, or severe throbbing pain. The daily headaches occur with variable intensity and may be exacerbated by certain foods, exercise, or menstrual periods. Failure to recognize the mixed character of these symptoms may often lead to incomplete treatment. Therapy may be initiated with tricyclic antidepressant agents, which may be combined with either beta blockers or calcium channel blockers to improve therapeutic efficacy. Resistant patients may respond to monoamine oxidase inhibitors. Relaxation therapy, biofeedback, or the dietary restrictions recommended for migraine may provide additional benefit.

Physicians should prescribe ergot derivatives with considerable caution. With these chronic headaches, there is a great risk of ergotamine dependency. Similarly, caffeine-containing preparations can be overused with resultant rebound headaches. Some of the more resistant patients may require further evaluation in a pain clinic, especially if they have concomitant medication abuse.

Other Types of Headaches

Temporal arteritis is characterized by inflammation of the superficial temporal and other cranial arteries. Most patients are over 55 years old and complain of nonspecific headaches that usually involve the temporal areas but may be generalized. Associated symptoms include fatigue, musculoskeletal pain and stiffness, low grade fever, weight loss, and jaw pain with mastication (jaw claudication). The most important complication of temporal arteritis is retinal artery occlusion with resultant blindness, which may occur abruptly. To prevent this complication, high dose corticosteroid therapy should be initiated immediately whenever the diagnosis is strongly suspected. The diagnosis is suggested by an elevated erythrocyte sedimentation rate (occasionally this test is normal) and a positive temporal artery biopsy. Because a temporal artery biopsy can be negative as result of discontinuous involvement, bilateral biopsies of long arterial segments may be required in some patients.

Structural lesions of the brain are uncommon causes of headaches in ambulatory care practice. A slowly growing brain tumor may present with progressive headaches in the absence of other neurologic signs or symptoms. A mass above the tentorium is more likely to cause frontal headaches, whereas posterior fossa tumors usually cause occipital pain. In hemispheric tumors, the pain sometimes overlies the mass lesion. Cough, straining, exertion, and position changes may worsen the pain of tumor-associated headaches. Subdural hematoma should be considered as a possible cause of headaches in alcoholic, older, or recently traumatized patients. A continuous headache from the date of injury is a characteristic clinical feature. A CT scan may be insensitive in the early phases of subdural hematoma development or in the rare cases of bilateral hematomas. Diagnosis can then be made by MRI scanning or angiography.

Exertional headaches may be precipitated by any type of physical activity, including sexual intercourse (benign orgasmic headaches). Most of these headaches are probably related to migraines. However, because exertional headaches may be an early symptom of intracranial mass lesions, CT or MRI scans should always be performed. If no structural lesions are present, these patients frequently respond to indomethacin or beta blockers administered before the exertion.

Subarachnoid hemorrhage is frequently precipitated by physical activity and causes a sudden, extremely severe headache associated with signs of meningeal irritation, focal neurologic deficits, and impaired consciousness. The major diagnostic difficulty occurs in recognizing smaller hemorrhages called sentinel leaks, which may precede a massive hemorrhage; these headaches may masquerade as benign exertional or orgasmic headaches. A lumbar puncture and angiography may be necessary to differentiate sentinel leaks from benign exertional headaches. Arteriovenous malformations or unruptured aneurysms do not generally cause chronic headaches.

Eye and sinus diseases infrequently precipitate headaches. Acute or subacute glaucoma can present with severe headaches associated with nausea and vomiting. Anterior uveitis or iritis causes orbital pain with associated photophobia and blurred vision. Astigmatism and oculomotor muscle imbalance cause eye strain and headaches. Refractive eye disorders, especially myopia, do not generally cause headaches. Acute sinusitis can cause severe headaches and is easily diagnosed by clinical examination and sinus radiography. Sinus pain is typically dull and aching and is improved by the patient's assuming a supine position. Chronic sinusitis is not a common cause of headache.

Bibliography

Dalessio D (ed). Wolff's Headache and Other Head Pain, ed 5. New York, Oxford University Press, 1987.
  Comprehensive review of aspects of diagnosis and treatment of headaches.
Dexter JD, Byer JA, Slaughter JR. The concomitant use of amitriptyline and propranolol in intractable headache. Headache 20:157, 1980.
  Decribes the therapeutic value of combined drug therapy for chronic headaches.
Friedman AP. Migraine. Med Clin North Am 62:481, 1978.
  Review of diagnosis and treatment of migraine.
Kudrow L. Cluster Headache. New York, Oxford University Press, 1980.
  Comprehensive review of aspects of diagnosis and treatment of cluster headaches.
Kumar K, Cooney T. Vascular headache. J Gen Intern Med 3:384–395, 1988.
  This article is an excellent, thorough review of the subject.
Kunkel RS. Complicated and rare forms of migraine, in Diamond S, Dalessio DJ (eds). The Practicing Physician's Approach to Headache, ed 4. Baltimore, Williams & Wilkins, 1986, pp 76–83.
  Review of infrequent forms of migraine.
Saper JR. Headache Disorders: Current Concepts and Treatment Strategies. Littleton, MA, PSG Publishing Co., 1983.
  Comprehensive review of aspects of diagnosis and treatment of headaches.
Wilkinson M. Treatment of the acute migraine attack: current status. Cephalalgia 3(1):61, 1983.
  Update on migraine treatment.

PART TEN

Prevention

41

✓ Periodic Health Examination for Adults

JOHN H. HOLBROOK, M.D.

Introduction

Ostensibly healthy patients frequently visit physicians for a checkup. With each such physician-patient encounter there are diverse concerns and expectations including those of the patient, the physician, and often a third party, such as an employer. For example, the patient may inquire about his or her health status; the physician may focus on cost-effective use of resources; and the employer may request clearance for the patient to perform a particular activity.

The emphasis of the checkup has been on disease prevention and more recently on health promotion. Although clinicians spend most of their time providing curative medical care, there is increasing physician interest in these other two aspects of care. Unfortunately, surveys have shown that practitioners frequently do not provide recommended preventive measures.

A consensus has emerged that the checkup should consist of a series of clinical interventions, which comprise the periodic health examination (PHE), that are individually tailored by the personal physician according to the patient's age, gender, and risk category. The PHE is offered to established patients who already have a comprehensive data base. Although components of the PHE may be incorporated into the initial diagnostic evaluation, the PHE should not be used as a substitute for the diagnostic evaluation of a new patient. The components of the PHE include the interim history, the basic physical examination, selected laboratory/diagnostic studies, an immunization update, and counseling.

This chapter outlines the purposes, scientific basis, and content of the PHE. The physician's role in designing, implementing, and managing the PHE is also discussed.

Purposes of the PHE

The principal purposes of the PHE are to prevent disease and promote health. The PHE also serves other useful functions such as facilitating patient-physician communication, updating medical data bases, and providing information to interested third parties such as insurance companies (Table 41–1).

Primary prevention, i.e., interventions that reduce the likelihood of disease, is the ultimate example of effective medical practice. Immunization is a proven but underutilized method to achieve this goal.

Secondary prevention, i.e., the detection and management of asymptomatic and remediable disease, holds much promise for the future. Some important chronic diseases such as breast cancer and hypertension may be detected before symptoms are noted. Early detection improves the likelihood of a cure and of minimizing complications.

Tertiary prevention refers to the medical

Table 41–1. Selected Purposes of the PHE ✓

Prevent disease, e.g., immunize against influenza
Detect asymptomatic disease, e.g., hypertension
Identify risk factors, e.g., hypercholesterolemia
Update comprehensive data base, e.g., allergic drug reaction
Facilitate patient-physician communication, e.g., review how to reach physician during an emergency
Counsel on unhealthy behavior, e.g., failure to wear seat belts
Promote healthy behavior, e.g., give exercise prescription
Provide data for third parties, e.g., respond to insurance company questionnaire

management of symptomatic disease with the goals of controlling disease progression, anticipating and avoiding complications, and reducing functional impairment. Prevention of pressure (decubitus) ulcers in high risk patients is an example of tertiary prevention.

Much of the current interest in the PHE stems from a better understanding of the natural history of chronic diseases such as atherosclerosis, cancer, and chronic obstructive lung disease, which account for most of the deaths in the United States. These chronic diseases also result in most of the ambulatory care problems in the United States. Increasingly, clinicians are attempting to reduce the morbidity and mortality of these disorders by identifying and treating antecedent risk factors. Proponents of this strategy emphasize that when chronic disease becomes clinically apparent, it may be far advanced, life-threatening, or untreatable.

Common, important risk factors can be identified through simple clinical tools. Surveys of adult Americans demonstrate that each of the following risk factors has a prevalence of 20% or more: hypertension, hypercholesterolemia, smoking, obesity, a sedentary lifestyle, alcohol/drug abuse, and failure to wear a seat belt.

The comprehensive patient data base may become outdated. Through the PHE the clinician can add important, new information concerning medical problems, hospitalizations, surgery, medication, allergic reactions, accidents, unhealthy behavior, occupational risks, hereditary disorders, psychosocial stresses, and family problems.

The PHE may enhance patient-physician communication. The patient who understands the purposes of the PHE and is an active partner in the ongoing process is more likely to volunteer important data, to make recommended lifestyle changes, and to contact the physician promptly concerning new developments.

Scientific Basis of the PHE

In 1964, the Kaiser Permanente Medical Care Program began the only large, long-term study of the PHE. The interventions in this study were much more complex and expensive than those currently recommended for the PHE. The follow-up reports now extend over a 16-year period. The mortality from hypertension and colorectal cancer was significantly less in the group receiving regular PHEs compared

with a matched control group. There was no difference in total mortality in the two groups.

The 1979 Canadian Task Force on the Periodic Health Examination developed a set of standardized criteria for evaluating scientific evidence on the effectiveness of preventive interventions. These criteria included the effectiveness of treatment or prevention for specific conditions, the burden of morbidity and mortality related to the conditions, and the quality of the screening procedures. The criteria have been used to develop recommendations for interventions to prevent specific diseases and unhealthy states. Other important reasons for performing PHEs (Table 41–1) were not considered in the development of the Canadian Task Force criteria.

Several other analyses of specific PHE interventions have been published, including those of the U.S. Preventive Services Task Force, the Institute of Medicine, the American College of Physicians, the American Cancer Society, the American Medical Association, and Frame. These analyses utilized various criteria for developing PHE guidelines. Some of the institutional guidelines have not been updated since the publication of important new studies. In many areas, there are inadequate data to support scientifically valid recommendations. Thus, it is not surprising that there is a lack of agreement among experts on what the PHE should include and how often it should be offered. Nonetheless, a consensus is developing that a streamlined, targeted PHE should be developed for the individual patient.

The following guidelines are based on the premise that there are several important reasons for performing PHEs (Table 41–1). The guidelines reflect the author's assessment of the current medical literature; however, they should be considered provisional and subject to modification as new data become available.

PHE Content

Interim History

The history remains the physician's most important source of data. The interim history (Table 41–2) differs from the initial history in that it is brief and focuses on events that have occurred since the patient's last visit.

New signs and symptoms should be noted. Direct, targeted questions are indicated for patients in high risk groups. For example, most adolescent deaths in the United States are due

Table 41–2. *Interim History*

1. Elicit new signs and symptoms
2. Obtain interval past history
    a. Hospitalizations
    b. Visits to other physicians
    c. Medication
    d. Allergic reactions
    e. Accidents
    f. Occupational and environmental exposures
    g. Unhealthy behavior
    h. Diet
    i. Exercise
    j. Sexual practices
    k. Contraception
    l. Social history
    m. Family history
3. Review and update problem list
4. Review screening tests and immunization checklist

to accidents, homicide, and suicide; hence, specific behavioral questions may be appropriate for patients in this age group. Inquiring about exertional chest pain is indicated in patients with coronary risk factors. Patients can also be instructed to report important abnormalities (e.g., postmenopausal vaginal bleeding) if they occur in the future.

The interval past history emphasizes contacts with other physicians, hospitalizations, use of medication (prescription and over the counter), allergic reactions, accidents, occupational and environmental exposures, and unhealthy behavior such as smoking. Information should also be obtained concerning diet, exercise, sexual practices, contraception, psychosocial problems, and hereditary problems. Intensely personal information such as alcohol use or sexual behavior may be revealed as the physician and patient become better acquainted.

Finally, the patient and physician should review and update the problem list. Screening tests and immunizations appropriate for the patient should also be reviewed (Table 41–3).

Basic Physical Examination

A basic physical examination (Table 41–4), consisting of approximately 50 maneuvers, can be completed by an experienced clinician in 10 to 15 minutes. This examination provides important data about common risk factors such as hypertension and obesity.

Most guidelines for structuring PHEs recommend screening for cancer of the breast, cervix, and colorectum; these objectives are realized in part through the basic physical examination. Although additional cancer screening is not of proven benefit and not widely recommended, the basic physical examination is a useful tool to screen for several types of cancer including oral, thyroid, prostate, testicular, lymphatic, and skin. Recent studies suggest that melanoma is a potentially curable cancer. Patients with the dysplastic nevus syndrome and those with blood relatives with this syndrome or melanoma should receive periodic screening.

Dental and gum pathology is common and readily identified via the physical examination. In older populations, screening for visual and auditory deficits may be of value.

Data generated through the interim history and basic physical examination may lead to a more detailed physical examination and to specific laboratory/diagnostic studies.

Laboratory/Diagnostic Studies

Numerous disorders have been mentioned as candidates for screening in the PHE. However, available data support laboratory/diagnostic screening for only a few conditions including breast cancer, cervical cancer, colorectal cancer, and hypercholesterolemia. Mammography, Papanicolaou's test, stool testing (guaiac) for occult blood, and the serum cholesterol determination are the only tests currently considered efficacious for screening of asymptomatic adult Americans. The recommendations for specific tests and the frequency of testing have changed and will continue to change. It is notable that many commonly ordered tests such as electrocardiography, the chest x-ray, urinalysis, and chemical profile are not recommended for inclusion in the PHE (see Chap. 45).

Mammography detects clinically occult disease and reduces mortality from breast cancer. It should be ordered in conjunction with a breast examination by the physician. Women between the ages of 40 and 50 should have a mammogram every 2 years; women over 50 years of age should receive annual mammograms (see Chap. 44).

There is considerable indirect evidence that Papanicolaou's test reduces cervical cancer mortality. Controversy continues concerning the frequency of this testing. According to the American Cancer Society, women should have annual tests beginning at the age of 20 years or before that time if the woman is sexually active. After two negative tests performed at a 1-year interval, Papanicolaou's test should

Table 41–3. The PHE: Content and Frequency*

Age (yr)	Examinations Needed at Intervals of				
	1 yr	2 yr	3 yr	5 yr	10 yr
20–39		BP Weight	Pap test†	Interim Hx Basic PE Chol	Td
40–49	BP Weight Breast examination Rectal examination	Mammography Stool guaiac	Interim Hx Basic PE Pap test†	Chol	Td
50–59	BP Weight Breast examination Rectal examination Mammography Stool quaiac	Interim Hx Basic PE	Pap test†	Chol	Td
60+	Interim Hx Basic PE Mammography Stool guaiac Influenza vaccine Pneumococcal polysaccharide		Pap test†	Chol	Td

Modified from Holbrook J. West J Med 141:828, 1984, with permission.
*Abbreviations: BP, blood pressure; PE, physical examination; Chol, serum cholesterol level; Td, tetanus-diphtheria booster; Hx, history.
†Three-year interval after two initial negative Pap tests at 1-yr interval. Six window tests for patients 65 years of age and older.

be repeated every 3 years. Women who are at increased risk for cervical cancer may require more frequent testing (see Chap. 44).

The six "window" stool guaiac test increases the likelihood of detection of early colorectal cancer. Studies are in progress concerning the effect of stool guaiac testing on colorectal cancer mortality. Based on available data, men and women between 40 and 50 years of age should submit guaiac cards every 2 years; after the age of 50, the cards should be submitted annually (see Chap. 44).

Studies have shown that lowering serum cholesterol levels reduces mortality from coronary heart disease. Initial screening for hypercholesterolemia should begin in men and women by the age of 20 years. Thereafter, testing should be repeated at 5-year intervals (see Chap. 15).

Immunization for Adults

U.S. childhood immunization programs are comprehensive and reach a high percentage of the intended population. In contrast, the number of immunization interventions routinely recommended for asymptomatic adult Americans is small, and a much lower percentage of adults receive recommended immunizations. For example, only 20% of high risk patients

in the United States receive influenza vaccinations, and only 50% of all individuals over the age of 60 in the United States have protective antibody titers against tetanus.

There is general agreement that all adults should receive a tetanus-diphtheria booster (adult) every 10 years and that all adults over the age of 65 should receive an annual influenza vaccination (Table 41–3). Younger individuals at increased risk for influenza may also benefit from vaccination.

There is controversy concerning the efficacy of the pneumococcal vaccine in protecting older patients against pneumococcal disease. Nonetheless, the American College of Physicians recommends its use in all adults over 65 years of age (Table 41–3). Others at increased risk for pneumococcal infections, e.g., asplenic patients, should receive the vaccine.

Women in the child-bearing age group are candidates for rubella vaccination unless there is evidence of immunity. The vaccine should not be given to a pregnant woman.

The hepatitis B vaccine provides effective protection against the virus. Individuals in high risk groups, e.g., selected health care workers, should receive this vaccine.

Counseling

Physicians have a unique opportunity to encourage patient involvement in protecting

Table 41–4. Basic Physical Examination

Minute	Activity
	Patient Sitting
1	Inspect general appearance
	Inspect hands, nails, skin, joints
	Palpate, compare, and count radial pulses
2	Measure blood pressure
3	Inspect face and head
	Test visual acuity
	Inspect conjunctiva and sclera
	Test pupillary reaction to light
	Perform ophthalmoscopy
4	Examine ears, externally and with otoscope
	Inspect nose
	Inspect mouth (gums and teeth)
	Test hearing
5	Test range of neck motion
	Palate neck for nodes and thyroid
6	Observe chest symmetry with deep breath
	Percuss and auscultate lung fields
	Patient Supine
7	Palpate breast and axillary nodes
	Inspect neck veins and palpate carotid arteries
	Inspect and palpate precordium
8	Auscultate heart
9	Inspect and palpate abdomen
	Palpate for liver and spleen
	Palpate inguinal nodes and femoral pulses
10	Inspect legs
	Check for edema
	Palpate dorsalis pedis pulses
	Test plantar flexion reflexes
	Patient Sitting
11	Inspect breast for asymmetry, retraction (in women)
12	Test nervous system: wrinkle forehead, show teeth, protrude tongue, test biceps, knee and ankle reflexes
	Patient Standing
13	Observe gait
	Examine male genitalia:
	Inspect and palpate penis, epididymis, testes, and inguinal canals for hernia
	Perform rectal and prostate examination
	Patient Supine
	Examine female genitalia
	Inspect external genitalia
	Inspect vaginal vault with speculum
	Palpate vagina, cervix, uterus, and ovaries
	Perform rectal examination

Modified from Hillman RS, et al. Clinical Skills. New York, McGraw-Hill Book Co., 1981, p 102, with permission.

and promoting their own health. When a risk factor is identified, the clinician can explain the specific health hazard in a personally relevant fashion and detail the benefits of risk reduction.

Although many physicians have not been trained in behavioral modification and are not comfortable in this role, there is a growing trend toward direct physician involvement in prescribing diets, exercise programs, and smoking cessation programs. Successful clinicians assist patients to reach specified goals and to maintain healthy lifestyle changes. Studies have shown that physicians can effectively help patients achieve behavioral change such as smoking cessation and use of seat belts.

The PHE in Clinical Practice

The practice of medicine requires that the physician function in several different roles. The primary care physician generates a comprehensive data base and manages the patient's overall care. Interaction with the health care system is directed and facilitated. Inappropriate therapy and unnecessary interventions are avoided. Complications of appropriate therapy are minimized by careful monitoring. Physicians can also help to minimize or prevent disabling psychosocial problems that often accompany illness. As the patient's counselor and advocate, the clinician should recommend PHEs for both asymptomatic patients and those with symptomatic disease.

Designing the PHE

The content of the PHE and how often it should be given are determined by the patient's age, gender, and risk category. In general, the PHE becomes more complex and should be given more frequently as patients grow older. Table 41–3 outlines specific recommendations.

Patients in the 20-to 39-year-old age group should have an interim history, a basic physical examination, and a serum cholesterol determination approximately every 5 years. During this 20-year interval, a tetanus-diphtheria booster should be given every 10 years. Papanicolaou's test should be performed every 3 years in women who have had two negative tests that were given at a 1-year interval. In this age group, weight and blood pressure should be checked every 2 years.

Individuals in the 40- to 49-year-old age group should have an interim history and basic physical examination approximately every 3 years. The tetanus-diphtheria booster should be given once during this 10-year interval, the serum cholesterol should be measured every 5 years, and women should continue to have Papanicolaou's test every 3 years. Beginning with this age interval, women should have a

PATIENT MONITORING FORM*

✓ Ordered   ✕ Completed

Patient Name _____   Date _____

Intervention								
Clinical:								
Interim history								
Basic physical examination								
Blood pressure measurement								
Weight								
Physician breast examination								
Digital rectal examination								
Laboratory:								
Pap test								
Mammography								
Stool guaiac								
Serum cholesterol								
Rubella titer								
Immunizations:								
Tetanus–diphtheria booster								
Influenza vaccination								
Pneumococcal vaccination								
Counseling:								
Smoking								
Diet								
Exercise								
Alcohol/drugs								
Seat belts								

Figure 41–1. Practical tool for monitoring periodic health examination compliance. *See Table 41–3 for recommended frequency of interventions.

mammogram every 2 years, and all patients should submit stool guaiac cards every 2 years. In this age group, the blood pressure, weight, breasts (women), and rectum should be examined each year.

The interim history and basic physical examination should be offered every 2 years in the 50- to 59-year-old age group. As described for younger age groups, the tetanus-diphtheria booster should be given once in the 10-year interval, the serum cholesterol should be meas-

ured every 5 years, and women should have Papanicolaou's test every 3 years. The blood pressure, weight, breasts (women), and rectum should be examined yearly. In this age group, women should have an annual mammogram, and all patients should submit guaiac cards once a year.

Patients who are 60 years of age or older should be scheduled for an annual interim history, basic physical examination, mammogram (women), and stool guaiac testing. As mentioned for younger age groups, the tetanus-diphtheria booster should be given every 10 years, the serum cholesterol should be measured every 5 years, and women should have a Papanicolaou test every 3 years. Beginning at the age of 65 years, patients should receive an annual influenza vaccination and a single pneumococcal vaccination.

Implementing the PHE

Studies have shown discrepancies between standard PHE guidelines and actual clinical performance. There are several explanations for this involving the physician, the patient, and the health care system.

Physicians tend to emphasize curative medicine rather than preventive measures. They may lack knowledge of PHE guidelines, or they may disagree with them. In the rush of clinical practice, preventive measures may be ignored. Also, physician reimbursement for PHE interventions is often inadequate.

Patients may not accept the PHE because of fears about testing, concerns about cost, and a desire to continue unhealthy behavior. The patient may also disagree with recommended PHE guidelines and request other interventions.

In general, the pluralistic U.S. health care system provides little reimbursement for outpatient preventive services. Some prepaid systems limit availability of or access to preventive services.

The clinician can overcome such problems and implement a successful PHE program by educating patients and incorporating the PHE into routine clinical encounters. Interested asymptomatic patients should be scheduled for recommended PHE follow-up visits.

Managing the PHE

The effective clinician knows his patients and manages their health care. In terms of the PHE, this means that the physician must monitor and remind patients about recommended interventions. Patient-monitoring forms (Fig. 41–1) and computerized reminder systems can assist both the physician and patient to keep recommended PHE interventions current. Prompt follow-up of abnormal results is essential. This allows the clinician to educate the patient about the significance of an abnormality and what can be done about it. Often this

is an ideal opportunity to assist the patient to change unhealthy behavior.

Bibliography

Caldroney RD. The periodic health examination. Hosp Pract 22:189, 194, 197, passim, 1987.
  A current clinical review of the periodic health examination.
Canadian Task Force on the Periodic Health Examination. The periodic health examination. Can Med Assoc J 121:1193–1254, 1979.
  The landmark study in which standardized criteria were developed to evaluate data on the effectiveness of preventive interventions.
Canadian Task Force on the Periodic Health Examination. The periodic health examination: 2. Can Med Assoc J 130:1278–1285, 1984.
  A 1984 update of the 1979 report, covering chlamydial genital infections, adult hearing impairment, hypertension, skin cancers, scoliosis, asymptomatic coronary artery disease and cervical bruits, testicular cancer, breast feeding, and hepatitis B immunization.
Canadian Task Force on the Periodic Health Examination. The periodic health examination: 2. Can Med Assoc J 134:724–729, 1986.
  A 1985 update covering breast cancer, smoking, and primary open angle glaucoma.
Canadian Task Force on the Periodic Health Examination. The periodic health examination: 2. Can Med Assoc J 138:618–626, 1988.
  A 1987 update covering unwanted teenage pregnancy, endometrial cancer, and postmenopausal osteoporosis and related fractures.
Cheney C, Ramsdell JW. Effect of medical records' checklists on implementation of periodic health measures. Am J Med 83:129–136, 1987.
  The utility of checklists for managing the PHE.
Committee on Immunization, American College of Physicians. Guide for Adult Immunization. Philadelphia, American College of Physicians, 1985.
  Authoritative guidelines on adult immunization.
Fletcher S. The periodic health examination and internal medicine: 1984. Ann Intern Med 101:866–867, 1984.
  An editorial surveying the state of the art of the PHE in internal medicine.
Frame PS. A critical review of adult health maintenance, parts 1–4. J Fam Pract 22:341–346, 417–422, 511–520, 1986; 23:29–39, 1986.
  Detailed review of screening in the PHE with some controversial recommendations.
Friedman GD, et al. Multiphasic health checkup evaluation: a 16-year follow-up. J Chronic Dis 39:453–463, 1986.
  A summary and 16-year follow-up report of the findings from the long-term Kaiser Permanente Medical Care Program study on the PHE.
Goldblood R, Battista RN. The periodic health examination. Can Med Assoc J 134:721–729, 1986.
  A 1985 update from the Canadian Task Force on the PHE.
Grundy SM. Cardiovascular and risk factor evaluation of healthy American adults. A statement for physicians by an ad hoc committee, American Heart Association. Circulation 75:1340A–1362A, 1987.
  Current recommendations from the American Heart Association on the PHE with an emphasis on cardio-

vascular disease. *Some recommendations are not supported by published data.*

Holbrook JH. Personal health maintenance for adults. West J Med 141:824–831, 1984.
An overview of the clinician's role in maintaining adult health.

Holbrook JH (ed). Disease Prevention and Health Promotion: A Handbook for Physicians. Philadelphia, Praeger Scientific, 1986.
A collection of papers on practical topics such as preventive health care for the elderly and physician involvement in counseling on smoking, diet, and exercise.

Horsburgh CR Jr, Douglas JM, LaForce FM. Preventive strategies in sexually transmitted diseases for the primary care physician. JAMA 258:814–821, 1987.
Specific recommendations from the U.S. Preventive Services Task Force on preventing sexually transmitted diseases.

Knight KK, Fielding JE, Battista RN. Occult blood screening for colorectal cancer. JAMA 261:586–593, 1989.
Specific recommendations from the U.S. Preventive Services Task Force on colon cancer screening.

Kottke TE, Battista RN, DeFriese GH, et al. Attributes of successful smoking cessation interventions in medical practice: a meta-analysis of 39 controlled trials. JAMA 259:2883–2889, 1988.
Specific recommendations from the U.S. Preventive Services Task Force on smoking cessation interventions.

LaForce FM. Immunizations, immunoprophylaxis, and chemoprophylaxis to prevent selected infections. JAMA 257:2464–2470, 1987.
Specific recommendations from the U.S. Preventive Services Task Force on immunization, immunoprophylaxis, and chemoprophylaxis for selected infections.

Lawrence RS, Mickalide AD. Preventive services in clinical practice: designing the periodic health examination. JAMA 257:2205–2207, 1987.
Introduction to a series of background papers to be released by the U.S. Preventive Services Task Force.

O'Malley MS, Fletcher SW. Screening for breast cancer with breast self-examination. JAMA 257:2196–2203, 1987.
Specific recommendations from the U.S. Preventive Services Task Force on breast cancer screening.

Polen MR, Friedman GD. Automobile injury—selected risk factors and prevention in the health care setting. JAMA 259:76–80, 1988.
Specific recommendations from the U.S. Preventive Services Task Force on counseling for automobile occupant protection.

Selby JV, Friedman GD. Sigmoidoscopy in the periodic health examination of asymptomatic adults. JAMA 261:594–601, 1989.
Specific recommendations from the U.S. Preventive Services Task Force on colon cancer screening.

42

Understanding and Improving Patient Compliance

STEPHEN A. ERAKER, M.D., M.P.H.
MARSHALL H. BECKER, Ph.D., M.P.H.
JOHN P. KIRSCHT, Ph.D.

Compliance with medical regimens is important for adequately treating many diseases and is the mutual responsibility of patient and physician. Compliance is the degree to which a person's actions follow medical advice. Compliance encompasses an entire range of behaviors including taking preventive action, taking medications, and keeping appointments. Common errors of compliance with taking medication include failing to take medicine, adding medications not prescribed, prematurely ending therapy, or taking an improper dosage.

Optimal efforts to modify compliance occur only when the physician understands the patient's health beliefs, preferences, experiences, knowledge, and environment. Only then can the physician effectively encourage patient compliance by communicating in a manner that responds to the patient's views and develops the patient's ability to follow treatment and advice. Although improving compliance should be a major goal of patient advocates and providers, there is a discernible lack of interest in the problem. This may result both from a failure to reimburse physicians adequately for their non–acute illness time and from a mistaken belief that physicians are not effective in changing behavior.

In this chapter, we discuss the magnitude of the problem of compliance and the ability of the physician to understand, detect, and improve it.

Significance of Noncompliance

Noncompliance may be the most significant problem facing medical practice today. For outpatients treated with short-term antibiotics for streptococcal pharyngitis or otitis media, compliance is 75% for the first few days but less than 25% for the 10-day course. Estimates of noncompliance average about 50% for chronic diseases. For example, up to 50% of patients with hypertension fail to follow referral advice; more than 50% drop out of care within 1 year, and only about two thirds of those who remain under care consume enough medication to adequately control their blood pressure. In one study, inpatients with bedside antacids consumed less than 45% of their prescribed regimen. Compliance with behavior modifications is an even more difficult task. Only 30% of patients comply with even minimal dietary advice and less than 10% of smokers without end-organ damage stop smoking.

Noncompliance has several consequences. The most obvious result is that the patient does not receive full benefit of treatment. The physician might incorrectly assume a lack of therapeutic response and increase the dosage of the medication, prescribe a more potent drug, or subject the patient to further diagnostic procedures. On the other hand, overuse of a medication increases the risk of adverse reactions. One study indicated that drug overutilization caused 65% of compliance problems. Another important problem is the interpretation of clinical trials. If only half of the patients take as little as 80% of prescribed medications, there is a vast increase in the number of patients needed to show a treatment's efficacy. More important, problems with noncompliance in clinical drug trials may affect the ability of investigators to establish the true rates of efficacy and toxicity of any given agent. Finally, the cost of medical care increases with noncompliance. Increased costs may be due to hospitalization from inadequately treated disease or toxic drug effects, use of more expensive drugs, or increased utilization of outpatient services.

Detection of Noncompliance

Clinical judgment, based on previous knowledge of the patient, does not reliably predict compliance. Physicians may utilize several methods to detect noncompliance:

- Ask the patient in a nonjudgmental manner.
- Ask family members.
- Identify patients who fail either to appear or to make follow-up appointments.
- Identify patients who fail to attain expected therapeutic goals.
- Check medication refills.
- Perform drug assays.

The easiest method is to ask the patient. Direct questioning, in a nonjudgmental manner, can detect 30 to 50% of noncompliant patients. Such a question can be phrased in the following way: "People frequently find it difficult to remember to take medications. Do you ever miss yours?" Those who admit their noncompliance can be believed and are more responsive to attempts to improve compliance. Failure to appear for follow-up outpatient visits is another clue to medication noncompliance. A third method is to assess a patient's response to treatment. The possibility of noncompliance should be investigated in all patients who fail to respond to what would usually constitute appropriate therapy. Pill counting, an important research tool for detecting noncompliance, has limited clinical utility. Patients may forget to bring in their pill bottles or may bring in only some of their unused pills. An alternative, but not always feasible, method is to determine the pattern of medication refills; failure to refill prescriptions at expected times raises the suspicion of noncompliance. Determining serum concentrations of drugs is generally the most accurate way of assessing compliance. Unfortunately, assays are expensive and are not available for many agents.

Understanding Noncompliance: The Patient's Perspective

After detection, the physician must attempt to understand the reasons for this behavior. Patients are continually exposed to descriptions (some accurate, some inaccurate) of various risks to their health and to the likely benefits and costs of medical testing and treatment. Patients are influenced by past therapeutic encounters that they have personally experienced, witnessed, or heard about. Many persons have had (or believe they have had) iatrogenic consequences from medications. One survey of 817 patients in a general practice found that 41% "certainly" or "probably" had experienced a reaction to prescription drugs. Patients may have difficulty perceiving the logic of some recommended behavior modifications because most risk factors (smoking, overeating, lack of exercise) do not result in readily observable illness in the short run, nor does every risk taker eventually become ill. It is therefore not surprising that patients have developed beliefs that affect their decisions about the necessity and desirability of following professional advice. By understanding the patient's health beliefs, the physician can better educate the patient, redesign the therapeutic regimen, and reinforce helpful behaviors.

Enhancing Patient Compliance

The Health Decision Model

There is a large body of empirically based literature suggesting that a patient's beliefs make substantial contributions to decisions about cooperation with treatment plans. Such health beliefs have been incorporated into various models that identify a particular set of beliefs that may explain a patient's health-related decision. According to the health decision model shown in Figure 42–1, the probability that advice will be followed is a function of the patient's perceptions of susceptibility to the disease, the likely severity (clinical and social) of the disease if contracted, and the benefits and barriers likely to be derived and encountered as a result of the recommended action. Although no all-purpose solution to the compliance problem has been discovered, enough practical knowledge has evolved to provide a foundation for attempts to improve cooperation with treatment. Beginning with

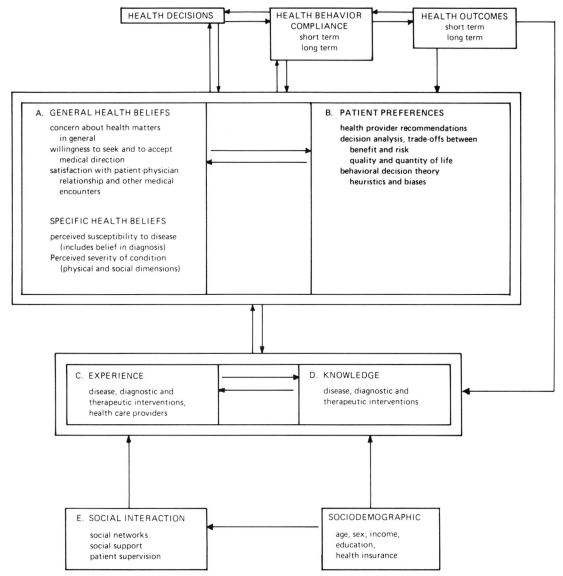

Figure 42–1. *The health decision model, which combines the health belief model and patient preferences, including decision analysis and behavioral decision theory. Reproduced, with permission, from Eraker S, Kirscht J, Becker M. Understanding and improving patient compliance. Ann Intern Med 1984; 100:258–268.*

the central health decision in Figure 42–1, we proceed from left to right and relate interventions to changing general and specific health beliefs, altering therapeutic recommendations to reflect patient preferences, modifying current experiences, enhancing knowledge, and manipulating social interaction factors.

General Health Beliefs

Health beliefs are opinions about illness that are shaped by personal, interpersonal, and cultural factors. General and specific health beliefs are an important determinant in patient decisions about cooperation with a treatment plan. The physician must first identify and assess these beliefs. Questions directed to the patient and phrased in a nonthreatening, open-ended manner should include the following points: (1) Does the patient agree with the diagnosis? This is a crucial issue because patients frequently have well-defined but erroneous health beliefs about medical diagnoses. (2) Does the patient have any particular fears about the illness? (3) What does the patient believe caused the illness? (4) What is the effect of this illness on the patient's life? (4) Does the patient have any particular fears about the illness? (5) Does the patient agree about the necessity of treatment? (6) Does the patient believe that the recommended treatment will work? (7) Does the patient believe that the treatment regimen will be difficult to follow or will cause significant side effects?

Once the patient's beliefs are determined the physician can inform the patient about points of uncertainty, correct erroneous beliefs, and reinforce beliefs that are appropriate. Patients who hold incorrect beliefs about their illness or treatment plan may be difficult to manage. Several methods can be used: pointing out the particular mistaken beliefs and providing adequate information; appealing to sources of information in whom the patient can develop considerable trust (such as individuals with the same illness who have responded to the recommended treatment); or using social pressure or social support (group discussions, family).

The quality of patient-physician interactions is an important determinant of general health beliefs. In general, a positive interpersonal relationship enhances patient compliance. Patients are generally more satisfied with physicians who fulfill a variety of expectations. These include physician friendliness, encouragement of patient questions and active involvement in their own care, response to patient complaints, and detection of and attention to underlying patient concerns. Congruence between the physician and the patient in their appreciation of the underlying illness and its management results in greater satisfaction and improved compliance.

PATIENT PREFERENCES

Altering treatment recommendations to reflect patient preferences can enhance compliance. For example, in considering selection of antihypertensive therapy a patient might be asked about willingness to incur the increased cost of a more expensive medication taken once a day, which would be easier to remember, as opposed to a less expensive medication that must be taken two times daily. Other clinical decisions characterized by greater uncertainty and the need to make value judgments are more difficult.

The incorporation of patient preferences regarding benefit and risk into health decisions depends on the ability of the patient and physician to determine and communicate those preferences. It is important to describe both immediate and long-term benefits and risks of treatment. Treatment options should be presented and considered in light of patient preferences.

EXPERIENCE WITH TREATMENT REGIMENS

Patients do not like treatment regimens that include multiple medications or that require frequent dosing. In patients with diabetes mellitus or congestive heart failure, medication errors were less than 15% when only one drug was prescribed and were 25% when two or three drugs were taken, but exceeded 35% when five or more drugs were taken. In another study, noncompliance doubled when the number of medications was increased from one to four or when the frequency of administration was increased from once daily to four times daily. Frequency of dosing may be a more important factor for compliance than the number of different medications taken at each dose interval. Treatment expense or regimens that require substantial alterations of lifestyle (diet, exercise, smoking abstinence) are additional impediments to patient compliance.

Various maneuvers can be used to improve compliance with treatment regimens, as indicated in Table 42–1. Physicians should regularly review and delete components of the treatment plan that are of little or questionable benefit. Physicians should avoid the routine prescription of medications such as vitamin supplements, bowel preparations, and tranquilizing drugs. By establishing priorities of elements of the regimen, the physician empha-

Table 42–1. *Measures for Improvement of Patient Compliance*

1. Simplify treatment regimen by continuing only cost-effective, essential drugs.
2. Change treatment gradually by establishing priorities, graduated implementation, or tailoring.
3. Decrease dosing frequency when possible.
4. Consider using contingency contracts.
5. Identify and encourage participation in support groups.
6. Enlist family members to supervise medication use or to reinforce certain behaviors.
7. Employ maneuvers initiated by health care personnel such as house calls, telephone calls, or more frequent outpatient visits.
8. Develop a good patient rapport.
9. Give clear, explicit instructions both verbally and written, and test the patient for comprehension of instructions.

sizes the need to adhere to particularly critical aspects of the treatment. Graduated regimen implementation divides the treatment plan into less complex stages that can be followed sequentially as each step is mastered by the patient. "Tailoring" the regimen matches the treatment schedule to the patient's regular daily activities to minimize inconvenience and forgetfulness. Physicians can decrease the frequency of dosing by using sustained-release preparations, transdermal delivery systems, or intramuscular injections. By using generic drugs and pricing medications at different pharmacies, patients can lower the expense of treatment. Lifestyle changes should be introduced over the course of several visits. If several alterations are necessary, they should be addressed one at a time, preferably in an order selected by the patient. Improvements in compliance should be reinforced before addition of further components of the therapeutic regimen.

An innovative method to improve patient compliance is use of a contingency contract. This contract, a written agreement between patient and physician, is a formal commitment outlining the obligations of each party during a specified time. An example of such a contract is as follows. A hypertensive patient with poorly controlled hypertension agrees to the daily ingestion of medications and to weekly blood pressure checks by a nurse in the physician's office. The physician agrees to call the patient weekly at a specified time and to spend more time with the patient at the regularly scheduled visits. The contract provides the patient with an opportunity to discuss potential problems and solutions and involves the patient in the treatment planning.

PATIENT KNOWLEDGE

Patients frequently have inadequate knowledge about their illness and its treatment. One can hypothesize that this ignorance leads to poor compliance, which can improve with adequate instruction. Studies have shown that compliance with short-term medical regimens is improved by careful instruction about the need to take all the drugs over a specified time or by giving both written and verbal instructions. However, there is no evidence that improving patient knowledge of the disease and its treatment increases compliance with long-term regimens.

Aside from the issue of compliance, physicians should educate patients about their illness and its treatment. Patients have an ethical right to be informed about their illness and must know the proposed regimen if they are expected to comply. There are, however, many problems that interfere with patient education. One study showed that physicians failed to state the regimen 17% of the time. When the regimen was both verbally given and written on the prescription container, the two statements were contradictory 20% of the time. Patients may fail to understand the regimen. A study showed that "every 6 hours" was correctly interpreted by only 36% of patients. Considerable variation has also been shown for understanding of the terms evening and with meals. A study from a neighborhood health center showed that physicians infrequently give indications regarding the duration of the regimen or often do not provide complete written instructions. Finally, patients frequently forget what physicians have instructed; up to one half of physician's statements are forgotten by the patient almost immediately.

To enhance the patient's understanding of instructions, the physician should remember the following points. Instructions should be clear, concise, and explicit, and the terms used should be understood by the patient. If fewer instructions are given, a greater proportion are remembered. Physicians should supplement verbal with written instructions, emphasize and repeat important features, and give the most important instructions first. When new or complex information is offered, the physician may wish to evaluate comprehension by asking the patient to repeat essential elements of the message, particularly the specific actions required by the treatment plan. Furthermore, categorization of new information increases recall. These categories may include explanations of the diagnosis, necessary diagnostic evaluation, effects of the illness, and treatment regimen.

SOCIAL INTERACTION

Manipulation of social interaction factors, such as support and supervision by family, group, or health care personnel, can improve compliance. Encouraging family involvement offers the advantages of compliance reinforcement in the patient's own home without the need of direct clinician supervision. Studies of weight control show that persons who received assistance from another family member in reinforcing proper eating behavior were more likely to lose weight and to maintain weight loss. Group discussions on self-help, including self-monitoring and self-selection of antihypertensive medications from a standard protocol, have resulted in improvement in medication compliance. In another study, group discussions on prevention of asthmatic attacks resulted in a short-term decrease in emergency room visits for acute asthma.

Practical recommendations for noncompliant patients include enlisting the help of family members to supervise medication intake and to inform physicians if difficulties with compliance arise. Dietary modifications (for hypertension, hyperlipidemia, diabetes mellitus, or obesity) can be discussed with both the patient and family. Group discussion to enhance compliance has been extensively used for patients who are obese (Weight Watchers or Overeaters Anonymous), alcoholics (Alcoholics Anonymous), and tobacco abusers (Five-Day Plan or programs sponsored by the American Cancer Society and the American Lung Association). Clinicians can improve monitoring by increasing the frequency of outpatient visits, performing home visits, providing continuity of care, making reminder telephone calls about the regimen or the follow-up visit, requesting that pill bottles be brought to the next visit, and instructing the patient to keep a record of which pills were taken each day and at what times.

Issues Involving the Enhancement of Compliance

Two important ethical questions arise when physicians must extend compliance-enhancing strategies beyond a simple office visit. They are: (1) To what extent is the provider responsible for noncompliance? (2) What are some of the ethical limits on efforts to improve compliance?

The physician's responsibility for noncompliance varies inversely with the degree of patient participation in health decisions. Physicians who do not involve patients in significant decisions assume considerable responsibility and put themselves in a difficult ethical position. Patient participation in medical decisions appears to be increasing, as are requirements for informed consent. Given the wide spectrum of attitudes held by patients toward both their treatment and physicians, it would seem that physicians should provide each patient with information regarding the risks and benefits of proposed medical interventions. Patients should learn that the low risk of adverse drug effects may be outweighed by the potential benefit of the treatment. Patient preferences regarding these benefits and risks should be discussed and incorporated into decisions regarding the prescribed treatment. In a patient-physician relationship where compliance is expected, there should be an ethic of freedom, mutual understanding, responsibility, and satisfaction. Physicians have a right to expect compliance, and departure from an expected standard without some reasonable justification can appropriately involve blame. However, patient noncompliance does not absolve the physician of further responsibility to the patient.

Patient-directed strategies for improving compliance must be limited by certain ethical constraints: any communicated information must be truthful, and any attempts at behavior modification should be noncoercive. Graphic descriptions of health consequences are not inherently wrong but should be accurate. Arousing fear about consequences of noncompliance does not consistently improve compliance and, in some situations, may hinder compliance. Virtually every message about health carries an implied threat and raises a subsequent need for reassurance. Education about compliance has two components: information necessary to make informed decisions, and behavioral skills necessary to act on that information. Health professionals have the right and obligation to provide information to an uninformed patient in such a manner that it is received and understood. Then, for the motivated patient who wishes to act on that knowledge, the physician is further obliged to provide instruction in behavioral skills that help to achieve the goals. It becomes an obligation of physicians to educate patients and to assist them in following instructions by using whatever ethical means available. For patients who subsequently do not wish to comply, it is inappropriate to attempt to change behavior.

The responsibility for compliance must be shared between physician and patient. The physician is in a unique position of responsibility and opportunity. It is hoped that our discussion of the serious problem of patient compliance has illustrated the issues and provided a basis for physician action that will ultimately lead to an improved quality of patient care.

Bibliography

Becker MH, Maiman LA. Strategies for enhancing patient compliance. J Community Health 6:113–134, 1980.

Eraker SA, Kirscht JP, Becker MH. Understanding and improving patient compliance. Ann Intern Med 100:258–268, 1984.

Haynes RB, Taylor DW, Sackett DL (eds). Compliance in Health Care. Baltimore, Johns Hopkins University Press, 1979.

Kern DE, Baile WF. Patient compliance with medical advice, in Barker LR, Burton JR, Zeive PD (eds). Principles of Ambulatory Medicine. Baltimore, Williams & Wilkins, 1986, pp 41–57.

Matthews D, Hingson R. Improving patient compliance, a guide for physicians. Med Clin North Am 61:879–889, 1977.

Mullen PD, Green LW, Persinger GS. Clinical trials of patient education for chronic conditions: a comparative meta-analysis of intervention types. Prev Med 14:753–781, 1985.

Sackett D, Haynes RB, Tugwell P. Compliance, in Clinical Epidemiology: A Basic Science for Clinical Medicine. Boston, Little, Brown & Co., 199–222, 1985.

43

Smoking Cessation: A Five-Stage Plan

STEPHEN A. ERAKER, M.D., M.P.H.
MARSHALL H. BECKER, Ph.D., M.P.H.
JOHN P. KIRSCHT, Ph.D.

Physicians have substantial ability to encourage patients to reduce or stop cigarette smoking. Although the overall prevalence of smoking has decreased since 1964, current estimates indicate that about one third of all adults smoke regularly. Although more than 90% of smokers would like to quit, only about 15% try to quit each year, and fewer than 10% of smokers attend formal treatment clinics. Because more than 75% of adults see their physician at least once per year, the importance of messages from the physician relates to their ability to reach a large number of smokers in an environment emphasizing health.

Although most physicians in a survey agreed with the benefits to be derived from stopping smoking, only 14% were optimistic about their ability to help patients to quit. Population surveys show that fewer than 44% of smokers report having ever been advised by their physician to stop. Evidence from randomized studies clearly demonstrates that considerable progress can result from as little as 3 minutes of well-organized time. Because 95% of successful ex-smokers quit on their own rather than by formal treatment, health care providers have a responsibility and an opportunity to persuade patients of the necessity of trying to quit. This chapter provides a five-stage plan, outlined in Table 43–1, for physicians to more effectively help patients to stop smoking.

Stage 1: Determine Smoking Habits

Smoking habits should be determined during every medical visit. Lighter smokers are more likely to succeed in quitting than are heavier smokers. Smokers of more than 26 cigarettes per day, particularly smoking within 30 minutes after awakening, are more dependent on nicotine and likely to experience severe withdrawal symptoms. On stopping, 90% of smokers experience an unpleasant withdrawal syndrome of variable duration (Table 43–2). The

Table 43–1. *Stages in an Antismoking Program*

Stage Number	Steps in Plan
1	Determine smoking habits
	Is light or heavy smoker
	Has made repeated efforts to quit
	Uses other drugs such as alcohol and caffeine
	Include survey of smoking habits of spouse and friends
2	Determine health beliefs about
	Susceptibility to disease
	Severity of disease if contracted
	Benefits and barriers likely to be derived and encountered
	Ability to quit (provide encouragement)
3	Motivate patient to quit
	Educate about risks of smoking
	Set date for quitting
	Sign a contract
	Enlist support of friends and relatives
4	Develop a cessation plan, which may include
	Self-help kits
	Nicotine chewing gum
	Aversive conditioning or behavioral techniques
	Organized group programs
5	Monitor patient's progress
	Schedule follow-up visits
	Use positive reinforcement
	Encourage subsequent attempts if initial one fails

Table 43–2. Characteristics of Nicotine Withdrawal

Parameter	Alteration
Physiologic changes	Decrease in blood pressure
	Drop in heart rate
	Decrease in basal metabolic rate
	Change in electroencephalographic rhythms
	Alterations in rapid eye movement sleep patterns
Symptoms	Inability to concentrate
	Irritability
	Drowsiness
	Tremors
	Fatigue
	Sleep disturbances
	Headache
	Nausea
	Alteration in bowel habits
	Palpitations
	Depression
	Nicotine craving
	Increased appetite

Table 43–3. Behavior Related to Smoking

Years smoked
Number of cigarettes per day
Type of cigarette smoked
High risk of nicotine dependence
  Smoke within 30 min of awakening
  Smoke while ill
  Inability to go more than 1 hr without smoking
Smoking-related symptoms
  Cough
  Dyspnea
  Sore throat
Smoking-related illnesses in self
Smoking-related illnesses in family and friends
Prior attempts to quit
  How long did they last?
  Why did they fail?

occurrence of withdrawal symptoms is often cited as the reason why new ex-smokers start smoking again. It is important for physicians to discuss potential nicotine withdrawal symptoms with patients and to inform them that controlled studies have shown that heavy smokers given nicotine chewing gum after quitting have fewer withdrawal symptoms and are less likely to resume smoking.

Repeated efforts to quit increase the likelihood of success. Users of other drugs, such as alcohol and caffeine, have more difficulty in stopping successfully. Although males have higher overall rates of smoking, they are more likely to stop and are less likely to go back to smoking than are females. Having a nonsmoking spouse increases the ability to quit, although the influence of smoking behavior of other family members, friends, or work associates is less clear. Pertinent historical data regarding smoking behavior are indicated in Table 43–3.

Stage 2: Determine Health Beliefs

Understanding a patient's health beliefs helps the physician to determine how to motivate the patient to quit. The health belief model has shown that compliance with advice from the physician depends on the patient's perceptions regarding susceptibility to a disease, severity of the disease if contracted, and the benefits and barriers likely to be derived and encountered, respectively, by undertaking a recommended action. The health belief model also recognizes the importance of other factors such as experience, knowledge, self-efficacy (self-confidence in ability to quit), and social and demographic variables.

Worry about susceptibility to disease is the most common reason given by former smokers for quitting. Former smokers indicate greater concern about symptoms such as sore throat, cough, and dyspnea, and less concern about their own susceptibility to more serious illness such as lung cancer or heart disease. It is possible for physicians to emphasize relationships between smoking and minor symptoms and to provide more realistic perceptions regarding susceptibility to disease. More than 80% of a national sample of 12,000 people agreed that smoking is detrimental to health. Such beliefs about the health hazard of smoking were stronger among ex-smokers than among either smokers or people who had never smoked regularly. A study of patients who had had a myocardial infarction found an overwhelming belief that smoking was of etiologic importance. Physicians' messages were even more effective when given to patients with smoking-related illness. Survivors of myocardial infarction given an antismoking message during hospitalization had a 63% rate of smoking cessation 1 to 3 years later compared with a 27% cessation rate for patients offered no special advice. Such messages are also more credible when given by physicians who are themselves good role models because they have quit smoking.

Belief in the ability to quit (i.e., self-confidence or "efficacy" expectation) has been shown to affect smoking cessation efforts dramatically. Smokers most likely to quit are those who expect to succeed and believe in their personal competence and security. In a prospective, randomized trial, an experimental group was given an efficacy-reinforcing message indicating that they had strong will power and great potential to control behavior and that they would completely stop smoking. After 14 months, the number of cigarettes smoked per day was reduced by 70% for the experimental group compared with 30% for the control group. Patients reporting high levels of both susceptibility and efficacy have been shown to have the highest rates of smoking cessation.

It is also important to explore perceived barriers to quitting. The patient's beliefs regarding barriers such as weight gain, nicotine withdrawal, peer pressure, and emotional stress need to be explored and considered when attempting to motivate the patient and develop a cessation plan.

Stage 3: Motivate by Educating About Risks of Smoking and Benefits of Quitting

Many patients seen for a variety of health reasons are often ambivalent about quitting. Unlike the situation in stop-smoking clinics (where smokers are ready to quit), the physician must make special efforts to motivate patients. The patient may move through stages, from being disinterested, to considering a change, to making an effort to quit.

The results of educating about risks of smoking depends on the patient's willingness to change established behavior. For patients interested in stopping immediately, the physician should move to stage 4 and establish a cessation plan. For patients not yet ready to stop, it is important to understand the reason why. At this stage, it may be useful to provide information about the risks of smoking (Table 43–4). Nearly all smokers are aware of the health hazards of smoking, but their perception of personal risk is usually hazy. Although some patients can be motivated to stop by providing a threatening message, this message must be considered in view of existing health beliefs. Excessively strong fear messages may trigger denial and other coping mechanisms and may actually interfere with adoption of health-facilitating behavior. For example, smokers who viewed a film about a lung cancer operation were found to be less likely to undergo chest radiography than smokers who did not see the film.

A smoking cessation contract signed by both

Table 43–4. Risks Associated with Smoking

Symptoms	Cough
	Shortness of breath
	Wheezing
	Chest pain/discomfort
	Sore throat
	Dyspepsia
Cancer	Respiratory
	Lung
	Larynx
	Gastrointestinal
	Oral
	Esophagus
	Pancreas
	Genitourinary
	Bladder
	Kidney
Cardiovascular	Coronary artery disease
	Angina
	Myocardial infarction
	Sudden death
	Vascular disease
	Peripheral vascular disease
	Stroke
	Thromboangiitis obliterans
	Aortic aneurysms
Other	Perinatal effects
	Peptic ulcer disease

the patient and the physician can be useful in motivating the patient to quit. Most studies indicate that making a contract provides additive benefits when used with other advice on quitting. This can be a formalized document or simply a handwritten statement on a prescription pad, a copy of which can be placed in the medical chart.

Describing benefits to be derived from quitting, as indicated in Table 43–5, is a very important component of the plan. Discussion

Table 43–5. Benefits of Quitting Smoking

Immediate
  Save money
  No ashtrays to empty
  No burn holes
  More employable
  Better and cheaper insurance
  Decreased social pressure of trying to smoke in public
Health symptoms
  Improved ability to breath
  Better sense of smell and taste
  Increased energy
  No tobacco stains on teeth, fingers
  Decreased heart rate and improved exercise tolerance
  Reduced perspiration
Health benefits
  Reduce significant coronary events by 50% if smoking ceases before age 65
  Reduce mortality by 50% if stop smoking after myocardial infarction
  Decrease lung cancer rate by 60% after 5 yr and by 90% after 15 yr of cessation
  Slow decrement in pulmonary function

of both health and nonhealth benefits provides positive reinforcement for the patient making an effort to quit.

It is important to relate risks and benefits to the patient's medical problems, smoking history, family history, social support, and interests. In addition to asking the patients about dyspnea and morning cough, a carboxyhemoglobin or pulmonary function test (although some studies have not indicated value) may demonstrate to the patient the adverse effects of smoking. The more specific the information, the clearer (and more personally motivating) the message to stop.

Stage 4: Develop a Cessation Plan

A well-developed cessation plan is based on what has been learned about the patient's smoking habits, health beliefs, motivation to quit, and perceived barriers likely to be encountered. There is a wide range of available cessation therapies, which are based on a variety of assumptions about why a person smokes.

Many smokers find it difficult to stop because of the psychologic reinforcement resulting from habitual behavior associated with smoking. Persons who smoke more from habit than from addiction to nicotine are more likely to benefit from programs that make them aware of environmental cues. The majority of smokers do not want to attend a formal treatment program, and self-help quitting guides are therefore recommended. Most guides are fairly similar in content and suggest alternatives to smoking. For example, a person who usually smokes during coffee breaks may take a walk instead or drink coffee in nonsmoking areas. Evaluation of the American Cancer Society's self-help manuals and other programs has found an 18% long-term cessation rate. A comparison of three self-help books under self-administered and therapist-administered conditions found that these books were more effective in getting smokers to quit or to reduce smoking when combined with therapist interventions.

The ability of a provider-initiated, minimal contact intervention to modify the smoking behavior of ambulatory clinic patients was recently reported. Smokers at two outpatient sites were assigned to one of three groups: provider intervention only, provider intervention plus self-help manual (Step-by-Step Quit

Table 43–6. *Self-Help Smoking Cessation Material and Sources*

Step-by-Step Quit Kit
  School of Public Health, Department of Health Behavior/Health Education, University of Michigan, 109 South Observatory Street, Ann Arbor, MI 48109
Calling It Quits
Quit It, A Guide to Help You Stop Smoking
For Good, A Guide to Living as a Non-Smoker
  Office of Cancer Communication (Room 10-A-18), National Cancer Institute, Bethesda, MD 20205; telephone 1–800–4–CANCER
Fresh Start
  American Cancer Society; contact local representatives

Kit), and a control group. The physician's message emphasized the patient's personal susceptibility, the physician's concern, and the patient's ability to quit (self-efficacy). The overall 6-month quit rate for intervention groups ranged from 15 to 25%. Participants receiving the self-help manual in addition to the physician's messages were between two and three times more likely to quit smoking during the study period than were participants in either of the other study groups.

Physicians or other health professionals should review one of the guides listed in Table 43–6 with the patient and direct the individual

Table 43–7. *Characteristics and Side Effects of Nicotine Chewing Gum*

General information
  Boxes with 96 pieces
  Cost: about $20.00
  Use only for smokers who have quit entirely
  8–10 pieces per day throughout the day
  Take for 2–3 mo, with gradual taper
  Physician instruction needed
Contraindications (or cautionary indications)
  Recent myocardial infarction
  Serious arrhythmia
  Vasospastic disease
  Pregnancy
  Lactation
  Severe angina
  Temporomandibular joint disease
Possible complications
  Peptic ulcer disease (or acid peptic disease)
  Hypertension
  Insulin-dependent diabetes
  Hyperthyroidism
Side effects
  Sore jaw
  Mouth irritation or ulcers
  Nervousness
  Dizziness
  Nausea and vomiting
  Intestinal distress (hiccups)
  Headache
  Excess salivation

to materials that address specific concerns such as weight gain.

There is also the pharmacologic influence of nicotine that provides a coping mechanism by achieving either a stimulant or a sedative effect. Cigarettes often help the smoker to cope better with stress, and smoking rates are higher among those experiencing a life crisis. Addiction to nicotine is one of the main reasons cited by smokers for not stopping.

Nicotine chewing gum contains 2 mg of nicotine bound to an ion exchange resin. The nicotine is released during chewing and is absorbed through the buccal mucosa. Although there are studies with both positive and negative results for the use of nicotine gum, the best studies indicate that it is effective when used in conjunction with physician counseling. Simply giving the patient a prescription for nicotine gum is probably useless. Heavy smokers given nicotine chewing gum report fewer withdrawal symptoms and are less likely to resume smoking. One-year cessation rates ranging from 30 to 50% have been reported. Nicotine gum is particularly appropriate for heavy smokers and only for those who have quit entirely. Although the average dose per day is usually 8 to 10 pieces, if smokers receive no instruction they tend to use too few pieces for too short a time.

Although nicotine chewing gum has been used for 15 years in Sweden and for a shorter time in other European countries, there continues to be concern about its short- and long-term safety, as indicated by the contraindications in Table 43–7. Side effects are often a result of overly vigorous chewing and rapid release of nicotine and include sore jaw, mouth irritation or ulcers, nervousness, dizziness, nausea, vomiting, hiccups, intestinal distress, headache, and excess salivation. To reduce these symptoms, smokers should chew the gum slowly. Best results are obtained when the gum is used in conjunction with a behavioral modification program or with self-help materials.

Mixed results have been obtained from a variety of aversive-conditioning techniques involving electric shock, rapid smoking, warm stale smoke, and nicotine fading. Although it appeared initially that rapid smoking could result in 100% cessation and 60% abstinence at 6 months, recent studies have documented rates of 20 to 30% abstinence. Because carbon monoxide levels may reach 17% saturation and impair myocardial and tissue oxygenation, rapid smoking techniques are not recommended for smokers with significant heart or lung disease.

A number of behavioral techniques, such as hypnosis and acupuncture, have not been adequately evaluated. Most studies assessing hypnosis have been uncontrolled, with results showing an abstinence rate of 25% at 6 months. A report utilizing tragus acupuncture achieved a success rate of 88% with a 34% attrition rate and 31% relapse rate at 2 years.

A variety of organized group programs are available, such as those sponsored by the American Cancer Society and the American Lung Association. However, they have not been adequately evaluated. SmokeEnders reports abstinence rates ranging from 70% at the end of the 8-week program to 27% after 4 years.

Stage 5: Monitor Patient Progress

It is essential to monitor progress during a smoking cessation program. For example, the smoker could be phoned on the designated quit day, and the patient could be seen again within 1 to 3 weeks. A return visit for follow-up counseling provides physicians with an opportunity to congratulate successful nonsmokers. It also allows the physician to remind smokers whose attempts to quit were unsuccessful that relapses occur. Studies have indicated that relapsing is as big a problem as quitting and that monitoring improves cessation rates. Most smokers succeed only after making several attempts to quit, and another attempt should be encouraged.

Conclusion

The effectiveness of advice given by primary care physicians to stop smoking was demonstrated in a study of general practitioners in London. Although the 5% increase over baseline in the rate of smoking cessation was small, it was statistically significant and confirmed that simple, routine advice given by physicians can effectively motivate some smokers to quit.

For patients not wishing to quit, the physician should provide a clear message with relevant information. It is important to respect the patient's wishes. The physician's concern for the patient's well-being, however, should motivate continuing efforts to discuss smoking cessation on every visit.

Bibliography

Eraker SA, Becker MH, Kirscht JP. Smoking behavior, cessation techniques and the health decision model. Am J Med. 78:817–825, 1985.
A review and intervention guide based on a model.
Fisher EB, Rost K. Smoking cessation: a practical guide for the physician. Clin Chest Med 4:551–565, 1986.
A good general review containing outlines for interventions and questionnaires useful in office counseling.
Greene HL, Goldberg RJ, Ockene JK. Cigarette smoking: the physician's role in cessation and maintenance. J Gen Intern Med 3:75–87, 1988.
A well-referenced practical guide to the consequences of smoking and approaches to cessation.
Health and Public Policy Committee, American College of Physicians. Methods for stopping smoking. Ann Intern Med 105:281–291, 1986.
An objective, critical review and series of practical and policy recommendations.
Janz NK, Becker MH, Kirscht JP, et al. Evaluation of a minimal-contact smoking cessation intervention in an outpatient setting. Am J Public Health 77:805–809, 1987.
Patients receiving a self-help smoking cessation manual were between two and three times more likely to quit smoking than patients in the usual care-control group.

Kottke TE, Battista RN, DeFriese GH, et al. Attributes of successful smoking cessation interventions in medical practice: a meta-analysis of 39 controlled trials. JAMA 259:2882–2889, 1988.
Recommendations from the United States Preventive Services Task Force. Emphasizes the critical role of repeated reinforcement by health professionals in the maintenance of smoking cessation.
Lam W, Sze PC, Sacks HS, et al. Meta-analysis of randomised controlled trials of nicotine chewing-gum. Lancet 2:27–29, 1987.
An analysis of 14 randomized controlled trials indicating that proper use of nicotine gum increases the cessation rate.
Rigotti NA. Smoking cessation techniques in primary care practice, in Goroll AH, May LA, Mulley AC (eds). Primary Care Medicine. Philadelphia, JB Lippincott, 1987, pp 243–249.
A well-organized, practical guide with innovative, helpful suggestions for physicians.
Tonnesen P, Fryd V, Hansen M, et al. Effect of nicotine chewing gum in combination with group counseling on the cessation of smoking. N Engl J Med 318:15–18, 1988.
Nicotine chewing gum is most effective when used properly with group counseling.

44

Cancer Prevention in Primary Care

WILLARD H. DERE, M.D.
RANDALL W. BURT, M.D.
BARRY M. STULTS, M.D.

A number of cancer preventive services may be included in the periodic health examination. Primary cancer prevention measures, such as smoking cessation, are designed to reduce the likelihood of cancer occurrence. Secondary cancer prevention includes measures for the early detection of treatable, asymptomatic malignancies and may be accomplished by screening large asymptomatic populations or by examining individual patients in the office (case finding). These maneuvers include Pap smears, mammography, clinical breast examinations, breast self-examinations, fecal occult blood testing, and sigmoidoscopy. The purpose of this chapter is to review the evidence concerning the utility of cancer prevention measures and to provide practical suggestions on how to perform and implement them.

Delivery of Cancer Prevention Measures

Cancer prevention measures are not sufficiently utilized by patients and their health care providers. Patients frequently fail to comply with cancer screening tests. Table 44–1 illustrates the relatively low levels of compliance, particularly among the elderly, in recent population screening trials offering free fecal occult blood testing and mammography. The reasons for low compliance rates have not been defined but may include inaccurate knowledge about cancer (e.g., beliefs that cancer cannot be diagnosed at a curable stage or that the treatment is worse than the disease), fear of the cancer screening maneuver (e.g., mammography), perceived physician indifference, misunderstanding of testing directions, lack of effective patient education materials, and cost.

Medicare, Medicaid, and most private insurance companies do not pay for cancer screening procedures. However, as demonstrated by Table 44–1, even provision of free cancer screening is not sufficient to guarantee good compliance.

Health care providers frequently fail to offer cancer prevention measures. Practitioners' estimates of their own performance generally fall short of American Cancer Society (ACS) guidelines (Table 44–2). Furthermore, practitioners seriously overestimate their actual performance of these maneuvers (Table 44–3). The causes of this poor physician performance are unknown. Postulated reasons include simple forgetfulness, lack of time, insufficient monetary reimbursement, patient discomfort or refusal, and confusion about recommendations because of the lack of consensus among experts. Potentially useful reminder systems and flow sheets for office use are discussed in Chapter 41.

Table 44–1. Compliance with Fecal Occult Blood Testing and with Mammography According to Age

	Compliance (%)	
Study	**Age 50–59**	**Age over 70**
FECAL OCCULT BLOOD TESTING		
Bat*	46	33
Jansen†	62	39
Klaaborg‡	75	52
MAMMOGRAPHY		
Tabár§	93	63
Verbeek‖	73	34

*Bat L, et al. Am J Gastroenterol 81:647, 1986.
†Jansen JH. Soc Sci Med 18:633, 1984.
‡Klaaborg K, et al. Scand J Gastroenterol 21:1180, 1986.
§Tabár L, et al. Lancet 1:829, 1985.
‖Verbeek A, et al. Lancet 1:1222, 1984.

Table 44–2. Physician Estimates of Their Own Cancer Screening Performance

Prevention Measure	Battista* (Quebec)	Gemson†	McPhee‡	Woo§
Clinical breast examination	99%	80%	81%	116%‖
Mammography	8%	20%	36%	32%
Pap smear	91%	92%	57%	146%‖
Fecal occult blood test	15%	48%	74%	100%
Sigmoidoscopy	—	41%	3%	9%
Rectal examination	—	79%	67%	81%

*Battista R. Am J Public Health 73:1036, 1983
†Gemson D, Ellison J. Am J Prevent Med 2:226, 1986.
‡McPhee S, et al. J Gen Med 1:275, 1986.
§Woo B, et al. JAMA 254:1480, 1985.
‖Frequency of performance exceeded that of recommendations.

Primary Cancer Prevention

Primary cancer prevention requires knowledge of the etiology and pathogenesis of individual cancers. This information is not available for most cancers. Potentially useful interventions include cessation of tobacco smoking, dietary modifications, and removal of colonic or cervical benign neoplasias (the latter is discussed in the section on secondary prevention).

Cigarette smoking accounts for 30% of all cancer deaths in the United States. Lung cancer accounts for the majority of these deaths. Other cancers associated with cigarette use include cancers of the bladder, stomach, pancreas, cervix, esophagus, larynx, and oral cavity; in the development of the last three neoplasms, alcohol acts synergistically with cigarette smoking. In middle-aged populations, smoking cessation decreases the risk of lung cancer by more than 50% within 5 to 9 years, and after 15 years the ex-smoker's risk begins to approximate that of the nonsmoker. (See Chap. 43 for office techniques to facilitate smoking cessation.)

Diet may play a role in as many as 35% of all cancers. Saturated and unsaturated fats, cholesterol, and smoked or cured foods containing nitrites are the most commonly impli-cated carcinogenic substances. Dietary fiber, cruciferous vegetables, and certain vitamins and minerals (e.g., vitamin A and selenium) may play a protective role. Dietary recommendations of the ACS are listed in Table 44–4.

Secondary Cancer Prevention Activities

Effective secondary prevention measures must fulfill several criteria: (1) The cancer to be detected must be common and treatable. (2) Randomized controlled trials should demonstrate that the use of the specific early detection measure decreases morbidity and mortality in the screened population. (3) The screening test must be relatively inexpensive, comfortable, safe, and convenient. There are currently no secondary cancer prevention measures that meet all these requirements. However, although data are insufficient to justify large scale screening programs in the community, sufficient evidence exists to recommend case-finding activities in the physician's office for cancers of the breast and cervix, and more controversially, for cancer of the colorectum. Recommendations for cancer screening from different expert panels are listed in Table 44–5.

Table 44–3. Comparison Between Physician Performance and Physician Estimation of Performance of Cancer Screening Procedures*

Procedure	Physician Performance (%)		Physician Estimation (%)	
	McPhee	Woo	McPhee	Woo
Clinical breast examination	39	76	81	116
Mammography	13	5	36	32
Pap smear	22	175	57	146
Fecal occult blood test	28	48	74	100
Sigmoidoscopy	0.3	14	3	9
Rectal examination	29	46	67	81

*Based on ACS recommendations. See Table 44–2 for references to McPhee and Woo.

Table 44–4. Dietary Recommendations
of the ACS

1. Avoid obesity.
2. Reduce total fat intake (no greater than 30% of daily caloric intake).
3. Eat more high fiber foods, such as whole grain cereals, fruits, and vegetables.
4. Include foods rich in vitamins A and C in the daily diet.
5. Include cruciferous vegetables, such as cabbage, broccoli, Brussels sprouts, turnips, and cauliflower, in the diet.
6. Be moderate in the consumption of alcoholic beverages.
7. Be moderate in the consumption of salt-cured, smoked, and nitrite-cured foods.

To effectively screen patients for cancer, physicians must know not only the published recommendations for screening and the proper diagnostic evaluation of a positive test but also the pitfalls of cancer screening. False-positive results occur with considerable frequency and their diagnostic evaluation may be quite costly (Table 44–6). False-negative results are also common (Table 44–6), and unless patients are properly counseled to continue regular participation in the screening program, such results may inappropriately reassure them about their long-term health status. Although not yet adequately defined, cancer screening may have short-term adverse psychologic effects on some patients who experience considerable anxiety during the screening period, especially if a test result is falsely positive. For others, misinterpretation of the screening process as an index of illness may diminish independence and functional status.

Cancer screening may not be warranted in persons with an already limited life expectancy and/or poor quality of life because of serious comorbid conditions. However, advanced age by itself is rarely a reason to avoid cancer screening. The elderly population over age 65 has the highest incidence of breast and colorectal cancer and a considerable incidence of invasive cervical cancer. In the absence of other serious comorbid illnesses, they tolerate surgery, chemotherapy, and radiation therapy for these malignancies as well as younger persons.

Breast Cancer

With an estimated 130,000 new cases and 42,000 deaths in the United States in 1988, breast cancer is the most common cause of cancer and cancer-related mortality in women.

Mortality correlates with the stage of disease at diagnosis. The 5-year survival for stage 1 disease (tumor < 2 cm in diameter with no evident axillary or distant metastases) is 80% compared with 25% for stage 4 disease (distant metastases).

The incidence of breast cancer increases with age; an 80-year-old woman has twice the risk of a 40-year-old woman. A past history of breast cancer confers a 1.8 to 5 times greater risk of developing a second breast malignancy. Breast cancer in a first-degree relative (e.g., mother, sister, or daughter) increases risk two- to three-fold. The risk appears to be greater if the relative had premenopausal or bilateral breast cancer. The lifetime risk for first-degree relatives of women with both premenopausal and bilateral breast cancer is estimated to be 30 to 50% compared with an average lifetime risk of 9% in the general American female population.

Mammography, in combination with a physical examination, has emerged as the best method of breast cancer screening. Two randomized, controlled trials with mammography as the primary test modality conclusively demonstrated a reduction in breast cancer mortality in women over age 50 years. The Health Insurance Plan of New York study employed an annual two-view mammography and physical examination in women aged 40 to 64 years and demonstrated a 30% reduction in breast cancer mortality that has been maintained through 18 years of follow-up. The Swedish WE study employed single-view mammography alone in women aged 40 to 74 years every 2 to 3 years and demonstrated a similar 31% reduction in breast cancer mortality in the screened group. Case-control studies from the Netherlands have noted 50 to 70% decreases in breast cancer mortality in women who had received prior mammography.

There is controversy about the merits of mammography for women between ages 40 and 49 years. The Health Insurance Plan study showed a statistically significant decrease in breast cancer mortality for this group 18 years later. Conversely, the initial results of the Swedish WE study demonstrated no beneficial effect for screened women aged 40 to 49; critics attribute the lack of benefit to a longer screening interval (24 months), the use of a less sensitive single-view mammography technique, and the exclusion of a physical examination. Any modest benefit of screening women in this age group must be balanced against financial costs, unnecessary surgery, and radiation risks.

Table 44–5. Recommendations for Cancer Screening from the ACS

Screening Test	Age (Yr)	Frequency	Comments*
Mammography	35–40 40–49 > 50	Baseline 1–2 yr Annually	NCI/USPSTF: annual mammography over age 50; high risk women (e.g., first-degree relative with premenopausally diagnosed breast cancer): annual mammography at an earlier age CTF: annual mammography for ages 50–59
Breast self-examination	> 20	Monthly	NCI/USPSTF/CTF: not recommended
Clinical breast examination	20–40	Every 3 yr	USPSTF: annual examination for age 40 and over CTF: annual examination for ages 50–59 NCI: annual examination age 50 and over
	> 40	Annually	
Pap smear test	> 18†	Annually; after three consecutive normal examinations, timing of further tests should be discussed with patient	CTF: annual examination ages 18–35; then every 5 yr until age 60
Stool guaiac slide test	> 50	Annually	UICC: no test as public policy
Sigmoidoscopy	> 50	Two-consecutive annual examination; if both are negative, every 5 yr	
Rectal examination	> 40	Annually	

*USPSTF, U.S. Preventive Services Task Force; CTF, Canadian Task Force on the Periodic Health Examination; NCI, National Cancer Institute; UICC, International Union Against Cancer.
†Begin earlier if the patient is or has been sexually active.

The potentially greater benefit of screening women with either a personal or family history of breast cancer may warrant annual screening of this subgroup during their fifth decade.

Mammography in the United States routinely employs two views (mediolateral and craniocaudal) for the breast image. The equipment in current use delivers only 0.1 to 0.2 rad to breast tissue, and as a result the risk of radiation-induced malignancy is negligible in centers using the optimal technique and technology. The sensitivity of mammography for detecting breast cancer is 75 to 85%. Unfortunately, the positive predictive value of mammography is relatively low, particularly in younger women. The overall ratio of benign

Table 44–6. Screening Tests for Cancer and Their Costs

Test	Cost ($)	% False-Positive (Neoplasia)	% False-Negative (Neoplasia)	Cost of False-Positive Test ($)
Pap smear	10	5–40	20–30	170*
Mammography	80	65–85	20	900†
Fecal occult blood test	8	50–75	30–75	820‡

*Colposcopy, cervical biopsy, and physician fees; University of Utah, 1988.
†Eddy D. JAMA 259:1512–1519, 1988.
‡Eddy D. In Levin B, Riddell R (eds). Frontiers in Gastrointestinal Cancer. New York, Elsevier Science Publishing Co., 1984, pp 203–219.

to malignant breast biopsies is 5:1, whereas in older women it declines to 2.7:1.

The clinical breast examination remains an important screening maneuver because 5 to 10% of breast cancers are detected by this examination but not by mammography in an ambulatory care setting. The denser breasts of younger women reduce the sensitivity of mammography, thereby increasing the importance of the clinical breast examination in this subgroup. In the Breast Cancer Detection and Demonstration Project, 13% of tumors in women between ages 40 and 49 years were detected by this examination but not by mammography, compared with 7% detected by examination alone in women between ages 50 and 59 years. The clinical breast examination also establishes a normal base line for women being instructed on breast self-examination.

The detection of breast lumps is dependent on the size and firmness of the tumor and the thoroughness of the examination. Both breasts should first be inspected for cutaneous evidence of malignancy such as dermatitis and peau d'orange (breast edema). The patient should assume a supine position; to make the breast as flat as possible, a towel or pillow should be placed under the scapula. The patient's ipsilateral hand should be raised above the head. Breast palpation is performed using pads (not tips) of the middle three fingers. The examiner should press down firmly and use a rotatory motion. Several patterns of examination have been recommended. The vertical strip method allows for the most thorough examination: the rectangular area bounded by the midaxillary line, sternum, clavicle, and lower costal margin is examined in vertical strips. Two other methods, the radial spoke method, which begins at the periphery and converges at the nipple, and the circular method, which employs concentric circles starting at the outer breast and ending at the nipple, are other recommended ways. The examination is completed by squeezing the nipples in an attempt to elicit discharge, and by palpating the axillae while the patient is upright.

The utility of a monthly breast self-examination has not been determined. No prospective, controlled trials are yet available concerning its effect on breast cancer mortality. Preliminary data from a prospective, controlled British trial suggest that it may increase the detection of lesions less than 2 cm in diameter (from 30 to 57%) and decrease the number of tumors with axillary node metastases (from 52 to 35%); however, any effects of this examination on breast cancer mortality in this trial will not be known for at least several years. The accuracy of breast self-examination in different age groups after training has not been adequately determined, nor are there sufficient data on the psychologic effects (positive or negative) or net costs of breast self-examination. The U.S. Preventive Services Task Force and the World Health Organization indicate that no specific recommendations can be made on whether to utilize this method in cancer screening programs. If health care providers choose to incorporate breast self-examination into the periodic health examination, they should instruct patients to visually examine the breast in front of a mirror in three positions: arms at sides, arms over the head, and hands on hips pressing down to tense chest muscles. Patients should look for swelling, puckering, or dimpling of the skin, and any changes in nipple color or shape. The manual examination should be performed as described above, with each breast examined by the contralateral hand. Powder or lotion on the finger pads reduces the friction between the skin of the hand and that of the breast and may facilitate deeper palpation of the breast parenchyma. The self-examination should be performed 1 week after the beginning of a menstrual period in premenopausal women; in postmenopausal women it should be performed at the beginning of each month. The woman should demonstrate breast self-examination for the physician and should repeat this demonstration on return visits. Women instructed in this method by a clinician are more likely to perform the procedure than those who learn from other methods.

Cervical Cancer

Cervical cancer has an annual incidence in the United States of 15,000 cases and is the fifth most common cause of cancer mortality in women. There is considerable evidence that cervical cancer may be sexually transmitted. Women with multiple sex partners or early age of onset of intercourse are at increased risk, whereas virgins have minimal risk. Recent studies suggest an association of cervical cancer with various sexually transmitted serotypes of papilloma virus. Heavy tobacco smoking may be another risk factor.

The natural history of cervical cancer makes it particularly suitable for early detection. The exocervix is composed of squamous epithelium and moves inward with aging, slowly replacing the columnar epithelium of the endocervix. The normal transformation at this squamocolumnar junction is called metaplasia, and this is the site of neoplastic transformation for cervical squamous cell cancer. The earliest neoplastic change is squamous dysplasia. Some dysplastic lesions naturally regress, but most progress to carcinoma in situ (CIS) during an average of 7 years, or sometimes more rapidly in younger women. The ages of peak incidence of CIS are 25 to 30. CIS persists for an estimated 8 to 30 years before progression to invasive cervical carcinoma (ICC). Ages of peak incidence of ICC are 50 to 55 years. Both dysplasia and CIS are detectable by screening, and resection of either lesion results in a 100% cure rate. In contrast, localized ICC has an 80% 5-year survival rate, which decreases to 40% with regional metastasis.

Cervical cancer screening includes obtaining a Pap smear and direct cervical visualization. Large scale, randomized, prospective trials have not been performed, but several lines of evidence strongly suggest that screening reduces the incidence and mortality of cervical cancer. Countries that have introduced well-organized screening programs have noted large decreases in cervical cancer mortality. Case-control studies have demonstrated a several-fold increased incidence of ICC in unscreened women. Finally, there appears to be an inverse relationship between the frequency of screening and the incidence of ICC, and screening every 1 to 3 years appears to afford greater protection than screening every 5 to 10 years.

The most appropriate interval between screening examinations is controversial. The different opinions emanate from two concerns. First, there are inherent limitations in the sensitivity of the Pap smear. Even when optimally performed, the Pap smear has a sensitivity of 79% and a specificity of 95% in detecting neoplastic cervical changes. Pregnancy, the use of oral contraceptives, and the menopausal state decrease the accuracy of Pap smears. Pregnancy and oral contraceptives decrease the cohesiveness of endocervical cells such that they are not seen in sheets on the smear, whereas menopausal women may have involution of the squamocolumnar junction, making proper sampling more difficult. In addition, estrogen deficiency may cause inflammation, which mimics dysplasia or even CIS. A second reason for disagreement on the interval be-

tween screening examinations is the occurrence of unusually rapid progression from CIS to ICC in less than 3 years in an estimated 5% of patients, most of whom are young. Mathematical analysis suggests that testing every other year confers benefits similar to those of annual testing, whereas extending the interval to 3 years decreases the benefits slightly. The Canadian Task Force on Cervical Cancer Screening Programs recommends annual screening for sexually active women between the ages of 18 and 35 years, then every 5 years to age 60 years. Previous American College of Obstetrics and Gynecology guidelines called for yearly screening in all sexually active women and all women over the age of 18 years. The 1988 American College of Obstetrics and Gynecology and ACS recommendations call for three consecutive annual screenings for women who are or have been sexually active or who have reached age 18 years. After three or more consecutive normal examinations, the Pap smear may be performed less frequently at the discretion of the physician; there is no recommendation for an upper age limit on testing.

Inadequate screening of elderly women is an important source of missed ICC diagnoses. Because the incidence of CIS is extremely low after age 60 years, most current recommendations eliminate screening after this age on the presumption that these women have had repeatedly normal prior Pap smears. However, an estimated 40% of elderly American women have never had a Pap smear. As a result, cervical cancer mortality in women aged 60 to 79 years has not significantly changed in countries following these screening recommendations, and it is as high or higher than mortality in women aged 50 to 59 years. Health care providers must determine the cervical cancer screening histories of their elderly female patients. Women over age 60 years who have had no Pap smears or women with fewer than two negative Pap smears in the previous 10 years should probably have annual smears for at least 2 years followed by a third and final smear 3 years later.

The use of the proper technique in obtaining a Pap smear is essential. A speculum lubricated only with water is inserted and the cervix is visualized. Any suspicious areas should be biopsied (usually by a gynecologist) even though the subsequent Pap smear may be negative. Excess mucus is swabbed from the cervix before the smear is taken because thick smears are unsuitable for microscopy. The largest prong of the spatula (wooden; Ayres) is inserted into the external os and rotated through 360°; the examiner should maintain firm pressure on the spatula. The examiner withdraws the spatula without touching the vaginal wall and with a circular motion spreads the cells from the spatula onto a slide. A cotton swab of the endocervix is then obtained and spread onto a slide. The slides are promptly fixed, most commonly by immersion in 95% ethyl alcohol. Failure to fix the smear before it dries out is the most important mistake in the handling of cytologic material. The slide should then be sent to a laboratory known for accurate cytopathology. If the slide is unsatisfactory, the clinical examination should be repeated. Patients with evidence of dysplasia, CIS, and ICC should be promptly referred to a gynecologist.

Clinicians, patients, and laboratory error are responsible for the failure to detect even greater numbers of neoplastic lesions. An estimated 50 to 70% of patients with ICC have not had a Pap smear within the 2-year period before diagnosis. Although many of these patients received medical care during this period, their clinicians did not provide cancer screening. Pap smears are frequently inadequate, failing to yield endocervical cells; smears from postmenopausal women have an especially low yield of 32%. For a variety of reasons, women often fail to comply with requests to obtain a Pap smear. Even in well-organized screening programs, compliance averages only about 70%. Misreading of smears and disagreements in interpretation of neoplastic changes are common laboratory errors. In one study, when two slides were taken from the same woman, cells showing CIS on one slide were missing from the other slide one third of the time; for dysplasia, the discrepancy occurred in one half of the cases. Considerable disagreement was found among 10 readers in 38% of CIS and 44% of ICC diagnoses.

Colorectal Cancer

Colorectal cancer is the second most common internal malignancy in the United States. In 1988, it is expected that there will be 148,000 new cases of this tumor and 60,000 deaths. There is a rapid increase in the incidence of colorectal cancer after age 40 years, with a peak incidence at age 65 years and a gradual decline thereafter. The prognosis of colorectal adenocarcinoma (which accounts for 95% of

colorectal cancers) is best associated with the Dukes's staging system. Dukes's staging quantifies the degree of invasion into four categories. Dukes's A, invasion into but not through the muscularis, and Dukes's B, invasion through but not beyond the muscularis, are associated with an 80 to 90% 5-year survival. Patients with Dukes's C, positive local lymph nodes, and Dukes's D, distant metastasis, lesions have a 20 to 30% 5-year survival. The overall 5-year survival rate for all stages is 53%.

Genetic and dietary factors appear to have roles in the etiology of this disease. First-degree relatives of individuals with colorectal cancer have a several-fold increased risk. Familial polyposis coli and Gardner syndrome are rare syndromes in which a highly penetrant autosomal dominant expression of colorectal cancer is observed in affected pedigrees. Women with uterine, ovarian, and possibly breast cancer likewise have a somewhat increased risk. Diets high in total fat are associated with an increased risk, whereas diets high in fiber or vegetables are associated with a decreased risk (see section on primary prevention).

Adenomatous polyps are considered to be the precursors for most, if not all, colorectal cancers. Several observations support this association: adenomatous polyps frequently harbor colorectal cancers; polyps of increasing size, atypia, and villous histology have correspondingly greater risks of containing cancer; almost all small and some large colorectal cancers contain remnants of benign adenomatous polyp tissue; there is a progressively increasing risk of colorectal cancer at the site of an adenomatous polyp that has not been removed; and a less than expected incidence of colorectal cancer is observed when adenomatous polyps are removed. Hyperplastic colonic polyps are usually less than 5 mm in diameter and are not thought to be related to adenomatous polyps or colorectal cancer.

Two features of colorectal cancer have been utilized in screening. First, this tumor often bleeds into the bowel lumen when it is small. Second, the adenomatous polyp is an identifiable benign precursor. Three screening procedures have capitalized on these characteristics: the digital rectal examination, the fecal occult blood test, and proctosigmoidoscopy.

A yearly digital rectal examination beginning at age 40 years is presently recommended as part of colorectal cancer screening. No formal studies have specifically addressed the validity of performing an annual rectal examination. However, this recommendation seems reasonable because the test is safe and inexpensive and because 5 to 10% of colorectal tumors occur within reach of the examining finger.

Current screening recommendations also include an annual fecal occult blood test, beginning at age 50 years. Studies have demonstrated that colon cancers found on the basis of a positive test are either Dukes's A or B in 60 to 80% of cases. Without screening, only 35% of colon cancers are in these localized stages. Patient compliance is much higher in motivated than in unmotivated subjects (80 compared with 15%). The rate of positive tests is 1 to 5%. Limited specificity is a serious problem with the fecal occult blood test. The predictive value for neoplasia in a positive test is 18 to 50%, with one fourth of true positive tests arising from cancer and the remainder arising from adenomatous polyps. The false-negative rate for this test may be as high as 30 to 75%.

Proper performance of the fecal occult blood test is important. The patient should begin a high fiber diet with no red meat 3 days before sampling stools and should continue this diet throughout sampling. Aspirin and other nonsteroidal anti-inflammatory drugs, vitamin C supplements (which cause a false-negative test), and iron pills (which cause a false-positive test) should be avoided during this same period. Samples should be taken for six stool smears (two from different portions of the stool from three successive bowel movements). Smears should be returned for development within 2 weeks of collection, and the guaiac cards should not be rehydrated before applying the developer. Evaluation should be undertaken if any one of the six smears is positive.

Because of the significant rate of both false-positive and false-negative stool occult blood tests, more sensitive and specific tests are being sought. The Hemoquant test detects stool porphyrins and may prove to be both more sensitive and more specific than the stool guaiac reagents. Tests specific for human hemoglobin are also under study. To improve patient acceptability, stool occult blood tests have been developed that are placed in the toilet after a bowel movement. The patient is instructed on observing an immediate result. Although this type of test has already been marketed, limited clinical experience makes the test results difficult to compare with standard stool occult blood tests.

Although clinical studies suggest that the fecal occult blood test may be effective as a screening tool, a decrease in mortality from screening has not yet been demonstrated in two large ongoing trials. Until these investigations are completed, large-scale population screening cannot be recommended. In addition, the cost effectiveness of screening has not been adequately studied. Present recommendations, therefore, are limited to case finding in the office. Individuals at increased risk should be encouraged to enter the medical system for standard screening, including first-degree relatives of persons with colorectal cancer and women who have had ovarian, uterine, or breast cancer. Persons who have had previous colorectal cancers and polyps should be followed more aggressively by periodic colonoscopy in addition to yearly stool guaiac tests. Individuals who belong to pedigrees affected with one of the rare inherited forms of colon cancer should have screening appropriate to the particular disease.

Proctosigmoidoscopy has been recommended by the ACS as a complementary case-finding tool to be performed every 3 to 5 years for individuals over age 50 years. It detects cancers in the distal colon and rectum and reliably identifies premalignant adenomatous polyps. One study employing rigid sigmoidoscopy has shown that individuals who had regular screening and removal of any detected polyps had a lower than expected incidence of rectosigmoid cancer. Despite this observation, screening by rigid sigmoidoscopy has been unsuccessful because of the lack of patient and physician acceptance. The introduction of flexible proctosigmoidoscopic instruments may be a solution to this problem. Studies consistently demonstrate a greater depth of insertion and a higher yield of neoplastic lesions with the flexible instruments. Patient comfort and physician acceptance have also been improved. Examination techniques with the 35-cm flexible instrument are quickly and easily mastered by the nonendoscopist. More training is required for facility with the 60-cm instrument, but a proportionately increased yield is also expected.

Other Malignancies

Rectal examination has an estimated sensitivity of 50% for detecting a potentially curable stage B prostate cancer, and examinations done by skilled examiners have an overall sensitivity of 69% and a specificity of 89% in detecting prostate cancer. The serum acid phosphatase assay is neither sensitive nor specific for detecting early disease and should not be used as a screening maneuver. At this time, there are no controlled data available as to whether an annual rectal examination in asymptomatic individuals leads to diagnosis of prostate cancer at an earlier pathologic stage or to reduced mortality.

The incidence of lung cancer increases with age, and there is evidence that the prevalence of potentially curable lung cancer also increases with age. Fifteen percent of patients under age 54 years, 22% between ages 65 and 74 years, and 25% over age 75 years have localized tumors. However, screening programs for lung cancer using both sputum cytology and chest radiographs every 4 months have failed to demonstrate improved survival. At this time, there is no role for lung cancer screening in asymptomatic individuals.

Bibliography

Baines CJ, Miller AB, Wall C, et al. Sensitivity and specificity of first screen mammography in the Canadian National Breast Screening Study: a preliminary report from five centers. Radiology 160:295–298, 1986.
The overall sensitivity and specificity of mammography for detecting histologically confirmed breast cancer were 69 and 94%, respectively. This sensitivity is significantly lower than that found in the Swedish two-county screening trial.

Battista R, Grover S. Early detection of cancer: an overview. Annu Rev Public Health 9:21–45, 1988.
In this up-to-date, well-written review, the authors thought that there was insufficient evidence to support the use of the fecal occult blood test and sigmoidoscopy in colorectal cancer screening.

Canadian Task Force. Cervical cancer screening programs: summary of the 1982 Canadian Task Force report. Can Med Assoc J 127:581–589, 1982.
This report updates the 1976 Task Force recommendations. Using the argument that women between ages 18 and 35 years are generally a high risk group (early age of sexual intercourse, several partners), the Task Force made a uniform recommendation of annual screening of all women in this age group. Thereafter, screening can be done every 5 years and can stop at age 60 years if the women had received regular screening previously.

Chamberlain J, Day NE, Hakama M, et al. UICC Workshop of the Project on Evaluation of Screening Programmes for Gastrointestinal Cancer. Int J Cancer 37:329–334, 1986.
This paper concisely reviewed important issues of colorectal cancer screening and concluded that there is presently insufficient evidence to support such screening as a public health policy. Mathematical models, which support the use of screening, cannot replace results from ongoing randomized controlled trials.

Desmond S. Diet and cancer—should we change what we eat? West J Med 146:73–78, 1987.
This is a concise review of potential dietary influences on the development of malignancy.

Eddy D. Appropriateness of cervical cancer screening. Gynecol Oncol 12:S168–187, 1981.
This is a thorough review of the natural history of cervical cancer, the risks and benefits of Pap smears, and the importance of proper interpretation of the smears. Using a mathematical model, the author concluded that annual screening has the potential of significantly increasing costs without a significant increase in benefit.

Eddy D. Cost-effectiveness of colorectal cancer screening, in Levin B, Riddell R (eds). Frontiers in Gastrointestinal Cancer. New York, Elsevier Science Publishing Co., 1984, pp 203–219.
The author used a mathematical model, modified from the model initially described in 1980, to assess the cost effectiveness of colorectal cancer screening. Fecal occult blood testing alone delivers about two thirds of the effectiveness achievable by annual occult blood testing and annual rigid sigmoidoscopy. Overall, annual screening should decrease mortality by about one third.

Eddy D, Hasselblad V, McGivney W, et al. The value of mammography screening in women under age 50. JAMA 259:1512–1519, 1988.
Using mathematical models, the authors estimated that screening mammography can be expected to reduce mortality from breast cancer in women aged 40 to 49 years. However, the costs of mass screening in this age group would be high, and the benefits would not be as great as those when women over age 50 years are screened.

Frank J. Occult-blood screening for colorectal carcinoma: the benefits, the risks, and the yield and the costs. Am J Prev Med 1(3):3–9, 1(4):25–32, 1(5):18–24, 1985.
This three-part article is an extensive review of the use of fecal occult blood testing for colorectal cancer screening. The author concluded that use of this test as a routine health maintenance maneuver cannot yet be justified.

Habbema JD, van Oortmarssen GJ, van Putten DJ, et al. Age-specific reduction in breast cancer mortality by screening: an analysis of the results of the Health Insurance Plan of Greater New York study. JNCI 77:317–320, 1986.
Screening by both mammography and physical examination decreased mortality in all age groups between 40 and 64 years after 14 years of follow-up. The greatest reduction in percent mortality occurred in women aged 40 to 44 years at the time of entry into the study.

Hamblin JE, Brock CD, Litchfield L, et al. Papanicolaou smear adequacy: effect of different techniques in specific fertility states. J Fam Pract 20:257–260, 1985.
This study revealed that (1) smears from postmenopausal women had the lowest yield of endocervical cells; (2) swabbing excess mucus from the cervix before scraping increased the yield of endocervical cells; and (3) use of Milex spatula (plastic) for postmenopausal women increased the yield of endocervical cells.

Howard J. Using mammography for cancer control: an unrealized potential. CA 137:33–48, 1987.
This article is an excellent review of the completed clinical screening trials and of the use and deterrents to the use of mammography.

Knight KK, Fielding JE, Battista RN. Occult blood screening for colorectal cancer. JAMA 261:586–593, 1989.

The U.S. Preventive Services Task Force concluded that there is insufficient evidence to recommend either for or against fecal occult blood screening for individuals aged 45 years and older.

Laara E, Day N, Hakama M. Trends in mortality from cervical cancer in the Nordic countries: association with organised screening programmes. Lancet 1:1247–1249, 1987.

Analysis of mortality data from five countries supports the belief that cervical cancer screening decreases mortality. The nationwide program in Iceland had the widest target age range for screening and had the greatest decrease in mortality (80%); in Norway only 5% of the population received organized screening and the nationwide decrease in mortality was only 10%.

Miller A. Screening for breast cancer: a review. Eur J Cancer Clin Oncol 24:49–53, 1988.

This concise review summarized the completed and ongoing screening trials and concluded that screening should be concentrated in women between ages 40 and 69 years.

Moskowitz M. Costs of screening for breast cancer. Radiol Clin North Am 25:1031–1037, 1987.

Cost-benefit analysis using data from the Health Insurance Plan of New York study showed that the costs of screening women are well within the cost-benefit range that is accepted for other areas of the medical care system.

O'Malley M, Fletcher S. Screening for breast cancer with breast self-examination. JAMA 257:2197–2203, 1987.

This critical review of the literature assesses the efficacy of self-examination as a screening test for breast cancer. The authors concluded that it is a potentially useful screening technique but that there is presently inadequate evidence to advocate its widespread use.

Rogers R, Hansell R. Evaluation of the uterine cervix for cancer. Indiana Med 81:393–397, 1988.

This is a concise discussion of the technique of obtaining a Pap smear, the potential importance of cytobrush and spatula sampling, and the importance of proper sample fixation.

Selby J, Friedman G, Collen M. Sigmoidoscopy and mortality from colorectal cancer: the Kaiser-Permanente Multiphasic Evaluation study. J Clin Epidemiol 41:427–434, 1988.

The authors analyzed the data from this randomized trial, which has been interpreted as demonstrating that screening sigmoidoscopy reduces mortality from colorectal cancer. They concluded that the lower mortality in the study group cannot be attributed to the use of screening sigmoidoscopy.

Selby JV, Friedman GD. Sigmoidoscopy in the periodic health examination of asymptomatic adults. JAMA 261:594–601, 1989.

The U.S. Preventive Services Task Force concluded that there is insufficient evidence to recommend either for or against periodic screening sigmoidoscopy in persons of average risk who are aged 40 or older. This group did recommend periodic screening sigmoidoscopy for patients at high risk for colorectal cancer (persons with hereditary polyposis syndromes, ulcerative colitis for more than 10 years, prior history of colorectal cancer or adenomatous polyps, or two or more first-degree relatives with colorectal cancer).

Simon J. Occult blood screening for colorectal carcinoma: a critical review. Gastroenterology 88:820–837, 1985.

This literature review concluded that fecal occult blood testing should not be performed in the absence of improved survival rates in screened individuals with colorectal cancer (154 references).

Stenkvist B, Bergström R, Eklund G, et al. Papanicolaou smear screening and cervical cancer. What can you expect? JAMA 252:1423–1426, 1984.

Women who received at least one Pap smear during a 10-year period had a 75% decrease in invasive cervical cancer.

Tabár L, Dean P. The control of breast cancer through mammography screening: what is the evidence. Radiol Clin North Am 25:993–1005, 1987.

This paper discussed the rationale for controlled screening trials, reviewed the randomized and nonrandomized screening trials, and noted the various features required to maintain high quality mammographic techniques. Of special note: the sensitivity of mammography in the Swedish two-county study was greater than 90%.

Tabár L, Faberberg CJ, Gad A, et al. Reduction in mortality from breast cancer after mass screening with mammography. Lancet 1:829–832, 1985.

This randomized, controlled trial demonstrated that single-view mammography alone decreases mortality from breast cancer in women over age 50 years.

Tabár L, Faberberg G, Day NE, et al. What is the optimum interval between mammographic screening examinations? An analysis based on the latest results of the Swedish two-county breast cancer screening trial. Br J Cancer 55:547–551, 1987.

The apparent lack of benefit of single-view mammography for women aged 40 to 49 years may emanate from the 2-year screening interval. The authors recommended annual two-view mammography in women between ages 40 and 49 years and biennial screening in women over age 50 years.

Winawer SJ, Prorok P, Macrae F, et al. Surveillance and early diagnosis of colorectal cancer. Cancer Detec Prev 8:373–392, 1985.

An excellent review of the subject is provided.

45

Routine Laboratory Testing in General Medical Practice

CLIFFORD JOHNSON, M.D.
ALVIN MUSHLIN, M.D., Sc.M., F.A.C.P.

Detecting and treating a disease early in its course are intuitively superior to treating a patient with advanced disease. However, the seemingly simple decision to use laboratory testing to screen for a disease can be complex. In this chapter, the theory behind screening is discussed, the potential benefits and harms that may occur are considered, and the empiric evidence to support or reject the recommendations regarding specific outpatient and inpatient screening tests is presented.

Two primary questions are addressed. First, in an apparently healthy, asymptomatic adult, what laboratory tests should be performed during an office visit to detect unknown disease and why? Second, what laboratory tests should be performed routinely on hospital admission and why? Only routine testing for nonmalignant diseases is considered in this chapter because cancer screening is discussed elsewhere in this book (see Chap. 44).

The natural history of a disease process is shown in the following equation[38]:

$$\text{Biologic onset} \rightarrow \text{early diagnosis possible} \rightarrow$$
$$\text{usual clinical diagnosis} \rightarrow \text{outcome}$$

Initially, an undetectable biologic process begins. As the pathologic process continues, disease may be detected if the asymptomatic patient is tested. As the disease progresses, symptoms occur and clinical diagnosis usually is possible. Treatment is then initiated. Screening is an attempt to detect disease when early diagnosis is possible but before the clinical diagnosis is usually made. If testing asympto-

matic patients is to be useful, not only must the disease or risk of disease be detected early, but therapeutic intervention must be more effective in the asymptomatic than in the symptomatic stage. Table 45–1 shows the criteria that must be met for a screening test to benefit patients.[17]

Potential Benefits of Screening

Many potential benefits of screening have been discussed in the medical literature. Benefits may include reduced mortality and morbidity, or increased mental health, quality of life, and well-being. All arguments for routine testing should be judged by these criteria. It is not enough to make new diagnoses if outcome is not improved. For example, in a study performed at Kaiser Permanente,[20] all patients had 20 blood tests performed. For half of the patients, the complete results were reported to the patient's physician; in the other half, only 8 of the 20 results were reported. The complete test group had more new diagnoses, more confirmation of existing diagnoses, and addi-

Table 45–1. Criteria for Useful Screening Tests

1. The disease must have a significant effect on quality or quantity of life.
2. Acceptable methods of treatment must be available.
3. The disease must have an asymptomatic period during which detection and treatment significantly reduce morbidity and/or mortality.
4. Treatment in the asymptomatic period must yield a therapeutic result superior to that obtained by delaying treatment until symptoms appear.
5. Tests must be available at reasonable cost to detect the condition in the asymptomatic period.
6. The incidence of the condition must be sufficient to justify cost of screening.

Supported in part by a grant from the Charles A. Dana Foundation.

tional follow-up visits, phone calls, tests, advice, prescriptions, and referrals. But no conclusions could be made regarding the usefulness of reporting the extra tests because benefits to the patient were not studied.

Very few routine tests have been shown to improve patient care, and thus other reasons for testing asymptomatic patients are often given. Obtaining a base line (e.g., electrocardiogram [ECG]) is a common practice. Also, physicians may think that patients want a test performed and that patients appreciate thoroughness. Others believe that there is a value in confirming health so that the patient and physician are reassured. But these and other justifications for routine testing are not sufficient if patient outcomes are not improved.

Potential Harms of Screening

Although the potential harms of screening may not be as obvious as the potential benefits, they can be substantial. One problem with the routine testing of asymptomatic individuals is that the low prevalence of disease causes most of the abnormal results to be false positives and few to be true positives. For example, suppose a test for disease X was abnormal in 80% of the patients with the disease and normal in 90% of healthy patients (sensitivity = 80% and specificity = 90%). This is represented in Figure 45–1, where 1000 patients are considered each to have a 5% likelihood of being diseased. A positive test in an individual who has a 5% probability of having disease X based on history and physical examination increases the probability of disease to 30% (40

of 135). This figure shows that 70% (95 of 135) of the abnormal tests are false positives, occurring in patients without the disease. For many illnesses, the tests are not as sensitive or specific as in the above example, and the prevalence is much less than 5%. This results in an even higher percentage of false-positive results. For instance, if a patient has a 1% probability of disease before testing and the test's sensitivity and specificity are both 75%, then a positive test increases the probability of disease to only 3%!

False-positive test results may be detrimental to patients in many ways. Patients may be required to undergo further testing, which may involve risks. For instance, if an asymptomatic person has an exercise stress test as part of an "executive physical" program, the possibility of a false-positive result exists. If this occurs, the person could have a cardiac catheterization performed, which has a small but definite complication rate. If a complication occurs in a normal person, screening would have led to more harm than good. There are also financial as well as emotional costs involved in pursuing a false-positive result. The fiscal and emotional costs of false-positive tests should be included in the costs of any screening program.

Another potential harm of screening is the false reassurance given to patients with false-negative results. Because the sensitivity of many screening tests is not very high, a disease or risk factor may not be detected when it exists. For instance, a resting ECG is often normal in patients with significant coronary artery disease. If this normal test reassures a patient, motivation to alter risk factors such as hypertension or hypercholesterolemia may be reduced. In addition, patients may delay seeking care if symptoms do develop.

Another concern is the labeling effect. In a Canadian study of steelworkers screened for hypertension, there was a dramatic 80% increase in absenteeism, particularly related to illness, when steelworkers were told they had hypertension.[22] This increase occurred whether or not patients were started on treatment and was thought to be the result of adopting a sick role image. Thus, it is extremely important to screen for disease only if early intervention improves patient's health because diagnosis without effective treatment may be more harmful then beneficial.

Ambulatory testing of asymptomatic individuals is unique. Patients come to their physician feeling well, with a low likelihood of having any specific disease, and an even lower likeli-

DISEASE X

		Present	Absent	Total
TEST	Positive	40	95	135
	Negative	10	855	865
	Total	50	950	1000

Assume: prevalence of disease = 5%
sensitivity of test = 80%
specificity of test = 90%

Figure 45–1. *Test results and disease classification of 1000 hypothetical patients.*

hood of having a serious disease that would respond favorably to an intervention. This is in contrast to the usual clinical setting where a symptomatic patient sees a physician for evaluation and therapy. The potential for doing harm (e.g., diagnostic false-positive results, labeling, or inappropriate therapy) is much greater in the asymptomatic individuals who, in general, do very well without any intervention. A physician has an obligation to ensure that any intervention initiated in a patient feeling well results in health improvement. This ethical consideration should make physicians cautious in testing asymptomatic patients unless they are confident that screening will benefit patient care.

The best method of considering all of these issues is to do a randomized trial, where a sample of the population is routinely tested, the remainder is not tested, and a follow-up determines the effect of the screening on mortality, morbidity, and other outcome measures. Only then can we be certain that patients benefit from screening. But as will be seen, most studies are not comprehensive randomized trials. The major studies concerning the usefulness of commonly ordered outpatient and inpatient routine tests will now be reviewed.

Outpatient Screening

Ambulatory Multiphasic Screening

Multiphasic screening uses multiple tests for screening purposes. There have been several randomized trials evaluating its effectiveness. More than 10,000 Kaiser Foundation Health Plan members were randomized to either a control group that received routine care or the study group that was urged to have a yearly battery of clinical and laboratory tests (including blood pressure, ECG, spirometry, chest radiograph, mammography for women over 48 years old, urinalysis, serum panel, Pap smear, and sigmoidoscopy).[9] Mortality from colorectal cancer and hypertension complications was diminished in the study group. Screening for these diseases was worthwhile, but the many other tests performed showed no demonstrable benefit. In another study, patients from two group practices were randomly assigned to the control group or the screening group (which underwent a physical examination, chest radiograph, pulmonary function tests, ECG, blood pressure, and assays for levels of hemoglobin, blood glucose, blood urea nitrogen, cholesterol, uric acid, and occult blood in stool).[27] The screening occurred initially and again 2 years later, and both groups were followed for a total of 5 years. There was no difference between the two groups in mortality or morbidity as measured by hospital admissions or sickness absentee rates, no difference in the prevalence of symptoms or level of functioning, and no difference in the reduction of cardiovascular risk factors (weight, cholesterol, or cigarette smoking). Similar results were found in a study of 574 families randomized to a screening or a control group.[34] After 1 year, there was no difference in health status or disability in the two groups. The only difference was an increase in number of nights hospitalized for screened patients.

In an observational study of multiphasic screening, more than 5000 patients had testing consisting of assays for levels of hemoglobin, blood glucose, cholesterol, thyroxine, calcium, alkaline phosphatase, serum glutamic-oxaloacetic transaminase, potassium, uric acid, and bacteria in the urine, and forced expiratory volume in 1 second, tonometry, audiography, and visual field tests.[3] The serum cholesterol and 1-hour postprandial blood glucose tests led to new diagnoses in approximately 2.5% of those screened. The other tests led to new diagnoses in less than 1% of participants. The number of patients who benefited from treatment of a previously undiagnosed condition was not studied but was certainly exceedingly small.

These studies have looked at large numbers of ambulatory patients, screened them with multiple tests, and found benefits only from the screening for colorectal cancer and hypertension. With the low prevalence of disease, the financial costs, the problem of false-positive and false-negative results, the potential harm of the labeling effect, and the lack of proven treatment efficacy for many asymptomatic illnesses, multiphasic screening of ambulatory patients cannot be recommended. It is possible that specific tests could be targeted to selected groups of patients (based on age, for example) to yield a benefit in patient care. This has been the approach recommended by the Canadian Task Force,[7] Frame,[13–16] Breslow and Somers,[6] and the American College of Physicians Medical Practice Committee.[2] The major studies examining the utility of specific tests for specific diseases will next be considered.

Complete Blood Count

The major reason for obtaining a routine complete blood count (CBC) in an asymptomatic patient is to detect silent underlying disease. In a study of 1080 women aged 20 to 64 years screened for anemia, 11% had a hemoglobin level less than 12 g/dl and 4.1% had a hemoglobin level less than 10 g/dl.[12] Although the women were not extensively evaluated, only one was found to have a serious underlying illness, a bronchial carcinoid found by chest x-ray and thought to be a coincidental finding. In another study, 18,740 Welsh women over age 21 years were screened for anemia and followed for 3 years.[11] The women with a hematocrit less than 36% had a greater chance of dying from cancer than women with higher hematocrit values. Nevertheless, only 1% of these anemic women actually died of cancer, and many of these very possibly had incurable tumors when they were screened. Thus, screening for anemia is an inefficient method of identifying underlying treatable disease. There are more effective methods that should be used to detect specific cancers (see Chap. 44). Likewise, there is no evidence that a routine white blood count or differential count is useful.[35] Thus, a routine CBC cannot be recommended for ambulatory asymptomatic adults.

Biochemical Profile

Screening outpatients by use of biochemical profiles (levels of serum electrolytes, blood glucose, blood urea nitrogen, creatinine) has not been very well studied. In the randomized study performed at the Kaiser Foundation mentioned earlier, no benefit was found from utilizing these tests. A recently published review of this topic also concluded that biochemical profiles were not warranted for ambulatory screening.[8] It is not surprising that screening electrolytes does not improve patient care, because the illnesses that cause these abnormalities (e.g., syndrome of inappropriate antidiuretic hormone, diabetes insipidus, hyperaldosteronemia) are rare and are usually symptomatic. It is possible that early detection of renal dysfunction (blood urea nitrogen or creatinine level) may be of benefit because low protein dietary treatment may alter the progression of renal dysfunction.[36] But before all patients are screened for mild renal insufficiency and are instructed to alter their diets

for the remainder of their lives, the evidence that early dietary treatment is beneficial in the asymptomatic stage needs to be further documented.

It is unknown whether early detection of asymptomatic glucose intolerance improves patient outcome. Patients with impaired glucose tolerance have mortality rates between normal subjects and overt diabetics. However, in one study, there was no difference in mortality if the patients were not treated, treated with diet, or treated with diet and tolbutamide.[39] The University Group Diabetes Program (UGDP) has led to considerable controversy but has raised the possibility that tolbutamide may increase the cardiovascular mortality in adult onset diabetics.[4] Although this remains a controversial topic, testing for early asymptomatic glucose intolerance cannot be recommended because early treatment has not been shown to reduce morbidity or mortality.

Electrocardiograms

ECGs might theoretically be of benefit to ambulatory asymptomatic patients for several reasons. Occult heart disease might be detected, patients might be reassured, and a base line might be obtained for future comparison. Nevertheless, problems limit the potential benefits from each of these considerations. The resting ECG lacks adequate sensitivity and specificity. In a population-based study comparing the accuracy of Q wave ECG abnormalities with autopsy-determined old myocardial infarction, the sensitivity was 43% and the specificity was 94%.[25] Thus, of the people who died and had autopsy evidence for a previous myocardial infarction, 57% had had ECGs without abnormal Q waves, and of those who died without autopsy evidence for an old infarction, 6% previously had abnormal Q waves. If, for example, the prevalence of an old myocardial infarction in asymptomatic adults is 1%, then an ECG with abnormal Q waves increases the probability of an old infarction to only 7%. Thus, 93% of all ECGs with abnormal Q waves would occur in people without heart disease! Figure 45–2 diagrams the ECG results of 10,000 asymptomatic patients undergoing testing, assuming that the prevalence of coronary artery disease is 1%, that its sensitivity is 43%, and that its specificity is 94%. Forty-three people are correctly diagnosed as having coronary artery disease,

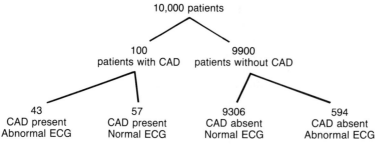

Figure 45–2. *The ECG results in 10,000 hypothetical asymptomatic patients.*

57 patients are incorrectly told they are free of heart disease (false negatives), and 594 patients are incorrectly diagnosed as having heart disease (false positives). A false-positive result would undoubtedly worry a patient needlessly, perhaps lead to further testing or therapy that is not indicated, and may lead to detrimental alterations in lifestyle such as an aversion to exercise. A false-negative result may also have adverse effects by falsely re-assuring a patient. The potential detrimental effects of these numerous false results may well offset the potential gain of identifying 43 people correctly. Thus, an ECG is a poor test to diagnose a previous myocardial infarction in an asymptomatic patient.

Could other forms of occult heart disease be diagnosed by an ECG? Rhythm or conduction disturbances may be documented, but the value of these findings in asymptomatic patients is questionable. Left ventricular hypertrophy may be diagnosed, but the ECG for this purpose also has many false-positive and false-negative results and is of limited utility in asymptomatic patients. Thus, the ECG is limited in its ability to detect occult heart disease. The false-positive and false-negative rates are too high for this test to be useful in asymptomatic outpatients.

The value of obtaining an ECG as a base line is also limited because its utility decreases with time. For instance, if a patient presents with chest pain, an ECG obtained 5 years ago or even 1 year ago may not be very helpful, whereas one obtained 1 week beforehand may be very useful. In the one study of the potential benefits of a base-line ECG in patients with chest pain going to an emergency room, decisions were made on the basis of clinical presentation and were infrequently influenced by the lack of a base-line ECG.[37] A few patients may have avoided admission by having an old

ECG available. If all patients have a base-line ECG so that a few might benefit by avoiding future admissions, a large number of false-positive and false-negative results would be obtained and may do more harm than good.

Chest Radiographs

Routine outpatient chest radiographs are not justified for lung cancer detection, even in high risk patients (i.e., smokers) because there is no evidence that survival is increased by screening. There is no empiric evidence suggesting that routine chest radiographs be performed to detect nonmalignant diseases.

Urinalysis

Routine urinalysis cannot be recommended for all outpatients. Although these assays are simple to perform, there are well-documented inaccuracies in the results.[18] Dales's study of multiphasic screening discussed earlier showed no benefit from this test.[9] In another study of 2600 outpatient screening urinalyses, only 13 new decisions for further laboratory testing or new treatment resulted.[19] Most of these abnormalities were glycosuria or trace proteinuria and did not affect clinical management. A recent review of this topic has reached similar conclusions.[29]

Serum Cholesterol

There is abundant evidence that elevated cholesterol levels predict increased cardiovascular disease and that the reduction of elevated low density lipoprotein cholesterol slows the progression of atherosclerotic vascular disease and reduces cardiac mortality. The Oslo study,[26] the National Heart, Lung, and Blood Institute Type 2 Coronary Intervention Study,[5] and the Lipid Research Clinics Coronary Primary Prevention Trial[32] all suggest a benefit from reducing elevated cholesterol levels. (This topic is covered in greater detail in Chap. 15.)

Many questions remain regarding the cost effectiveness of screening, compliance with dietary recommendations in a general medical practice, the "best" test for screening (i.e., total cholesterol, low density lipoprotein cholesterol, high density lipoprotein cholesterol level, or some combination of these), the optimal screening interval, and the cholesterol level indicating that treatment is needed. Nevertheless, screening all adults by use of a nonfasting total cholesterol assay appears to be indicated. Elevated values should be confirmed, and a high density lipoprotein cholesterol and triglyceride analysis should be considered for calculation of the low density lipoprotein cholesterol level. Dietary or drug therapy for those patients with persistently elevated total or low density lipoprotein cholesterol levels should be individualized.

Of the many possible screening tests for nonmalignant diseases discussed earlier, only a serum cholesterol level is indicated for asymptomatic, ambulatory adult patients. The yield of the other tests is low; the possible benefits are usually offset by the frequent false-positive and false-negative results and the inability of early detection to alter the disease processes.

Inpatient Screening

There are several important differences between routine outpatient screening and inpatient testing. The purpose of ambulatory screening is to detect silent treatable conditions. Often the potential benefit is not seen for years, as in the treatment of hypercholesterolemia to prevent coronary artery disease. In contrast, the goal of routine inpatient testing is more immediate: to detect conditions that may adversely affect the current hospitalization. Another difference is that inpatients usually have a higher prevalence of underlying diseases than asymptomatic outpatients, so that routine tests should more often be positive and the predictive value of a positive test should be higher. Thus, one might believe that routine testing would be useful for inpatients

in detecting unsuspected disease and that the benefits would occur during the hospitalization. As will be shown, the data do not support this belief. As with outpatient screening, the yield of unsuspected abnormalities is low, the number of new diagnoses and treatments is even lower, and benefit to patient care is rare. In addition, false-positive results can be problematic and can lead to a delay in indicated treatment, to unnecessary testing, and sometimes to inappropriate care.

The heterogeneity of inpatients makes it difficult to have general recommendations regarding routine testing for asymptomatic disease. The benefits of a screening test may be different in elective preoperative patients, emergent preoperative patients, and medical patients. Even among medical patients, someone with one illness may benefit from a test, whereas another patient with a different illness may not. Most studies have looked at all preoperative patients or all medical patients. Thus, there may exist subsets of patients who would benefit from a test that is not indicated for all patients admitted to the hospital. The utility of routine testing of medical inpatients will now be considered. (Routine preoperative testing is discussed in Chap. 54.)

Multiphasic Testing

Several studies have examined the usefulness of a routine multiphasic battery of tests for patients being admitted to the hospital. Because these patients are sick enough to require hospitalization, it is not surprising that many abnormal laboratory results are found. But an abnormal result is not in itself beneficial to a patient. For a routine test to be beneficial, a condition neither previously known nor previously suspected should be detected, and a new treatment should be prescribed and result in an improved patient outcome. Studies that have examined patient outcomes have found little benefit from most routine inpatient testing.

In a prospective Australian trial of admission screening, 500 study patients were given a multiphasic battery of tests.[10] These patients were compared with 1000 control patients who did not receive these tests. There was no significant effect on mortality, length of stay in the hospital, disability, speed at which therapy was begun, distress suffered by patients, or patient satisfaction despite 25% more consultations and 78% more laboratory tests in the study group.

In another Australian study, patients were screened on admission to a teaching hospital with a CBC, erythrocyte sedimentation rate, sequential multiple analyses (SMA-6 and SMA-12), ECG, chest radiograph, urine culture, prothrombin time, and several other tests.[23] In the control group, the results of these tests were not made available until discharge or death, whereas in the study group, the results were available to the physician caring for the patient. Although there were only 50 patients per group, no difference in death rate, state of health at discharge, disability, length of stay, hospital cost, or extent of nursing or medical care provided between the two groups was detected.

These are the only controlled trials of routine inpatient testing. Both show no benefit for the group screened despite more consultations and further investigations, although there was no long-term follow-up in either study.

Similar conclusions were found in a study of 1000 adult patients admitted to a community hospital and screened with 20 laboratory tests. Only 1% of all results led to new diagnoses, and only one patient was judged to have benefited.[30] Multiphasic screening of medical admissions does not appear to be indicated.

Complete Blood Count

A CBC is indicated (and thus not considered screening) at admission for many patients. Infection, bleeding, hematologic diseases, and planned surgery associated with more than minor blood loss are obvious indications for a CBC. If no indication is present, the CBC is rarely of benefit. Although no study has specifically evaluated the CBC as a routine test for medical admissions, the studies of multiphasic screening discussed earlier found the CBC to have no attributable benefit.

Chest Radiographs

Many hospitalized patients have pulmonary symptoms or signs; a chest x-ray would be indicated based on these findings. Reasons for obtaining this study in patients without respiratory problems by history or physical examination include detection of occult disease and obtaining a base line. As with most other routine tests, the yield is low, and the benefits are exceedingly small and are offset by the potential harm that may occur.

There are high false-positive and false-negative rates in the interpretation of chest x-rays, which are in part the result of interpreter variability. These rates have been documented to be as high as 25%.[24, 40] Two interpreters have disagreed with each other up to one third of the time and with themselves when rereading the films up to one fifth of the time.[40] Thus, the potential for missing important lesions and for reading an abnormality when none exists is significant. Of course, identifying true abnormalities on a chest x-ray is not uncommon, but finding an abnormality does not justify the examination. Changes in patient management with improvement in outcome need to be considered.

In a study of patients admitted to a Veterans Administration hospital's medical service, only 4 of 294 routine chest x-rays showed new or worsening abnormalities.[28] Three of these four patients probably would have had historical or physical evidence of their disease found during hospitalization and thus would have received a chest x-ray if one had not been done routinely on admission. The fourth patient had a lung cancer detected, and he died of this disease despite screening. Although a large number of x-ray abnormalities were found, the findings were predominantly chronic and stable, and their impact on patient care was small. When chest disease is not clinically suspected, chest radiographs add little to the management of these medical patients.

Electrocardiograms

Admission ECGs for medical patients without known heart disease are performed to detect silent heart disease that may influence a patient's hospital course or to provide a base line. In a study of 1410 patients admitted to a general medical ward, 1% of screening ECGs added information not obtained by the history or physical examination.[33] Some of the abnormal ECGs suggested diagnoses that proved to be incorrect. The presence of cardiac abnormalities by history or physical examination was the single most important predictor of an ECG's providing new information. Also, the older the patient, the greater the likelihood of obtaining new information. In this study, there was no admission ECG that was indispensable to the care of patients who subsequently developed symptoms during their admission. Thus, the utility of the ECG overall was low, especially in younger patients without evidence of heart disease. Little benefit from using the ECG as a base line could be documented.

Routine ECGs for all patients admitted to the hospital are not indicated. Patients who have symptoms or signs of heart disease receive the most benefit. Also, men older than age 45 years and women older than age 55 years may benefit from routine ECGs. Although not specifically studied, other subsets of patients may benefit as well. These include patients with a high probability of electrolyte disturbances, those with diabetes or peripheral vascular disease, or those taking drugs that may cause cardiac toxicity. Clinical judgment should guide the use of ECGs.

Urinalysis

Although inpatients often have no indications for a urinalysis, it is a frequently obtained routine admission test. In one study, only 10 of 746 routine admission urinalyses affected patient management.[31] Asymptomatic urinary tract infections were the diagnosis in most of these cases. In another study of 123 routine admission urinalyses, only one patient probably benefited.[1] This patient also had a urinary tract infection. Clinical judgment, not routine practice, should guide the ordering of the admission urinalysis.

Conclusions and Recommendations

Current medical literature does not support the widespread use of outpatient or inpatient screening for detecting nonmalignant disease. If an illness is unsuspected after a history and physical examination, patient care usually is not affected by routine testing. Detrimental effects of screening are poorly documented, although the potential harm may be substantial. This may be a fruitful area for future research.

The data reviewed in this chapter support a nonfasting serum cholesterol determination as the only outpatient screening test for nonmalignant disease in the general population. Other tests may be indicated in special subgroups, such as a rubella titer in young women. This is in agreement with some, but not all, of the previously published recommendations. The conclusions by Frame[13–16] agree with ours. Breslow and Somers[6] recommend screening tests for certain age groups, includ-

ing tests for syphilis, gonorrhea, anemia, diabetes, and hypercholesterolemia. They also recommend routine outpatient ECGs. The Canadian Task Force on the Periodic Health Examination[7] did not recommend screening for hyperlipidemia; tests recommended by Breslow and Somers were also not recommended unless patients were in a high risk subgroup. A recent American Heart Association position statement has recommended routine ECGs at ages 20, 40, and 60 years, and a routine chest radiograph at age 40 years.[21] No justification for these recommendations is given.

Uniform recommendations regarding admission screening cannot be made because of the heterogeneity of inpatients. Further clinical studies are needed to better define populations that may benefit. Although testing for a disease unsuspected after a history and physical examination is seldom helpful, certain tests may be of value for specific subgroups of patients. For example, ECGs may benefit men older than 45 years and women older than 55 years. There are no recommendations in the medical literature from an authoritative group regarding inpatient screening. The consensus opinion of such a group could help establish admission screening guidelines.

References

1. Akin BV, Hubbell FA, Frye EB, et al. Efficacy of the routine admission urinalysis. Am J Med 82:719–722, 1987.
   This retrospective analysis of routine admission urinalyses indicated a very small impact on patient care.
2. American College of Physicians Medical Practice Committee. Periodic health examination: a guide for designing individual preventive health care in the asymptomatic patient. Ann Intern Med 95:729–732, 1981.
   This concise review of previous recommendations regarding periodic health examinations concluded that routine annual checkups be replaced by a selective approach determined by age and gender of patient.
3. Bates B, Yellin JA. The yield of multiphasic screening. JAMA 222:74–78, 1972.
   Multiphasic screening was performed on more than 5000 patients, and results were sent to their physicians. Most abnormalities were not confirmed, new diagnoses were infrequently made, and management was seldom altered. Patient outcomes were not assessed.
4. Bradley RF, Dolger H, Forsham PH, et al. Settling the UGDP controversy? JAMA 232:813–817, 1975.
   The UGDP controversy was discussed.
5. Brensike JF, Levy RI, Kelsey SF, et al. Effects of therapy with cholestyramine on progression of coronary arteriosclerosis: results of the NHLBI type 2

coronary intervention study. Circulation 69:313–324, 1984.

Patients with coronary artery disease and elevated low density lipoprotein cholesterol were randomized to either cholestyramine or placebo. Coronary angiography initially and 5 years later showed less progression of coronary disease in the cholestyramine-treated group.

6. Breslow L, Somers AR. The lifetime health-monitoring program. A practical approach to preventive medicine. N Engl J Med 296:601–608, 1977.

A proposal was presented of desirable preventive health goals and professional services based on a patient's age.

7. Canadian Task Force on the Periodic Health Examination. The periodic health examination. Can Med Assoc J 121:1193–1254, 1979.

This landmark review of prevention and treatment effectiveness for 78 conditions provided recommendations for a lifetime program of periodic health assessment based on age.

8. Cebul RD, Beck JR. Biochemical profiles. Applications in ambulatory screening and preadmission testing of adults. Ann Intern Med 106:403–413, 1987.

The utility of the biochemical profile in ambulatory and admission testing was reviewed.

9. Dales LG, Friedman GD, Collen MF. Evaluating periodic multiphasic health checkups: a controlled trial. J Chronic Dis 32:385–404, 1979.

This large controlled study showed a decrease in deaths related to hypertension and colorectal cancer by use of periodic health examinations. No decrease was found in overall mortality.

10. Durbridge TC, Edwards F, Edwards RG, et al. An evaluation of multiphasic screening on admission to hospital. Med J Aust 1:703–705, 1976.

This large Australian controlled study showed no beneficial effect of admission multiphasic screening.

11. Elwood PC, Waters WE, Benjamin IT, et al. Mortality and anaemia in women. Lancet 1:891–894, 1974.

Routine hemoglobin and hematocrit tests were done for more than 18,000 women. After 3 years, there was a small increase in deaths in women with hematocrits < 36%, but only 1% of these anemic women died from neoplastic disease.

12. Elwood PC, Waters WE, Green WJ, et al. Evaluation of a screening survey for anaemia in adult nonpregnant women. Br Med J 4:714–717, 1967.

Community-based screening detected anemia in a significant percentage of women, but there was an apparent absence of serious treatable disease and an absence of benefit in those treated with iron.

13. Frame PS. A critical review of adult health maintenance. Part 1: prevention of atherosclerotic disease. J Fam Pract 22:341–346, 1986.

This detailed review of atherosclerosis prevention recommended screening for, and reduction of, risk factors including tobacco use, elevated serum cholesterol level, and hypertension.

14. Frame PS. A critical review of adult health maintenance. Part 2: prevention of infectious diseases. J Fam Pract 22:417–422, 1986.

This detailed review of infectious disease prevention recommended influenza and pneumococcal vaccine in high risk groups, tetanus-diphtheria booster every 10 years, rubella vaccine in susceptible women of childbearing age, and syphilis screening in high risk groups.

15. Frame PS. A critical review of adult health maintenance. Part 3: prevention of cancer. J Fam Pract 22:511–520, 1986.

This detailed review of cancer prevention recommended reduction of tobacco use, stool occult blood testing, self-breast examinations, physician breast examinations, mammograms, Pap smears, the teaching of reporting postmenopausal bleeding, and the teaching of mouth, neck, skin, and testes self-examination.

16. Frame PS. A critical review of adult health maintenance. Part 4: prevention of metabolic, behavioral and miscellaneous conditions. J Fam Pract 23:29–39, 1986.

This detailed review of metabolic, behavioral, and miscellaneous disease prevention recommended clinical evaluation of menopausal women for osteoporosis risk, obtaining patients' weight, and encouraging seat belt use.

17. Frame PS, Carlson SJ. A critical review of the periodic health screening using specific screening criteria. Part 1: selected diseases of respiratory, cardiovascular, and central nervous systems. J Fam Pract 2:29–36, 1975.

This is similar to the above reviews.

18. Fraser CG. Urine analysis: current performance and strategies for improvement. Br Med J 291:321–323, 1985.

A discussion, with literature review, of the inaccuracies in urine protein, glucose, bilirubin, blood, and nitrate analysis was presented.

19. Fraser CG, Smith BC, Peake MJ. Effectiveness of an outpatient urine screening program. Clin Chem 23:2216–2218, 1977.

Routine outpatient urinalyses (2600) added to costs without significant patient benefit.

20. Friedman GD, Goldberg M, Ahuja JN, et al. Biochemical screening tests. Effects of panel size on medical care. Arch Intern Med 129:91–97, 1972.

Patients at Kaiser Permanente (8446) were randomly assigned to have either 20 or only 8 automated biochemical test results reported. In the first group, the intensity of medical care was increased. Patient benefit was not studied.

21. Grundy SM, Greenland P, Herd A, et al. Cardiovascular and risk factor evaluation of healthy American adults. A statement for physicians by an ad hoc committee appointed by the steering committee, American Heart Association. Circulation 75:1340A–1362A, 1987.

Recommendations were provided from the American Heart Association regarding cardiovascular prevention.

22. Haynes RB, Sackett DL, Taylor DW, et al. Increased absenteeism from work after detection and labeling of hypertensive patients. N Engl J Med 299:741–744, 1978.

Canadian steelworkers (245) had hypertension found on screening. These men subsequently had increased absenteeism from work.

23. Hecker R. Medical practice and multiphasic screening. Med J Aust 2:398–401, 1975.

Pilot randomized study of multiphasic admission screening showed no benefit from a battery of blood, urine, and x-ray tests.

24. Herman PG, Gerson DE, Hessel ST, et al. Disagreements in chest roentgen interpretation. Chest 68:278–282, 1975.

Admission radiographs (100) were independently reviewed by five radiologists; 41% of reports contained false-positive or false-negative results, and 25% of important findings were omitted.

25. Hiyoshi Y, Omae T, Hirota Y, et al. Clinicopathological study of the heart and coronary arteries of autop-

sied cases from the community of Hisayama during a 10 year period. Part 5. Comparison of autopsy findings with electrocardiograms—Q.QS items of the Minnesota code. Am J Epidemiol 121:906–913, 1985.

Population-based autopsy series of men with previous ECGs showed Q waves on ECG to have sensitivity of 32 to 43% and a specificity of 94 to 95% in identifying previous myocardial infarctions.

26. Hjermann I, Byre KV, Holme I, et al. Effect of diet and smoking intervention on the incidence of coronary artery heart disease. Lancet 2:1303–1310, 1981.

The Oslo study of 1232 hypercholesterolemic cigarette smoking men randomized to an intervention group (diet and smoking cessation advice) or a control group showed that the intervention group had 47% lower incidence of myocardial infarction and sudden death.

27. Holland WW, D'Souza M, Swan AV. Is mass screening justified? Tijdschr Soc Geneeskd 56:22–25, 1978.

In a large randomized British trial of screening a general practice population aged 40 to 64 years, 5-year follow-up showed no effect of screening on various outcome measures.

28. Hubbell FA, Greenfield S, Tyler JL, et al. The impact of routine admission chest x-ray films on patient care. N Engl J Med 312:209–213, 1985.

Four of 294 routine Veterans Administration hospital admission chest radiographs identified abnormalities not suggested by clinical findings. Three of these four patients probably would have had a chest radiograph performed anyway because of historical or physical evidence of disease during their hospitalization.

29. Kiel DP, Moskowitz MA. The urinalysis: a critical appraisal. Med Clin North Am 71:607–624, 1987.

Role of the routine urinalysis in ambulatory practice was critically reviewed.

30. Korvin CC, Pearce RH, Stanley J. Admissions screening: clinical benefits. Ann Intern Med 83:197–203, 1975.

In multiphasic screening (20 tests) of 1000 patients admitted to a community general hospital, 1% of results led to new diagnoses, mostly hepatobiliary disease and mild diabetes; one patient was judged to have benefited from the routine testing.

31. Kroenke K, Hanley JF, Copley JB, et al. The admission urinalysis: impact on patient care. J Gen Intern Med 1:238–242, 1986.

Only 1.3% of routine admission urinalyses affected patient therapy, and the majority of the results showed asymptomatic bacteriuria.

32. Lipid Research Clinics Program. The lipid research clinics coronary primary prevention trial results. 1. Reduction in incidence of coronary heart disease. JAMA 251:351–364, 1984.

Men with low density lipoprotein cholesterol levels > 175 mg/dl after diet were randomized to either cholestyramine or placebo. There was a 24% reduction in coronary heart disease deaths in the treatment group after 7.4 years. This is considered the best evidence for lowering elevated cholesterol levels.

33. Moorman JR, Hlatky MA, Eddy DM, et al. The yield of the routine admission electrocardiogram. Ann Intern Med 103:590–595, 1985.

Only 1% of admission ECGs added additional information after a history and physical examination. Information was added more often for patients 45 years or older and for patients with clinical evidence of heart disease.

34. Olsen DM, Kane RL, Proctor PH. A controlled trial of multiphasic screening. N Engl J Med 294:925–930, 1976.

Randomized study of multiphasic screening showed an increase in nights hospitalized in those tested. There was no difference in health status or disability between groups.

35. Rich EC, Crowson TW, Connelly DP. Effectiveness of differential leukocyte count in case finding in the ambulatory care setting. JAMA 249:633–636, 1983.

No clinically inapparent disease was discovered by 474 outpatient routine white blood cell counts with differential counts. Most abnormalities were not noted by the physicians.

36. Rosman JB, Wee PMT, Meijer S, et al. Prospective randomized trial of early dietary protein restriction in chronic renal failure. Lancet 2:1291–1295, 1984.

Prospective randomized trial of patients with various renal diseases concluded that early moderate dietary protein restriction retarded the development of end-stage renal failure.

37. Rubenstein LZ, Greenfield S. The baseline ECG in the evaluation of acute cardiac complaints. JAMA 244:2536–2539, 1980.

Study of 236 patients presented to an emergency room with chest pain and no prior cardiac history. Only a small percentage of patients might have benefited from a previous routine ECG, and the benefit would have been avoidance of a possibly unnecessary admission.

38. Sackett DL, Haynes RB, Tugwell P. Clinical Epidemiology: A Basic Science For Clinical Medicine. Boston, Little, Brown & Co., 1985.

This is an excellent textbook of clinical epidemiology, with a good discussion of routine testing.

39. Sartor G, Scherstein B, Carlstrom S, et al. Ten year follow-up of subjects with impaired glucose tolerance. Diabetes 29:41–49, 1980.

In this trial of diet, no treatment, or tolbutamide in patients with impaired glucose tolerance, although tolbutamide appeared to lower the rate of progression to diabetes, there was no difference in mortality between groups after 12 years.

40. Yerushalmy J. The statistical assessment of the variability in observer perception and description of roentgenographic pulmonary shadows. Radiol Clin North Am 7:381–392, 1969.

This article documents a high degree of observer variability in the interpretation of chest radiographs.

PART ELEVEN

Pulmonary

PART ELEVEN

Urinary

46

Evaluation and Management of Chronic Cough

ARTHUR S. BANNER, M.D.

Cough commonly accompanies a wide variety of pulmonary disorders. When cough occurs in the context of an identified pulmonary condition, it is rarely a source of concern to either the patient or the physician. Patients seek medical advice when the basis for the cough is obscure or when the cough is attended by other symptoms. The muscular effort associated with a cough may give rise to traumatic complications such as rib fractures, pulled abdominal muscles, hernias, and injuries to the airways or larynx. The high intrathoracic pressures that are generated during a cough may interfere with cerebral perfusion, and syncope may result. Cough of prolonged duration may result in alarming constitutional symptoms such as fatigue, anorexia, and weight loss. The psychologic consequences of a chronic, unexplained cough may be considerable and are characterized by anxiety, depression, and fears of loss of control. The psychologic burden of waiting for the next cough paroxysm may lead to lifestyle changes such as avoidance of theaters and restaurants. The fact that even an innocuous cough may have a major impact on a patient's life dictates an aggressive approach to diagnosis and management. Unfortunately, the work-up for cough is not standardized, and it is often difficult to establish the basis for a cough even after an extensive evaluation. Equally important, a troublesome cough may be amazingly resistant to all forms of antitussive interventions. The following remarks are meant to guide the physician in the often difficult task of evaluation and treatment of a cough. The manner in which cough is managed may differ among physicians but should always be guided by a knowledge of cough physiology, good clinical judgment, and a genuine concern for the psychologic welfare of the patient.

Physiology of Cough

Cough is one of a group of respiratory reflexes that have as their primary function the defense of the integrity of the respiratory system. Cough not only defends the lungs from inhaled injurious agents but also serves to cleanse the airways of products of inflammation. In addition, cough has been termed the watchdog of the lungs in that the cough reflex serves to warn the individual of the presence of abnormal conditions within the respiratory system.

The afferent component of the cough reflex involves a variety of sensory receptors that are located for the most part within the airway epithelium; they are also found in airway smooth muscle and in extrapulmonary locations such as the larynx, tympanic membranes, ear canals, hypopharynx, and perhaps the pleura, pericardium, and diaphragm. The connections to the brain are contained almost exclusively in the vagus nerve. The afferent signals accumulate within areas of the medulla, where the efferent response of the cough reflex is coordinated and modulated. The efferent component of the cough reflex consists of the motor act of cough, which comprises a coordinated interaction of the muscles of respiration and the larynx. Additional efferent responses consist of airway smooth muscle contraction, secretion of mucus from submucosal bronchial glands, and responses from the cardiovascular system, including tachycardia and constriction of systemic vessels. It should be noted that most coughs are probably a consequence of an interaction of many stimuli on a variety of receptors. We know, for instance, that cough receptors respond to many chemical and mechanical stimuli and that these stimuli probably act synergistically to produce a cough. For instance, there is experimental evidence that airway smooth muscle contraction (a mechanical stimulus) lowers the threshold of cough receptors to a number of chemical agents. Furthermore, every cough probably involves more than one class of receptors, and multiple reflexes interact with each other to effect a cough response. Thus, although the receptors primarily responsible for a cough lie in airway epithelium, other receptors, such as those situated in airway smooth muscle, make the cough possible. There is also experimental evidence that stimulation of receptors at one location makes receptors situated at other locations more susceptible to tussive stimuli. Animal experiments have shown that irritation of the pleura lowers the threshold of cough receptors in the trachea. It must also be kept in mind that the cough reflex is subject to considerable modulation within the central nervous system. A tendency to cough varies among individuals and is determined by levels of arousal and probably by genetic factors related to respiratory control.

Evaluation of the Patient with an Unexplained Cough

There is no standardized approach to the evaluation of a cough. In recent years, several clinicians have suggested a systematic approach to cough evaluation. They base their counsel on the notion that a cough arises from stimulation of specific sensory receptors and that the work-up ought to be directed at identifying the involved receptors and the stimuli responsible for their discharge. Although such an approach is intellectually satisfying, it is unrealistic to expect that one can accomplish such goals because of the complex manner in which a cough may be elicited.

The complexity of the cough mechanism and the multiplicity of conditions that lead to cough dictate an operational approach to evaluation. The work-up should be guided by a knowledge of cough physiology but should also be tempered by acknowledgment that our understanding of cough is incomplete. Our functions as physicians are to identify serious underlying disease that may have resulted in the cough, to treat the trivial conditions that may aggravate the symptom, and to provide reassurance that the patient's bothersome symptom is not a manifestation of a disorder that may be life-threatening. Common findings of an evaluation

for a cough of obscure etiology include postinfectious conditions, asthma or airway hyperreactivity, rhinitis, postnasal drip, bronchitis (smoking), gastroesophageal reflux, and left ventricular failure. It should be noted that the diagnostic criteria for many of these conditions are poorly delineated. Consequently, the frequencies with which each of these conditions is encountered in patients with cough are variable. Two groups of investigators have published their experience with cough evaluation. Both Irwin and colleagues and Poe and colleagues agree that asthma or airway hyperreactivity is associated with a cough in approximately 40% of patients. On the other hand, Irwin and coworkers attributed cough to postnasal drip in 46% of patients, whereas Poe and colleagues identified this condition in only 5% of their patients. Similarly, Poe and coworkers concluded that 25% of their patients' coughs were postinfectious, whereas Irwin and colleagues failed to consider this condition in any of their subjects. Both groups of investigators agreed that cardiac disease, cancer, and gastrointestinal disease are unusual causes for a cough of obscure etiology.

Components of a Cough Evaluation

History

A cough evaluation starts with an appropriate history (Table 46–1). Such a history begins with identifying the duration of the cough. In the absence of other symptoms, cough should

Table 46–1. *Components of History Related to Cough*

1. Duration of cough
2. Cough antecedents, i.e., upper respiratory tract infections, pneumonia, noxious inhalants, smoking, allergies
3. Symptoms suggestive of upper respiratory tract disease, i.e., hoarseness, rhinitis, throat clearing, sinusitis, hearing impairment
4. Symptoms suggestive of asthma, i.e., wheeze or dyspnea with upper respiratory tract infections, after coughing or sneezing, or after exercise in cold weather
5. Symptoms suggestive of malignancy, i.e., hemoptysis, chest pain, weight loss, cigarette addiction
6. Symptoms suggestive of esophageal disease, i.e., heartburn, sour eructations, nocturnal cough or choking spells, cough exacerbated by theophylline
7. Symptoms suggestive of left ventricular failure, i.e., nocturnal cough, paroxysmal nocturnal dyspnea, nocturia

persist for at least 1 month before a rigorous evaluation is initiated. Patients who smoke should be counseled to abstain. Abstinence from smoking for at least 3 months results in alleviation of the cough in the majority of such individuals. The history should then be directed at discerning how the cough began. Prolonged cough after an upper respiratory tract infection is exceedingly common and is responsible for at least 25% of the cases of cough of obscure etiology. This type of cough may begin after the initial symptoms of the infection have resolved. Many patients report that a cough initially accompanied a typical upper respiratory tract infection but then resolved spontaneously, only to recur a week or two later. The physiologic basis for this type of cough is unknown. Although airway hyperreactivity may arise with such infections, these coughs rarely respond to bronchodilators.

At least two studies have concluded that asthma or airway hyper-reactivity is responsible for the majority of cases of unexplained cough. Airway reactivity refers to the tendency of airways to constrict. This characteristic is measured by a laboratory test termed bronchoprovocation. A bronchoprovocation test consists of serial measurements of airway flow after the administration of airway smooth muscle agonists. Usually methacholine or histamine is administered by inhalation in serially increasing concentrations; the test is concluded when forced expiratory volume in 1 second is observed to fall by 20%, or until a predetermined dose of agonist is administered. It is pertinent to note that asthma may present solely with a cough and that the only evidence for asthma may be airway hyper-reactivity evidenced by bronchoprovocation. Historical evidence for asthma in a patient who denies asthmatic attacks is a childhood history of asthma or allergic rhinitis or chest tightness occurring under certain conditions. For instance, some patients complain of dyspnea or slight wheezing only during upper respiratory tract infections or after coughing or sneezing. A common manifestation of subclinical asthma is excessive dyspnea with wheeze under conditions that lead to increased heat or water loss from the airways. Thus, patients should be questioned about their respiratory responses to exertion in cold weather. A report of mild wheezing under such conditions is good evidence for asthma. On the other hand, a cough after exercise is common in a normal population and is not discriminating for asthma.

Nasal congestion appears to be common in individuals with cough, and there may be a causal link between the two conditions. Many clinicians believe that nasal secretions that drip down the posterior oropharynx may elicit a cough through direct stimulation of receptors within the oropharynx or larynx. A report of a sensation of something dripping down the posterior oropharynx has been termed postnasal drip. This condition is thought to result from sinusitis, nonallergic perennial rhinitis, or allergic rhinitis. Although a complaint consistent with postnasal drip is common in patients who have a cough, there is considerable disagreement as to whether and how this condition may predispose to cough. Some physicians believe that nasal congestion leads to a cough by interfering with the normal conditioning of air that takes place within the nose. With the nostrils occluded, patients must resort to mouth breathing. This mode of breathing results in drying of the mucosa of the oropharynx and larynx; a cough may then occur because of discharge of receptors at these sites. Thus, it is important to know whether the patient suffers with nasal congestion and can sense secretions within the oropharynx. Patients should also be questioned about their hearing because nasal congestion is often associated with obstruction of the eustachian tubes. Difficulty in hearing may also be a consequence of cerumen or foreign bodies within the ear canals, which may also serve as cough stimuli.

Cancer appears to be an unusual cause for cough of obscure etiology. In the report of Irwin and colleagues, only 1 patient out of 49 was found to have cancer. Similarly, Poe and coworkers found 1 patient with lung cancer out of 109 patients with an isolated symptom of cough. Although an unexplained cough is rarely related to cancer, the consequences of failing to correctly diagnose such a condition may have dire results. In addition, most patients with an unexplained cough harbor a suspicion that their cough may be due to malignancy. They must therefore be reassured that their physician has carefully considered such a possibility and has made an appropriate effort to exclude the diagnosis. When the history is obtained, it is appropriate to indicate to the patient which aspects of the history are relevant to a diagnosis of cancer. A careful smoking history should be obtained. If patients have stopped smoking, it is essential to ascertain when they stopped and for what reason. Many patients stop smoking after an episode of hemoptysis. Patients should be questioned specifically about chest pain, weight loss, a change in the quality of a chronic cough, or arthritic symptoms, which may be a manifestation of pulmonary osteoarthropathy. Patients should also be questioned about hoarseness. Although hoarseness is common in individuals with a cough, it can be a manifestation of glottic tumors or tumors of the airways because the latter may metastasize to the ductus nodes beneath the aortic arch and thereby give rise to hoarseness through involvement of the recurrent laryngeal nerve.

In some patients, cough is due to conditions involving lung parenchyma rather than to disorders of the airways. Cough receptors are stimulated as a result of a decrease in lung compliance. These conditions are manifested by symptoms such as shortness of breath, particularly on exertion, and other symptoms related to the underlying pathologic process. Thus, the history must be directed at excluding such disorders as sarcoidosis, collagen disease, and pneumoconiosis. An occupational history should include a listing of every type of work the patient has ever done and all possible exposures.

Published experiences attribute an unexplained cough to left ventricular failure in 6% of patients. The precise mechanism by which left ventricular failure leads to cough is unknown but may relate to changes in lung compliance or to activation of nervous receptors in the lung. Thus historical data should be obtained that aids in the evaluation of left ventricular function. In particular, it should be determined whether the cough occurs at night or during exercise and whether the patient suffers with paroxysmal nocturnal dyspnea or nocturia.

In recent years, there has been an increasing awareness that esophageal dysfunction may lead to respiratory dysfunction, including restrictive lung disease, wheezing, and cough. Proposed mechanisms include gastroesophageal reflux, wherein a cough is induced by aspiration of stomach contents, or by reflexes elicited by acid in the midesophagus. Pertinent historical data include whether the patient has ever been diagnosed as having a hiatal hernia or whether heartburn, sour eructations, nocturnal cough, or nocturnal choking spells occur. Effects of bronchodilator medications on the cough should also be ascertained. It has been shown that agents such as theophylline and terbutaline result in relaxation of the gastroesophageal sphincter and thus lead to an increase in nocturnal cough.

A complete cough history should also include inquiries about medications. A number of drugs have been reported to have adverse respiratory effects, including dyspnea, bronchospasm, and presumably cough. Cough has been noted specifically with amiloride, nifedipine, enalapril, and captopril. The best documented are the angiotensin-converting enzyme inhibitors. It has been postulated that such agents produce a cough by interfering with the breakdown of bradykinin, a known tussive mediator.

Physical Examination

A careful physical examination should be performed for all patients with cough (Table 46–2). Special attention should be paid to the respiratory system, but it must be recalled that a cough may arise from conditions outside the respiratory tract, including the cardiovascular system, and from the upper respiratory tract. The nose should be examined to exclude rhinitis. Some authors have observed that an examination of the oropharynx may reveal evidence of postnasal drip, such as the presence of secretions and a cobblestone appearance of the mucosa. The ears should be examined for the presence of cerumen, foreign bodies, and hairs abutting the tympanic membranes. The sinuses should be percussed for tenderness, which might indicate acute sinusitis. For those skilled in indirect laryngoscopy or for those with access to a flexible laryngoscope, an examination of the cords should be performed. When hoarseness is present, this examination is mandatory and is best performed by an otolaryngologist. The lungs should be examined for wheezes or rhonchi, and one should listen over the larynx for inspiratory sounds that would indicate laryn-

Table 46–2. Components of Physical Examination for Patients with Cough

1. Head and neck, i.e., nasal turbinates; appearance of posterior oropharynx, ear canals, and tympanic membranes; appearance of larynx (laryngoscopy); stridor
2. Chest, i.e., wheezes (localized or diffuse), rhonchi, rales
3. Cardiovascular system, i.e., signs of congestive failure
4. Abdomen, i.e., organomegaly
5. Extremities, i.e., arthritis, clubbing
6. Neurologic system, i.e., weakness, particularly of muscles of respiration
7. Other, i.e., acoustic quality of cough, general appearance of patient

geal disease. Special attention should be paid to the presence of a unilateral wheeze, which may result from localized airway obstruction. During rapid respirations, obstructions may also give rise to a peculiar sound, not unlike that of an accordian. A careful cardiovascular examination is also important to rule out left ventricular failure. In addition to the above examinations, one should seek ancillary evidence for the presence of malignancy such as evidence of weight loss, organomegaly, or digital clubbing.

If at all possible, one should also witness the cough and note its qualities. A great deal of throat clearing is suggestive of rhinitis and postnasal drip. A loose or brassy cough suggests large airway disease. A muffled, nonresonant cough is said to be typical of vocal cord injury, whereas a whistling cough is associated with laryngeal stenosis.

Laboratory Examination

The minimal laboratory evaluations for all patients with cough should include a chest radiograph (posteroanterior and lateral), spirometry, complete blood count (including differential count), and erythrocyte sedimentation rate.

For a good quality chest radiograph, high kilovoltage technique, a wide latitude film, and preferably a grid should be used. Such a film reveals detail of the mediastinum, airways, and lung fields.

Spirometry should be performed in every case. When no etiology for cough is uncovered, additional pulmonary function tests may be helpful. These would include measurements of lung volume and diffusing capacity. A measurement of diffusing capacity is indicated because some restrictive disorders may be associated with minimal decrements in lung volume but major decreases in diffusing capacity. Similarly, pulmonary vascular disease is typically associated with normal lung volumes but with decreased diffusing capacity. A normal examination effectively excludes obstructive and restrictive lung disease and usually the presence of significant vascular disease of the lungs.

Examination of the blood should include a complete blood cell count and differential count to rule out the presence of eosinophilia, a sign of bronchial asthma or allergic disease. The erythrocyte sedimentation rate is also helpful in excluding a variety of systemic disorders including malignancy, infections, and

collagen disease. Although this last test is rarely diagnostic of any disorder, a normal value is reassuring to the worried physician. When the sedimentation rate is elevated or if a systemic disorder is suspected, additional blood tests may be indicated.

Additional Investigations

An algorithm for cough evaluation is given in Figure 46–1. Once the history, physical examination, and basic laboratory work are obtained, a tentative diagnosis may be evident and treatment may be initiated. Published experiences suggest that more than 90% of patients with chronic cough can be adequately evaluated with a thorough history, a minimal laboratory investigation as described earlier, and a trial of bronchodilators and corticosteroids. The decision to pursue further investigations should be based on the response to therapy, the severity of the impairment, the probability of uncovering serious underlying disease, and the likelihood that further investigation will yield clinically important and relevant data. Additional studies that are indicated in some patients with cough are shown in Figure 46–1. One needs to be aware that most conditions that are thought to predispose to cough are common in asymptomatic individuals. To increase the likelihood that the findings consequent to additional investigations are relevant to the cough symptom, one should avoid a "fishing expedition" approach to diagnosis. The tests chosen should be based on the observed clinical findings.

In recent years, there has been a great deal of attention paid to the relationship of cough to asthma and airway hyper-reactivity. Some clinicians routinely perform bronchoprovocation for patients with a cough and normal pulmonary function, with the intention of uncovering "hidden" asthma. Reported studies suggest that asthma is a frequent predisposition for cough and that bronchodilators are antitussive in patients with proven airway hyper-reactivity. However, a number of factors limit the clinical utility of this test. The majority of patients with a cough exhibit a degree of reactivity that is intermediate between normal and asthma. The clinical significance of a modest increase in reactivity is unknown. In particular, no controlled studies have examined the relationship between airway reactivity and the antitussive efficacy of bronchodilators and non-bronchodilator drugs such as corticosteroids

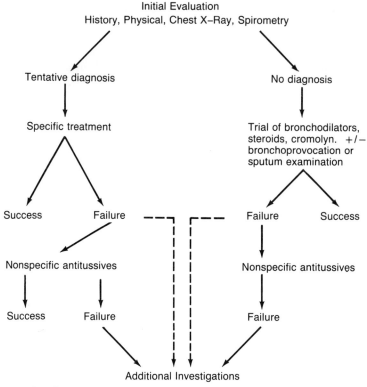

Initial Evaluation
History, Physical, Chest X–Ray, Spirometry

Tentative diagnosis

No diagnosis

Specific treatment

Trial of bronchodilators, steroids, cromolyn. +/– bronchoprovocation or sputum examination

Success   Failure — — — — — Failure   Success

Nonspecific antitussives

Nonspecific antitussives

Success   Failure

Failure

Additional Investigations

1. Complete pulmonary function tests.
   Indication: All subjects with undiagnosed cough who fail to respond to therapy

2. Sinus films. Indication:
   Persistent rhinitis, postnasal drip

3. Bronchoscopy +/– transbronchial biopsy.
   Indication: Abnormal chest x-ray. History suggestive of carcinoma. Abnormal pulmonary function tests.

4. Gastrointestinal contrast study.
   Indication: History suggestive of reflux but unresponsive to antireflux measures. History or x-ray suggestive of aspiration

5. 24–h pH monitoring. Indication: Consideration for antireflux surgical procedures

6. Echocardiography, cardiac catheterization.
   Indication: History suggestive of cardiac disease

Figure 46–1. *Algorithm for evaluation of chronic cough. The dashed lines indicate an optional pathway if clinically indicated.*

and sodium cromoglycate. In most cases, the need for bronchoprovocation can be obviated by an examination of the sputum for eosinophilia or simply by a trial of bronchodilators and corticosteroids. Bronchoprovocation would be indicated in situations where there is a relative contraindication for bronchodilator or steroid therapy or when patients insist on a diagnosis before treatment. Bronchoprovocation with histamine may also be useful in excluding psychogenic cough. It has been shown that patients with a cough invariably exhibit a marked tussive response to histamine, which is related to the magnitude of provoked bronchoconstriction. It would appear unlikely that patients with psychogenic cough would exhibit the same phenomenon.

The role of bronchoscopy in the routine evaluation of unexplained cough has been evaluated recently by Poe and colleagues. These investigators have shown that routine bronchoscopy in all patients with a cough is not cost effective. They suggest that bronchoscopy should be reserved for the suspicious case in which other causes for the cough have been eliminated. However, bronchoscopy, especially when combined with transbronchial lung biopsy, may be very useful in establishing a diagnosis of diffuse disease of the lung, such as that occurring with sarcoidosis or interstitial pneumonitis. However, in such cases, radiographic or functional abnormalities usually suggest that such disorders are likely. In the absence of such findings, it would seem reasonable to reserve bronchoscopy for the older patient with a smoking history who has symp-

EVALUATION AND MANAGEMENT OF CHRONIC COUGH / 465

toms or radiographic evidence suggesting airway neoplasm. Although younger, nonsmoking subjects may on occasion suffer with low grade malignancies of the airways, i.e., carcinoid tumors, such individuals eventually experience hemoptysis or exhibit radiographic evidence of atelectasis. Thus, careful follow-up of such young patients may obviate the need for bronchoscopy. The role of cytologic sputum analysis in the evaluation of cough is at present undefined. There is probably no indication for this analysis in younger patients because carcinoid tumors do not exfoliate. Although examination of sputum for malignant cells may be indicated in older patients who smoke, such efforts are probably not cost effective, and a negative examination would provide a false sense of security for the patient suspected of harboring a malignancy. In such individuals, bronchoscopy is indicated irrespective of the results of sputum analysis.

The importance of esophageal disease in patients with chronic cough is unknown. In two published series, cough was attributed to gastroesophageal reflux or aspiration in 7 to 10% of patients. Gastroesophageal reflux is thought to lead to a cough by either of two mechanisms: aspiration of stomach contents or a reflex mechanism initiated by acid in the midesophagus. It is actually quite difficult to prove the association in individual subjects. When the history suggests a reflux-induced cough, a trial of antireflux measures should be instituted and an upper gastrointestinal examination may be obtained. Antireflux therapy includes dietary manipulations, cimetidine or antacids, and elevation of the head of the bed. Surgical procedures should be considered only if medical therapy fails and if there is suggestive evidence of aspiration such as recurrent pneumonia. Before surgical intervention, radiographic documentation of reflux is necessary, and 24-hour esophageal pH monitoring should be obtained. Because a cough can induce reflux, it is advisable for patients to maintain a diary of symptoms while esophageal pH is being monitored so that the relationship between the cough and reflux episodes can be established.

Treatment

When a presumed etiology for cough has been uncovered, the underlying condition should be treated. Therapy should also be directed at easily remedied conditions that may exacerbate a cough. Thus, nasal congestion ought to be treated to improve the conditioning of inspired air. Similarly, environmental manipulations should be attempted, such as home humidification and avoidance of irritating inhalants such as cigarette smoke or perfumes. Because our knowledge of how cough arises is limited, it is prudent to avoid excessively invasive, dangerous, or expensive interventions. One must estimate a degree of certainty concerning the cause of the cough and the likelihood that any intervention will be effective. For example, a patient with a chronic cough and gastroesophageal reflux is ill served by an antireflux surgical procedure that relieves heartburn but has no ameliorative effect on cough.

When a specific etiology for cough cannot be identified and the above measures are ineffective, a trial of antitussive medication should be considered. Such therapy is especially indicated when the cough is nonproductive and is associated with adverse consequences such as syncope or rib fractures. Codeine, dextromethorphan, and diphenhydramine have been shown to be safe and effective antitussive agents. Bronchodilating agents may occasionally be helpful, as are corticosteroids and sodium cromoglycate. There are unfortunate patients for whom no diagnosis is obtained and for whom no therapy is effective. Such individuals need to be reassured that they have no serious underlying illness and that most coughs either resolve spontaneously or at least remit in intensity for unpredictable periods of time.

Bibliography

Banner AS. Cough: physiology, evaluation and treatment. Lung 164:79–92, 1986.
> *A comprehensive review of cough covering physiology, cough evaluation, and therapy, including the use of antitussive agents.*

Braman S, Corrao WM. Cough: differential diagnosis and treatment. Clin Chest Med 8:177–188, 1987.
> *A comprehensive review of cough with particular emphasis on differential diagnosis.*

Corrao WM, Braman SS, Irwin RS. Chronic cough as the sole presenting manifestation of bronchial asthma. N Engl J Med 300:633–637, 1979.
> *The seminal article linking cough to airway hyperreactivity. These authors suggest that bronchoprovocation be included in the work-up of patients with unexplained cough and normal lung function.*

Coulter DM, Edwards IR. Cough associated with captopril and enalapril. Br Med J 294:1521–1523, 1987.
> *A description of cough related to angiotensin-converting enzyme inhibitors in a large number of patients*

derived from a postmarketing surveillance system in New Zealand.

Irwin RS, Carrao WM, Pratter MR. Chronic persistent cough in the adult: the spectrum and frequency of causes and successful outcome of specific therapy. Am Rev Respir Dis 123:413–417, 1981.

A list of diagnoses obtained in a group of patients with unexplained cough. The authors based their diagnostic protocol on the anatomy and distribution of cough receptors. The authors claimed that by using this approach they were able to obtain a specific diagnosis in each case and that therapy based on their findings was invariably successful.

Korpas J, Tomori Z. Cough and other respiratory reflexes. Prog Respir Res 12:1–356, 1979.

An encyclopedic review of cough dealing mainly with human and animal physiologic studies. Of particular value is the international scope of this review, providing descriptions of work previously available only in the non-English literature.

Leith DE. Cough in Respiratory Defense Mechanisms, Part 2. New York, Marcel Dekker, 1977, pp 545–592.

A well-referenced review of the physiology of cough, which concentrates on cough mechanics.

Poe RH, Israel RH, Utell MJ, et al. Chronic cough: bronchoscopy or pulmonary function testing. Am Rev Respir Dis 126:160–162, 1982.

A list of diagnoses obtained in patients with unexplained cough. The important point of this paper is that bronchoscopy has a limited role in the routine evaluation of patients with cough.

Widdicombe JG. Respiratory reflexes and defense, in Brian JD, Proctor DF, Reid LM (eds). Respiratory Defense Mechanisms, Part 2. New York, Marcel Dekker, 1977, pp 593–630.

A well-referenced review of a variety of respiratory reflexes including cough. This chapter deals mainly with animal research and is written from a neurophysiologic point of view.

47

Practical Prescription of Home Oxygen Therapy

JOHN WADE SHIGEOKA, M.D.

Introduction

Home therapy with oxygen has increased dramatically during the past two decades because it is beneficial and because the prevalence of lung disease is high. The rising cost of this expensive therapy has alarmed governmental and third-party health care payers who now require detailed information about the need for and the use of home oxygen therapy. Although this simply seems to be just another burdensome cost containment maneuver, it is best to remember that physicians are the most qualified to decide when and what form of oxygen therapy is appropriate for their patients. Physicians are more objective and altruistic than profit-motivated vendors and economy-minded payers when making these important decisions. Furthermore, the general internist and the pulmonologist will share the responsibility for prescribing home oxygen therapy as it becomes more widely used.

Rationale for Chronic Home Oxygen Therapy

The benefits of chronic home oxygen therapy have been established in controlled studies of hypoxemic patients with chronic obstructive pulmonary disease. These include improved survival, improved neuropsychologic function, and amelioration of polycythemia, pulmonary hypertension, and right-sided heart failure (cor pulmonale). Chronic oxygen therapy halves the annual mortality of patients with chronic obstructive pulmonary disease with cor pulmonale and is the only therapy known to do this. Additional, less well-established benefits include improved endurance during exercise,

reduced exercise-related dyspnea, reduced number of days in the hospital, and the ability to resume gainful employment.

The disadvantages of chronic home oxygen therapy include high cost (typically $300 to $500 per month), inconvenience imposed by limited supplies and heavy equipment, and potential adverse effects such as injury from equipment, burns if the plastic tubing catches fire, and *minimally* accentuated retention of carbon dioxide.

Background

The current recommendations for providing chronic oxygen therapy are based on pathophysiologic mechanisms, clinical observations, and technology. The shape of the hemoglobin-oxygen dissociation curve is a helpful mnemonic to explain these recommendations (Fig. 47–1). Arterial oxygen tensions (Pa_{O_2}) in the range of 55 to 60 torr (mm Hg) identify the *shoulder* of this curve that corresponds to arterial oxygen saturations (Sa_{O_2}) of 88 to 91% under normal conditions. When Pa_{O_2} drops acutely to this range, it is common to see abnormal neuropsychologic function (impaired short-term memory and judgment), physiologic responses (hyperventilation, tachycardia, and pulmonary arterial vasoconstriction), and the *initiation* of chronic compensatory responses (secondary polycythemia).

Below the shoulder lies the *steep part* of the curve where a small drop in Pa_{O_2} produces a large drop in oxygen saturation and blood oxygen content (ml O_2/100 ml blood). When Pa_{O_2} is in this range, the risk is high for developing cor pulmonale during exacerbations of bronchitis. Of course, decompensation

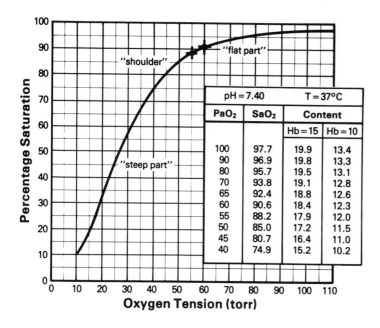

Figure 47–1. The normal hemoglobin-oxygen dissociation curve at normal temperature and pH: note the three parts of the curve: (1) the steep part where a small change in oxygen tension (P_{O_2}) causes a large change in saturation (S_{O_2}) and oxygen content; (2) the flat part where a large change in P_{O_2} causes a small change in saturation and content; and (3) the intervening shoulder. The crosses mark the P_{O_2} criteria used by Medicare (at 55 and 60). In the columns to the right of the curve, note the deleterious effect of anemia on oxygen content.

may occur at higher levels of Pa_{O_2} when there are known aggravating conditions, e.g., anemia or left-sided heart failure, and unknown reasons (heightened sensitivity).

Above the shoulder lies the *flat part* of the dissociation curve where a large rise in Pa_{O_2} causes a small rise in Sa_{O_2} and oxygen content. When Pa_{O_2} exceeds 65 torr (Sa_{O_2} of 92%), there is increased risk for suppressing the hypoxic ventilatory drive; when Pa_{O_2} exceeds 70 torr (Sa_{O_2} of 94%), there is little gain in oxygen content.

In summary, the shoulder of the dissociation curve identifies an important range of Pa_{O_2} and Sa_{O_2} values. As Pa_{O_2} drops below the shoulder, there is a greater likelihood for the adverse effects of hypoxemia, and as Pa_{O_2} rises above the shoulder, there is a greater likelihood for side effects and the wasting of oxygen. Raising Pa_{O_2} just over the shoulder of the dissociation curve with supplemental oxygen achieves a maximum increase in oxygen content with the greatest economy and a minimum of side effects.

The hypoxemia of chronic obstructive lung disease usually responds well to low flow oxygen therapy. Although low flow refers to delivery flows of less than 5 L/min, most patients need less than 3 L/min, and the majority need 2 L/min or less. These low flows are tolerated well when delivered through nasal cannulae (prongs), they do not commonly aggravate alveolar hypoventilation (seen as a significant rise in Pa_{CO_2}), and they are easily provided at home with current equipment.

The aim of therapy is to provide sufficient supplemental oxygen to raise Pa_{O_2} into the ideal range of 61 to 70 torr. The oxygen flow that accomplishes this at rest is raised empirically by 1 L/min during sleep and exercise because these activities commonly worsen hypoxemia.

Patient Selection

Almost all the experience with home oxygen therapy has been obtained from patients suffering with chronic obstructive lung disease who are hypoxemic at rest. It is reasonable to follow the same general approach for less well-studied hypoxemic conditions, such as pulmonary fibrosis, kyphoscoliosis, pneumoconiosis, pulmonary carcinomatosis, and chronic left-sided heart failure, and when hypoxemia occurs only with exercise or sleep.

In general, experts agree that oxygen therapy is indicated for patients suffering with lung disease when Pa_{O_2} is 55 torr or less while sitting and breathing air. Oxygen therapy is also indicated when hypoxemia is less severe (Pa_{O_2} is less than 60 torr) if there is evidence of cor pulmonale (jugular venous distention, liver engorgement, or edema), polycythemia, or electrocardiographic changes of "P pulmonale" (P wave exceeds 3 mm in leads II, III, and aV_F). These were the entry criteria for the Nocturnal Oxygen Therapy Trial and have been adopted by Medicare for reimbursement of home oxygen services (Table 47–1).

Table 47–1. *Selection Criteria for Chronic Home Oxygen Therapy*

1. Stable severe chronic lung disease: obstructive diseases (bronchitis, emphysema, bronchiectasis), pulmonary fibrosis, kyphoscoliosis, pneumoconiosis, and pulmonary carcinomatosis

   or

   hypoxemia-related symptoms or findings: pulmonary hypertension, recurrent congestive heart failure from chronic cor pulmonale, erythrocytosis, impaired cognitive processes, and hypoxemia associated with sleep or exercise
2. Optimum medical therapy provided: bronchodilators, antimicrobials, corticosteroids, smoking cessation, congestive heart failure treatment
3. Documented hypoxemia on air (one of the following):
   a. $Pa_{O_2} < 55$ torr (or $Sa_{O_2} < 85\%$) at rest
   b. $Pa_{O_2} < 55$ torr (or $Sa_{O_2} < 85\%$) during sleep or exercise*
   c. $Pa_{O_2} < 60$ torr ($Sa_{O_2} < 90\%$) and one of the following:
      i. Cor pulmonale (edema, liver engorgement, venous distention)
      ii. Electrocardiographic abnormalities: P pulmonale
      iii. Polycythemia (hematocrit $> 56\%$)

*Oxygen use is approved only under these conditions.

Some patients become severely hypoxemic only during exercise or sleep, so most experts prescribe oxygen therapy during those activities. Some experts also prescribe oxygen for patients who have less severe degrees of hypoxemia and evidence of end-organ impairment, e.g., angina, mental confusion, or pulmonary hypertension, if oxygen therapy can be shown to have clinical benefit.

Until recently, Pa_{O_2} was the sole test that could determine the presence of hypoxemia. Now that finger and pulse oximeters allow reasonably accurate *noninvasive* measurements of Sa_{O_2}, Medicare accepts the following measurements as equivalent: 85% Sa_{O_2} and 55 torr Pa_{O_2} (note: this is based on a right-shifted dissociation curve because Sa_{O_2} is normally 88% when Pa_{O_2} is 55), and 90% Sa_{O_2} and 60 torr Pa_{O_2} (normal curve).

Patients should receive the benefit of optimum medical therapy, including the stopping of smoking, appropriate use of bronchodilators, antimicrobials, and corticosteroids, and treatment of problems known to aggravate hypoxemia such as congestive heart failure and massive obesity. There are three important reasons to stop smoking. First, smoking aggravates chronic obstructive lung disease, the most common cause of hypoxemia. Second, smoking raises the blood carboxyhemoglobin level, reduces oxyhemoglobin saturation, and reduces oxygen-carrying capacity, i.e., it essentially negates the improved blood oxygen content provided by oxygen therapy. Finally, smoking may result in burns or smoke inhalation injury if the plastic oxygen delivery tubing catches fire. Common sense dictates that patients using oxygen should not smoke.

The Nocturnal Oxygen Therapy Trial verified that lung disease should be stable before starting chronic home oxygen therapy. Nearly half the patients who initially qualified for home oxygen therapy improved sufficiently after a month of medical treatment that oxygen therapy could be stopped. Most candidates for home oxygen therapy are discovered during hospitalization for an exacerbation of lung disease. It is reasonable to start home oxygen therapy when the patient is discharged, to provide optimal medical treatment, and, after 1 month, to evaluate the need to continue therapy.

Basic Technical Considerations

The three basic *systems* of equipment for delivering oxygen therapy at home include compressed oxygen cylinders, liquid oxygen, and oxygen concentrators. *Stationary* forms are used in the home and *portable* are used outside during ambulation. The choice of system depends on needs, availability, and cost. In general, patients with hypoxemia at rest need both stationary and portable equipment, those with hypoxemia during sleep need only stationary equipment, and those with hypoxemia during exercise need only portable equipment. The regional variation in availability and cost of equipment is considerable, so it is best to compare prices, e.g., liquid oxygen may be available only in large cities and may cost three times more in one part of the country compared with another part. Although economy and convenience are important considerations (discussed later), reliable *service* is probably the most important. The vendor is expected to do the following: educate the patient and family about the proper and safe use of equipment, perform maintenance and repair service (including emergency), conduct follow-up visits to ensure the continued proper use and function of equipment, and discuss any problems and recommendations with the physician.

Compressed oxygen cylinders are well-known and ubiquitous. Unfortunately, cylinders are made from heavy steel alloy and hold small volumes of oxygen under very high pressure (up to 2200 psi). A typical stationary system consists of a large (size H or K) cylinder, regulator (control valve with pressure and flow gauges), and stand or cart (dolly) to support and move the cylinder safely. An H/K cylinder is about 5 ft tall, weighs 150 lb, holds 6900 liters when full, and provides oxygen at 1 L/min continuously for about 4 to 5 days (1 L/min $\times$ 60 min/h $\times$ 24 h/day = 1440 L/day and 6900 L/1440 L/day = 4.8 days). A portable system consists of a small (size E) cylinder, regulator with yoke connector (not compatible with the threaded connecter on large cylinders), and small dolly. It weighs about 20 lb, contains 600 liters, and at 1 L/min lasts about 10 hours. Half-size versions of H/K and E cylinders (M and D) are more convenient but less available. Compressed oxygen cylinders can be filled only from other high pressure cylinders or special pumps, usually by the distributor or vendor. It is not recommended that patients fill small cylinders unless they receive special training because of the dangers imposed by the high pressures.

Liquid oxygen (LOX) is most convenient for active, ambulatory patients because it is very compact, i.e., 1 liter of LOX is equal to about 860 liters of gas. It is very cold (below $-297°F$ or $-180°C$), so it must be stored in special insulated Dewar reservoirs (thermos vacuum bottles). Ambient heat causes LOX to boil slowly and to form gaseous oxygen. In contrast to compressed cylinders, LOX equipment operates under low pressures, either 20 or 50 psi. A typical stationary reservoir resembles a drum 3 ft tall, weighs about 40 lb empty, has a built-in flow regulator, and is usually mounted on a wheeled platform with scales for weighing contents. Reservoir capacity depends on the manufacturer and is described confusingly by LOX volume, equivalent gas volume, and, most practically, LOX weight (1 liter = 2.5 lb). There are usually two sizes: large stationary LOX reservoirs hold between 30 and 40 liters (25,800 to 34,400 liters of gas or 75 to 100 lb), and small reservoirs hold between 16 and 20 liters (13,800 to 17,200 liters of gas or 40 to 50 lb). Miniature (portable) reservoirs usually come in two sizes: standard portable LOX reservoirs hold about 2.5 to 3 lb (about 860 to 1032 liters of gas) and weigh about 8 to 10 lb full, and small portable reservoirs hold roughly half the amount (about 350 to 500 liters of gas) and weigh only 5 to 7 lb full. LOX is routinely and easily transferred from the stationary to the portable reservoir. Unfortunately, LOX may be available only in large cities and boils away continuously, i.e., an unused reservoir losing 1 to 2 lb a day will be empty after a month.

The oxygen concentrator is economical because it obtains oxygen from the air with a zeolite molecular sieve. Oxygen is delivered at more than 95% concentration, but the concentration may drop to as low as 80% at high delivery flows. A typical concentrator looks (and sounds) like a small refrigerator, weighs 60 to 75 lb, and has wheels for moving around the house. The oxygen enricher is similar but more compact and quiet because it uses a semipermeable membrane to provide 40% oxygen. To compensate, nearly triple the gas flow is used (the flow meter is usually calibrated in terms of pure oxygen). This flow may become disagreeably high when it exceeds the equivalent of 2 L/min oxygen. Patients needing continuous therapy also require cylinder oxygen for ambulation and emergencies (power failure or equipment malfunction). A small cylinder system is usually adequate for both, but an additional large cylinder emergency system may be needed in areas where there are long delays in restoring power or providing repair services and by patients who use high flows that quickly exhaust a small cylinder. This requirement for cylinder oxygen reduces the economy of concentrators and enrichers (which operate under low pressure and cannot fill the cylinders). The cost of electricity (roughly $50 a month) is not covered by health insurance.

Based on this background, the advantages and disadvantages of the oxygen delivery systems become clear (Table 47–2). The compact nature of LOX is ideal for ambulatory patients. For example, a typical patient who receives oxygen continuously at 2 L/min and ambulates an average of 3 hours a day uses 20,160 liters (17,640 liters stationary, 2520 liters portable) or nearly three H/K and four E cylinders per week. Patients object to having this many cylinders in the house and a limited (5-hour) portable supply when they wish a longer outing. This may force the supplier to make two deliveries a week. A 30-lb LOX stationary reservoir easily holds this supply of oxygen (this allows a weekly delivery schedule) and a standard portable reservoir lasts for more than 8 hours. On the other hand, concentrators are ideal for nonambulatory patients. Those confined to a room or two may use a long (50-ft) extension hose when moving about, whereas those in wheelchairs may ask a helper to move the concentrator to different rooms. In Salt Lake City, ambulatory patients find that LOX is competitively priced with concentrators, nonambulatory patients find that concentrators

Table 47–2. Comparison of Oxygen Equipment Systems

System	Advantages	Disadvantages
Compressed gas	Widely available No loss when off	Heavy cylinders Small oxygen volume
Liquid oxygen	Lightweight Large oxygen volume Best for ambulation	Limited availability Oxygen loss even if off
Concentrator or enricher	Low cost Best for house-bound patients	Requires electricity High maintenance Not portable

are most economical, and both find that compressed cylinders are simply too expensive for most situations (Table 47–3).

The typical monthly costs of oxygen therapy charged to Medicare patients in Salt Lake City are shown in Table 47–3. Patients pay an annual deductible charge of $75 and 20% of the listed costs; Medicare pays 80%. The charges to Blue Cross/Blue Shield patients are similar. Patients with major medical benefits pay 20% of the monthly charges until the accumulated monthly charges reach a "stop amount" ($2,500 or $5,000, depending on the policy). Then, Blue Cross/Blue Shield pays the entire amount of the allowable monthly charges for the rest of the year, i.e., the maximum annual out-of-pocket cost is either $500 or $1,000. Through competitive bidding, the contract prices for health maintenance organizations, the Veterans Administration, and Medicaid are substantially lower than those shown in Table 47–3.

Prescribing Home Oxygen Therapy

Medicare certification and prescription are discussed here because the requirements

(based on the recommendations of experts) are so comprehensive. Medicare requires the following: (1) a physician's statement that optimal medical therapy has been provided; (2) the diagnosis of severe lung disease *or* the symptoms and signs related to hypoxemia that may be expected to improve with oxygen therapy; (3) laboratory evidence of hypoxemia (quote the arterial blood gas or oximetry results); (4) specific orders concerning oxygen concentration (usually pure oxygen), dosage (flow), and duration of therapy (14 to 24 hours/day; "as needed" is not acceptable); (5) an estimated period of usage (1 month to lifetime); (6) if portable oxygen is needed, activities for which it is needed, therapeutic purpose, and whether performance is improved; and (7) a statement that the physician has examined the patient recently and will supervise the oxygen therapy. Fortunately, most carriers (the local Medicare administrator, often Blue Cross/Blue Shield) provide special forms to expedite this process. A facsimile is shown in Figure 47–2.

The criteria used by Medicare for initiating oxygen therapy are given in Table 47–1. The following stipulations should be noted. First, if hypoxemia occurs only during sleep or ex-

Table 47–3. Monthly Cost of Oxygen Therapy*

Flow (L/min)	Nocturnal			Stationary			Ambulatory		
	CGO	LOX	CON	CGO	LOX	CON	CGO	LOX	CON
1	*120*	146	250	222	*200*	292	329	*243*	382
2	*220*	221	250	372	330	292	534	*372*	462
3	295	*247*	250	522	459	292	774	*501*	552
4	395	373	*250*	672	587	292	989	*631*	642
5	495	448	*250*	847	713	292	1229	760	*732*

*Typical monthly cost in dollars for oxygen therapy charged to Medicare in Salt Lake City, UT (March 1987). Nocturnal refers to therapy with oxygen only during sleep for 14 h/day; stationary to continuous therapy for nonambulatory patients (emergency back-up included); ambulatory, to continuous therapy with an average of 3 h spent outside each day; CGO, to compressed gas oxygen; LOX, to liquid oxygen; and CON, to concentrator oxygen. The most economical costs appear in italics. For nocturnal or stationary therapy, compressed gas oxygen is economical only at low flows (< 2 L/min); otherwise, concentrator therapy is the most economical. However, for ambulatory therapy, LOX is the most economical except at the highest flow. For out-of-pocket costs, see text.

Medicare Part B Oxygen Form (Facsimile)

Mr. B. Bloater
PO Box 111B
Salt Lake City, UT 84148

HIC-123-45-6789A
claim—87-5-07701

Dear Beneficiary:

Medicare regulations require from the prescribing physician a certification form that oxygen is medically necessary.
Please have your physician complete the following:

Date oxygen was prescribed: ___*31 May 87*___. What other forms of treatment have been tried?
Please explain: *metaproterenol sulfate (Alupent), theophylline, corticosteroids*

Diagnosis	Equipment	Usage (not PRN, not indefinite)	
✓ COPD	__ Stationary	✓ Continuously	__ ____ Months
✓ CHF due to	__ Portable	__ 20 h/day	__ 1 year
__ Cor pulmonale	✓ Both	__ 16 h/day	✓ Lifetime
__ Widespread pulmonary neoplasm		__ __ h/day	__ Other: ____
__ Sleep apnea			
__ Cystic fibrosis			
__ Other: ____			

Prescribed flow	How delivered	Place used	Prognosis
2 L/min	✓ Nasal cannula	✓ Home	✓ Fair
	__ Mask	__ Nursing home	__ Guarded
	__ Other: ____	__ Other: ____	__ Poor

Are hypoxemia-related symptoms improved by oxygen? ✓ yes __ no
Please supply us with results of blood gas studies and note the conditions under which tests were obtained:

A { *57* PO$_2$ — ✓ Room air — ✓ At rest — __ Exercise
  { *83%* Saturation — __ Asleep — __ With oxygen at____ L/min

B { *66* PO$_2$ — __ Room air — ✓ At rest — __ Exercise
  { *93%* Saturation — __ Asleep — ✓ With oxygen at *2* L/min

Test date: _____   Test location: _____

For portable oxygen:

A. Patient activities or exercises that require a portable system:

✓ Walking   ✓ Housekeeping   __ Bathing   ✓ Ambulation
__ Other (please explain): _____

B. Therapeutic purpose served by a portable system that cannot be met by a stationary system:

__ Increase mobility   ✓ Ambulation to increase exercise tolerance   ✓ Maintain tissue oxygenation
during ambulation

C. Does the use of portable oxygen result in a clinical improvement in the patient's ability to perform the activities
and/or exercises described in A above? ✓ yes __ no

Will you be indirectly supervising the use of this oxygen? ✓ yes __ no

Date when you last saw this patient: ___*3 July 87*___

Prescribing Physician (please print): *JW Shigeoka M.D.*
Signature: *John W Shigeoka M.D.*   Date: *9 June 87*

Figure 47–2. *Medicare Certification-Prescription form for home oxygen therapy. This is a facsimile of the current form produced by the Salt Lake City carrier: the physician checks the appropriate responses and supplies the requested material. Any additional comments and explanations (not shown) should be written on a separate sheet of paper and submitted with this form.*

ercise, then oxygen therapy is covered only during those activities. Also, repeat tests (Pa$_{O_2}$ or Sa$_{O_2}$) that demonstrate the relief of hypoxemia with oxygen during sleep or exercise are required. Second, if Pa$_{O_2}$ is 60 torr or higher or if Sa$_{O_2}$ is 90% or higher, *the carrier is required to presume that oxygen therapy is not necessary and rebut the claim.* On appeal, the carrier's medical staff must review and approve the claim. This rebuttal, appeal, and review may cause inordinate delays. Third, Medicare regulations *exclude* oxygen therapy for the following: angina pectoris without hypoxemia, breathlessness without hypoxemia or cor pul-

monale, peripheral cyanosis related to vascular disease only, and terminal illnesses that do not affect the lungs.

Physicians should anticipate problems when their patients do not meet the usual criteria because Medicare claims are reviewed by non-physician personnel. Physicians should write a concise, lucid explanation, provide supportive information, and request a review by the carrier's *medical staff* who must grant specific approval before the claims are reimbursed. The following four patients with stable chronic lung disease and a Pa$_{O_2}$ of 61 torr probably would have their claims rebutted under current policies: patient A has angina pectoris that improves with oxygen; patient B has severe anemia from chronic renal failure; patient C lives at an altitude 5000 ft higher than that of the blood gas laboratory; and patient D, who has used oxygen therapy for several years, was given oxygen at 3 L/min when the Pa_{O_2} was measured. The claims reviewers probably would rebut the claims simply because the Pa_{O_2} is "too high" (patient A also has a diagnosis, angina pectoris, that is "specifically excluded"). These nonmedical reviewers would not understand that angina may be aggravated by moderate hypoxemia and can be ameliorated by oxygen (patient A), that anemia reduces oxygen-carrying capacity (B), that going to a higher altitude lowers the Pa_{O_2} (C), or that stopping supplemental oxygen lowers Pa_{O_2} (D).

Physicians should remember that the guidelines used by Medicare are based on past recommendations provided by experts. By their very nature, guidelines cannot consider the unique problems of individual patients and cannot evolve as quickly as medical knowledge. Physicians must work with the carrier's medical staff whenever their patients are affected by atypical situations or when new indications arise. In some instances where the guidelines are clearly unreasonable, the implementation has been quite practical: the guidelines require documentation of the activities that require a portable oxygen system and that portable oxygen results in a clinical improvement in the ability to perform those activities. As noted earlier, the local carrier expedited the process by providing a check list (Fig. 47–2) and accepts the physician's word that there is a clinical improvement. (If for incomprehensible reasons, the carrier requires formal documentation of clinical improvement with portable oxygen, the physician could simply measure the ambulatory time [seconds] or distance [yards] with and without supplemental oxygen. As an alternative, the physician could arrange to have portable oximeter readings taken during ambulation with and without supplemental oxygen.)

Supervising Home Oxygen Therapy

Medicare has instructed each carrier to conduct periodic reviews of continued medical necessity for oxygen therapy. At this writing, the local carrier has not determined the appropriate interval for review. The author usually assesses his patients after 1 and 4 months of oxygen therapy, and then, if stable, every 6 months. The following are evaluated (Table 47–4): (1) stability of the lung disease (bronchospasm, infection) and any aggravating conditions (anemia, congestive failure); (2) control of cor pulmonale (weight gain, edema, hepatic enlargement) and polycythemia (hematocrit or hemoglobin); (3) medical therapy (dosage of bronchodilators, antimicrobials, corticosteroids, and diuretics, and compliance); (4) oxygen therapy (oxygen flow, duration, and compliance); and (5) a blood gas test on the prescribed amount of oxygen. Ideally, Pa_{O_2} should be between 61 and 65 torr (at the most 70 torr), which corresponds to Sa_{O_2} between 90 and 92% (at the most 94%). The percent blood carboxyhemoglobin—measured with many blood oximeters—should be normal (< 2%) if the patient has stopped smoking (for comparison, this value is approximately 5% in patients who smoke one pack of cigarettes per day). If Pa_{O_2} is out of range, the oxygen flow is adjusted accordingly and the tests are repeated. If Pa_{O_2} is unusually high on very small amounts of oxygen, it is possible that oxygen therapy may be discontinued. Tests should be repeated after air breathing for 20 minutes. The oxygen vendor and payer should be notified of changes in the oxygen prescription.

Table 47–4. *Follow-up Evaluations of Home Oxygen Therapy**

1. Schedule of evaluations: after 1 and 4 mo of therapy, then every 6 mo
2. Stability of underlying lung disease
   a. Control of bronchospasm and infection
   b. Compliance with pulmonary therapy
   c. Cessation of smoking (carboxyhemoglobin)
3. Stability of other aggravating medical problems
   a. Control of left-sided heart failure and anemia
   b. Compliance with general medical therapy
4. Control of cor pulmonale
   a. Stable weight, absence of edema, hepatic enlargement, venous distention
   b. Absence of polycythemia (hematocrit or hemoglobin)
5. Adequacy of oxygen therapy
   a. Compliance, complaints, interactions with vendor
   b. Blood gas test on prescribed flow and conditions
      i. PO_2 between 61 and 65 torr (< 70) or
      ii. SO_2 between 90 and 92% (< 94)
      iii. No significant rise (> 8 torr) in PCO_2
   c. Notify vendor and carrier of changes in oxygen prescription

*Recommended by author; current Medicare policy is unclear concerning follow-up.

Additional Practical Points

There may be problems with compliance because oxygen therapy is inconvenient and expensive. Education and encouragement may improve compliance. Offer hope by emphasizing the preventive value of therapy. Patients enjoy learning that oxygen prevents "heart strain" and improves survival and mental function (mood, the ability to balance checkbooks, and reaction time when driving). Some states require physicians to report conditions that impair driving ability, such as severe hypoxemia, and the possibility of losing their license may encourage some patients to comply with therapy. Avoid negative comments, e.g., "You need oxygen because your lungs have deteriorated," because they generate denial and resentment, e.g. "I don't want to become addicted to oxygen; anyway, it's only for the sick and dying, not me!" Patients may use inadequate amounts of oxygen if they have difficulty affording the 20% copayment. They must understand that this is counterproductive because oxygen therapy may reduce the need for hospitalization, i.e., the copayment is a bargain compared with hospital bills. Finally, patients should be informed that exertional dyspnea is caused by the underlying lung disease and a lack of relief is not a failure of oxygen therapy. Educational material is available from vendors and other sources. Pulmonary rehabilitation programs and support groups may help patients and families learn to cope with their illness.

Traveling long distances with oxygen requires careful planning. Experienced vendors may provide valuable advice and arrange oxygen supplies along the route. The altitude of the route should be considered (see later part of chapter). When traveling by automobile, the concentrator or enricher system is probably the most convenient because the easily replenished small oxygen cylinders may be used on the road and the concentrator in the motel. LOX is less convenient because refills may be hard to find and the stationary reservoir is large and heavy (weighing nearly 100 lb full). In general, large oxygen cylinders are impractical (some ingenious patients have installed racks to hold these unwieldy cylinders in their trucks).

Air travel is made difficult by Federal Aviation Administration regulations that forbid the use of personal oxygen equipment. Not all airlines offer in-flight oxygen service, and oxygen service, equipment, and policy vary considerably among airlines. Attempts are being made to formulate more modern, uniform policies. Until then, the following recommendations are offered. Patients should inquire about oxygen service in advance. Most airlines require medical clearance; this may be a simple telephone call or a physician's written statement about the medical condition, prognosis, and oxygen requirements. The itinerary is important because flight time cannot exceed oxygen supply time and there must be a reserve to cover delays and route changes. Patients must use the airline's oxygen equipment on the aircraft and personal equipment must be carried empty (LOX) or nearly empty (maximum of 50 psi in cylinders) in the baggage hold. Patients must make separate arrangements with a vendor to have oxygen equipment waiting at the destination.

The cabin pressure drops as commercial jets climb to cruising altitude. In a jet flying at 35,000 to 40,000 ft, the cabin pressure may be equal to the barometric pressure at 5000 to 7000 ft. Patients starting a trip at sea level may have to increase their oxygen flow, whereas those from Salt Lake City or Denver (altitude about 5000 ft) probably do not. Of greater concern are patients with hypoxemic chronic lung disease who ordinarily do not use oxygen. In general, if Pa_{O_2} exceeds 68 torr at rest on air at sea level, the Pa_{O_2} exceeds 55 torr at 5000 ft. To estimate the effect of altitude, patients may breathe hypoxic gas mixtures (high altitude simulation test), or Gong's prediction equation may be used:

$$\text{predicted } Pa_{O_2} = 22.8 - 2.7x + 0.68y$$

where x is the equivalent altitude in the cabin (in thousands of feet) and y is the Pa_{O_2} at sea level. What is a patient's Pa_{O_2} in a jet cruising at 40,000 ft if the sea level Pa_{O_2} is 60 torr ($y = 60$)? At the cruising altitude, the cabin pressure is equal to an altitude of 7000 feet ($x = 7$), so Pa_{O_2} is about 45 torr (severe hypoxemia), i.e., this patient will benefit from inflight oxygen therapy.

New and Future Developments

Clinical (ear and finger pulse) *oximeters* measure arterial oxygen saturation noninvasively using the principle of dual wavelength absorption photospectroscopy. Medicare accepts these measurements as an alternative to Pa_{O_2} when assessing patients for oxygen therapy. Oximeters may be especially helpful for assessing patients at home and those with exercise- and sleep-related hypoxemia. For example, patients receiving continuous oxygen therapy are instructed to increase oxygen flow by an additional 1 L/min during sleep or exercise. Oximeters may determine if this empiric recommendation is necessary and adequate. However, clinical oximeters may not work well in the presence of peripheral vascular disease, dark skin pigment, and high levels of carboxyhemoglobin or blood lipids. Finally, limited accuracy (approximately ± 3 to 5%) may cause problems. For example, a reading of 89% may lead to inappropriate oxygen therapy if Sa_{O_2} is really 94% (Pa_{O_2} of 70 torr), and a reading of 91% might lead to denial of therapy even if Sa_{O_2} is really 86% (Pa_{O_2} of 52 torr).

Equipment is improving rapidly and becoming more convenient. Aluminum cylinders that are nearly 30% lighter than standard cylinders are becoming more widely available. Patients who carry very small cylinders (sizes A, B, and D) appreciate the lighter weight, whereas those who push their E cylinders on carts notice little difference. New, smaller, and lighter (35 to 40 lb) oxygen concentrators are now available. Recently, two manufacturers announced briefcase-sized, battery-powered concentrators that weigh less than 10 lb. The long-term reliability of these new small concentrators has not been determined. As noted above, most portable LOX reservoirs now come in a small (half standard) size. Even smaller pediatric 1-lb reservoirs are planned.

The development of *oxygen-conserving devices* is an exciting technological advancement. Conventional therapy wastes up to 75% of oxygen by providing flow during expiration and flow to dead space. These devices—the transtracheal oxygen catheter, reservoir cannula, and pulsed dose demand valve—reduce oxygen waste, reduce overall use of oxygen (by a substantial 50 to 70% in laboratory studies), and allow the use of smaller, more convenient portable equipment. Unfortunately, experience with these devices is limited and long-term reliability has not been evaluated. However, the near future may see an oxygen conserver used with a 1-lb pediatric LOX reservoir or book-size concentrator.

Addendum

Recent congressional legislation (Public Law 100-203, Section 4062) instructs Medicare to use standard rates starting in 1989 to reimburse the cost of home oxygen therapy. The rates will be based on flow and ambulatory requirements; will be modified only for extremes of flow, inflation, and regional differences in costs; and will no longer consider delivery methods, i.e., the same rate will be used for cylinder, liquid, and concentrator oxygen. Standard rates will favor the least costly delivery method and will force both physician and supplier to review more carefully the needs of each patient. Systems that are both economical and convenient include a concentrator with small portable cylinder, a liquid oxygen system with large stationary reservoir that reduces delivery costs, and a liquid oxygen system with demand valve or other conserving device that minimizes waste.

Bibliography

AMA Commission on Emergency Medical Services. Medical aspects of transportation aboard commercial aircraft. JAMA 247:1007–1011, 1982.
> *An excellent summary of the effect of hypobaria encountered aboard commercial aircraft on a variety of medical conditions; cardiorespiratory problems are emphasized.*

Christmas Seal League of Southwestern Pennsylvania. Self-help: Your Strategy for Living with COPD. Palo Alto, CA, Bull Publishing Co., 1983.
> *An excellent 26-page booklet for patients and their families that discusses many aspects of caring for chronic obstructive pulmonary disease; good use of charts and diary entries.*

Conference on Home Oxygen Therapy Report. Problems in prescribing and supplying oxygen for Medicare patients. Am Rev Respir Dis 134:340–341, 1986.
> *Criticisms of Medicare policies and recommendations made by a panel of expert pulmonary clinicians.*

Department of Health and Human Services Health Care Financing Administration. Medicare program: coverage of oxygen for use in a patient's home. Fed Regist 50:13,742–13,750, 1985.
> *The official, detailed announcement of the home oxygen policy now used by Medicare.*

Fulmer JD, Snider GL. ACCP-NHLBI national conference on oxygen therapy. Chest 86:234–247, 1984.
> *A summary of recommendations concerning acute and chronic oxygen therapy; includes an excellent bibliography for the scientific basis of oxygen therapy.*

Gong H Jr, Tashkin DP, Lee Ey, et al. Hypoxia-altitude simulation test. Am Rev Respir Dis 130:980–986, 1984.
> *Simulation of the effects of altitude on Pa_{O_2} by use of hypoxic gas mixtures; a nomogram can be used to predict the effects of altitude.*

Medical Research Council Working Party. Long term domiciliary oxygen in chronic hypoxic cor pulmonale complicating chronic bronchitis and emphysema. Lancet 1:681–686, 1981.
> *A landmark controlled study complements Nocturnal Oxygen Therapy Trial Group study; see annotation for that study for details.*

Nocturnal Oxygen Therapy Trial Group. Continuous or nocturnal oxygen therapy in hypoxemic chronic obstructive lung disease. Ann Intern Med 93:391–398, 1980.

A landmark controlled study; complements Medical Research Council Working Party study; patients who received no oxygen (MRCWP controls) suffered from premature death; those who received oxygen for 12 to 16 hours (MRCWP study group, NOTT controls) had improved survival; and those who received oxygen "continuously" (20 hours/day, NOTT study group) had the best survival.

Petty TL. Ambulatory Oxygen. New York, Thieme-Stratton, 1983.

An excellent monograph for professionals by the "father" of LOX therapy.

Second Conference on Long-term Oxygen Therapy Report. Further recommendations for prescribing and supplying long-term oxygen therapy. Am Rev Respir Dis 138:745–747, 1988.

Eleven recommendations were made recently to help clarify patient activities while receiving therapy, documentation of medical necessity, standards for quality assurance, education of physicians, and reimbursement.

Skorodin MS. Current oxygen prescribing practices—problems and prospects. JAMA 255:3283–3285, 1986.

A blunt commentary concerning the recent changes in oxygen reimbursement policies adopted by Medicare, the limitations of our scientific knowledge, and the economics of prescribing oxygen.

Timms RM, Khaja FU, Williams GW, et al. Hemodynamic response to oxygen therapy in chronic obstructive pulmonary disease. Ann Intern Med 102:29–36, 1985.

Detailed study of the cardiac catheterization data generated by the NOTT study; improvement was found in pulmonary vascular resistance, pulmonary artery pressure, and stroke volume index. Also, the greater the hemodynamic improvement, the better the survival.

PART TWELVE

Rheumatology

48

Management of Regional Low Back Pain

ROBERT J. QUINET, M.D.
LEONARD H. SEREBRO, M.D.

Most people have at least one episode of low back pain during their lifetime, and it is the most common painful condition seen by physicians. The natural history of these attacks is that the majority are self-limited, with 60% resolved after 1 week and 90% resolved after 2 months. Less than 5% of acute episodes of low back pain require surgery.

There are many different causes of back pain (Table 48–1). More than 80% of low back pain is due to mechanical factors involving one or more of a multitude of structures such as ligaments, muscles, disks, facets, or nerve roots.

We are unable to differentiate these various causes of mechanical back pain accurately, but the management is similar whichever structure or combination of structures is affected. Even when nerve root involvement accompanies mechanical pain, initial management is the same unless there is evidence of severe or progressive neurologic deficit (in which case urgent neurosurgical consultation is required).

The diagnostic challenge in cost-effective evaluation of low back pain is to select the minority of patients who require more intensive (and expensive) testing from the majority who require little or no initial testing. Careful history-taking and physical examination enable us to select patients: (1) with significant neurologic involvement who may require surgery and need neurosurgical evaluation; (2) with *extraspinal* disease or *nonmechanical* intraspinal disease, because knowledge of the cause may influence therapy; (3) with possible litigation, who may need studies for medicolegal reasons; (4) with marked emotional overlay that may predict poor response to therapy and possible need for psychologic evaluation.

History

A detailed history is essential.

Onset

Did low back pain start gradually or suddenly? Is the pain acute or chronic? A gradual onset of pain of several months' duration that improves with exercise and worsens after rest and at night, associated with severe morning stiffness, suggests possible inflammatory spondylitis. Mechanical back pain improves with recumbency and is worse after activity or prolonged sitting. Nonmechanical pain not related to inflammation is usually continuous and is not aggravated by exercise.

Is there a history of trauma? (If so, is litigation a possibility?) Did pain begin at work (compensable?) Is this the first attack, or have there been previous episodes? (If so, note the duration, management, and response to therapy.)

Is There Neurologic Compromise?

Describe the location of the pain:
1. Is it confined to the back, or are there leg symptoms suggestive of cauda equina syndrome or radiculopathy?
2. Does pain radiate down one or both legs? (If so, which part of the leg is involved? True radicular symptoms have a dermatome distribution [Table 48–2].) Ask specifically about numbness and paresthesias, weakness in legs, or difficulty in walking (falling).
3. Are bowel or bladder symptoms present?

Table 48-1. Causes of Low Back Pain

Intraspinal (97%)		Extraspinal (3%)
Mechanical (81%)	**Nonmechanical (16%)**	**Referred Pain**

1. Nonspecific lumbar strain
2. Herniated disks
3. Facet (apophyseal) osteoarthritis
4. Fractures
5. Spinal stenosis
6. Multilevel degenerative disk disease (spondylosis) (severe)
7. Spondylolisthesis (severe)
8. Scoliosis (severe)
9. Kyphosis (severe)
10. ? Spondylolysis
	1. Infection
	  a. Osteomyelitis
	  b. Septic diskitis
	  c. Epidural abscess
	  d. Paraspinous abscess
	  e. Bacterial endocarditis
	2. Neoplasia
	  a. Metastatic disease
	  b. Multiple myeloma
	  c. Lymphoma and leukemia
	  d. Primary: skeletal or spinal cord tumors (benign or malignant)
	  e. Retroperitoneal tumors
	3. Inflammatory spondyloarthritis (often HLA B27 positive)
	  a. Ankylosing spondylitis
	  b. Reiter's disease
	  c. Psoriasis
	  d. Inflammatory bowel disease
	4. Metabolic
	  a. Osteoporosis (with compression fracture)
	  b. Osteomalacia
	  c. Paget's disease
	  d. Hyperparathyroidism
	  e. Cushing's disease
	5. Other
	  a. Iatrogenic (steroids with compression fracture)
	  b. Scheuermann's disease (osteochondritis)
		1. Pelvic organs
		  a. Prostatitis
		  b. Endometriosis
		  c. Chronic pelvic inflammatory disease
		2. Renal disease
		  a. Stones
		  b. Pyelonephritis
		  c. Perinephric abscess
		  d. Cystitis
		3. Aortic aneurysm (abdominal)
		4. Gastrointestinal disease
		  a. Pancreatitis
		  b. Cholecystitis
		  c. Penetrating ulcer
		  d. Colorectal pathology (pilonidal sinus)
		5. Hip pain
		6. Trochanteric bursitis
		7. Ischial bursitis
		8. Fat herniation of lumbar space

From Deyo R. J Gen Intern Med 1:328–338, 1986, with permission.

Table 48-2. Lumbar Radicular Syndromes

Nerve root	Cauda equina L4–5 >L5–S1	S1	L5	L4
Disk level	Central herniation	L5–S1	L4–L5	L3–L4
Pattern of pain (all may affect low back and buttocks)	Perineum (both legs; may be unilateral)	Posterior leg (unilateral)	Lateral leg and thigh (unilateral)	Posterolateral leg (unilateral)
Motor defect	Unilateral or bilateral leg weakness	Unilateral weak plantar flexion foot; toe walking difficult	Unilateral weak dorsiflexion foot; heel walking difficult	Unilateral quadriceps weakness
Sensory deficit	Decreased buttocks, perineum Low back Thighs, legs, feet (may be saddle anesthesia)	Decreased lateral foot and posterolateral calf	Decreased lateral calf and between first and second toes	Decreased knee and distal anterior thigh
Reflex depressed	Ankle jerk	Ankle jerk	0	Knee jerk
Action taken	Urgent neurosurgical consultations for decompression	Treat conservatively unless severe or progressive neurologic deficit; if so, consult neurosurgeon		

Cauda equina compression from a midline disk herniation or tumor may cause incontinence, difficulty in walking, and bilateral saddle anesthesia. The pain related to a cauda equina tumor is typically worse when the patient lies down at night, and the patient may sleep in a chair or pace the floor to seek relief. These symptoms should trigger a detailed neurologic examination (Table 48–2), including a rectal examination.

4. Does coughing or straining at stool worsen pain? If so, this suggests dural irritation from disk herniation.

Is There Systemic or Visceral Disease?

Nonspecific mechanical low back pain tends to occur most frequently in the third to fourth decades. Patients over 50 years of age have a greater incidence of specific and more serious causes of back pain.

Always ask about recurrent fever, chills, and night sweats. These symptoms suggest the possibility of infections like osteomyelitis, septic diskitis, or epidural abscess (intense pain). Infective endocarditis may be characterized by nonspecific back pain with fever (ask about heart murmurs and drug abuse). Febrile illness may suggest retroperitoneal or renal abscess, prostatitis, cystitis, or tuberculosis. Local causes of fever include infected pilonidal cyst or infected sebaceous cyst. Recent weight loss or a history of previous malignancy suggests the possibility of neoplasia. Alcoholism may be a clue to referred pain from pancreatitis or a duodenal ulcer, especially if abdominal symptoms are present.

Studies of several large series of patients have shown that tumors, infections, and inflammatory spondyloarthropathies *together* comprise less than 2% of cases. The exact percentage in an individual physician's practice depends on the age of the patient population (with a higher incidence of tumors and infections in a predominantly geriatric population). Physicians spend much time and effort to detect these rare patients because of the severity of their illness and the need for specific diagnosis and therapy where possible.

Intensity of Pain

The most severe back pain comes from acute compression fractures, which may occur spontaneously in osteoporotic older patients (frac-

tures are more common in the thoracic than the lumbar spine). An epidural abscess (usually febrile), neoplastic disease, or large central disk herniation also causes very intense pain. Pain severe enough to wake the patient from sleep suggests one of the above or inflammatory spondylitis (younger patients), penetrating peptic ulcer, or dissecting aortic aneurysm (older patients). Occasionally, pain related to trochanteric bursitis, which is often present in patients with mechanical back pain with or without radiculopathy, can be severe enough to awaken them if they turn in their sleep to lie on the affected side. Patients with intense pain usually need a more detailed evaluation before initiation of therapy (Fig. 48–1).

Pseudoclaudication

Spinal stenosis is a condition with narrowing of the spinal canal often caused by a combination of a congenitally narrowed canal and disk protrusion and osteophytes. This condition occurs in older patients who describe symptoms of pain, numbness, or weakness, usually of both buttocks or of the thighs and legs (may be asymmetric or unilateral). The pain occurs on standing or walking and worsens the more the person walks. It is completely relieved within a few minutes by rest, especially with flexion of the lumbar spine, and tends to have an insidious onset and slow progression. These symptoms should be differentiated from true claudication by careful vascular evaluation and confirmation of spinal stenosis by computed tomographic scan if surgery is contemplated.

Medication: Drug and Alcohol Abuse

What medications is the patient taking? Present or past corticosteroid use may be a clue to a compression fracture. Is there a history of drug abuse, alcohol abuse, or past or present significant depressive illness? The physician must also take into account which medications, both prescription and over the counter, the patient is taking because of possible interaction with drugs that may be prescribed.

The standard review of systems and medical history, including operative and family history (cancer, arthritis), may provide important additional data.

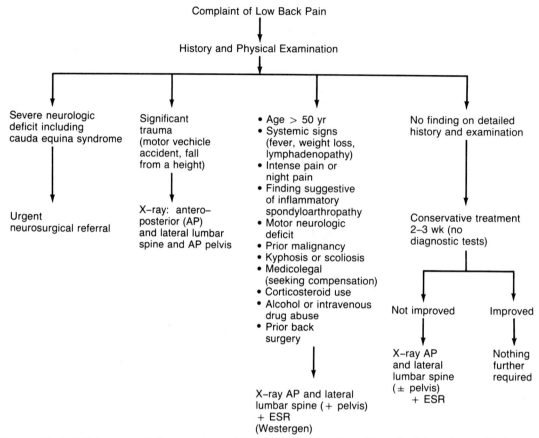

Figure 48–1. Initial approach for a patient with low back pain. From Deyo R. J Gen Intern Med 1:328–338, 1986, with permission.

Physical Examination

A detailed general physical examination should consider vital signs (to rule out fever); evaluation of thyroid gland, lymph nodes, breasts, prostate, rectum, and female pelvis (to help rule out cancer); and evaluation of the abdomen (for neoplasm, aneurysm, pancreatitis), heart (for murmurs, endocarditis), chest (for infection, e.g., tuberculosis; decreased chest expansion in spondylitis), and femoral and pedal pulses (to exclude vascular disease).

Local examination of the back should include a search for lesions (e.g., infected pilonidal sinus) and obvious structural abnormalities (e.g., kyphosis, scoliosis). Although these findings may not be related to the pain, they may indicate the need for x-rays. An unusual prominence of a spinous process may suggest spondylolisthesis or a compression fracture, which could be confirmed radiologically.

A detailed neurologic examination is required to localize affected nerve roots (if any) and define the severity of any neurologic change. Evaluation of reflex and muscle strength, as well as careful sensory testing, is needed. This evaluation also serves as a base line (Table 48–2). More than 90% of disk herniations occur at the L4–L5 or L5–S1 levels, so the neurologic examination should focus on these nerve roots.

About 90% of surgically proven disk herniations are associated with an impaired ankle reflex or weak foot dorsiflexion or plantar flexion. Sensory deficits of the L5 and S1 roots occur in the posterior and lateral aspects of the leg and are more difficult to establish on examination than motor defects because of their subjectivity. Only 5% of patients with proven disk herniation have impaired knee reflexes because herniation above L4–L5 is rare.

The straight leg raising test, when positive, produces back pain at an elevation of 60° or less. Gentle dorsiflexion of the foot at the onset of the painful arc should increase the discomfort if there is true nerve root irritation.

Positive results with this test should be confirmed by leg extension in the seated position. The straight leg raising test is one for the L5 and S1 nerve roots. It is a sensitive test in that it is positive in 95% of patients who prove to have a herniated disk at surgery. It is nonspecific in that it is also positive in 89% of surgical patients with negative exploratory surgery. If the straight leg raising test is positive for both legs, the specificity is greatly increased, with a likelihood of a true disk herniation in more than 90% of the patients.

The femoral stretch test, performed by flexing the knee with the patient in the prone position, may be positive in the rare L4 root syndrome.

Chest expansion and lumbar flexion may be decreased in spondyloarthritis. Shober's test measures flexion between two points 10 cm apart on the lumbar spine, the bottom point being drawn through the dimples of Venus (posterior superior iliac spine) in the erect position. After forward flexion, the distance between these points should increase at least 4 cm. This test is not specific for ankylosing spondylitis, but if it is reduced (i.e., less than 4 cm) in a patient with inflammatory symptoms, an x-ray examination of the pelvis is warranted to evaluate the sacroiliac joints.

Hip motion, especially internal and external rotation, should be tested. Internal rotation is often painful and is decreased if there is hip joint disease, e.g., osteoarthritis. Pain on external rotation only may suggest trochanteric bursitis. The greater trochanters and the ischial tuberosities should be palpated as part of the examination of the back to detect bursitis, which may respond to local therapy if it is a significant cause of symptoms. Despite extensive examination, in the vast majority of patients one finds only nonspecific lumbar or sacral tenderness or mildly limited motion of the back—findings that are not diagnostically helpful. Nearly all patients have elements of both psychogenic and organic pain. The presence of three of five of these elements (Table 48–3) suggests an important nonorganic component, which may identify patients who will prove difficult to manage.

Tests That Should Be Ordered

Initial Visit—When to X-ray (Fig. 48–1)

Patients under age 50 years with an acute episode of regional, nonspecific, mechanical

Table 48–3. *Five Signs Suggesting a Major Psychogenic Overlay or Malingering*

Neurologic deficits without anatomic correlation (e.g., decreased sensation on whole leg rather than dermatome distribution)
Tenderness unrelated to anatomic structures (e.g., tenderness to light touch to the skin in a wide distribution)
Over-reaction during examination (e.g., collapsing, sweating, tremor, or excess verbalization)
Positive straight leg raising test results in the supine position but negative in the sitting position
Pain produced by tests to simulate spine loading or rotation without causing the simulated effect

back pain and a history and physical examination negative for nonmechanical factors need no further study before initiating 2 to 3 weeks of conservative therapy. The majority of patients recover after this time, and the minority who do not can have further studies performed, including x-rays.

Lumbar spine x-rays are expensive and nonspecific and may show abnormalities unrelated to the cause of the back pain (Table 48–4). These x-rays expose patients to high doses of radiation for a low yield of useful findings and should be ordered selectively only if evaluation suggests infectious, neoplastic, inflammatory, or traumatic diseases (Fig. 48–1).

Anteroposterior and lateral views of the lumbar spine are sufficient (omit oblique views unless specifically indicated). Anteroposterior views of the pelvis are needed if hip or sacroiliac joint involvement is suspected or if there is pelvic trauma.

Laboratory Tests

Laboratory tests are not helpful in patients with mechanical back pain and are not required. Like x-rays, these tests are used for the initial evaluation of patients whose clinical features suggest an underlying neoplastic, infectious, or inflammatory process. The erythrocyte sedimentation rate is more sensitive than the white blood count in screening for these conditions.

Other laboratory tests, including urinalysis, should be tailored to the specific findings of the patient being studied; for example, in an elderly patient with low back pain and significant weight loss who has a change in bowel habits, evaluation of the colon and rectum is indicated to rule out malignancy.

Table 48–4. Indications for X-rays for Low Back Pain

Indications for Lumbar Films	Causes of Backache That May Be Specifically Diagnosed by X-ray	Nonrelevant X-ray
1. Serious trauma	1. Disk space infection	1. Spondylosis
2. Prior back surgery	2. Osteomyelitis	2. Facet osteoarthritis
3. Intense pain	3. Sacroiliitis	3. Disk degeneration (single)
4. Radicular signs/symptoms	4. Metastatic tumor	4. Diffuse idiopathic skeletal
5. Fever	5. Myeloma	hyperostosis
6. Weight loss	6. Fracture	5. Transitional lumbosacral
7. Age over 50	7. Spondylolisthesis	segment
8. History of prior neoplasm	(> 25% slippage)	6. Schmorl's nodes
9. Symptoms or signs of malignancy	8. Primary bone tumor	7. Spina bifida occulta
on history or physical examination	9. Mild scoliosis	8. Mild kyphosis
10. History of prior back disease	10. Osteopenia	9. Increased lumbosacral angle
11. History of significant	11. Multilevel disk degeneration	10. Spondylolysis (?)
corticosteroid therapy	12. Scheuermann's osteochondritis	
12. Symptoms of inflammatory disease		
(prolonged morning stiffness)		
13. Significant night pain		
14. History of intravenous drug abuse		
15. Medicolegal reasons (e.g.,		
compensation, disability)		
16. Hostile patient		

Other Studies

Bone Scan. A radionuclide bone scan is valuable in the diagnosis of suspected metastatic disease, occult vertebral fracture, osteomyelitis, or metabolic bone disease, even before definite x-ray changes. Bone scans are useful in evaluating back pain associated with fever, weight loss, and increased erythrocyte sedimentation rate.

Electromyography/Nerve Conduction Studies. These studies are not part of the initial evaluation for acute back pain even if radicular symptoms are present because they take 10 to 14 days after onset of nerve compression to become abnormal. These studies should be reserved for patients with radicular symptoms who fail to respond adequately to an initial 2 to 4 weeks of conservative therapy and in whom confirmation of nerve irritation is required for medicolegal or prognostic reasons.

Computed Tomographic Scan. In general, this expensive test ($350 to $600) is reserved for evaluation of patients for whom surgery is being considered. Demonstration of a herniated disk or spinal stenosis becomes important if neurologic deficits are present and have not responded adequately to conservative therapy. When the clinical neurologic findings correspond to those of the scan, finding a causal relationship is likely. Unselected use of the scan gives many false-positive results: up to 34% of asymptomatic people may have "abnormal" findings.

Magnetic Resonance Imaging (MRI). This procedure is even more expensive ($600 to $800) than the computed tomographic scan. Magnetic resonance imaging may be useful for selected patients, such as those who have had multiple previous back surgeries, or for presurgical evaluation.

Myelography. This test is the gold standard of presurgical evaluation. Cost is approximately $2,000 including hospitalization.

Minnesota Multiphasic Personality Inventory. This psychologic test may indicate major psychopathology in selected patients with chronic back pain.

Management of Regional Low Back Pain

The following discussion applies to the majority of patients with regional low back pain who do *not* have a neoplasm, infectious process, referred pain, spondyloarthropathy, specifically treatable metabolic process, or either of the two absolute surgical indications, cauda equina syndrome or marked progressive muscle weakness. Therefore, the majority of patients have a *nonsurgical* disease, either a nonspecific lumbar backache or a lumbar radicular syndrome (most commonly affecting the L5 or S1 nerve root).

Management of Acute Low Back Pain

Pain confined to the low back is initially managed in a similar fashion whether or not there are associated radicular symptoms, in the absence of cauda equina or progressive motor weakness, which would necessitate immediate surgery.

The natural history of acute low back pain is benign. Sixty percent of patients are better at 1 week, 80% at 2 weeks, and 90% by 6 weeks of illness, no matter what therapy is given. Encouragement and postural advice are crucial. With such a good natural history, it has been difficult if not impossible to improve it with current therapy.

BED REST AND BACK PROTECTION

The prescription of bed rest is aimed at allowing healing to take place by minimizing biomechanical stress. This is the mainstay of conservative management. Recumbence should take place on a firm-hard mattress, perhaps with a ¾-in plywood board between mattress and box spring, or on the floor. Two pillows, a *small* one under the head and another behind the knees, are permitted. Lying on the side in a fetal posture is also acceptable, but lying prone is prohibited. A short walk to the bathroom or *brief* sitting for meals is allowed; however, bedpans are best avoided in hospitalized patients.

For a backache with sciatica, bed rest may be needed for as little as a few days to as long as several weeks. The patient should gradually ambulate as symptoms permit. For a simple backache, bed rest for 2 to 3 days is usually adequate. Bed rest longer than absolutely necessary produces osteoporosis and disuse muscle atrophy and is to be avoided, particularly in the elderly.

The patient should be mobilized during a 7- to 10-day period, with frequent rest periods in the supine position. A fitted lumbosacral corset or abdominal binder should be used if necessary for a low backache. A thoracolumbar corset with shoulder straps or an extension brace may be used for the patient with thoracolumbar compression fractures. Prolonged sitting or standing for longer than 30 to 45 minutes should be avoided during this time, and all bending, stooping, lifting, and carrying are also best avoided.

This is an excellent time to introduce the concept of back protection, body mechanics, and ways to avoid stress in the low back. This information is best provided by the physician and, if possible, should be reinforced with printed literature (e.g., booklets obtainable from the Arthritis Foundation, Atlanta, GA,

for a nominal fee, or the excellent series of booklets published by the Patient Information Library, Krames Communications, Daly City, CA). Certain patients may benefit from the more formal educational program of a "back school."

DRUG TREATMENT

Analgesics are provided for symptomatic relief, and although they decrease pain they do not affect a patient's return to work. Non-narcotic analgesics are preferred. Narcotics, if used, are best restricted to short-term use (3 days or less). None of the available nonsteroidal anti-inflammatory agents or analgesics are demonstrably more efficacious than aspirin, and therefore enteric-coated aspirin is recommended (325 mg, two to three tablets three or four times a day, after meals and at bedtime, as tolerated), until symptoms improve. Aspirin in anti-inflammatory doses or other nonsteroidal anti-inflammatory drugs are preferable to simple analgesics. All of the available muscle relaxants produce significant depression of the central nervous system and have not been shown to relax striated muscles independent of their sedative-hypnotic effects.

SPINAL MANIPULATION

Spinal manipulation is not widely available or practiced in the United States, and when it has been studied formally it has not been shown to have any long-term, clinically meaningful benefit. Further study of this approach may yield subsets of patients with acute low back pain who might benefit, as some studies do demonstrate short-lived relief.

TRACTION

Standard Buck's pelvic traction requires 30 kg of traction force in the average patient to appreciably reduce lumbar intradisk pressure. Formal studies of lumbar traction on a table with a mobile lower segment (Tru-Trac), Autotraction, or gravity inversion have not produced convincing evidence of efficacy. Gravity inversion is usually associated with major elevations of systolic and diastolic blood pressure and is thus contraindicated for many patients. In patients with refractory symptoms, however, a trial of supine pelvic traction with a Tru-Trac table may be given and is sometimes worthwhile. If it does nothing else, traction serves to keep the patient in bed!

PHYSICAL THERAPY

There is no evidence to support the use of therapeutic exercise, shortwave diathermy, ultrasound, or biofeedback for *acute* low back pain. A hot bath or Thermaphore moist heating pad may provide palliative relief of muscle spasm, as may ice packs or ice massage in selected patients. Exercises are best withheld until *after* the acute episode has subsided.

EPIDURAL STEROIDS

Some data support the use of epidural steroids in patients with low back pain and sciatica who have not responded to a more conservative program of therapy. This approach may simply defer surgery to a later date, as no long-lasting benefit has been demonstrated.

CHEMONUCLEOLYSIS

This technique of intradisk injection of chymopapain has not proved to have any real advantages compared with available neurosurgical procedures for acute disk herniation and in fact is more expensive, is associated with the *production* of backache and anaphylaxis, and produces less than optimal results on long-term follow-up. We do not refer our patients for this procedure.

SURGERY

As indicated, the cauda equina syndrome and progressive, important motor weakness are the only two absolute indications for surgery. Most back specialists recommend taking advantage of the natural history of this illness and deferring surgery until 2 to 3 months of conservative management have been accomplished. However, it is wise to hospitalize patients with severe intractable pain or neurologic symptoms or signs to enforce appropriate rest, provide adequate analgesia, and follow neurologic examination closely. Failure to improve while in the hospital suggests the need for appropriate diagnostic imaging and surgical consultation. Except for the two conditions mentioned, there is no evidence that this delay compromises the functional result. By the end of this period, many patients are better without surgery. Repeat surgery for low back pain is usually unrewarding unless there is documented new disk herniation or herniation at a level different from the site of the original operation.

SUMMARY

Rest and analgesics or nonsteroidal anti-inflammatory agents are the cornerstones of therapy, and the overwhelming majority of patients respond positively to them and to simple explanations and education regarding back protection. In patients whose leg pain or radicular symptoms fail to improve, definition of the problem with computed tomography, magnetic resonance imaging, or lumbar myelography with a view to possible surgery is indicated. Careful serial back and neurologic examinations can be correlated with the patient's symptoms to help assess improving or worsening symptoms. Conservative therapy usually provides relief of symptoms, restores activity and mobility, and at the same time avoids invasive therapy with its attendant morbidity.

Management of Chronic Lumbar Backache (Tables 48–5 and 48–6)

EXERCISES

Exercises are nearly always indicated for patients with chronic low back pain as well as for patients recently recovered from an episode of acute pain. The limited activity consequent to chronic pain or to the rest prescribed for acute backache results in disuse atrophy and diminished flexibility. We recommend (1) knee-chest exercises, (2) pelvic tilts, (3) quadricep and hamstring strengthening, and (4) isometric abdominal strengthening exercises. These should be performed as a routine once or twice daily, 3 to 20 repetitions each, after a hot bath or shower. We also recommend walking, swimming, and biking (with use of traditional nonracing type handlebars) as excellent general exercises that are not particularly stressful to the lumbar spine. Aerobics, "jazzercise," vigorous calisthenics, and racket sports are more likely to aggravate a backache and are therefore best avoided. It often helps to have a physical therapist take the patient through each exercise and review proper body mechanics to be sure that the patient does the exercises properly and understands their rationale. Maintenance of optimal weight is also important.

CORSETS

The use of an abdominal binder may be temporarily useful for the patient with abdom-

Table 48–5. *Advice Concerning Posture for Patients with Chronic Lumbar Backache*

Do's	Don'ts
1. Use good lumbar support when seated or driving. Sit close to steering wheel. Use headrest.	1. Avoid driving with seat pushed back and lumbar spine relatively extended.
2. Sit on hard chair. May prop up feet so knees are higher than hips. Use armrests when seated and use them to help push up when rising.	2. Avoid stooped shoulders or swayback posture.
3. Stand erect with back and pelvis straight.	3. Avoid stooped or bent forward posture, especially when lifting.
4. Lift by bending the knees. Lift close to the body. Let the quadriceps do the work.	4. Avoid sleeping prone (on stomach).
5. Sleep supine or in fetal position on firm mattress, with or without bed board (¾-in plywood).	5. Avoid high heels.
6. Use rubber or crepe soles or ripple soles with low or normal heel, arch supports if needed.	6. Avoid aerobics, "jazzercise," racket sports, running, contact sports.
7. Do isometric lumbar, abdominal, and thigh-strengthening exercise. Swimming, upright cycling, walking are best.	7. Avoid obesity.
8. When standing still for a long time, prop one leg up on small stool or ledge.	8. Avoid racing handlebars when biking and toe touches, windmills, sit-ups, straight leg raises when exercising.
9. Bend knees rather than back when making bed, using low sink, vacuuming, or mopping.	
10. Get into car feet first.	
11. Get out of bed by first swinging legs off the side and pushing to seated position.	
12. Use stepladder or stool to reach into high shelf or cabinet.	
13. Maintain ideal body weight.	
14. Stop or modify painful exercise.	

inal obesity until an exercise program corrects this. By reinforcing proper posture, decreasing stress on the lumbar spine at rest and during lifting, and limiting adverse movements, a formal corset may also be useful temporarily. Neither a binder nor a corset should be prescribed in the absence of an appropriate set of abdominal exercises, which allow eventual discontinuation of the support. If these supports are continued for long periods, the patient's intrinsic muscles may weaken further. Some patients find it helpful to keep a corset available to use if back symptoms return.

Table 48–6. *Conservative Therapies (Based on Medical Literature) for Chronic Lumbar Backache*

Definitely useful (proven)
  None
Probably useful (not proven)
  Bed rest
  Drugs: aspirin, naproxen, piroxicam, diflunisal, carisoprodol
  Autotraction (Lind)
  Exercise (isometric, flexion type)
Possibly useful (not proven)
  Spinal manipulation in *acute* backache for *short-term* relief (benefit)
  Corsets
  Transcutaneous electrical nerve stimulation
  Supine traction (Tru-Trac)

TRANSCUTANEOUS ELECTRICAL NERVE STIMULATION

This is a safe and often effective way to control acute or chronic pain and is useful if a trial in physical therapy demonstrates efficacy. A unit may be rented for temporary use or may be purchased. It should always be tried in patients heavily dependent on analgesics to help decrease the amount of medication they need.

DRUG THERAPY

In addition to the modalities already mentioned, patients with chronic pain should take non-narcotic analgesics (acetaminophen), salicylates, or other nonsteroidal anti-inflammatory drugs in preference to narcotic analgesics. Tricyclic antidepressants have proved efficacious in rather small doses for chronic low backache, even in the absence of clinical depression. Patients who are addicted should take acetaminophen, nonsteroidal anti-inflammatory drugs, and a tricyclic antidepressant, as well as use transcutaneous electrical nerve stimulation, as part of a basic program to decrease narcotic analgesic intake. Patients who remain dependent on narcotics despite this approach should be considered for admission to a pain unit for a multidisciplinary approach to their serious problem. In general, medications should be de-emphasized in the management of chronic regional low back pain, and proper body mechanics, a positive attitude, and back and general exercises should be promoted.

LOCAL THERAPY

As for acute low back pain, local moist heat or ice packs may provide palliative, temporary relief and may be utilized as necessary.

INJECTIONS

Epidural steroids appear to provide only temporary relief of sciatic symptoms. In selected patients in whom the facet or apophyseal joint appears to be the source of their backache, a block or local anesthetic-corticosteroid preparation injected into the joint under fluoroscopic visualization is sometimes but not consistently helpful. Again, relief tends to be short-lived, and subsequent injections may be necessary. When formally studied, acupuncture was not shown to be superior to placebo for chronic low backache, but it is relatively safe and could be tried for a rare patient who is resistant to other nonsurgical approaches.

SURGERY

Surgery is best avoided in most instances of chronic low backache. It has no role in chronic backache alone, although in rare instances it may be necessary for recurrent or persistent sciatica. However, surgery should be contemplated only when a surgically remediable anatomic abnormality has been demonstrated. Exploratory or diagnostic surgery is to be absolutely avoided and should not be necessary with the availability and accuracy of current imaging techniques.

Denervation procedures, particularly of facet joints, are done only rarely and in exceptional patients, with equivocal results.

Lumbar fusion is of no help in the absence of demonstrable and significant instability. The pros and cons of this procedure have been debated for 50 years and have not yet been resolved.

PSYCHOLOGIC EVALUATION

In patients with chronic pain of any type, secondary or reactive psychologic abnormalities supervene—particularly depression and anxiety. In patients with back symptoms of more than 6 months' duration, formal psychologic testing commonly reveals evidence of anxiety, depression, hysteria, and hypochondriasis. Usually, in addition to the education and physical manner outlined, these psychologic issues need to be addressed, either with supportive or formal psychotherapy or by psychopharmacotherapy. If these issues do not receive attention, back symptoms tend to persist despite optimal medical management. The role of our work and legal environment in the development and persistence of chronic backache is addressed in detail in several of the references.

SUMMARY

In summary, the major goal in the management of chronic backache is to encourage patient control and responsibility for symptoms in the absence of a more specifically treatable medical or surgical back disorder. Medication should be used sparingly, and specific back exercises, general conditioning exercise, proper body mechanics, and possibly the use of a corset or transcutaneous electrical nerve stimulation unit should be emphasized. Proper attention should be given to reactive psychologic issues as well as to a frank discussion of social, legal, and occupational issues if a complete approach to the individual patient is to be provided.

Bibliography

Bell GR, Rothman R. The conservative treatment of sciatica. Spine 9:54–56, 1984.
   A reasoned interpretation of current management practices.
Deyo RA. Conservative therapy for low back pain: distinguishing useful from useless therapy. JAMA 250:1057–1062, 1983.
   A detailed review of therapy of lumbar backache.
Deyo RA. Early diagnostic evaluation of low back pain. J Gen Intern Med 1:328–338, 1986.
   A review of cost-effective approaches to diagnosis.
Deyo R, Diehl A. Cancer as a cause of back pain. J Gen Intern Med 3:230–238, 1988.
   Factors significantly associated with low back pain from cancer include age greater than 50, previous history of cancer, duration of pain for more than 1 month, failure of pain to improve with conservative therapy, elevated erythrocyte sedimentation rate, and anemia. The authors propose an algorithm for the cost-effective use of spine radiographs.
Deyo RA, Diehl AL, Rosenthal M. How many days of bed rest for acute low back pain—a randomized clinical trial. N Engl J Med 315:1064–1070, 1986.

A well-conceived study, which is an example of what basic "tenets" need to be scientifically explored.

Frymoyer JW. Back pain and sciatica. N Engl J Med 318:291–300, 1988.

Recent review of low back pain.

Hadler NM. Regional back pain. N Engl J Med 315:1090–1092, 1986.

Editorial presenting a comment on back disease as an individual and societal "predicament."

Nachemson A. Recent advances in the treatment of low back pain. Int Orthop 9:1–10, 1985.

A general overview of this field today, and what to expect in the near future.

Quinet RJ, Hadler NM. Diagnosis and treatment of backache. Semin Arthritis Rheum 8:261–287, 1979.

A detailed review of lumbar backache.

Wiesel SW, Cuckler JM, DeLuca F, et al. Acute low-back pain: an objective analysis of conservative therapy. Spine 5:324–330, 1980.

A good study documenting the effect of rest and analgesics.

49

✓ Diagnosis and Management of Shoulder Pain

RICHARD H. WHITE, M.D.

Introduction

Pain in and around the shoulder joint is a very common complaint that primary care physicians should know how to evaluate and treat. Although the list of causes of shoulder pain is extensive (Tables 49–1 and 49–2), only a few relatively easy to diagnose conditions make up the majority of cases. The evaluation process is straightforward and depends principally on historical and physical examination findings, with highly technical diagnostic tests playing a very minor role.

Shoulder Anatomy

To assess a patient with shoulder pain accurately, it is essential to know normal shoulder anatomy and understand the functional inter-relationships between the important elements (Fig. 49–1). Motion of the shoulder actually involves five different joints all working in concert. Disease in any one of these joints can cause shoulder pain with abnormal shoulder motion. In addition to three major diarthrodial joints, the glenohumeral, the sternoclavicular, and the acromioclavicular joints, there are two very important "functional" joints: (1) scapular motion over the thorax and (2) the subacromial apparatus. The latter is bounded superiorly by the undersurface of the acromion and the tough coracoacromial ligament, and inferiorly by the mobile rotator cuff tendons that overlie and insert onto the humeral head. Interposed is the subacromial bursa, which can be thought of as a simplified joint space (Fig. 49–2). Shoulder pain caused by inflammation in the subacromial region is extremely common.

The head of the humerus is held firmly against the glenoid fossa and the surrounding fibrocartilaginous labrum by several small but important glenohumeral ligaments, by the joint capsule, and by the tonic action of the four rotator cuff muscles: the subscapularis, which originates on the anterior surface of the scapula and inserts anteriorly on the lesser tuberosity; the supraspinatus, which originates on the superior rim of the scapula before passing under the acromion to insert on the greater tuberosity; the infraspinatus, which originates on the posterior aspect of the scapula below the scapular spine and inserts posteriorly on the greater tuberosity; and the teres minor, which originates and inserts parallel to and just below the infraspinatus. The subscapularis is responsible for internal rotation, the supraspinatus depresses the head of the humerus and acts as an abductor, and the infraspinatus and teres minor are external rotators.

The vascular supply to a portion of the rotator cuff is quite tenuous, particularly that region of supraspinatus and infraspinatus tendons proximal to where they insert on the humeral head (Fig. 49–3). The poor blood supply to this critical region may explain why this area appears to be prone to inflammation, degeneration, and rupture. This portion of the cuff also happens to be the area where calcium hydroxyapatite crystal deposition builds up in certain individuals.

Approach to the Patient

Given the relatively large number of potential causes of shoulder pain, certain epidemiologic facts should be kept in mind as one begins the evaluation of a patient with shoulder

Table 49–1. *Differential Diagnosis of Shoulder Pain Caused by Nontraumatic Disease Intrinsic to the Shoulder Apparatus*

Disorder	Incidence	Clinical Features
Rotator cuff lesions		
Rotator cuff tendinitis	Very common	Subacute onset; night pain, aching over shoulder and midhumerus; painful arc of abduction 40°–120°; improvement in pain and motion after injecting 8 ml 1% lidocaine into subacromial region
Complete rotator cuff tears	Rare	Acute onset after lifting, pulling, or other similar activities; profound weakness; normal passive range of motion
Acute calcific tendinitis	Occasional	Abrupt onset; excruciating pain; local redness, heat, and tenderness; ± bursal effusions; large calcific mass in rotator cuff seen on plain x-rays
Bicipital tendon lesions		
Tendinitis	Occasional	Usually associated with rotator cuff tendinitis; anterior tenderness over bicipital groove; painful resisted flexion and supination
Rupture of long head	Rare	Obviously flaccid mass of biceps muscle on flexion
Dislocation	Rare	Clicking and pain on internal or external rotation
Frozen shoulder	Common	Pain minimal to moderate; motion reduced in *all* planes; external rotation less than 30°; no improvement after 8 ml 1% lidocaine injected into subacromial region
Arthritis		
Septic	Rare	Fever; excruciating pain during minimal motion; effusion palpable
Osteoarthritis		
Acromioclavicular joint	Occasional	Local acromioclavicular joint tenderness; high painful arc of abduction 140°–170°; osteoarthritis evident on x-ray
Glenohumeral	Rare	Diffuse pain; ± crepitance; joint space narrowing, especially inferiorly, with osteophyte formation
Systemic arthritis (rheumatoid arthritis, pseudogout, and others)	Common	History and signs of systemic arthritis; local joint effusion; often coexisting inflammation in the subacromial bursa with signs of rotator cuff tendinitis
Aseptic necrosis	Rare	Pain; normal range of motion; bone scan diagnostic early; plain radiographs diagnostic later
Instability (nontraumatic)	Rare	Generalized joint laxity

pain. First, rotator cuff tendinitis (also called the shoulder impingement syndrome or the painful arc syndrome) is the most common cause of nontraumatic shoulder pain, with frozen shoulder, myofascial pain, and acute calcific tendinitis being responsible for the majority of the remaining cases. Second, the physical examination provides the most valuable diagnostic information, and physical findings alone are diagnostic in most cases.

A pragmatic approach to the diagnosis of shoulder pain is to first elicit essential historical information and then proceed quickly to the physical examination. If the diagnosis is not immediately apparent, a more detailed history and further diagnostic testing can then be done. Important historical information includes (1) a description of the onset and character of the pain, (2) the presence or absence of a past history of shoulder pain or trauma, including excessive occupational stress, (3) factors that exacerbate or relieve the pain, and

Table 49–2. Differential Diagnosis of Shoulder Pain Caused by Disorders Extrinsic to the Shoulder

Disorder	Incidence	Clinical Features
Neurologic disorders		
Cervical radiculopathy	Occasional	Neck pain; paresthesias; focal neurologic findings, positive electromyogram; motion normal
Brachial neuritis	Rare	Full range of passive motion; isolated weakness of muscle groups (e.g., scapular winging); positive electromyogram
Suprascapular nerve entrapment	Rare	Posterior shoulder pain; electromyogram infra- and supraspinatus atrophy; positive electromyogram; history of trauma to scapula or heavy backpacking
Vascular disorder		
Thoracic outlet syndrome	Rare	Vague shoulder, arm pain; symptoms or signs consistent with vascular insufficiency in arm; positive positional arteriogram showing osseous or nonosseous compression of vascular tree
Myofascial pain		
Isolated trigger point	Common	Local pain in muscle at discrete point; unilateral; most often in rhomboid or midtrapezius
Fibromyalgia	Very common	Diffuse aching; poor, nonrestorative sleep; diffuse symmetric trigger points; skin roll tenderness over midtrapezius
Tumors		
Primary bone or metastatic	Rare	Bone tenderness; plain x-rays showing defect or cortical erosions; bone scan positive; shoulder motion normal or strikingly abnormal
Referred pain		
Abdominal or thoracic source	Occasional	Pain from diaphragm referred to superior aspect of scapula; normal shoulder motion; myocardial pain often radiating along inner aspect of arm, not over shoulder

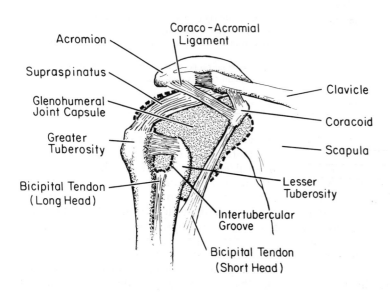

Figure 49–1. Anterior view of the shoulder showing the important bony landmarks, the glenohumeral joint capsule, and the position of the most superior rotator cuff muscle, the supraspinatus.

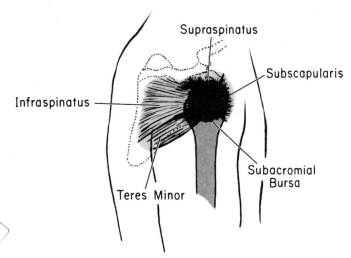

Figure 49–2. *Illustration showing the relative areas of insertion of the rotator cuff muscles on the humeral head and the overlying subacromial bursa.*

(4) the presence of any other systemic or musculoskeletal symptoms. A history of shoulder trauma followed by the abrupt onset of pain suggests a major orthopedic problem, such as fracture or dislocation, a major rotator cuff tear, acromioclavicular joint separation, or fracture of the glenoid labrum. Abrupt onset of shoulder pain in the absence of trauma suggests acute calcific tendinitis, acute inflammatory arthritis (e.g., pseudogout), or an acute septic arthritis. Local soft tissue disorders frequently begin insidiously over days to weeks, with pain often referred distally toward the middle of the humerus near the point of insertion of the deltoid. Very chronic shoulder pain may be felt in the distribution of the C4 dermatome extending down to the thumb. Motion of the shoulder intensifies the pain

associated with local bony and soft tissue problems but does not intensify the pain associated with more distant problems, such as myocardial infarction or acute cholecystitis.

Physical Examination

Because the physical examination is the most important step in the evaluation process, every patient should be draped so that both shoulders are fully exposed, allowing easy comparison of the shoulders. *Inspection* may reveal swelling, redness, atrophy, or signs of recent or remote trauma. Redness suggests infection or an acute inflammatory process, whereas atrophy certainly indicates a more chronic problem. In a systematic fashion, the acromio-

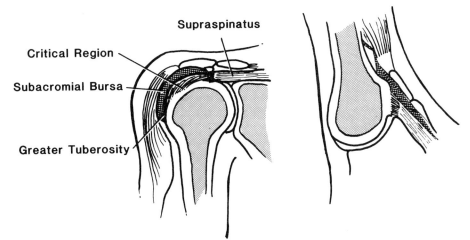

Figure 49–3. *Schematic cross-section of an anterior view of the shoulder showing the subacromial bursa and the proximity of the greater tuberosity to the undersurface of the acromion during abduction.*

clavicular joint should be *palpated*, followed by the glenohumeral joint, which is best felt just inferior and lateral to the coracoid process, followed by the greater tuberosity, which lies laterally just below the acromion (Fig. 49–4). The bicipital groove is best appreciated with the arm externally rotated (thumb out). The anterior and lateral aspects of the rotator cuff are frequently very tender in patients with acute calcific tendinitis or rotator cuff tendinitis.

The *active range of motion* should be carefully analyzed while standing behind the patient. Motion of the scapula relative to the humerus and the thoracic wall should be scrutinized during active abduction (with the arm externally rotated and the thumb out). Normally there is smooth and coordinated upward rotation of the scapula relative to the thorax from approximately 30° abduction to 180° abduction, so-called scapulothoracic rhythm. Most derangements "in" the shoulder, such as rotator cuff tendinitis, glenohumeral arthritis, frozen shoulder, and acute calcific tendinitis, lead to painful abduction and abnormal scapulothoracic rhythm. Instead of fluid-like integrated motion, there is usually rather coarse shrugging of the shoulder, with tilting of the torso away from the affected shoulder. This maneuver allows a patient to elevate the arm without actually moving the humerus relative to the scapula. In patients who have full range of motion, a painful arc of abduction between 40° and 120° during either elevation or lowering the arm from 180° suggests rotator cuff tendinitis (Fig. 49–5). It is during this particular arc that an inflamed or damaged rotator cuff comes into close contact with the cora-

coacromial arch (see Fig. 49–3). Patients with brachial neuritis or a nerve entrapment syndrome may show weakness of specific muscle groups (e.g., winging of the scapula with long thoracic nerve involvement). Patients with myofascial pain or referred pain usually have normal scapulothoracic rhythm.

Active flexion usually reveals findings similar to those of active abduction, albeit less pronounced. Internal rotation should be tested by asking the patient to reach behind his or her hip and touch as high as possible on the back. The hand can usually reach the lower portion of the thoracic vertebrae. External rotation is measured with the elbow flexed at 90° and held firmly against the side (iliac crest) as a fulcrum, with rotation of the forearm away from the body. Normal external rotation is between 45° and 80°. External rotation less than 30° strongly suggests the diagnosis of frozen shoulder, although patients with a major rotator cuff tear or acute calcific tendinitis may have markedly restricted motion secondary to severe pain.

Testing the passive range of motion is important if the active range of motion is abnormal. Frozen shoulder is characterized by markedly restricted active and passive range of motion in *all* planes. In patients with very large rotator cuff tears, the passive range of motion may be much greater than the active range of motion.

The impingement sign is popular among orthopedic surgeons. The elbow (and arm) is passively elevated and internally rotated, which forces the antecubital fossa of the elbow joint to nearly touch the forehead. During this maneuver, the greater tuberosity passes close

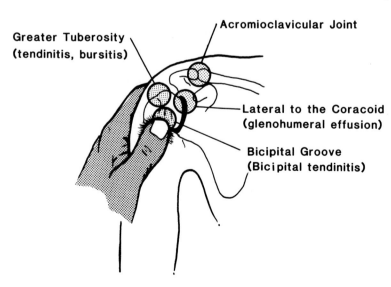

Greater Tuberosity
(tendinitis, bursitis)

Acromioclavicular Joint

Lateral to the Coracoid
(glenohumeral effusion)

Bicipital Groove
(Bicipital tendinitis)

Figure 49–4. *Important areas to palpate when examining the shoulder.*

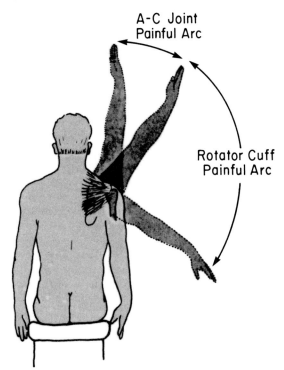

A-C Joint
Painful Arc

Rotator Cuff
Painful Arc

Figure 49–5. *Tendinitis of the rotator cuff is classically associated with a painful arc of abduction between 40° and 120°, whereas pain caused by degenerative disease in the acromioclavicular (A-C) joint usually causes a high painful arc of abduction between 120° and 180°.*

to the undersurface of the acromion. Moderate to severe pain correlates with abnormal pathology in the rotator cuff.

Ancillary Tests

When rotator cuff tendinitis, acute calcific tendinitis, or frozen shoulder is suspected, the most useful ancillary test is a therapeutic trial of local (subacromial) injection of 8 to 9 ml of 1% lidocaine. Significant reduction in pain with improved range of motion is characteristic of the response of patients with rotator cuff tendinitis or acute calcific tendinitis. No improvement in range of motion is characteristic of patients with frozen shoulder.

Figure 49–6 illustrates how to inject the subacromial region by the lateral approach. The injection should be made somewhat anterior to the midline, approximately 2 cm below the top of the acromion, which is readily palpable. After placing the index finger of the right hand over this approximate area and applying pressure with the finger tip, the examiner should passively abduct the patient's

arm back and forth between 0° and 30° while holding the patient's flexed elbow with the left hand. At the correct location, the index finger can be felt to "fall" into the space between the lower border of the acromion and the humerus as the elbow is abducted. The correct spot for injection can be marked by applying pressure to the skin by using the fingernail. A small amount of 1% lidocaine should then be placed intradermally. Using at least a 25 gauge needle (or preferably a 27 gauge needle), insertion should proceed at approximately a 45° angle, gently advancing the needle tip through the deltoid muscle until reaching some resistance. Frequently one feels actual bone, but most commonly the tougher tissue of the rotator cuff is felt. The depth of the injection varies considerably from one individual to another. Obese or muscular patients require injection near the hilt of the needle, whereas other, very thin patients may require injection less than 1 cm from the skin surface. The injection should not be made into the tendon. By retracting the needle a very short distance after meeting resistance, one can be confident that the bevel of the needle is in the correct plane. Injecting the needle along too horizontal a plane should be avoided because often the needle advances tangential to or even through the supraspinatus tendon.

If septic arthritis or a septic subacromial bursitis is suspected, one must attempt to aspirate joint or bursal fluid to make the diagnosis. The glenohumeral joint should be approached anteriorly with the needle inserted just lateral to and slightly below the coracoid process.

Plain radiographs of the shoulder rarely add significant diagnostic information for patients who clinically have rotator cuff tendinitis or frozen shoulder. Plain films are useful in excluding uncommon disorders. Erosion of bone suggests a local infection or metastatic tumor. Severe glenohumeral joint space narrowing with inferior osteophyte formation is consistent with degenerative arthritis of the glenohumeral joint. Narrowing of the distance between the humeral head and the acromion (distance should be greater than 0.6 cm) suggests chronic rotator cuff disease. Calcification of the articular cartilage is consistent with calcium pyrophosphate deposition disease (pseudogout). To confirm the diagnosis for patients with suspected acute calcific tendinitis, plain films are needed, which should show a large hydrated mass of calcium in or around the rotator cuff tendons (Fig. 49–7).

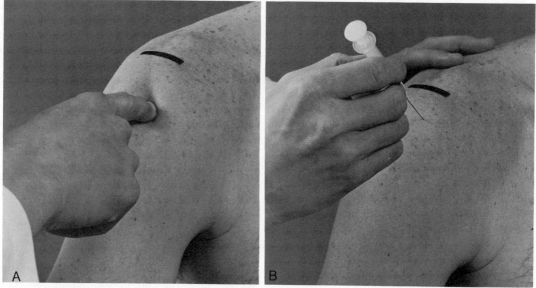

Figure 49–6. Photographs illustrating how to inject the subacromial region by the lateral approach. The black tape runs along the top of the acromion. A: Placing the tip of an index finger somewhat anterior to the midline 2 to 3 cm below the top of the acromion, one can feel the space between the acromion and the humeral head by passively abducting the humerus and feeling the finger tip dimple inward. B: At this spot one inserts a needle at approximately a 45° angle and injects just as the tip meets resistance after passing through the deltoid muscle.

Arthrography is indicated for any patient with a suspected acute major rotator cuff tear or for a patient with persistent pain related to rotator cuff tendinitis who is a candidate for orthopedic surgery. More recently, ultrasound study of the rotator cuff has been shown to be useful in detecting large rotator cuff tears and may replace arthrography in the future. An

arthrogram that shows contrast material passing from the glenohumeral space into the subacromial bursa is diagnostic of a complete tear that is either large or small.

In some centers, arthroscopy of the shoulder is being done more routinely and may be a valuable aid in the diagnosis of difficult cases of persistent shoulder pain. The arthroscope

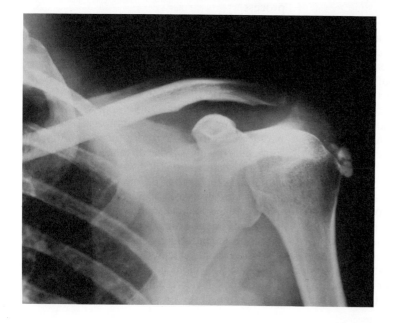

Figure 49–7. Plain radiograph demonstrating a large area of calcification in the region of the supraspinatus tendon. This finding is consistent with asymptomatic calcific periarthritis or symptomatic acute calcific tendinitis.

can be placed in both the glenohumeral joint and the subacromial space, which allows direct visualization of the rotator cuff, the glenoid cartilage, and the labrum.

Diagnosis and Treatment of Specific Shoulder Disorders

The most common causes of shoulder pain caused by disorders intrinsic to the shoulder and distant from the shoulder are given, respectively, in Tables 49–1 and 49–2. Although a discussion of all causes of shoulder pain is beyond the scope of this chapter, the clinical findings and treatment of the most common causes of shoulder pain are discussed.

Rotator Cuff Tendinitis (Impingement Syndrome, Supraspinatus Tendinitis, Subacromial Bursitis, Painful Arc Syndrome)

The term rotator cuff tendinitis includes a spectrum of pathologic findings ranging from mild inflammatory lesions in the rotator cuff tendons and in the overlying bursa to complete tears of the cuff. Younger individuals who stress their shoulders (e.g., swimmers, throwers, and heavy laborers) rarely tear the cuff but may traumatize it, which leads to an inflammatory response. Individuals over the age of 60 years frequently sustain minor tears in the critical zone of the cuff even after minimal stress, such as lifting a small load. Chronic stress to the shoulder caused by prior occupational or sporting activity appears to predispose to rotator cuff tendinitis. Most individuals with rotator cuff tendinitis, however, give no history of excessive shoulder use.

Patients generally present with significant shoulder discomfort often described as a dull or boring pain that has become maximal over a period of hours to days. Although patients frequently cannot recall a specific time or event associated with the onset of the pain, some do recall a minor stress, such as lifting or pulling with the shoulder just before the onset of pain. The location of the pain is highly variable, with more acute onset pain felt in and around the humeral head. Over time, the pain may move down the outer aspect of the arm to the midhumeral region, and long-standing pain may be felt as distally as the thumb. Some pain may radiate proximally at all stages. The pain is particularly bothersome at night, and

individuals have a difficult time sleeping on the affected shoulder.

The physical examination usually reveals no swelling, redness, or local heat. Atrophy of the deltoid or supraspinatus, if present, indicates rather long-standing dysfunction. Tenderness may be elicited either anteriorly over the lesser tuberosity, including the bicipital groove, or laterally over the greater tuberosity. The classic finding is a painful arc of abduction between approximately 40° to 120° with abnormal scapulothoracic rhythm (shrugging and tilting of the torso). The severity of abnormal motion varies from subtle shrugging of the shoulder with minimal pain to severe pain and inability to abduct beyond 60° to 80°. Internal rotation is frequently abnormal, with the patient unable to touch his or her sacral area or even the iliac crest without causing excruciating pain. External rotation is normal. The impingement sign is positive and correlates well with the severity of the abnormal arc of abduction.

Instillation of 8 or 9 ml of 1% lidocaine into the region of the subacromial bursa usually results in a dramatic reduction in pain after 10 minutes (greater than 50% reduction) and a modest to impressive improvement in the arc of abduction (generally greater than 20° to 30° improvement). Absolutely no improvement in pain or motion after lidocaine suggests a frozen shoulder or glenohumeral joint disease. Lidocaine relieves the pain of rotator cuff tendinitis for only several hours. However, the therapeutic efficacy of the injection may last significantly longer because the patient is reassured that the pain can be relieved and that motion can be improved.

Treatment of rotator cuff tendinitis consists of (1) the initial diagnostic lidocaine injection, (2) analgesic and anti-inflammatory therapy in the form of a potent nonsteroidal anti-inflammatory agent such as indomethacin 100 to 150 mg/day for at least 1 month, (3) avoidance of all activities that stress the shoulder, such as lifting or overhead work, and (4) range of motion exercises designed to maintain and gradually improve shoulder motion, which should be started immediately. The principal physical therapeutic exercises are (1) Codman's pendulum exercises, which are performed by asking the patient to bend forward and dangle the affected shoulder in gravity traction and swing the arm back and forth in the sagittal and frontal planes as far as possible without provoking intense pain, and (2) the finger-up-the-wall exercise, which involves slowly inching the arm up the wall until it is held at 180° abduction or the maximal height is reached, followed by slowly lowering the arm down using the wall as a friction pad, which functionally reduces the tension in the rotator cuff muscles. Referral to a physical therapist for local ultrasound therapy as well as closely supervised shoulder exercises, including use of pulleys, may speed the rate of resolution.

Approximately 60 to 70% of patients who are treated in this fashion improve significantly in 6 to 8 weeks. Injection of a long-acting corticosteroid preparation into the region of the rotator cuff tendons should be avoided because these preparations cause tendon degeneration and may increase the likelihood of eventual rupture. Subacromial instillation of aqueous dexamethasone 4 to 6 mg mixed with 2 ml of 1% lidocaine is a therapeutic option because it is safe and free of major side effects. Although there are no unequivocal data to show that use of dexamethasone hastens the healing process, if improvement is minimal at 4 weeks, such an injection is recommended and can be repeated 4 to 6 weeks later if clinically indicated.

Rotator cuff tendinitis that persists after 3 to 6 months of medical therapy and that causes the patient significant pain and/or dysfunction is an indication to make an orthopedic referral, if the patient is willing to consider surgery. Most orthopedic surgeons label the problem as chronic impingement. Options at this stage are (1) ordering an arthrogram to look for evidence of a complete rotator cuff tear, (2) moving directly to glenohumeral plus subacromial arthroscopy to visualize the entire shoulder and cuff, with arthroscopic debridement of cuff tears and arthroscopic decompression of the coricoacromial arch, or (3) open surgical exploration of the cuff with repair of a cuff tear and, if needed, acromioplasty and sectioning of the coricoacromial ligament. The decision to proceed with arthroscopic surgery versus an open procedure depends on the technical expertise and experience of the orthopedic surgeon. Although operative interventions generally result in a significant reduction in pain, motion may not always dramatically improve.

Rotator Cuff Tears

Clinical signs of a small tear are identical to those of rotator cuff tendinitis. Major rotator cuff tears are easy to diagnose. The patient gives a history of the abrupt onset of pain and weakness after using the shoulder. Active shoulder abduction is weak, with a markedly limited range of motion; after subacromial injection of 1% lidocaine, the passive range of motion may be improved but shoulder weakness remains, with most patients being unable to hold the arm at 90° abduction. A patient with an acute major rotator cuff tear should be referred immediately to an orthopedic surgeon for definitive surgical treatment.

Acute Calcific Tendinitis

For unclear reasons, a small percentage of individuals over the age of 25 years have the gradual build-up of a substantial amount of calcium hydroxyapatite in one of the rotator cuff tendons, usually in the critical zone. Often the process is bilateral, and joints other than the shoulder may be affected in a process termed calcific periarthritis. The majority of these individuals are asymptomatic and remain so for years. If modest shoulder trauma irritates the crystalline material, it may become hydrated and expand, with eventual rupture of the material into the overlying subacromial bursa. The clinical picture is striking and almost diagnostic. An otherwise asymptomatic person suddenly develops excruciating shoulder pain after minimal shoulder stress (e.g., gardening, lifting). The deltoid area becomes red, hot, and swollen, with marked local tenderness and with such severe pain that the arm is splinted to the side, with the patient reluctant to have the physician examine the shoulder. The picture may suggest an acute septic arthritis or septic bursitis. Plain radiographs taken with internal and external rotation views generally reveal a very large hydrated calcific mass in or near the rotator cuff tendons. The clinical picture plus the radiographic findings makes the diagnosis. Because hydroxyapatite crystals may be resorbed over several days to weeks, radiographs may be normal several weeks after the acute onset of pain.

Treatment of acute calcific tendinitis consists of giving adequate analgesia, which should include local subacromial injection of 8 ml of 1% lidocaine together with oral indomethacin 150 to 200 mg/day and additional analgesia with acetaminophen and codeine as needed. Pain on motion of the shoulder is so intense that this is one instance when short-term shoulder immobilization in a sling is indicated. Active physical therapy should commence only after the severe pain is controlled. Local injection of aqueous dexamethasone 4 to 6 mg mixed with 2 ml of 1% lidocaine is recommended in patients with clinically severe calcific tendinitis. Persistent symptoms may be an indication for attempting to "needle" the crystalline material by using ultrasound guidance. This may allow release of the crystalline material and more rapid resolution of the symptoms. Surgery is rarely if ever indicated. The long-term prognosis is excellent, with rare recurrence of these symptoms in the affected shoulder.

Bicipital Tendinitis

Inflammation limited to the biceps tendon is clinically quite rare. Most cases called bicipital tendinitis are actually rotator cuff tendinitis with involvement of the supraspinatus tendon *plus* the biceps or subscapularis tendon. In a few cases, all of the signs point to involvement of the long head of the biceps tendon only. Classically, patients who repetitively stress the shoulder (e.g., repeated pulling, tugging, throwing) may get anterior shoulder pain and tenderness over the bicipital groove. The range of motion is generally full, but there is often slightly abnormal scapulothoracic rhythm. Painful resisted flexion and painful resisted supination of the forearm (Yergason's sign) are usually present in patients with definite bicipital tendinitis. Anterior shoulder tenderness in and around the bicipital groove is a nonspecific finding.

Improvement in pain after local injection of 2 to 5 ml of 1% lidocaine into the cuff around the bicipital tendon helps to confirm the diagnosis. Treatment of bicipital tendinitis is similar to treatment of rotator cuff tendinitis. Local injection of a depocorticosteroid preparation should be avoided.

Frozen Shoulder

The term frozen shoulder, synonymous with adhesive capsulitis, is a disorder unique to the shoulder joint. The cause of the disorder is unknown, but it is seen after minor shoulder trauma, after prolonged immobilization, and after a stroke, and it is more common in patients with diabetes. Patients present with the subacute onset of mild to moderate shoulder pain and/or inability to use the shoulder

normally. The diagnosis can be made rapidly because the range of shoulder motion is severely restricted in all planes. Active abduction is usually no more than 40° and external rotation is limited to no more than 30°. When passively moving the shoulder, one senses that the limited motion is due to a tight or frozen shoulder and not to pain or reluctance of the patient to move the shoulder. The diagnostic step of injecting 8 ml of 1% lidocaine into the subacromial region results in minimal or no improvement in motion. Pathologically, the capsule becomes shrunken and fibrotic, and this limits shoulder motion. Therapeutically, one must stretch the capsule (by using aggressive physical therapy) or tear the capsule physically by using either a surgical approach or injection of a large quantity of fluid into the glenohumeral joint under pressure (brisement). The natural history of frozen shoulder is for the joint to "thaw" in approximately 2 years. Injection of a local corticosteroid preparation into the subacromial bursa or glenohumeral joint provides no benefit.

Other Conditions

Other shoulder disorders that are occasionally seen and that deserve comment are reflex sympathetic dystrophy and brachial neuritis.

Reflex sympathetic dystrophy is a rare disorder that presents as frozen shoulder *plus* pain and often tenderness distally in the forearm and hand, signs or symptoms of vasomotor instability in the hand, swelling of the hand with dystrophic skin changes, and, radiographically, extensive osteopenia in the extremity. Although the cause is unknown, neuroregulatory dysfunction of the autonomic nervous system is thought to play a role. Early in the course of reflex sympathetic dystrophy, a burst and taper of corticosteroid therapy (prednisone 60 mg/day tapering over 4 to 6 weeks) may be beneficial.

Brachial neuritis is an uncommon but interesting disorder that affects men and women of all ages. It is thought to be a postviral or immune-mediated process. Various portions of the brachial plexus can be involved, with a resultant spectrum of findings, including pain, weakness, and sensory loss in the involved extremity. Pain can be sudden and intense, with weakness developing over days. The active range of motion reflects the region of the plexus involved. Commonly there is winging of the scapula (long thoracic nerve) and supraspinatus or infraspinatus weakness. The passive range of motion is normal and does not provoke pain. The prognosis is generally good, with pain subsiding and patients beginning to recover strength in weeks to months. Ninety percent of patients recover completely during a 3-year period.

Bibliography

Bland JH, Merrit JA, Boushey DR. The painful shoulder. Semin Arthritis Rheum 7:21–47, 1977.
  A long but well-written summary of the topic of shoulder pain.
Bulgen DY, Binder AI, Hazleman BL, et al. Frozen shoulder: prospective clinical study with an evaluation of three treatment regimens. Ann Rheum Dis 43:353–360, 1984.
  An article focusing entirely on the natural history and treatment of frozen shoulder.
Halpern AA, Horowitz BG, Nagel DA. Tendon ruptures associated with corticosteroid therapy. West J Med 127:378–387, 1977.
  One of numerous articles showing the hazards associated with injecting a long-acting corticosteroid next to or into tendons.
Kessel L, Watson M. The painful arc syndrome. J Bone Joint Surg 59B:166–172, 1977.
  Outline of the approach of two highly respected orthopedic surgeons toward diagnosing and managing rotator cuff tendinitis.
Kozin F, Ryan LM, Carerra GT, et al. The reflex sympathetic dystrophy syndrome (RSDS). Am J Med 70:23–30, 1981.
  A well-written article that discusses the diagnosis and management of reflex sympathetic dystrophy syndrome, with extensive reference list.
Master R, Weisman MH, Armbuster TG, et al. Septic arthritis of the glenohumeral joint. Arthritis Rheum 20:1500–1506, 1977.
  A good discussion of septic arthritis in the shoulder joint.
Neer CS. Anterior acromioplasty for the chronic impingement syndrome in the shoulder. J Bone Joint Surg 54A:41–50, 1972.
  The first description of the now standard surgical approach to decompress the coracoacromial arch in patients with long-standing rotator cuff tendinitis.
Neer CS. Impingement lesions. Clin Orthop 173:70–77, 1983.
  A review of rotator cuff tendinitis by a premier orthopedic surgeon.
Neviaser RJ (ed). Management of shoulder problems. Orthop Clin North Am 18:343–487, 1987.
  A good overview of shoulder problems from the orthopedic perspective.
Resnick D. Shoulder pain. Orthop Clin North Am 14:81–97, 1982.
  Discussion by a world renowned bone radiologist of shoulder pain and associated radiographic findings.
Simon WH. Soft tissue disorders of the shoulder. Orthop Clin North Am 6:521–539, 1975.
  A detailed discussion of acute calcific tendinitis and bicipital tendinitis included.
Tsairis P, Kych PJ, Mulder DW. Natural history of brachial plexus neuropathy: report on 99 patients. Arch Neurol 17:109–117, 1972.
  A classic discussion of brachial plexus neuritis.
White RH. The painful shoulder, In Leek JL, Gershwin ME, Fowler WM (eds). Principles of Physical Medicine and Rehabilitation in the Musculoskeletal Diseases. Orlando, FL, Grune & Stratton, 1986, pp 335–367.
  Extensive discussion of the causes and treatment of shoulder pain by the author of this chapter.
White RH, Paull DM, Fleming KW. Rotator cuff tendinitis: comparison of subacromial injection of a long-acting corticosteroid versus oral indomethacin therapy. J Rheum 13:608–613, 1986.
  A study showing no short-term advantage of a corticosteroid injection into the subacromial region for treatment of rotator cuff tendinitis.

50

Renal Complications of Anti-Inflammatory Therapy

DAVID M. CLIVE, M.D.

Introduction

In 1977, Kimberly and coworkers reported the occurrence of acute renal insufficiency in patients with lupus erythematosus who were receiving aspirin. Shortly thereafter, they observed similar phenomena in patients treated with other nonsteroidal anti-inflammatory drugs (NSAIDs). In the decade that followed, a variety of untoward renal responses to NSAIDs have been documented. Today, these compounds are recognized as an important cause of iatrogenic renal disease; this is hardly surprising considering the enormous consumption of NSAIDs in the Western world.

A large number of NSAID products are currently in common use (Table 50–1). All of the NSAID-related renal disorders reflect the effects of these drugs on the metabolism of prostaglandins. This family of biologically active lipids was first described more than 30 years ago. More recently, science has begun to gain an understanding of their biochemistry and physiology. Several generalizations can be made about prostaglandin physiology: (1) their pharmacologic half-lives are short; (2) they are not stored but rather are synthesized on demand; (3) they function as autacoids, i.e., their action is exerted at the site of synthesis. There is little evidence that they circulate to other sites of action.

Prostaglandins are synthesized from a fatty acid precursor, arachidonic acid. The central step in their biosynthesis is catalyzed by the enzyme cyclo-oxygenase. Arachidonic acid can be metabolized along other pathways as well; collectively, the prostaglandins and other derivatives of arachidonic acid are referred to as eicosanoids or arachidonates.

Although prostaglandin synthesis occurs in virtually every cell in the body, the kidney is an especially active site of production. A variety of physiologic actions have been defined for renal prostaglandins including (1) vasodilation, (2) modulation of tubular ion transport, (3) stimulation of renin release, and (4) modulation of water reabsorption. Studies with animals have proved the ability of cyclo-oxygenase–inhibiting drugs to impair these functions.

The renal side effects of NSAIDs comprise a series of well-recognized syndromes that include (1) acute renal failure, (2) acute interstitial nephritis often accompanied by proteinuria, (3) sodium retention with edema and impaired responsiveness to diuretic and antihypertensive therapy, (4) hyperkalemia, and (5) water retention. The actual incidence of renal side effects of NSAID therapy is unknown. Estimates based on retrospective analyses of hospitalized populations are variable. It is hoped that prospective data will accrue and shed further light on this issue in the near future. In the meantime, clinicians must recognize the factors that place particular patients at increased risk of these reactions. In the following sections, each of these reactions is considered.

Acute Renal Failure

Hemodynamic Type

Inhibition of cyclo-oxygenase is the major pharmacologic effect of NSAIDs. Numerous studies with humans and animals have shown that intact organisms challenged with cyclo-oxygenase–inhibiting drugs experience no adverse effects on renal physiology. This suggests that under normal circumstances the mammalian kidney is not dependent on prostaglandin availability for maintenance of function. However, when NSAIDs are administered to animals in the setting of reduced cardiac output, hypovolemia, or hypotensive hemorrhage, significant reductions in renal blood flow and glomerular filtration rate may be demonstrated. In humans, too, most reported instances of NSAID-associated renal disease have occurred in patients with heart failure, cirrhosis, or volume depletion. These patients ordinarily have a degree of prerenal azotemia. Their susceptibility to further reduction in renal function when exposed to NSAIDs is likely related to contraction of the effective circulatory volume, which leads to the release of vasoconstrictor hormones (i.e., the renin-angiotensin and catecholamine systems). These hormones maintain systemic arterial perfusion pressure but could threaten renal blood flow by raising renovascular resistance. Locally produced vasodilatory renal prostaglandins regulate against these constrictor substances, thus helping to maintain renal function in these states (Fig. 50–1).

As Kimberly's studies of patients with lupus erythematosus have revealed, giving NSAIDs to patients with chronic parenchymal renal disease may also have adverse effects on renal hemodynamics, even though the systemic circulation may be normal. The acute decline in renal function engendered by nonsteroidals agents is likely a consequence of the imbalance in the relative activities of vasodilator and vasoconstrictor substances at the level of the glomerular arterioles, which occurs when prostaglandin synthesis is suppressed.

In the above-mentioned forms of acute renal failure, the effect of NSAIDs is to cause alterations in the renal microcirculation rather than to exert direct cytotoxic actions. Prostaglandins are not stored but rather are synthesized on demand at their site of action. Their biologic half-life in vivo is short. Therefore, prostaglandin depletion rapidly ensues when their synthesis is interrupted. Reduction of renal function probably occurs within hours of NSAID administration to patients dependent on prostaglandins for maintenance of optimal renal hemodynamics.

A renal biopsy in affected patients would be expected to show no specific lesion because acute renal failure is essentially prerenal in etiology. If renal ischemia is severe or prolonged, changes consistent with acute tubular necrosis may occur. In most cases, as is typical of hemodynamically mediated phenomena, the syndrome is rapid in onset after exposure to the drug, and resolution occurs within days of drug withdrawal.

Nonhemodynamic Types

Many NSAIDs, like the prototypic compound aspirin, are uricosuric. In rare cases, the presentation of copious amounts of uric acid to the distal nephron leads to transient oligoanuric renal failure from tubular obstruction, a situation analogous to the nephropathy caused by acute uric acid blockade occasionally

Table 50–1. NSAIDs Commonly Used in the United States as of 1987

Drug Family	Generic Name	Trade Name
Salicylates	Aspirin	
	Choline magnesium trisalicylate	Trilisate
	Salsalate	Disalcid
	Diflunisal	Dolobid
	Choline salicylate	Arthropan
	Sodium salicylate	Pabalate
Propionic acids	Ibuprofen	Motrin, Advil, Nuprin
	Naproxen	Naprosyn, Anaprox
	Fenoprofen calcium	Nalfon
	Suprofen	Suprol*
Indoleacetic acids	Indomethacin	Indocin
	Sulindac	Clinoril
	Tolmetin sodium	Tolectin
	Zomepirac sodium	Zomax*
Anthranilic acids	Meclofenamate	Meclomen
	Mefenamic acid	Ponstel
Pyrazolones	Phenylbutazone	Butazolidin
Oxicams	Piroxicam	Feldene

*No longer distributed.

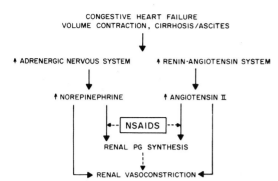

Figure 50–1. *Prostaglandins counter-regulate the vasoconstrictor actions of pressor hormones on the kidney. NSAIDs prevent this compensatory mechanism. Reprinted with permission from The New England Journal of Medicine (310;563–572, 1984).*

seen in patients after induction chemotherapy for hematologic malignancy. This complication was originally reported in association with phenylbutazone more than 30 years ago. With the newer NSAID suprofen, acute uric acid nephropathy occurred with sufficient frequency to lead to removal of the drug from the market. Fortunately this complication is rare enough in patients receiving other NSAIDs, including phenylbutazone, that such measures as allopurinol prophylaxis and urinary alkalinization are unnecessary.

Acute renal failure can also occur in the NSAID user as part of a syndrome of acute interstitial nephritis. This rare disorder varies in two important ways from the classic allergic-type interstitial nephritis seen, for example, in penicillin-treated patients. (1) Eosinophils are not prominent in the urinary sediment, peripheral blood, or cellular infiltrate in the kidney. Rather, the cellular infiltrate is composed of T-lymphocytes. (2) Patients with this disorder are likely to have nephrotic proteinuria, a remarkable feature because the pathologic changes in the kidney are predominantly in the interstitium rather than the glomerulus, which manifests a minimal change lesion (i.e., foot process fusion only).

NSAID-induced interstitial nephritis is more idiosyncratic than other NSAID-related renal syndromes, i.e., its risk factors are more obscure. It occurs in association with a number of the agents, most often fenoprofen. Its pathogenesis is poorly understood but probably revolves around suppression of prostaglandin synthesis. It is thought that inhibition of cyclooxygenase causes shunting of arachidonic acid into alternative metabolic pathways, particu-

larly the lipoxygenase system. Some products of this enzyme are lymphokines; others increase capillary permeability. Thus, the alteration by NSAIDs of renal eicosanoid balance may explain both the lymphocytic infiltrate and the proteinuria.

The course of NSAID-induced interstitial nephritis resembles that of the other form of drug-related acute interstitial disease in its variability. The time of drug exposure preceding the appearance of the syndrome may range from days to months. Similarly, the time from withdrawal of the agent to resolution of symptoms may vary considerably, although most patients get better within weeks. The efficacy of steroids in shortening the course of the disease has never been proved in a controlled fashion, probably because the syndrome is so rare as to prohibit a meaningful trial.

Course and Prognosis of NSAID-Related Acute Renal Failure Syndromes

It may be quite difficult to establish which of the above processes is responsible for acute renal failure in a patient receiving NSAID therapy. Hemodynamically mediated renal dysfunction is the most common of the syndromes discussed above. The risk factors for development of this disorder include cirrhosis, congestive heart failure, and chronic renal insufficiency. Patients with these diagnoses should be closely monitored (i.e., blood chemistry should be analyzed every few weeks) for the duration of NSAID exposure. Nephrotic range proteinuria suggests the occurrence of acute interstitial nephritis in azotemic patients receiving anti-inflammatory drugs. Fulminant onset, oligoanuria, and bilateral flank pain are features suggestive of uric acid crystal nephropathy.

Regardless of which mechanism is responsible, when a patient develops acute renal failure while receiving NSAIDs, the most important therapeutic maneuver is immediate discontinuation of the drug. No specific recommendations can be made regarding fluid therapy; because of the antinatriuretic effects of NSAIDs (see later sections), many patients are overloaded with fluid at the time of presentation with azotemia. Diuretics may be of use in this setting. Other patients may be volume depleted and benefit from the administration of isotonic fluids. In patients with profound renal failure or a particularly protracted course of the illness, interim dialysis may be indicated.

NSAIDs as a Cause of Chronic Renal Disease

A controversial issue is whether NSAIDs can produce chronic renal injury, especially when taken over a long period. Analgesic nephropathy remains an important worldwide cause of chronic renal disease in the 1980's. There is no doubt that the most culpable analgesic agent is phenacetin. Some authors, however, believe that aspirin may enhance phenacetin-induced injury, and others have speculated that aspirin by itself can produce the characteristic lesions of chronic interstitial nephritis and papillary necrosis. Cyclo-oxygenase–inhibiting drugs may induce papillary necrosis because they are known to induce ischemia of the renal medulla. In experimental models, a sustained period of medullary ischemia can be shown to lead to necrosis of the renal papilla.

There are a number of accounts in the literature of patients receiving long-term therapy with NSAIDs, including ibuprofen, indomethacin, and mefenamic acid, who developed chronic renal disease. Mefenamic acid appears to be the agent most often implicated. From these reports, it is impossible to determine the magnitude of the risk of irreversible renal damage from NSAIDs. The number of reports of papillary necrosis in NSAID users is certainly minuscule compared with the large number of patients receiving long-term therapy with these drugs for chronic rheumatologic disease. Furthermore, we know of no conclusive evidence that NSAID therapy has ever led to end-stage renal disease. The most prudent approach would still be to limit periods of NSAID exposure to the shortest possible course needed for the desired therapeutic result.

Sodium Retention, Edema, and Hypertension

The most common renal side effect of NSAID use is sodium retention, which occurs in up to 25% of patients regardless of other risk factors. Many patients with no underlying renal or circulatory disease may develop mild edema when given these agents. In normal individuals, prostaglandins exert natriuretic effects. Logically, removing these effects by suppressing prostaglandin synthesis would be expected to cause sodium retention. In individuals dependent on intact prostaglandin synthesis for the maintenance of normal glomerular filtration rate and renal blood flow (e.g., in cirrhosis or heart failure), NSAIDs can further reduce sodium excretion by lowering the filtered load of sodium. Patients in this category have been reported to suffer severe fluid overload within days of starting treatment with NSAIDs.

The natriuretic and vasodilatory actions of prostaglandins have led some investigators to postulate a pathogenetic link between prostaglandin deficiency and hypertension. Although there is no substantive evidence that NSAIDs can induce hypertension in normotensive people, it has been established that they mitigate the therapeutic efficacy of antihypertensive drugs including beta blockers, thiazide and loop diuretics, captopril, and prazosin.

In cases of severe sodium retention caused by NSAIDs or of exacerbation of underlying hypertension, judicious therapy begins with discontinuing the drug. Dietary sodium restriction and diuretics may have a role in accelerating the reversal of the untoward effects.

NSAID-Related Hyperkalemia

Hyperkalemia is a well-described phenomenon in NSAID-treated patients. In one study it occurred in 46% of hospitalized patients receiving indomethacin. In general, patients at risk for this complication have predisposing factors, usually chronic renal insufficiency. Although NSAIDs may decrease the glomerular filtration rate in such patients, the degree of hyperkalemia exceeds that expected on this basis alone, i.e., the reduction in filtered load of potassium cannot entirely account for the severe hyperkalemia. In these patients, a direct tubular effect of NSAIDs must be operative.

The currently favored hypothesis concerning the pathophysiology of NSAID-induced hyperkalemia centers on the ability of these drugs to suppress renin release. Prostaglandins are potent stimulators of renin release; drugs that inhibit prostaglandin biosynthesis markedly reduce plasma renin activity even in normal individuals. The reduction in plasma renin in turn lowers angiotensin II production, thus removing a stimulus for aldosterone synthesis. The usual clinical picture in patients with NSAID-induced hyperkalemia is similar to that of other forms of hyporeninemic hypoaldosteronism; a mild metabolic acidosis (type IV renal tubular acidosis) may be present. It is of note that prostaglandin deficiency has been observed in patients with spontaneously occurring hyporeninemic hypoaldosteronism.

Hyponatremia Related to NSAIDs

Prostaglandins normally promote free water excretion by counter-regulating the effects of antidiuretic hormone on the collecting tubule. NSAIDs impair water diuresis in normal individuals, although water retention great enough to cause hyponatremia occurs only in individuals with pre-existing impairments of water

excretion, e.g., patients with renal insufficiency, heart failure, volume contraction, diuretic therapy, and cirrhosis. Water restriction (750 to 1500 ml/day depending on the degree of hyponatremia) for several days after the withdrawal of the NSAID accelerates return of the serum sodium concentration to normal.

Therapeutic Implications

Virtually all the renal, fluid, and electrolyte disorders occurring with NSAID use appear attributable to the ability of these agents to suppress prostaglandin synthesis. With rare exceptions, only individuals with underlying renal disease or abnormal systemic hemody-

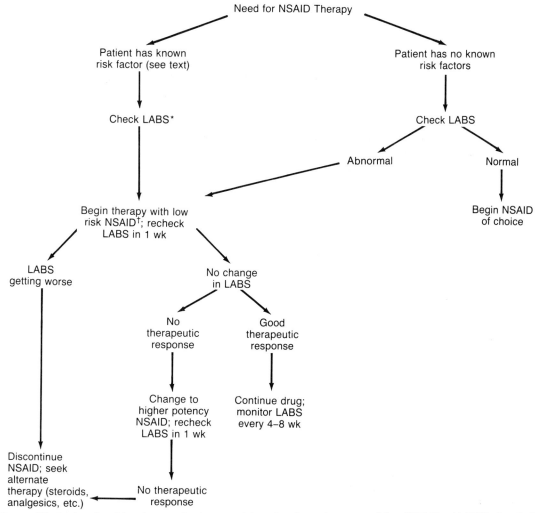

Figure 50–2. An algorithm for monitoring renal function in patients receiving NSAIDs. *LABS stands for blood urea nitrogen, creatinine and electrolyte tests, and urinalysis. †Low risk NSAIDs include sulindac or nonacetylated salicylates. Note: This algorithm represents a general set of guidelines. Drug therapy must always be individualized to suit the particular needs of each patient.

Table 50–2. NSAIDs with Data for Dose Adjustment in Special Patient Groups

Drug	Dose Adjustment
Elderly	
Etodolac	None
Ibuprofen	None
Ketoprofen	Half of normal dose or less
Naproxen	Half of normal dose
Oxaprozin	Half of normal dose
Piroxicam	Uncertain (probably none)
Cirrhosis	
Azapropazone	Mild: half of normal dose
	Severe: avoid
Carprofen	Uncertain
Ibuprofen	Uncertain
Naproxen	Half of normal dose
Sulindac	One fourth of normal dose
Renal insufficiency	
Azapropazone	Mild: half of normal dose
	Moderate: one fifth of normal dose
	Severe: one tenth of normal dose
Diclofenac	None
Diflunisal	None
Etodolac	None
Naproxen	Half of normal dose
Oxaprozin	Half of normal dose

From Brater DC. Am J Med 80(1A):62–77, 1986, with permission.

namics are at risk. The most important therapeutic maneuver in any of the above syndromes is to stop the rise of the NSAID. Because pharmacologic suppression of renal prostaglandin synthesis is generally short-lived, recovery from these syndromes may be complete within a few days after drug withdrawal. In acute renal failure resulting from NSAID-related interstitial nephritis, or in cases of hemodynamically mediated renal failure where renal ischemia is severe enough to cause acute tubular necrosis, the course may be more protracted, and interim dialytic support is occasionally required.

NSAIDs should be used with extreme caution in patients with the following risk factors:

1. Volume contraction (e.g., dehydration, diuretic use)

2. Congestive heart failure

3. Hepatic cirrhosis

4. Any form of chronic renal parenchymal disease

5. Hypertension

6. Previously documented fluid or electrolyte abnormalities (e.g., hyponatremia or hyperkalemia)

7. Age greater than 65 years

In these settings, patients should be monitored clinically and with blood chemistry tests for the duration of drug therapy. In addition, having the patient keep a daily record of body weight may provide an early warning of fluid retention. A suggested scheme for following renal function in patients given NSAIDs is shown in Figure 50–2. Clinicians should recall that ibuprofen is now available in several over-the-counter preparations and must advise high-risk patients against taking these without supervision.

For patients with these risk factors who have strong indications for anti-inflammatory drug therapy, there is some evidence to suggest that the safest agents may be sulindac and the newer nonacetylated salicylate compounds such as choline magnesium trisalicylate or salsalate, although these compounds may not always be the most therapeutically effective from a rheumatologic standpoint. They must not be considered unconditionally harmless, and the same guidelines for monitoring therapy should be applied.

Pharmacokinetics of some NSAIDs are altered in liver disease, renal insufficiency, or old age. Suggested dosage modifications for these situations are shown in Table 50–2.

Bibliography

Carmichael J, Shankel SW. Effects of nonsteroidal anti-inflammatory drugs on prostaglandins and renal function. Am J Med 78:992–1000, 1985.
This good review of data collected from the literature delineates epidemiologic aspects of the various syndromes.

Ciabattoni G, Cinotti G, Pierucci A, et al. Effects of sulindac and ibuprofen in patients with chronic glomerular disease. N Engl J Med 310:279–283, 1984.
Effects of NSAIDs on kidneys of patients with chronic glomerulonephritis and lupus nephritis are studied in depth. Authors characterize the relative extent to which NSAIDs alter vasoconstrictor and vasodilatory prostaglandins in these patients.

Clive DM, Stoff JS. Renal syndromes associated with nonsteroidal anti-inflammatory drugs. N Engl J Med 310:563–572, 1984.
This review defines each of the NSAID-related renal syndromes, with a concentration on pathophysiology.

Favre L, Glasson PH, Riondel A, et al. Interaction of diuretics and non-steroidal anti-inflammatory drugs in man. Clin Sci 64:407–415, 1983.
This article demonstrates how NSAIDs can blunt the natriuretic effect of diuretics.

Favre L, Glasson P, Vallotton MS. Reversible acute renal failure from combined triamterene and indomethacin. A study in healthy subjects. Ann Intern Med 96:317–320, 1982.
This article makes the same point as that of Muther et al. In this case diuretic-treated normal individuals had marked reductions in glomerular filtration rate when given indomethacin.

Finkelstein A, Fraley DS, Stachura I, et al. Fenoprofen nephropathy: lipoid nephrosis and interstitial nephritis:

a possible T-lymphocyte disorder. Am J Med 72:81–87, 1982.

This is a good clinical report of the interstitial nephritis-lipoid nephrosis syndrome with speculations about its immunopathogenesis.

Garella S, Matarese RA. Renal effects of prostaglandins and clinical adverse effects of nonsteroidal anti-inflammatory agents. Medicine 63:165–181, 1984.

This is a broad review of the NSAID-induced renal disorders with extensive analysis of clinical data culled from case reports.

Kimberly RP, Gill JR Jr, Bowden RE, et al. Elevated urinary prostaglandins and the effects of aspirin on renal function in lupus erythematosus. Ann Intern Med 89:336–341, 1978.

Adverse effects of NSAID on kidneys of patients with lupus are reported.

Muther RS, Potter DM, Bennet WM. Aspirin-induced depression of glomerular filtration rate in normal humans: role of sodium balance. Ann Intern Med 94:317–321, 1981.

This report demonstrates that NSAIDs have no effect on normal kidneys but can induce significant changes in renal function after dietary sodium restriction.

Stoff JS. Prostaglandins and hypertension. Am J Med 80(1A):56–61, 1986.

Relationship of prostaglandin metabolism to development of hypertension and mechanisms by which NSAIDs may interfere with antihypertensive therapy are reviewed.

Tan SY, Shapiro R, Franco R, et al. Indomethacin-induced prostaglandin inhibition with hyperkalemia. A reversible cause of hyporeninemic hypoaldosteronism. Ann Intern Med 90:783–785, 1979.

This clinical metabolic study documents induction by indomethacin of hyporeninemic hypoaldosteronism in a young woman with chronic renal disease.

Walshe JJ, Venuto RC. Acute oliguric renal failure induced by indomethacin: possible mechanism. Ann Intern Med 91:47–49, 1979.

This important case report illustrates how indomethacin may cause renal decompensation in the setting of severe heart failure.

Zimran A, Kramer M, Plaskin M, et al. Incidence of hyperkalaemia induced by indomethacin in a hospital population. Br Med J 291:107–108, 1985.

In this prospective study of 50 hospitalized patients receiving indomethacin, hyperkalemia was observed in 23 patients.

51

Gastrointestinal Complications of Nonsteroidal Anti-Inflammatory Agents

KEVIN SOMERVILLE, M.B., F.R.A.C.P.

The widespread use of nonsteroidal anti-inflammatory drugs (NSAIDs), both over the counter and by prescription, presumably is a tribute to their usefulness. However, concern and controversy are increasing about the frequency and clinical importance of a variety of adverse gastrointestinal effects possibly induced by these agents.

For two decades, animal and human studies have consistently demonstrated that short-term administration of NSAIDs may induce gastroduodenal erosions and increase fecal occult blood loss. Although these agents also cause dyspepsia in about 10 to 20% of patients, there is a poor correlation of upper gastrointestinal symptoms with visible mucosal abnormalities; 20% of patients with NSAID-induced dyspepsia have normal endoscopic examinations, and one half or more of patients with gastroduodenal erosions are asymptomatic. On the basis of these experimental studies and from clinical impressions, NSAIDs are believed by many physicians to cause and/or exacerbate chronic peptic ulcer and its associated complications of upper gastrointestinal bleeding (UGIB) and perforation. Recent case studies also suggest that NSAIDs may predispose patients to peptic esophageal strictures and to inflammation, hemorrhage, and perforation of the small and large bowels. Some NSAIDs (e.g., the controlled-release indomethacin preparation Osmosin, in Britain) have been withdrawn from the market because of the purported gastrointestinal adverse drug reactions (ADRs). However, the scientific evidence linking NSAIDs to clinically significant gastrointestinal ADRs is scanty and contradictory. Many rheumatologists, whose patients are proportionally the

heaviest users of these agents, remain unimpressed by their gastrointestinal toxicity. These discrepant viewpoints and the reasons for them are reviewed in this chapter, along with current clinical implications for primary care physicians.

NSAIDs and Peptic Ulcer Disease

Several types of evidence, including epidemiologic observations, experimental data, and observational studies, have linked the use of NSAIDs with chronic peptic ulcer disease and its complications.

Epidemiologic Observations

Despite an almost linear increase in NSAID prescriptions during the last 25 years, hospital admission and mortality rates for peptic ulcer disease have declined in Britain and the United States during the same period. However, this is due primarily to a steep decline in hospital admissions among persons under age 65 years; hospital admission rates and mortality from ulcer perforation have remained stable in elderly men and have more than doubled in elderly women. Although the numbers of prescriptions for NSAIDs have increased in younger age groups, a more impressive increment has occurred among the elderly, who are the heaviest users of these agents. On average, each person aged 65 years and older in Britain received one NSAID prescription in 1985. It is thus tempting to speculate that this differential trend in peptic ulcer mortality between the age groups may in part reflect different NSAID use. However, to confirm a causative role for NSAIDs in chronic peptic ulcer disease, we must refer to experimental and observational studies.

Experimental Studies

Short-term administration of either aspirin or nonaspirin NSAIDs (NANSAIDs) to animals and humans induces gastric erosions and microscopic bleeding in a significant proportion of subjects. With continued dosing for more than 24 hours, the gastric mucosa somehow adapts and the extent and pattern of injury decline. The available evidence suggests that NSAIDs cause such damage predominantly by impairment of mucosal defense mechanisms, reducing the mucous–bicarbonate acid defense barrier and possibly increasing the permeability of the gastric mucosa to acid. The mechanism for NSAID toxicity probably involves a reduction of mucosal prostaglandin synthesis, although direct topical irritancy occurs with salicylates and possibly also with indomethacin.

There is no experimental evidence, however, that NSAID-induced gastric erosions progress to chronic peptic ulcer or clinically important gastrointestinal hemorrhage. Caruso and Bianchi-Porro administered NSAIDs (and corticosteroids) to 249 patients with arthritis of various types. During a 1-year follow-up period, 31% of the patients developed endoscopically confirmed gastroduodenal lesions. However, only two patients developed new chronic ulcers, and 46% of patients with a prior history of peptic ulcer had a recurrence. These figures are not significantly different from those expected for patients not taking NSAIDs. Unfortunately, because of their poor ability to detect important but infrequent adverse events, experimental studies of this type do not definitively rule out a causative role for NSAID therapy in chronic peptic ulcer disease.

Observational Studies

Observational studies have the potential to discover a possible association between NSAIDs and chronic peptic ulcer disease, but such studies are frequently marred by spurious association, confounding, and bias. Several case series have demonstrated that a high proportion of patients hospitalized with a hem-

orrhage or perforation from peptic ulcer were users of NSAIDs. These case series may be misleading because of the lack of appropriate matched controls and the use of retrospective reviews of case notes for the identification of drug exposure (a source of bias because of the widely believed ulcer-NSAID association). Spontaneous ADR reports also may not accurately reflect the gastrointestinal toxicity of these agents. Such reporting seems dependent on whim and fashion, as evidenced by the recent increase in ADR reports for all drugs since 1982 and the tendency of such reports to follow a pattern, with a consistent rise in report rates to a peak 2 to 3 years after drug release, followed by a marked decline over the subsequent 3 years.

The most productive observational approaches are case-control and historical cohort studies. The latter studies arise from planned drug surveillance studies such as the Boston Collaborative Drug Surveillance Program. During the past few years, several investigations of these types have attempted to determine whether NSAIDs are associated with chronic peptic ulcer and UGIB.

Aspirin

Chronic, heavy aspirin intake has a consistent relationship with gastric ulcer and UGIB. The Boston Collaborative Drug Surveillance Program found a link between heavy (at least four aspirin tablets per week for 12 weeks) aspirin use and gastric ulcer; there was no association with lighter aspirin use, nor was there a correlation between aspirin use and duodenal ulcer. Case-control studies from Australia, a country where women are renowned for their analgesic intake, show similar results. Our case-control study from Nottingham, Britain, found a link between aspirin use in the preceding week and both gastric and duodenal ulceration, although the association was not strong.

Estimates of the strength of the association of aspirin and UGIB are variable. The Boston Collaborative Drug Surveillance group found that chronic heavy aspirin use increased the risk of acute UGIB from gastritis and gastric ulcer by 15 per 100,000 regular users each year. There is an association of short-term, casual use of aspirin to acute UGIB, but the relationship is probably not always causal. In another Nottingham study of patients admitted with UGIB, only one third of aspirin intake could be linked to UGIB. The remainder could be accounted for by reference to a control group or to aspirin used to treat simultaneously occurring gastrointestinal symptoms. Although the risk of UGIB to an individual user is low, the extensive over-the-counter use of aspirin may result in a substantial number of hospital admissions.

Nonaspirin NSAIDs

The data sets relating NANSAIDs to peptic ulcer and its complications are more contradictory. The most convincing association between NANSAID use and chronic peptic ulcer disease has been shown in our Nottingham case-control study. Patients over age 60 years hospitalized during a defined period with UGIB from peptic ulceration and their matched hospital and community controls were questioned about antecedent drug use. The 230 patients with UGIB were two to four times more likely to have been NANSAID users than their matched controls; if aspirin use was included, the relative risks and 95% confidence limits were not significantly changed at 3.5 (2.5 to 5.4) and 3.3 (2.2 to 5.2), respectively. Assuming causality and considering the background use of NANSAIDs in the community at risk, it was estimated that NANSAIDs could be responsible for a quarter of bleeding peptic ulcer admissions in the age group over 60 years. Because community use of NANSAIDs is so extensive (15% of community controls in this study had used an NANSAID in the preceding week), the absolute risk of UGIB to an individual user is small, e.g., probably one patient with UGIB from more than 25,000 patients exposed to an NANSAID in any 1 week.

A recent report from the University of Pennsylvania analyzing Medicaid data shows a significant but lesser relative risk of 1.5 (95% confidence interval of 1.2 to 2.0) for UGIB within 30 days after filling the NANSAID prescription. The risk appeared to increase with duration of therapy and dose of NANSAID. This association persisted when potential confounding by other factors (e.g., age, gender) was allowed for. These investigators estimated that only 4% of the UGIB could be attributed to NANSAIDs.

An earlier case-control study from Britain by Collier and Payne found an association of NANSAIDs with ulcer perforation. In a consecutive series of 168 elderly patients with perforated ulcers, 48% were NANSAID users compared with 7% of a surgical control group. The estimated relative risk of ulcer perforation for NANSAID users was 11! This figure is probably exaggerated by the use of retrospective case note review, in which the patients were more likely to be closely questioned about NANSAID use than were the controls. In addition, use of NANSAIDs by the control group was less than one half that found in other community-based surveys.

A contrary view of the relationship between NANSAIDs and peptic ulceration arises from two investigations carried out by the Group Health Cooperative of Puget Sound. In one study, they found that elderly persons who collected a prescription for NANSAIDs within the previous 90 days were no more likely to be admitted with UGIB than those who did not obtain such a prescription. Admission rates were 4.8 and 3.4 per million person-days for NANSAID prescription presenters and non-presenters, respectively. Although this difference is small and thought by the investigators to be "incompatible" with an important increase in risk, the data presented do not definitively exclude a two-fold increase in relative risk. The Group Health Cooperative also found that peptic ulcer perforation was no more frequent in the cohort prescribed NANSAIDs than in the subjects who were not prescribed these agents; the relative risk ratio for the NANSAID group was 1.2 (95% confidence limits of 0.8 to 2.8). However, although there was no further breakdown by age with regard to NANSAID use, the proportion of patients admitted with perforations who were prescription recipients (6 of 48 or 12.5%) is markedly lower than that in other series. Furthermore, when short-term use of less than 1 year was considered in this study, the relative risk ratio was higher at 2.6, with wide 95% confidence limits (0.86 to 8.1).

NANSAIDs and Ulcer Healing

There are studies showing reduced numbers of erosions or microbleeding with NSAIDs if subjects are concurrently administered H_2 receptor antagonists or prostaglandins such as misoprostol. On occasion, endoscopically observed erosions are mislabeled as ulcers, and inferences are drawn as to the prevention and healing of chronic active ulcers by such agents. The assumption that a reduction of erosions would parallel a reduction of chronic ulcer complications is not necessarily valid.

A recent Danish trial compared peptic ulcer healing rates in patients randomized to continue or discontinue NANSAID therapy. Of 62 patients (treated with either ranitidine or sucralfate), 23 of 30 (77%) who continued NANSAIDs had their ulcers heal compared with 29 of 32 (91%) who discontinued NANSAIDs, a nonsignificant difference. Among the patients whose ulcers healed, about one half in each group either resumed or discontinued NANSAID use in the following year for unspecified reasons; 14 patients had symptomatic ulcer recurrences, with the numbers equally distributed between those continuing or stopping NANSAIDs. Unfortunately, this study could not detect what could be a substantial difference in healing rates, and there was a higher proportion of ulcers healing in patients discontinuing NANSAIDs.

NANSAIDs: Differential Toxicity?

The relative gastrointestinal toxicity of different NSAIDs cannot be adequately determined from available data. A further study from the Puget Sound Group Health Co-operative suggests that differential prescribing of NANSAIDs occurs for cimetidine users (who presumably have a history of dyspepsia or ulceration) compared with cimetidine non-users. There was a preference for newly introduced NANSAIDs for the former but not for the latter, and it is possible that those at greatest risk of ulcer complications or UGIB are more often prescribed the latest anti-inflammatory drugs. If such a practice is widespread, attempts to determine the differential toxicity for NANSAIDs by a case-control approach would be undermined. For example, the Medicaid data analyzed by Carson and colleagues from the University of Pennsylvania suggested that sulindac may be more frequently associated with UGIB than indomethacin, naproxen, fenoprofen calcium, or tolmetin sodium. Compared with the other drugs in this study, the average daily dose of sulindac was closest to the maximum dose recommended by the manufacturer, perhaps partly explaining this difference. It is also possible that sulindac was used more frequently for those at greater risk of UGIB.

On the basis of anecdotal reports, some authorities have suggested that piroxicam causes unacceptable gastrointestinal ADRs and have called for its withdrawal from the market. However, there is no adequate scientific evidence that piroxicam has more gastrointestinal toxicity than other NSAIDs for which the association with peptic ulcer disease is equally brittle. Finally, enteric coating of aspirin does reduce the number of gastric mucosal erosions, but whether this translates to a reduction in peptic ulceration or its complications remains unproved.

NSAIDs and Fecal Occult Blood Testing

Short-term administration of NSAIDs frequently results in increased occult fecal blood loss as documented by microscopic bleeding techniques. On this basis, some physicians may attribute a positive fecal occult blood test (e.g., Hemoccult) obtained during colorectal cancer screening to the upper gastrointestinal irritant effects of the NSAID. They may transiently withdraw the drug, repeat the test, and if negative, avoid undertaking further bowel investigation. Recent studies suggest that this approach may be unwise. In a large colorectal cancer screening trial, 50 subjects concurrently taking NSAIDs were found to have positive tests. With colonoscopy or barium enema–sigmoidoscopy, 10 subjects (20%) proved to have colonic neoplasia (three carcinomas and seven adenomas larger than 1 cm); this detection rate was not significantly different from that in patients with a positive fecal occult blood test who were not taking NSAIDs. Because bleeding from colonic neoplasms may be intermittent, a negative test after NSAID withdrawal may provide false reassurance. For the purposes of such screening, the use of NSAIDs should be ignored.

NSAIDs and Other Gastrointestinal ADRs

NSAIDs may also damage other sites in the gastrointestinal tract. Patients with peptic esophageal strictures in one study were two- to three-fold more likely to be NSAID users than their age- and gender-matched controls. If possible, these drugs should be avoided by patients with reflux esophagitis.

NSAIDs are suspected by some investigators to cause small and large bowel inflammation, which may result in hemorrhage or perforation. They are well recognized to produce small intestinal ulceration, perforation, and death in experimental animals. In a recent case-control study, patients with intestinal hemorrhage and perforation were two to three times more likely than hospital control patients to be NSAID users. In Britain, a slow-release formulation of indomethacin (Osmosin) has been withdrawn from the market because of its purported association with multiple intestinal perforations. Long-term administration of NSAIDs to patients with rheumatoid arthritis leads to subclinical inflammation of the terminal ileum (detected by accumulation of indium-labeled leukocytes) in nearly two thirds of patients; a few of these patients develop radiographic changes, and occasionally patients have been reported with ulceration, stricture, or bile acid malabsorption. There are anecdotal reports of NSAIDs promptly exacerbating quiescent inflammatory bowel disease; whether these agents are causative or represent an epiphenomenon in this situation is uncertain.

NSAIDs and Peptic Ulcer Disease: Recommendations

Are the risks of peptic ulcer and its complications increased by NSAID use? There is good evidence linking aspirin use to gastric ulcer and UGIB and some evidence linking it to duodenal ulcer. The data are more contradictory for NANSAIDs. However, the confidence limits for relative risk in these studies are wide, and overall the data are consistent with a doubling of the rate of peptic ulceration and its complications. Risk may be greater for elderly persons over age 60 years and for patients taking higher doses of NANSAIDs. Whether risk varies with the duration of therapy, with the particular NANSAID utilized, or with concurrent peptic ulceration or alcohol consumption has not been determined. Although the absolute risk of peptic ulcer disease to an individual NSAID consumer is low, the extraordinarily wide use of these drugs may well be responsible for substantial morbidity and mortality in the general population.

How may the primary care physician reduce the upper gastrointestinal ADRs apparently produced by these agents? First, NSAIDs should not be routinely prescribed as the initial therapy for self-limiting conditions that may respond satisfactorily to safer analgesics such as acetaminophen. If NSAIDs are required, the lowest effective dose should be used; ibuprofen appears as safe as any NSAID and has the benefit of a wide dose range. In the elderly,

the maximal dose of NSAIDs should be adjusted to reflect any age-related alterations in pharmacokinetics for a given agent (see Chap. 50, Table 50–2). Pending further data, physicians may wish to caution patients against concurrent tobacco and alcohol consumption. Whether sucralfate or H_2 receptor antagonists reduce the frequency of NSAID-induced gastric erosions is controversial. However, there is currently no evidence that prophylactic antiulcer therapy prevents peptic ulcer or its complications in NSAID-treated patients. On the other hand, the withdrawal of NSAIDs from patients with peptic ulcer disease must be considered an individual decision rather than a total prohibition. Some arthritis patients have been subjected to a frozen, painful existence because of thoughtless discontinuation of NSAIDs. Seventy-five per cent of ulcers in NSAID-treated patients may heal despite continued NSAID use.

Conclusion

Whether prescriptions for NSAIDs should carry a government health warning is controversial. These agents probably do increase the risk of peptic ulcer and its complications, but the risk to the individual user is small. The problem is primarily a reflection of the widespread use of NSAIDs when less toxic alternatives are as efficacious. The association of NSAIDs with other gastrointestinal disorders has not yet been clarified. In the future, there may be better ways of detecting patients at greatest risk of gastrointestinal toxicity, and there may be ulcer-healing agents for such patients. At the moment, recommendations must be guarded, but the increasing development of slow-release preparations to bypass the upper gut could present gastroenterologists with a new set of problems in the lower gastrointestinal tract. The arguments in favor of pro-drugs, which attempt to avoid topical irritancy on the upper gut mucosa, are plausible but unproved.

Bibliography

Avila MH, Walkes AM, Romieu I, et al. Choice of nonsteroidal antiinflammatory drug in persons treated for dyspepsia. Lancet 2:556–559, 1988.
   This article suggests that elderly dyspeptic patients are more likely to use analgesics and that reports of an NANSAID-ulcer association would be artefactual.

Also, cimetidine users were more likely to be prescribed newly introduced NANSAIDs.

Beard K, Walker AM, Perera DR, et al. Nonsteroidal anti-inflammatory drugs and hospitalization for gastroesophageal bleeding in the elderly. Arch Intern Med 147:1621–1623, 1987.
Elderly subjects who had received a prescription for NSAIDs were not significantly more likely to be admitted with gastroesophageal bleeding than those who had not.

Bjarnason I, Zanelli G, Smith T, et al. Nonsteroidal antiinflammatory drug–induced intestinal inflammation in humans. Gastroenterology 93:480–489, 1987.
Occult small bowel inflammation may occur in more than half of those using anti-inflammatory agents.

Carson JL, Strom BC, Morse L, et al. The relative gastrointestinal toxicity of the nonsteroidal anti-inflammatory drugs. Arch Intern Med 147:1054–1059, 1987.
In this cohort study from Pennsylvania, those exposed to NSAIDs had 1.5 times the frequency of bleeding than those unexposed. Some differences were observed between the various anti-inflammatory drugs.

Carson JL, Strom BC, Soper KA, et al. The association of nonsteroidal anti-inflammatory drugs with upper gastrointestinal tract bleeding. Arch Intern Med 147:85–88, 1987.

Caruso I, Bianchi-Porro G. Gastroscopic evaluation of anti-inflammatory agents. Br Med J 280:75–78, 1980.
Approximately one third of NSAID users developed mucosal lesions.

Coggan D, Langman MJS, Spiegelhalter D. Aspirin, paracetamol and haematemesis and melaena. Gut 23:340–344, 1982.
Short-term aspirin use seems to carry an increased risk but is causal in only one third of aspirin users admitted to a hospital with bleeding.

Collier DSJ, Pain JA. Non-steroidal anti-inflammatory drugs and peptic ulcer perforation. Gut 26:359–363, 1985.
Elderly NSAID users were 11 times more likely to be admitted to a hospital with perforations than controls. The study has some difficulties and this is almost certainly an overestimate.

Jick H. Effects of aspirin and acetaminophen in gastrointestinal hemorrhage. Results from the Boston Collaborative Drug Surveillance Program. Arch Intern Med 141:316–321, 1981.
An association between heavy aspirin use and gastrointestinal hemorrhage was shown.

Jick SS, Perera DR, Walker AM, et al. Non-steroidal anti-inflammatory drugs and hospital admission for perforated peptic ulcer. Lancet 2:380–382, 1987.
Perforation rates were not altered by NSAID use in this cohort study from the Group Health Cooperative of Puget Sound.

Kurata JH, Elashoff JD, Grossman MD. Inadequacy of the literature on the relationship between drugs, ulcers and gastrointestinal bleeding. Gastroenterology 82:373–376, 1982.
This article is a useful analysis of the pitfalls of experimental and observational studies.

Langman MJS, Morgan L, Worrall A. Use of anti-inflammatory drugs by patients admitted with small or large bowel perforations and haemorrhage. Br Med J 290:374–379, 1985.
Anti-inflammatory users had two to three times the likelihood of lower bowel problems than nonusers.

Manniche C, Malchow-Moller A, Andersen JR, et al. Randomised study of the influence of non-steroidal anti-inflammatory drugs on the treatment of peptic ulcer in patients with rheumatic disease. Gut 28:226–229, 1987.
This article suggests that withdrawal of NSAIDs does not significantly increase the chances of ulcer healing.

Pye G, Ballantyne KC, Artimitage NC, et al. Influence of non-steroidal anti-inflammatory drugs on the outcome of faecal occult blood tests in screening for colorectal cancer. Br Med J 294:1510–1511, 1987.
Of 10,931 patients screened, 455 had occult blood tests that were positive. Fifty of these were using NSAIDs and 10 (20%) had neoplastic disease, as did 129 (32%) of those not using NSAIDs.

Roth SH, Bennett RE. Nonsteroidal anti-inflammatory drug gastropathy: recognition and response. Arch Intern Med 149:2093–2100, 1987.
It is argued that chronic peptic ulcer represents one extreme of a continuum of gastric mucosal reaction to anti-inflammatory drugs. This remains controversial, as does the suggestion that "cytoprotective rather than H_2-receptor antagonists are more effective healing agents for NSAID-associated ulcers."

Somerville KW, Faulkner G, Langman MJS. Non-steroidal anti-inflammatory drugs and bleeding peptic ulcer. Lancet 1:462–464, 1986.
Elderly patients admitted with peptic ulcer bleeding were three to four times more likely to be NANSAID users than matched controls.

Walt RP, Katchinski B, Logan R, et al. Rising frequency of ulcer perforations in elderly people in the United Kingdom. Lancet 1:489–492, 1986.
Whereas peptic ulcer perforation has declined in the young in recent years, it has increased in elderly women. The possible explanations are discussed.

PART THIRTEEN

Medical Care of Surgical Patients

52

Preoperative Assessment of Cardiac Patients Undergoing Noncardiac Surgery

ALLAN S. DETSKY, M.D., Ph.D., F.R.C.P.C.
HOWARD B. ABRAMS, M.D., F.R.C.P.C.

Approximately one third of the referrals to the general medical consultation service in our hospital concern the preoperative assessment of a patient with cardiac disease. There are several ways in which these assessments can help in patient care. The first is to enable the surgeon to weigh the potential benefits of the planned procedure against one particular risk. The second is the opportunity to alter the risk if the patient's condition can be improved by preoperative intervention. The third benefit is the information that the anesthesia team may use to prepare for the procedure and perhaps alter its approach. The last benefit is that preoperative cardiac assessment may help clinicians to be more explicit in describing risks when patients are deciding to undergo surgery and giving informed consent.

In this chapter, we review an approach to preoperative assessment of patients with cardiac disease. We describe a four-step process for assessing patients, which we derived after studying 455 consecutive patients seen by our service at Toronto General Hospital in 1983–1984.[1,2] This study tested the predictive validity of a modified version of the multifactorial risk index derived by Goldman and colleagues[3] in a study of 1001 consecutive patients undergoing noncardiac surgery at the Massachusetts General Hospital. We also comment on the difficulties in applying this index to patients with peripheral vascular disease, on an approach to patients with hypertension, and on

Supported in part by the National Health and Research Development Program (Canada) through a National Health Scholar Award to Dr. Detsky.

the indications for perioperative invasive monitoring with arterial lines and pulmonary artery catheters.

Estimating Risk of Cardiac Events for Individual Patients

This technique involves four steps. The approach is Bayesian in nature in that pretest probabilities (average risks of developing cardiac complications for groups of patients undergoing specific surgical procedures) are converted into post-test probabilities (risks for individual patients) by using a clinical index that reflects the clinical characteristics of those patients.

Step 1: Determining Average Risk for Surgical Procedures in Your Clinical Setting

The average risk of developing cardiac complications for patients undergoing noncardiac surgery varies according to the type of surgical procedure. Different surgical procedures have different stresses on the cardiovascular system, and one would expect these variations in stress to be reflected in variations in the risk of developing perioperative cardiac complications. For example, patients undergoing a repair of an abdominal aortic aneurysm have a higher chance of developing a cardiac complication than those undergoing a cataract extraction. Before considering individual patient characteristics, the average risk or pretest probability for the procedure should be assessed. Table 52–1 shows the pretest probabilities for patients with suspected cardiac disease referred to the general medical consultation service at our hospital, a large tertiary facility. The sample on which these estimates are based was not a consecutive series of all patients undergoing surgery, and therefore our pretest probabilities are higher than those found in such series (e.g., the study by Goldman and colleagues.[3] Because the cardiology service at our hospital refers virtually all preoperative risk assessments to the general medical consultation service, we believe that these patients are similar to those who may be seen by cardiologists and internists in other tertiary hospitals, and we expect that the same pretest probabilities (average risks) may apply. However, readers should note that the risks in their own institutions may vary considerably from those reported here.

In addition, readers should note that the pretest probabilities reported here are based on a finite sample of patients and thus have confidence limits associated with them as shown in Table 52–1.

Those involved in performing preoperative cardiac risk assessments should consider studying a sample of their own patients over time to calculate local pretest probabilities. Table 52–1 can provide a base-line set of pretest probabilities that should be revised according to local experience.

Step 2: Calculating Individual Risk Scores

Table 52–2 shows the variables and weighting scheme for our multifactorial risk index.

The variables are divided into seven groups. The first group concerns history and symptoms of coronary artery disease. The variables concerning a history of myocardial infarction are self-explanatory, although judgment is required when the direct evidence (creatine kinase–MB elevations or electrocardiographic changes) is not available at the time of the consultation. The angina classes included in our index are based on the Canadian Cardiovascular Society system. Class III angina is defined as angina that occurs when the patient walks one to two blocks on a level surface or climbs one flight of stairs under normal conditions and at a normal pace. Class IV angina is defined as an inability to carry on any physical activity without discomfort. Angina may or may not be present at rest. Unstable angina includes crescendo angina (more severe, prolonged, or frequent angina superimposed on an existing pattern of relatively stable exertion-related angina), coronary insufficiency syndrome, new onset angina (within 1 month) brought on by minimal exertion, and angina brought on at rest as well as with minimal exertion. We do not consider atypical, variant, or Prinzmetal's angina (i.e., angina that occurs mostly when the patient is at rest and not when the patient exerts himself or herself) to be unstable angina, although some cardiologists do. In addition, patients who have atypical angina are not considered as having class IV angina under the Canadian Cardiovascular Society system. If a patient had both class IV angina and crescendo unstable angina in the period just before admission, he or she would receive 20 points for the former and 10 points for the latter. If a patient had crescendo angina 2 months before admission

Table 52–1. *Pretest Probabilities for Types of Surgery, from the General Medical Consultation Service, Toronto General Hospital*

Type of Surgery	No. (%) Severe Cardiac Complications*	95% Confidence Limits
Major Surgery		
Vascular	10/76 (13.2)	6.5–19.7
Aortic	5/32 (15.6)	6.5–32.9
Carotid	4/27 (14.8)	5.6–33.9
Peripheral	1/17 (5.8)	0.8–32.9
Orthopedic	9/66 (13.6)	6.0–21.2
Intrathoracic/intraperitoneal	7/88 (8.0)	3.4–13.6
Head and neck	1/38 (2.6)	0.3–16.4
Minor Surgery		
(e.g., transurethral prostatectomies, cataracts)	3/187 (1.6)	0.5–1.6

From Detsky AS. Arch Intern Med 1986, 146:2131–2134, Copyright 1986, American Medical Association.
*Cardiac death, nonfatal myocardial infarction, or nonfatal alveolar pulmonary edema.

Table 52–2. *Modified Multifactorial Index*

Variable	Points
Coronary artery disease	
Myocardial infarction within 6 mo	10
Myocardial infarction more than 6 mo	5
Canadian Cardiovascular Society angina	
Class III	10
Class IV	20
Unstable angina within 3 mo	10
Alveolar pulmonary edema	
Within 1 wk	10
Ever	5
Valvular disease	
Suspected critical aortic stenosis	20
Arrhythmias	
Sinus plus atrial premature beats or rhythm other than sinus on last preoperative electrocardiogram	5
More than five ventricular premature beats per minute documented at any time before surgery	5
Poor general medical status*	5
Age over 70 yr	5
Emergency operation	10

From Detsky AS. Arch Intern Med 1986, 146:2131–2134, Copyright 1986, American Medical Association.
*Oxygen pressure < 60 mmHg; carbon dioxide pressure > 50 mmHg; serum potassium < 3.0 mEq/L (< 3.0 mmol/L); serum bicarbonate < 20 mEq/L (< 20 mmol/L); serum urea nitrogen > 50 mg/dl (> 18 mmol/L); serum creatinine > 3 mg/dl (> 260 mmol/L); aspartate aminotransferase, abnormal; signs of chronic liver disease; and/or bedridden from noncardiac causes.

but had a reduction in symptoms either spontaneously or because of an intensification of medical therapy, he or she would receive only 10 points for unstable angina.

A history of alveolar pulmonary edema results in the addition of either 5 or 10 points to the index score depending on its timing, as shown in Table 52–2. For recent pulmonary alveolar edema, we require chest x-ray documentation. If the patient's episode of pulmonary edema was remote, we accept a convincing clinical history in the absence of a chest x-ray.

Twenty points are added to the index score if the patient is suspected of having critical aortic stenosis. Although clinical assessment of this entity is difficult, we consider patients who have classic features of critical aortic stenosis in their history (near syncope, exertional angina, or recurrent congestive heart failure) in the setting of other signs (pulsus parvus et tardus, a thrusting left ventricular impulse in the presence of low blood pressure, and left ventricular hypertrophy) as having suspected critical aortic stenosis. Because the validity and reliability of these clinical features for predicting critical aortic stenosis are ques-

tionable,[4] we recommend the use of Doppler echocardiography to assess the gradient across the aortic valve.[5]

Two kinds of arrhythmias are included in the index: (1) on the last electrocardiogram obtained before the planned surgery, sinus rhythm with atrial premature beats or a rhythm other than sinus (e.g., atrial fibrillation) and (2) at any time before surgery, a history of more than five premature ventricular contractions per minute. An individual patient may be assigned five points both for atrial arrhythmias just before surgery and for documentation of more than five ventricular premature beats a minute at any time before surgery if he or she exhibits both characteristics. The latter characteristic includes a history of ventricular tachycardia or fibrillation at any time before surgery.

Poor general medical status is defined in a manner similar to that described by Goldman and coworkers[3] and is shown in Table 52–2.

A surgical procedure is designated an emergency operation if the patient must be taken to the operating room before his or her medical management can be optimized (adjustment of medication, correction of electrolyte or fluid imbalance).

Step 3: Using Nomogram to Convert Average Risk for Procedure (Pretest Probability) to Average Risk for Individual Patient (Post-test Probability)

The individual patient characteristics as summarized in the risk index score can be used to convert the pretest probability for patients undergoing a given surgical procedure into a post-test probability for the specific patient. The technique involves the use of likelihood ratios as described in our previous publications.[1, 2] The reader should note that scores that are associated with likelihood ratios less than 1 imply that the individual patient's risk of suffering from a cardiac complication is lower than the average risk for all patients undergoing that procedure, whereas a score associated with a likelihood ratio greater than 1 implies that the patient's risk is higher than the average risk for patients undergoing that procedure. Thus, for patients with scores of 0 and 5 that are associated with likelihood ratios less than 1, the risk of developing perioperative cardiac complications is lower than average, whereas for index scores greater than or equal to 15, the estimated risk is higher than average because the likelihood ratios are greater than 1. An index score of 10 is associated with a likelihood ratio of 1.1, and patients with this score have average risks. The legend for Figure 52–1 describes the use of this nomogram.

Three kinds of cardiac complications are predicted by using this system: cardiac death, nonfatal myocardial infarction, and nonfatal alveolar pulmonary edema, as described previously.[1] In our series of 455 patients, 30% of these events were cardiac deaths. Thus, one can convert the post-test probability estimates for developing cardiac complications into an estimate of cardiac case-fatality rates by multiplying the post-test probability by 30%. Those involved in assessing cardiac risk should validate this 30% figure for their own institutions in addition to estimating the risk of pretest probabilities. In a recently performed multicenter study of elective aortic aneurysm resection performed by vascular surgeons throughout Canada, the risk of developing perioperative cardiac complications was 15% (similar to the pretest probability in our study), and the proportion of these complications that were fatal was also approximately 30%, as found in our study (Johnston KW, personal communication).

Step 4: Adjusting for Other Patient Characteristics Not Considered by Index

Patients occasionally present with unusual characteristics that are either not included in or not adequately considered by the index. For example, our index does not consider conditions that were seen infrequently by our service, such as severe mitral stenosis or regurgitation. In addition, our index may not adequately reflect the interaction between some comorbid conditions, such as severe chronic obstructive pulmonary disease or diabetes, and the variables included in the index. To do so, our previous studies would have required extremely large sample sizes or a highly unusual sample of patients. Similarly, our index cannot adequately account for the patient whom we sometimes encounter who has minimal objective criteria on which one would base an estimate of high risk, but nevertheless "appears" to be a poor risk candidate. Last, the index may be difficult to use for patients from whom the historical variables

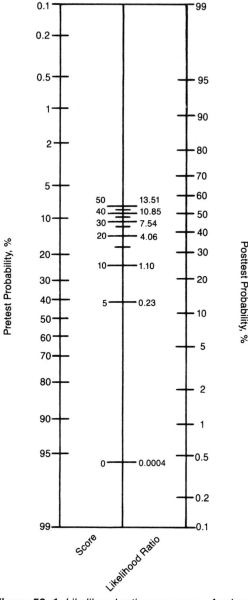

Figure 52–1. Likelihood ratio nomogram. Anchor a straight edge at the value on the pretest side of the nomogram determined by the surgical procedure. Direct the straight edge through the point in the middle column reflecting the patient's index score and associated likelihood ratio. The point at which the straight edge meets the right-hand column denotes the patient's post-test probability, i.e., the risk of perioperative cardiac complication. From Detsky AS. Arch Intern Med 1986, 146:2131–2134, Copyright 1986, American Medical Association.

included in our index, such as myocardial infarction or angina pattern, are difficult to elicit (e.g., no previous records, poor historian, or language barrier). The estimates of post-test risk should be adjusted in these circumstances. We emphasize that our multifactorial index is merely a model or starting point for clinicians who should not hesitate to make revisions in appropriate circumstances.

Patients with Coexisting Peripheral Vascular Disease

Patients with severe peripheral vascular disease may be difficult to assess by using the cardiac risk index because of their inability to ambulate to the point where they suffer from angina. Similarly, patients with severe debilitating diseases such as rheumatoid arthritis may also be difficult to assess. We pointed out in our previous study[1] that our clinical risk index was quite specific but may not be sensitive enough to rule out a clinically important risk of suffering from cardiac complications in patients with low scores of 5 or 10 who are undergoing peripheral vascular surgery.

As a result of these considerations, some consultants have recommended the use of supplementary diagnostic strategies for identifying a high risk subgroup among these kinds of patients. Tests that involve exercise are probably inappropriate for the same reasons that our clinical index cannot be used, that is, patients are unable to ambulate to the point where they suffer from angina. An algorithm combining certain clinical characteristics with dipyridamole-thallium scanning has been evaluated by Eagle and colleagues[6] who studied 111 patients referred for such scans before undergoing peripheral vascular surgery. The first 61 patients were used to derive the diagnostic algorithm and a subsequent 50 patients were used to test (validate) the algorithm. A low risk group was identified that exhibited none of the following screening characteristics: a history of angina, myocardial infarction, congestive heart failure, diabetes mellitus, or a Q wave on the electrocardiogram. Eagle and coworkers suggested that these low risk patients require no further testing. Among those who exhibit at least one of those screening characteristics, dipyridamole-thallium scans may be helpful for further stratifying patients. Among those patients in their study who exhibited at least one of the screening characteristics and had reversible defects on the scan,

the risk of suffering a postoperative ischemic event (cardiac death, myocardial infarction, ischemic pulmonary edema, or unstable angina) was high (15/33 or 45%). Only 2 of 26 (7.6%) patients with one or more of the clinical features given earlier but no reversible scan defects had postoperative cardiac events. Unfortunately, the cardiac risk index scores for those patients were not reported in their paper. Therefore, we cannot tell whether the dipyridamole-thallium scan added predictive power greater than the previously described multifactorial index for patients with low scores (e.g., 5 or 10), although we suspect that it did.

It seems reasonable that high risk patients identified either by the use of the multifactorial index described in this chapter or by the algorithm described by Eagle and colleagues[6] may benefit from coronary angiography and a revascularization procedure (coronary angioplasty or bypass surgery) if appropriate anatomic lesions are demonstrated angiographically. On the other hand, Leppo and coworkers[7] showed that among 11 patients with a strongly positive dipyridamole-thallium redistribution (out of 100 consecutive patients admitted for elective abdominal aortic or limb vascular surgery) who subsequently underwent coronary angiography, 6 suffered major complications (stroke, myocardial infarction, or death) after angiography, coronary bypass surgery, or vascular surgery. Thus, the ultimate clinical utility of pursuing coronary angiography before vascular surgery needs further study, and it would be inappropriate to provide firm recommendations regarding its use. Research groups should consider performing a randomized trial of coronary angiography and coronary bypass surgery for patients identified as high risk by either our clinical risk index or the algorithm suggested by Eagle and colleagues.

We can report that our group rarely (in fact almost never) recommends perioperative coronary angiography or either method of revascularization as a way to protect the patient against cardiac complications at the time of the primary (noncardiac) surgery unless the patient's cardiac condition would warrant these procedures independently of the need for surgery. That is, we rarely recommend coronary angiography unless the patient has a specific indication for this procedure, such as suspected critical valvular stenosis, an unacceptable amount of angina on maximal medical therapy, or early postinfarction angina with an early positive stress test suggesting high grade left main or proximal left anterior descending stenosis. We do alert the anesthesiologist that perioperative invasive hemodynamic monitoring should be considered for these high risk patients.

As a method of summarizing the preceding review of evidence and discussion about patients with peripheral vascular disease, we propose the algorithm shown in Figure 52–2.

Hypertension

We use a rough rule of thumb for postponing elective surgery in patients with hypertension: delaying surgery for those with diastolic blood pressures higher than 110 mmHg because we know that the anesthesiologists in our institution are reluctant to use anesthesia if the pressure is above that level. (We are not aware

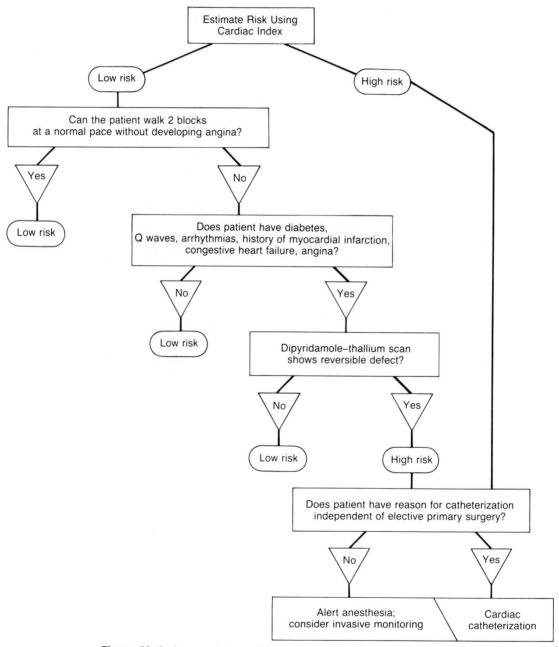

Figure 52–2. Approach for patients with peripheral vascular disease.

of clinical studies to support the 110 mmHg cutoff.)

The original study by Goldman and colleagues[3] suggested that stable hypertension was probably not a major independent risk factor for suffering from cardiac complications. In a subsequent publication,[8] Goldman and Caldera showed that both perioperative hypertension and intraoperative hypotension requiring an intravenous fluid bolus or adrenergic agent occur in roughly one quarter of all hypertensive patients. In their study, which involved 157 patients with treated or untreated hypertension, they could not detect a relationship between the degree of preoperative control and risk of developing either of these kinds of blood pressure complications. Most authors (including ourselves) recommend continuation of antihypertensive medications up to the time of surgery, with reinstitution of these medications (particularly beta blockers) as soon as possible after surgery.[9]

When patients are seen before surgery with unacceptably high blood pressure readings, we caution against aggressive administration of antihypertensive agents during the immediate preoperative period in an attempt to quickly reduce blood pressure. Often, patients have fairly high blood pressures on admission to hospital, which fall spontaneously during the subsequent 12 to 24 hours. In addition, we are concerned about the vigorous administration of diuretics and vasodilators immediately before surgery as these agents may predispose the patient to intraoperative hypotension, a known risk factor for subsequent myocardial infarction.[10] If a patient's blood pressure is too high to proceed with surgery as planned, we recommend a gentle introduction of antihypertensive therapy over a period of time rather than acute intensive efforts to rapidly lower blood pressure to the point acceptable to the anesthesiologist. With the trend toward performing surgery in ambulatory or outpatient units, the problem of treating patients with labile hypertension who have very high blood pressures on admission may increase because clinicians will not have the option of letting the patient settle overnight.

Invasive Hemodynamic Monitoring

The use of invasive hemodynamic monitoring during the perioperative period has been justified by observation of an apparent reduc-

tion in cardiac complication rates for patients with previous myocardial infarctions after use of these monitoring techniques had disseminated widely. For example, Rao and coworkers[11] demonstrated a reduction in perioperative myocardial infarction rates during 1977–1982 to 1.9% compared with a rate of 7.7% for patients who had undergone surgery during 1973–1976. The later period reflects the time when anesthesiologists in their institution commonly used invasive hemodynamic monitoring, whereas the earlier period represents a time when invasive monitoring was rarely performed. Unfortunately, conclusions based on comparisons of innovative treatment strategies with historical controls are tenuous. On the other hand, several investigators have reported the increased risk of perioperative infarctions associated with substantial intraoperative hypotension (e.g., a blood pressure decrease of 33% or more maintained for 10 minutes or longer), and it thus seems logical that invasive monitoring may help anesthesiologists avoid this problem. The use of invasive hemodynamic monitoring often requires utilization of postoperative intensive care unit services because some have recommended continuation of monitoring for 48 hours after surgery.

However, rigorous evaluations of the effectiveness of intra-arterial or pulmonary artery catheters for reducing the risk of cardiac complications have not yet been done. Nevertheless, these interventions are currently used for virtually all patients undergoing procedures associated with high average risks such as vascular surgery involving the aorta. Our group often recommends their use for patients with high risk scores who are undergoing procedures where their use is not routine (e.g., peripheral vascular surgery, intra-abdominal surgery), despite the lack of high quality evidence of their effectiveness. We are particularly likely to recommend invasive monitoring for patients who we believe cannot tolerate abnormally high or low systemic or pulmonary pressures during the perioperative period. For example, patients with critical aortic stenosis may develop irreversible cardiac complications such as ischemia if the systemic or left ventricular filling pressures decrease too much, whereas patients without aortic stenosis may tolerate these pressure changes well. Other kinds of patients who may fall into this group are those with unstable angina indicative of critical coronary artery stenosis, other critical valvular lesions, or severely impaired left ventricular function (e.g., cardiomyopathy, aneurysm). We point out that where strong evidence from clinical trials is lacking, clinicians must rely on judgment based on a knowledge of pathophysiology and its interaction with the perioperative environment that alters that physiology (e.g., medications, blood loss, assisted ventilation). However, we recommend that such trials be undertaken.

Discussion

In this chapter, we have discussed an approach for assessing cardiac patients before they undergo noncardiac surgery. In addition, special attention has been paid to patients with hypertension, peripheral vascular disease, and the role of invasive hemodynamic monitoring.

We emphasize that the method of assessment is a model that allows clinicians to focus on the components of risk in a systematic fashion. Like all models, it contains simplifications and limitations. It does not allow for a full risk/benefit assessment in that it clearly does not incorporate the benefits of the planned procedure. We also point out that, unlike some epidemiologic studies of operative risks,[12] most of the published studies testing the validity of these indexes do not cover cardiac events that may occur after the patient has been discharged from the hospital,[12] which also limits the use of the indexes in a full risk/benefit analysis.

At the beginning of the chapter, we outlined several potential uses of cardiac risk assessment. Throughout the chapter we have emphasized that there exists little high quality evidence to support the most obvious potential use of the index, that is, identifying methods for reducing risk through interventions or monitoring. In using the index, our group classifies the potentially reversible characteristics into three groups. The first group contains factors that could be corrected and where it seems highly likely that risk will fall (delay surgery until 6 months beyond a myocardial infarction or 3 months beyond an episode of unstable angina; full evaluation of suspected critical valvular lesion and surgical replacement if present; correction of severe fluid or electrolyte imbalances). The second group concerns factors that may change with therapy but for which there is really no evidence that overall risk will fall despite the logic of the approach (increasing medical therapy for angina, cardiac catheterization and revascularization). The third group contains factors that are clearly

not reversible (age, emergency surgery, history of remote myocardial infarction or of premature ventricular beats).

Finally, we point out that internists may differ in the method by which they communicate this information to the patient, the patient's family, the anesthesiologist, and the surgeon. Our consultation notes frequently follow the four steps outlined in this chapter: (1) statement of average risk for the procedure for patients referred to the consultation service at our hospital; (2) components of risk score, notation of potential for reversal, and total score; (3) estimate of post-test risk of a severe cardiac complication, and multiplication of this risk by 0.30 to give an estimate of risk of cardiac death; and (4) consideration of other patient characteristics that may not be well captured by the process. Some of our surgical colleagues have objected to the use of specific numbers, sometimes because they believe that the numbers are too high or give a false sense of precision. Some surgeons prefer the use of likelihood ratios because they are familiar with what the numbers represent and convey the notion that the patient's risk category was below average, average, or above average. For some services and frequently for families, we compare the patient's risk estimate to the average by using the terms above average (likelihood ratio > 1) and below average (likelihood ratio < 1). In addition to repeating our strong suggestion that clinicians should determine the pretest probabilities in their own clinical setting to judge the generalizability of the approach to their patients, we suggest that consultants try different approaches in communicating information to determine which approach works best for them.

References

1. Detsky AS, Abrams HB, McLaughlin JR, et al. Predicting cardiac complications in patients undergoing non-cardiac surgery. J Gen Intern Med 1:211–219, 1986.

   This paper describes the study that tested the predictive properties of a cardiac risk index, which was based on the hypothesis-generating study of Goldman et al. (see reference 3) and modified by the staff of the Medical Consultation Service at the Toronto General Hospital. The paper describes the methods used to validate the index and most of the primary data.

2. Detsky AS, Abrams HB, Forbath N, et al. Cardiac assessment for patients undergoing noncardiac surgery: a multifactorial clinical risk index. Arch Intern Med 146:2131–2134, 1986.

   This paper describes the cardiac risk index that was

tested in reference 1 and instructs clinicians in its use. *Some clinical examples are described.*

3. Goldman L, Caldera D, Nussabaum SR, et al. Multifactorial index of cardiac risk in non-cardiac surgical procedures. N Engl J Med 197:845–850, 1977.

   This is the original classic paper describing the hypothesis-generating study that developed the original multifactorial cardiac risk index. The paper describes the experience of the Medical Consultation Team on several of the surgical services at the Massachusetts General Hospital.

4. Lombard JT, Selzer A. Valvular aortic stenosis. Ann Intern Med 106:292–298, 1987.

   This paper describes the lack of sensitivity and specificity for various clinical features in predicting the degree of aortic stenosis.

5. Currie PJ, Saward JB, Reeder GS, et al. Continuous wave Doppler echocardiography assessment of severity of calcific aortic stenosis: a simultaneous Doppler-catheter correlative study in 100 adult patients. Circulation 71:1162–1169, 1985.

   This paper describes the accuracy of Doppler techniques in echocardiography for predicting the severity of aortic stenosis.

6. Eagle KA, Singer DE, Brewster DC, et al. Dipyridamole-thallium scanning in patients undergoing vascular surgery. JAMA 257:2185–2189, 1987.

   This paper describes the derivation and testing of a method of predicting patients who are at high risk of suffering from cardiac complications during vascular surgery. The method involves the use of clinical variables to screen patients who should then undergo dipyridamole-thallium scans to detect reversible ischemia.

7. Leppo J, Plaja J, Giomet M, et al. Noninvasive evaluation of cardiac risk before elective vascular surgery. J Am Coll Cardiol 9:269–276, 1987.

   This paper describes the use of dipyridamole-thallium scans for detecting patients who are at high risk of suffering from a cardiac complication during elective vascular surgery. It also demonstrates, however, that a policy of cardiac catheterization and possible revascularization may not reduce the risk of suffering a complication.

8. Goldman L, Caldera DL. Risks of general anesthesia and elective operation in the hypertensive patient. Anesthesiology 50:285–292, 1979.

   This paper examines the risk of hypertension for patients undergoing general anesthesia using the same patient sample described in the study that derived the multifactorial risk index (reference 3). The paper suggests that the degree of control of blood pressure before undergoing surgery is not predictive of intraoperative or postoperative difficulties related to blood pressure control.

9. Goldman L. Cardiac risks and complications of noncardiac surgery. Ann Intern Med 93:504–513, 1983.

   This paper is a review article on the subject and summarizes a great deal of literature.

10. Goldman L, Caldera DL, Southwick FS, et al. Cardiac risk factors and complications in non-cardiac surgery. Medicine 57:357–370, 1978.

    This paper is a secondary analysis of the data presented in reference 3. In addition to reviewing the patient's specific factors that predict risk of suffering from cardiac complications, the paper reviews other data, such as degree of hypotension that occurs intraoperatively, as risk factors for cardiac complications.

11. Rao TLK, Jacobs KH, El-Etr AA. Reinfarction following anesthesia in patients with myocardial infarction. Anesthesiology 39:499–505, 1983.

    This paper demonstrates a lower cardiac complication rate for patients with a history of myocardial infarction compared with earlier studies that demonstrated substantially higher risks.

12. Wennberg JE, Roos N, Sola L, et al. Use of claim data systems to evaluate health care outcomes. JAMA 257:933–936, 1987.

    This paper describes the use of medical claims data bases for health services research. In particular, it shows how morbidity and mortality after discharge from hospital can be detected in contrast to most of the studies reviewing the cardiac complication rates, which detected only in-hospital events.

53

Preventing Pulmonary Problems after Surgery

H. WILLIAM BONEKAT, D.O.
JOHN WADE SHIGEOKA, M.D.

Introduction

"Forewarned, Forearmed"

The lung is a common site for complications after surgery. To reduce the morbidity and mortality of pulmonary complications, general internists are often asked to assess risk and help plan perioperative care. When forewarned of increased risk, the health care team, consisting of the internist, surgeon, anesthesiologist, nurse, and respiratory therapist, may correct reversible factors, watch the patient more closely, and provide aggressive therapy to reduce pulmonary complications.

The presurgical pulmonary assessment is challenging because surgery is now performed on patients previously considered too old or too ill. Also, health insurers have increasingly pressured physicians to reduce the costs of added therapy and extra hospital days caused by pulmonary complications. Finally, the literature on perioperative pulmonary care is confusing and conflicting. It is difficult, if not impossible, to compare studies that differ markedly in design (prospective versus retrospective, controlled versus uncontrolled), definition of complication (clinical versus radiographic versus blood gas), type of patient (otherwise healthy versus having multiple medical problems), or type of surgery (elective versus emergency, upper abdominal site versus all sites). Comparisons are also difficult if they include studies that were performed decades ago when techniques and care differed from current practice. Sadly, because of logistics and great expense, it is unlikely that new, large, prospective, scientifically valid clinical studies concerning perioperative pulmonary care will be performed.

This chapter concisely reviews the pathophysiologic changes and common pulmonary problems that accompany surgery, the preoperative pulmonary assessment, and currently recommended measures for preventing pulmonary complications.

Changes in Lung Function Associated with Surgery

Otherwise normal patients experience changes in lung function during general anesthesia. There are altered shape and motion of the chest wall and diaphragm, reduced resting lung volume (functional residual capacity), reduced lung compliance, increased mismatching of ventilation to perfusion, and impaired gas exchange (oxygen uptake and carbon dioxide elimination). Inhibition of cough and diminished mucociliary clearance permit retention of airway secretions. Retained secretions in turn aggravate the loss of compliance and impaired gas exchange that result from breathing at low lung volumes. Ordinarily, this lung dysfunction is transient and clears in about 2 hours after surgery. An *exception* is when surgery involves the thorax or abdomen: lung function worsens progressively for 1 day and then gradually returns to normal in 7 to 10 days. After abdominal or thoracic surgery, diaphragmatic dysfunction, pain, splinting, analgesic medicines, bandages, abdominal distention, and confinement in bed are all thought to contribute to the following abnormalities of lung function: reduced lung volumes (vital capacity, total lung capacity, and functional residual capacity), rapid shallow breathing pattern, loss of sighs (physiologically important

Table 53–1. *Changes in Respiratory Function Associated with Surgery under General Anesthesia**

Initiators	Changes	Sequelae
Anesthetic	1–3, 6–8	A–D
Analgesic medications	1–3, 5, 6	A–D
Dry inhaled gases	7, 8	D
Diaphragmatic dysfunction	2–5	A–D
Distended abdomen	2–5	A–D
Muscle relaxant	2–5	A–D
Pain	1–5	A–D
Restrictive bandages	2, 3, 5	A–D
Supine position	2, 3	A, C

*Initiating factors, changes in lung function, and sequelae that typically occur during and after surgery on the upper abdomen under general anesthesia. Key for lung function changes: 1 = loss of sighs; 2 = loss of compliance; 3 = low lung volumes; 4 = rapid breathing; 5 = shallow breathing; 6 = diminished gag/cough reflexes; 7 = bronchial irritation; 8 = impaired mucociliary clearance. Key for sequelae: A = atelectasis; B = hypoventilation; C = hypoxemia; D = retained secretions.

periodic hyperinflations that normally occur about 10 times an hour), inability to inspire deeply, reduced effectiveness of cough, retained airway secretions, airway closure in dependent lung regions, and abnormal gas exchange of variable severity, i.e., from a large alveolar-arterial oxygen tension difference to systemic hypoxemia (Table 53–1).

Pulmonary Complications

In general, pulmonary complications are exaggerations of the lung dysfunction seen intra- and postoperatively. For convenience, there are four groups of pulmonary complications (Table 53–2).

Atelectasis. Atelectasis is the collapse of pulmonary alveoli. The term macroatelectasis is used when there are linear or plate-like radiographic densities and microatelectasis is used when there are no densities (the radiograph may show only decreased lung volume or poor inspiratory effort). Frequently, atelectasis is detected by abnormal oxygenation that ranges from a large alveolar-arterial oxygen tension difference (discussed later) to profound hypoxemia. Hypoxemia may manifest as a major organ dysfunction (e.g., confusion, angina) or damage (e.g., stroke, myocardial infarction) but may be difficult to detect clinically. Atelectasis may also mimic pneumonia, i.e., fever, rales, and tubular or absent breath sounds may be noted.

Infection. Pathogenic microbes rapidly colonize the mouth, respiratory tract, and stomach after surgery. Aspiration of oral flora (pathogenic or normal), reduced cough, and decreased mucociliary clearance predispose to infection (either acute bronchitis or pneumonia). Postoperative pneumonia has high morbidity and mortality, and the lung may act as a source of sepsis.

Airway Obstruction. Aspiration, retained secretions, bronchospasm, and dynamic airway collapse (especially in patients with emphysema) may lead to airway obstruction. Obstruction causes abnormal gas exchange (alveolar hypoventilation or hypoxemia) and increased work of breathing. When obstruction occurs during intra- or postoperative mechanical ventilation, the high driving pressure required to maintain ventilation may adversely reduce cardiac output, produce pneumothorax, and hinder weaning from the ventilator.

Miscellaneous. There are several uncommon yet preventable complications. The prolonged action of neuromuscular blockers, e.g., succinyl choline and pancuronium, and certain antimicrobials, e.g., aminoglycosides, polymyxin, and clindamycin, may precipitate ventilatory failure in patients with neuromuscular conditions (myasthenia gravis, myotonic dystrophy, Eaton-Lambert syndrome). During endotracheal intubation, patients with rheumatoid arthritis or ankylosing spondylitis affecting the cervical spine may suffer subluxation, quadriplegia, and acute ventilatory failure. Rheumatoid involvement of the laryngeal cricoarytenoid joints may make endotracheal in-

Table 53–2. *Pulmonary Complications after Surgery*

Complication	Consequence
Atelectasis	Poor gas exchange (hypoxemia)
	Pneumonia-like symptoms
Infection	Acute bronchitis
	Pneumonia
	Sepsis
Airway obstruction	Hypoxemia
	Increased work of breathing
	Ventilatory failure
Miscellaneous	
Prolonged neuromuscular blockade	Ventilatory failure
Cervical subluxation	Ventilatory failure, quadriplegia
Glottic edema	Stridor
Diaphragm dysfunction	Ventilatory failure, hypoxemia
Venous thrombosis	Pulmonary embolism

tubation most difficult and cause stridor post-operatively. Patients who breathe primarily by diaphragmatic activity, e.g., those with ankylosing spondylitis, kyphoscoliosis, or quadriplegia, may develop ventilatory failure after abdominal surgery. Finally, deep venous thrombosis and pulmonary thromboembolism are well-known postoperative complications (they are mentioned for completeness and are not discussed further).

Risks

The two most important risks for postoperative pulmonary complications are obstructive lung disease and the type of surgery. Other risks such as history of smoking, advanced age, obesity, long duration of anesthesia, and recent respiratory infection are somewhat controversial (Table 53–3). On the one hand, these conditions are often associated with abnormalities of pulmonary function, so it seems likely that they would predispose to complications. On the other hand, these conditions frequently coexist with known risks, so it is unclear if they represent truly independent risks.

Obstructive Lung Disease. Patients with obstructive lung disease have the highest risk of postoperative complications, up to 70%, in contrast with 1 to 5% for those with normal pulmonary function. In general, risk increases as pulmonary function worsens. Unfortunately, there is no best pulmonary function test that predicts complications, so several measures are used. When the forced expiratory vital capacity (FEVC), 1-second forced expiratory volume (FEV_1), or maximum voluntary ventilation (MVV, formerly called maximum breathing capacity or MBC) drops below 70% of predicted, there is *increased* risk of postoperative pulmonary complications. When these test results drop below 50% predicted, there is a *high* risk of complications.

Type of Surgery. The highest rates of pulmonary complications (up to 60%) follow thoracic and upper abdominal surgery, the lowest (up to 13%) follow surgery on the extremities, and intermediate rates (up to 33%) follow low abdominal and pelvic surgery. Complications appear to be related to the marked drop in lung volume: vital capacity drops by more than half and functional residual capacity by one fourth after upper abdominal and thoracic surgery. For comparison, the vital capacity drops by 25% and functional residual capacity changes little after nonabdominal, nonthoracic surgery, and the changes are intermediate after low abdominal surgery. As noted earlier, pain, splinting, abdominal distention, diaphragmatic dysfunction, supine position, and analgesic medications appear to contribute to the marked drop in lung volume after upper abdominal and thoracic surgery.

History of Smoking. Patients who smoke heavily (30 or more cigarettes a day) have more than four times the pulmonary complication rate of nonsmokers. This has been attributed to known effects of smoking such as hypersecretion of mucus, impaired mucociliary clearance, and inefficient oxygenation. The increased risk may also be explained by the high prevalence of obstructive lung disease (bronchitis and emphysema) in smokers. However, patients who smoke less heavily (10 cigarettes a day) and those without evidence of gross obstruction by spirometry have double the complication rate.

Advanced Age. Patients over age 70 years are reported to have increased risks because of the effect of age on the respiratory system,

Table 53–3. Risks for Postoperative Pulmonary Complications*

Factor	Comments
Obstructive lung disease	Risk is increased when FEV_1 and FEVC < 70% of predicted and is high when tests < 50% of predicted or when Pa_{CO_2} > 45.
Operative site	Risk is high with upper abdominal or thoracic surgery and is increased with lower abdominal surgery.
Smoking history†	Risk is doubled with 10 cigarettes per day and quadrupled with > 30 per day, possibly because of OLD.
Advanced age (> 70)†	Risk may be related to concomitant disease such as OLD and CVD.
Obesity†	Reported complications are often minor, e.g., hypoxemia and atelectasis.
Duration of anesthesia†	Risks may be related to type of surgery, e.g., abdominal and thoracic procedures.
Type of anesthesia†	There is no adverse pulmonary effect with regional anesthesia, but general anesthesia may be required; intubation allows better airway control.
Upper respiratory infection†	Risk is associated with bronchial hyper-reactivity and bronchospasm.

*OLD, obstructive lung disease; CVD, cardiovascular disease; FEV_1, 1-s forced expiratory volume; FEVC, forced expiratory vital capacity.
†Controversial risks.

including loss of elastic recoil, reduced maximal flows, less efficient gas exchange, and diminished cough and gag reflexes. However, appropriate statistical analysis indicates that most (if not all) of the increased pulmonary complication rate can be explained by the presence of chronic obstructive lung disease, a disease of middle-aged and elderly patients. Similarly, the increased surgical mortality seen in the elderly population can be attributed to underlying medical conditions such as cardiovascular disease.

Obesity. It is difficult to find support for the hypothesis that obesity itself increases postoperative pulmonary complications. Obesity is associated with low resting lung volume (functional residual capacity), early airway closure, and ventilation-perfusion abnormalities. Spirometric lung volumes (vital capacity, expiratory reserve volume) may also be reduced, but the difference is usually not significant until obesity is massive, i.e., when the weight/height ratio exceeds 1 kg/cm (this ratio is approximately 0.3 in nonobese patients) or when weight exceeds 250% of the ideal. Often, hypoxemia accompanying obesity depends on position and may be seen only in the supine or head-down position. Obstructive sleep apnea occurs more frequently in obese individuals; sedative and analgesic medications may worsen the episodes of profound hypoxemia that occur during sleep in these subjects.

Duration of Anesthesia. Long operations (exceeding 2 or 3 hours) are reported to increase pulmonary complications. However, it is likely that the increased complication rate may be explained by the operative site; long operations tend to involve the upper abdomen and chest (e.g., aortic aneurysm repair, cholecystectomy, pancreatectomy).

Type of Anesthesia. A common misconception is that spinal, epidural, and regional forms of anesthesia are safer than general anesthesia. This may have arisen from the observation that general anesthesia causes changes in respiratory function (discussed earlier), whereas regional anesthesia does not, and from a few reports that the pulmonary complication rate is higher after surgery under general anesthesia. The following should be noted. First, the anticipated surgery may require deep levels of general anesthesia, so regional anesthesia may not be possible. Second, the postoperative pulmonary complication rate is more likely to be related to the type of surgery (discussed earlier) than to the type of anesthesia. Third, endotracheal intubation may offer *better con-*

trol of airway secretions, ventilation, and oxygenation in some patients with an increased risk for pulmonary complications. Finally, it is best to remember that the *anesthesiologist*, not the internist, is responsible for selecting the appropriate form of anesthesia.

Upper Respiratory Infections. There are anecdotal reports that upper respiratory infections increase the risk of pulmonary complications. A proposed explanation is that inflammation of the upper respiratory tract induces reflex bronchial hyper-reactivity, which may lead to intra- and postoperative bronchospasm, retained respiratory secretions, gas exchange abnormalities, and their sequelae.

The Evaluation

History. Unsophisticated, denying, or sedentary patients may provide an initial medical history that is falsely negative. Very specific inquiries must be made about smoking (current and past, amount), cough and sputum production, exercise tolerance (ability to walk distances, climb stairs, and accompany healthy peers), past respiratory illness (childhood asthma, pneumonia, bronchitis), other medical conditions (neuromuscular disease, arthritis, stiff jaw and neck, hoarseness), and use of medications (present or past, bronchodilators, including over-the-counter drugs; theophylline; corticosteroid).

Physical Examination. The physical examination is more sensitive than the chest radiograph for detecting obstructive lung disease, yet it is curious that the physical examination continues to be neglected and the radiograph overused (see Chap. 54). The use of accessory breathing muscles, increased anteroposterior dimension, hyper-resonance, wheezing, and prolonged expiratory time provide strong evidence for substantial obstructive lung disease. Prolonged time for expiration (exceeding 5 seconds) and wheezing only during forced expiration indicate more subtle obstructive disease. A hoarse voice, prolonged time of *inspiration* (exceeding 3 seconds), and loud breathing sounds over the anterior neck may indicate laryngeal obstruction.

Musculoskeletal problems, clubbing, or end-inspiratory crackles suggest restrictive lung disease. Limited chest expansion related to a bellows problem, e.g., ankylosing spondylitis, kyphoscoliosis, and quadriplegia, indicates reliance on diaphragmatic or belly breathing. It is easier to recognize belly breathing when the patient is supine: there is outward abdominal motion during inspiration. Depending on the cause of limited chest expansion, there may be paradoxical inward chest wall motion during inspiration (quadriplegia) and forceful abdominal contraction during expiration (ankylosing spondylitis). In general, interstitial fibrosis does not constitute a substantial surgical risk until it is advanced, when there are problems with hypoxemia, limited cardiac output, and increased work of breathing. In contrast, some patients with neuromuscular conditions, e.g., myasthenia gravis, may appear to be normal before surgery.

Arthritic involvement may be suggested by a limited range of motion of the neck and mandible.

The presence of cor pulmonale (loud pulmonic component of the second heart sound, hepatomegaly, and peripheral edema) is worrisome because it usually indicates advanced parenchymal (emphysema or fibrosis) or vascular (recurrent thromboemboli or vasculitis) lung disease.

Pulmonary Function Tests. Spirometry (FEVC and FEV_1) and arterial blood gas measurements are simple, inexpensive, and widely available tests that provide important, objective, quantifiable information. These tests identify patients with an increased risk for pulmonary complications and may be used to follow the response to therapy.

Spirometry. Spirometry is more sensitive than the physical examination for detecting pulmonary disease. Like most medical tests, spirometry is nonspecific and has a relatively low predictive value, i.e., not everyone with abnormal spirometry results suffers postoperative pulmonary complications. This limited predictive value does not justify diagnostic nihilism. The health care team is more likely to react to abnormal spirometry results than to the all too common moniker chronic obstructive pulmonary disease.

Arterial Blood Gas Tests. Arterial blood gas tests provide important information about the overall status of gas exchange. The clinical examination is notoriously insensitive for detecting either hypoventilation (hypercarbia) or hypoxemia. Hypercarbia ($Pa_{CO_2} > 45$) in the presence of obstructive lung disease is ominous because it usually indicates advanced disease: the FEV_1 is less than 30% of the predicted value (roughly 800 ml for an adult of average size). Less ominous reversible causes of hypercarbia include concomitant metabolic alkalosis (often from diuretic therapy), hypothyroidism,

a "lazy" ventilatory center, or superimposed acute obstruction. Hypoxemia ($Pa_{O_2} < 80$ at sea level, < 70 at 1400 m) is nonspecific; it identifies the need to evaluate and treat possible underlying lung disease and to provide supplemental oxygen therapy. More subtle gas exchange abnormalities may be detected by calculating the alveolar-arterial oxygen tension difference. This is a simple three-step procedure:

1. Determine alveolar oxygen tension (PA_{O_2}):

$$PA_{O_2} = PI_{O_2} - 1.2(Pa_{CO_2})$$

where PI_{O_2} is the inspired oxygen tension, typically 150 torr breathing air at sea level and 126 at intermediate altitude (1400 m); and Pa_{CO_2} is the measured value of carbon dioxide tension in the blood sample.

2. Subtract oxygen tension measured in the blood sample (Pa_{O_2}): $PA_{O_2} - Pa_{O_2}$

3. Compare the result with the normal value. The upper normal limit may be estimated by dividing the age by 4, i.e., 5 torr for a 20-year-old person, 20 torr for an 80-year-old person.

Calculating the alveolar-arterial oxygen tension difference *for room air* helps to account for alveolar ventilation. Hyperventilation may cause Pa_{O_2} to rise transiently and mask hypoxemia. For example, at first glance, a Pa_{O_2} of 81 torr at sea level in a 50-year-old patient appears to be low normal. However, if Pa_{CO_2} is 32, the alveolar-arterial oxygen tension difference is 31 torr. This exceeds the estimated normal limit of 13 and indicates abnormal oxygenation. In other words, if the patient had not been hyperventilating, the Pa_{CO_2} would have been higher and Pa_{O_2} would been abnormally low.

Other Tests. The MVV is a popular test among surgeons because it is affected by ventilatory function (obstructive and restrictive diseases) and intangible factors such as stamina and cooperation. The test is performed by having patients breathe hard and fast to move as much air as possible. Although measured on a spirometer, the MVV is usually requested separately from simple spirometry. The MVV should probably be reserved for patients with obstructive lung disease when resection of lung tissue is planned; it is an excellent predictor of mortality after pneumonectomy. Otherwise, the MVV offers little compared with simple spirometry. The evaluation of patients about to undergo pneumonectomy is beyond the scope of this review. Consulting a pulmonary specialist is recommended because predicting postoperative pulmonary function may be difficult.

Tests for small airway disease, e.g., measurement of closing volume and frequency dependence of compliance, are not recommended because they do not improve the predictive value of simple spirometry.

The electrocardiogram is not recommended as a screening test for lung disease because it is too insensitive. Electrocardiographic changes, e.g., P pulmonale and right ventricular hypertrophy, appear late in the course of cor pulmonale.

Patients with the first three risks given in Table 53–3, namely, obstructive lung disease, surgery involving the abdomen or thorax, and cigarette smokers, should receive spirometry and arterial blood gas tests before surgery. Whether patients with the remaining risks should also receive these tests is controversial and depends on the clinical setting. Until sufficiently large (multicenter), prospective, randomized, controlled studies are performed, this controversy will persist.

Prevention of Complications

When the risks appear to outweigh the benefits of elective surgery, it is the *surgeon's* responsibility to postpone or cancel it. When the decision has been made to proceed with surgery, all members of the health care team must be alerted so that they may take appropriate action to prevent these complications. Nearly two decades ago, prospective clinical studies demonstrated the ability of preventive therapy to reduce the pulmonary complication rate from 60 to 20%. Preventive therapy may be divided conveniently into three phases (Table 53–4).

Preoperative Phase

Patients should be trained to participate actively in their treatment. They should stop smoking before surgery to allow bronchitis to improve. The evidence that stopping smoking reduces pulmonary complications is circumstantial; pulmonary function tests improve *4 to 6 weeks* after stopping smoking. Stopping smoking just 1 or 2 days before surgery allows blood carboxyhemoglobin levels to return to normal and improves blood oxygen-carrying capacity.

Table 53–4. Measures for Reducing Postoperative Pulmonary Complications*

Recommendations	Maneuvers
Preoperative Phase	
Educate and train	Stop smoking
	Practice deep breathing, coughing, incentive spirometry
Treat reversible problems	Give bronchodilators
	Correct electrolyte imbalance
	Treat infection
Alert anesthesia service	Avoid preoperative sedatives
	Give supplemental oxygen
Intraoperative Phase	
Take special precautions	See text
Maintain oxygenation	Give supplemental oxygen, check arterial blood gas level
Give bronchodilators	Inhaled, +/− intravenous
Maintain airway control	Remove secretions
Maintain volume control	Sigh (hyperinflate) intermittently
Postoperative Phase	
Maintain ventilation	Support ventilation until awake
Maintain control of airway	Extubate when wide awake
Maintain control of secretions	Aspirate secretions
Maintain oxygenation	Check arterial blood gas level or arterial oxygen saturation
Maintain lung volumes	Exhort to breathe deeply and cough, stir up, incentive spirometry or continuous positive airway pressure
Maintain control of pain	Use analgesics judiciously

*This is a partial list of maneuvers to reduce postoperative pulmonary complications. Indications vary according to the needs of each patient.

Experienced surgical nurses and respiratory therapists should train patients to increase lung volumes. The object is to prevent the development of low lung volume and associated physiologic abnormalities (Table 53–1). One method for increasing lung volumes, sustained maximal inspiration therapy, emulates normal sighing. The patient is taught to take and hold deep inspirations, usually from 500 to 2000 ml for 3 to 5 seconds. An *incentive spirometer* helps patients monitor the depth of each breath. A *volume* type of spirometer (bellows or electronic turbine style) is easier to use because the volume is registered directly. Some instruments also have a light that signals when the desired volume has been achieved and a counter that records the number of breaths. The small, disposable *flow*-type incentive spirometers are more difficult to use. The patient must inhale at a certain steady flow (indicated by a floating ball) for a sufficient time to ensure an adequate inspired volume. Untrained patients mistakenly take short rapid inhalations to make the ball hit the top of the spirometer. This improper use of the flow-type incentive spirometers actually encourages the abnormal rapid shallow breathing pattern that predisposes to atelectasis! Because it is effective, less expensive, and has fewer adverse effects (barotrauma), incentive spirometry has replaced intermittent positive pressure breathing in many hospitals.

Deep breathing and coughing exercises are a second way to increase lung volumes. Patients learn to splint abdominal or thoracic wounds, inhale deeply, and cough. An advantage is that direct attempts are made to clear retained secretions.

The classic "stir up" method has patients learn to turn, sit, and stand properly to minimize both wound discomfort and gravity-dependent atelectasis. It is often used with incentive spirometry or deep breathing and coughing. The old-fashioned "blow bottle" therapy has been abandoned because it promotes lung *deflation*.

Bronchodilators are recommended for patients with obstructive lung disease. Inhaled beta$_2$-adrenergic drugs are the mainstay of therapy. Powered nebulizers deliver bronchodilators equally well as intermittent positive pressure breathing machines at a lower cost and without the risk of barotrauma. Recent studies suggest that metered dose inhalers also deliver bronchodilators efficiently and with fewer side effects because lower doses are administered. An additional advantage is that patients may use their metered dose inhalers as needed and do not have to rely on respiratory therapists or nurses. A few patients lack sufficient coordination to activate the inhaler or are unable to inhale deeply or long enough to ensure adequate delivery of medication. Adding a spacer reservoir may allow these exceptional patients to use metered dose inhalers.

In the past decade, the enthusiasm for theophylline has waned because of its weak bronchodilator action, numerous side effects, and frequent interaction with other drugs (including anesthetic agents). In general, we avoid using theophylline and rely on inhaled bronchodilators. When theophylline must be used, changing from an oral sustained-release preparation to a short-acting form 1 week before surgery and then to an intravenous form (aminophylline) during the evening before surgery is recommended to avoid potential problems with drug absorption. Blood theophylline levels should be monitored carefully.

Empiric antimicrobial therapy, e.g., with trimethoprim/sulfamethoxazole, tetracycline, or ampicillin, may be given to patients producing purulent sputum. It may be prudent to postpone surgery until the volume and consistency of sputum improve.

Corticosteroid therapy may be indicated for two reasons. First, corticosteroids should be given to patients who stopped chronic therapy within the past year (often with the help of inhaled corticosteroids) to avoid acute adrenocortical insufficiency. Second, corticosteroids may be given to treat bronchospasm in patients with chronic obstructive lung disease, so-called asthmatic bronchitis, and with asthma refractory to inhaled bronchodilators. These patients are hospitalized frequently for exacerbations of bronchospasm, may have blood eosinophilia, and demonstrate spirometric improvement with corticosteroid therapy (often at high doses). Because these patients can be challenging to treat, it may be prudent to postpone elective surgery if there has been a recent exacerbation of bronchospasm.

Intraoperative Phase

When forewarned, anesthesiologists take appropriate steps to minimize the risk of pulmonary complications. Some examples are given here. Routine preoperative sedative medications may be avoided to reduce the risk of suppressing ventilation en route to the surgical suite. Supplemental oxygen may be provided to patients with hypoxemia or inefficient oxygenation during transportation to and from the surgical suite. When there is cervical spine or mandibular disease, endotracheal intubation may be performed by the nasal route, which avoids the need to extend the neck or open the mouth. A fiberoptic laryngoscope and smaller than usual endotracheal tube may be used when there are glottic problems. Arterial blood gas levels may be monitored more frequently in hypoxemic patients who require supplemental oxygen. Alternative methods of induction, deeper levels of anesthesia, and less irritating anesthetic gases may be used to avoid bronchospasm in patients with asthma. Muscle relaxants may be used at lower doses in patients with neuromuscular disease.

Postoperative Phase

Again, patients identified to have increased risks may benefit from special attention. Patients at increased risk for ventilatory failure, e.g., with severe obstructive lung disease whose FEV_1 and FEVC are less than 50% of the predicted level and with neuromuscular problems, should remain intubated and using a mechanical ventilator in the recovery room or surgical intensive care unit until they have awakened completely. Before extubation, these high risk patients should demonstrate an adequate level of consciousness, return of the gag reflex, and adequate ventilation and oxygenation by blood gas analysis. Repeat blood gas tests help assess continued adequate ventilation and oxygenation. Continuous pulse oximetry is a useful noninvasive alternative to arterial blood gas tests when only oxygenation must be assessed.

Patients must be exhorted to breathe deeply and cough while residual effects of general anesthesia reduce alertness and motivation. It may be necessary to aspirate copious respiratory secretions (nasotracheal suctioning via a nasal trumpet) when the cough is ineffective. Inhaled bronchodilators, via either nebulizer or metered dose inhaler, may be used to treat bronchospasm.

As noted earlier, sustained maximal inflations (deep breathing) emulate the normal sigh mechanism and are intended to reduce atelectasis. Cooperation is poor when the patient is either overly sedated or suffering excessively from pain, i.e., analgesics must be used cautiously to maintain that delicate balance. In theory, deep breathing must be performed 10 times an hour (every 6 minutes) to be effective. Preoperative education, training, and frequent encouragement by the family members, therapists, nurses, and physicians improve the patient's cooperation.

Continuous positive airway pressure therapy delivered by a face mask is a fairly new alternative to incentive spirometry. Low pressures (less than 10 cmH_2O) force the patient to breathe at larger lung volumes, reduce airway closure, and prevent atelectasis. The advantage is that the patient is not required to perform frequent inspiratory maneuvers. Disadvantages include the discomfort of a tight-fitting mask, a sensation of smothering, and aerophagia with abdominal distention and emesis. To prevent aspiration of vomitus or respiratory secretions, candidates for this type of therapy should be alert, should have a good gag reflex, and may require decompression with a nasogastric tube.

More aggressive application of preventive measures (incentive spirometry, deep breathing or coughing, inhaled bronchodilators) may treat atelectasis effectively. Bronchoscopic aspiration of secretions from the lower airway may be helpful if these maneuvers fail and atelectasis worsens.

Early ambulation and continued cautious use of analgesics are recommended when patients return to their rooms.

Bibliography

Celli BR, Rodriguez KS, Snider GL. A controlled trial of intermittent positive pressure breathing, incentive spirometry, and deep breathing exercises in preventing pulmonary complications after abdominal surgery. Am Rev Respir Dis 130:12–15, 1984.
One of the first contemporary studies to compare the newer treatments. All treatments halved the complication rate from 48% in control group, but intermittent positive pressure breathing had side effects.

Craig DB. Postoperative recovery of pulmonary function. Anesth Analg 60:46–52, 1981.
A lucid review.

Geiger K, Hedley-Whyte J. Preoperative and postoperative considerations, in Weiss EB, Segal MS, Stein M (eds). Bronchial Asthma: Mechanisms and Therapeutics, ed 2. Boston, Little, Brown & Co., 1985, pp 892–907.
A complete discussion of how patients with asthma can be challenging during surgery. A rapid and deep induction can minimize bronchospasm induced by endotracheal intubation.

Glass GD, Olsen GN. Preoperative pulmonary function testing to predict postoperative morbidity and mortality. Chest 89:127–135, 1986.
The most recent review. There still is no best test—the Holy Grail for pulmonologists.

Latimer RG, Dickman M, Day WC, et al. Ventilatory patterns and pulmonary complications after upper abdominal surgery determined by preoperative and postoperative computerized spirometry and blood gas analysis. Am J Surg 122:622–632, 1971.
A well-written report of a prospective study that showed how frequently spirometric and blood gas abnormalities occur after upper abdominal surgery. The major difficulties encountered with attempting to compare reports of postoperative pulmonary complications are reviewed.

O'Donohue WJ Jr. Prevention and treatment of postoperative atelectasis—can it and will it be adequately studied? Chest 87:1–2, 1985.
Yet another plea for better-designed prospective multicenter studies.

Pasulka PS, Bistrian BR, Benotti PN, et al. The risk of surgery in obese patients. Ann Intern Med 104:540–546, 1986.
A concise review of this controversial risk factor. The limitations of published reports, including small numbers, lack of statistical significance, and dearth of prospective studies, are noted.

Pierson DJ (chairperson). Perioperative respiratory care.

Part 1. Part 2. Respiratory Care 29:459–549, 603–683, 1984.

> A collection of 17 articles from a conference on perioperative respiratory care attended by experts. The limitations of the current data base, new directions, and practical considerations are reviewed. Although the journal is aimed at respiratory therapists, the articles are informative for the entire health care team.

Poe RH, Kallay MC, Dass T, et al. Can postoperative complications after elective cholecystectomy be predicted? Am J Med Sci 295:29–34, 1988.

> Report questioning whether pulmonary function tests can identify patients with increased risk for postoperative pulmonary complications in a cost-effective manner. This study adds more controversy to the literature because respiratory therapy methods (aerosol and physiotherapy), frequency (only four times a day), and costs ($15 per treatment) may vary considerably among medical centers.

Pontoppidan H. Mechanical aids to lung expansion in nonintubated surgical patients. Am Rev Respir Dis 122(5, pt 2):109–119, 1980.

> A critical review of methods to prevent and treat postoperative atelectasis and the difficulties in conducting clinical trials in surgical patients. Incentive spirometry and continuous positive airway pressure appear to be useful whereas blow bottle therapy does not. More rigorous studies of the value of these methods are recommended.

Rehder K. Anaesthesia and the respiratory system. Can Anaesth Soc J 26:451–462, 1979.

> A complete discussion of the physiologic disturbances produced by general anesthesia.

Stock MC, Downs JB, Gauer PK, et al. Prevention of postoperative pulmonary complications with CPAP, incentive spirometry, and conservative therapy. Chest 87:151–157, 1985.

> Study suggesting that frequency and supervision may be more important than type of therapy. A persistently high prevalence of minor abnormalities despite treatment is characteristic of contemporary studies. In this study, all patients had reduced lung volumes and up to 40% had macroatelectasis. The prevalence of major complications was low—only 3% developed pneumonia.

Tisi GM. State of the art: preoperative evaluation of pulmonary function. Am Rev Respir Dis 119:293–310, 1979.

> A review aimed at pulmonologists. It emphasizes that there is no best pulmonary function test to predict postoperative morbidity and mortality in high risk pulmonary patients.

Tisi GM. Preoperative identification and evaluation of the patient with lung disease. Med Clin North Am 71:399–412, 1987.

> Review emphasizing the bedside pulmonary examination.

Wahba WM. Influence of aging on lung function—clinical significance of changes from age twenty. Anesth Analg 62:764–767, 1983.

> A lucid review of the physiologic changes that accompany aging and their effect on intra- and postoperative gas exchange.

Yellin A, Benfield JR. Surgery for bronchogenic carcinoma in the elderly. Am Rev Respir Dis 131:197, 1985.

> Editorial reviewing how in the past decade the mortality rate after resectional surgery for lung cancer in carefully selected patients over age 70 years has dropped from 20% to less than 6%. It takes the position that the risk of lung resection in the elderly is now acceptable and provides a short bibliography of recent surgical series.

54

Preoperative Evaluation of the Healthy Patient

JOHN A. ROBBINS, M.D.

Introduction

The usual patient being considered for surgery is not typified by the 80-year-old grandmother with multiple medical problems. Most of the 30 million patients who are operated on annually in the United States are young and healthy. Fifty-seven percent of patients hospitalized for surgery are less than 50 years old. The bulk of outpatient surgery is also performed on younger individuals. Approximately half of patients who are operated on are classified by the American Society of Anesthesiologists as class I physical status: "no disease other than the surgical pathology, no systemic disturbances." The risk of death related to surgery for these patients when they undergo low risk surgical procedures is on the order of 1 per 3000 operations. The mortalities for very common surgeries such as inguinal hernia repair and cervical dilatation and curettage are reported as 1 per 10,000. It is this very large population for whom we must consider the risks and benefits of performing various preoperative evaluations. Major high risk surgical procedures such as pneumonectomies or craniotomies are more life-threatening and require more elaborate preoperative evaluation.

Avoidance of the use of tests produces relatively small savings in cost per patient; however, this translates into a major cost saving because of the enormity of the population under consideration. Kaplan and coworkers[7] suggested that a $4,170 cost savings per abnormal test resulted from a relatively conservative limit on preoperative testing. They arrived at this figure from their study, which suggested that only 23 *potentially* significant abnormalities would have been missed had $100,000 worth of laboratory tests not been ordered for

8600 patients admitted for surgery. Blery and colleagues[2, 3] reported reducing the use of laboratory tests by half by the initiation of a standard protocol to evaluate some routine preoperative screening tests. Savings also accrue from the elimination of unnecessary follow-up of false-positive tests and the costs of surgical delay.

In this chapter, I consider multiple forms of evaluation that are routinely recommended in many surgical and anesthetic textbooks but that may not be necessary. Wherever possible, judgments are based on clinical studies from the literature. When no studies exist or when their quality is poor, it may be necessary to make suggestions based on theoretical grounds. In 1979, Mushlin and I identified a number of theoretical criteria necessary to select a test for preoperative screening[10]:

1. The condition tested for must be asymptomatic and not obvious from a routine history and physical examination.

2. The condition must significantly affect the morbidity or mortality of surgery or must represent significant risk to those associated with the patient's care.

3. A preoperative diagnosis must be more beneficial to management of the patient than a diagnosis established in the perioperative or postoperative period.

4. Tests must be available of sufficient specificity and sensitivity to allow for detection of the condition.

5. The prevalence of the condition must be high enough so that efficient detection of an asymptomatic patient with the condition is possible.

If these criteria are met, one should include the test as part of the routine preoperative evaluation.

When considering the theoretical basis for

Table 54–1. Usefulness of a Test Based on Predicted Prevalence*

Prevalence (%)	50	10	5	1	0.1
Predictive value of a positive test (%)	95	68	50	16	2
False-positive rate (%)	5	32	50	84	98

*Specificity and sensitivity are 95%.

deciding how to evaluate a preoperative patient, it is important to pay special attention to criterion 5. The prevalence of a condition, or what is sometimes referred to as prior probability, has a major effect on the predictive value of a test. The usefulness of a test is defined by its sensitivity, or the percentage of individuals with a condition identified by the test, and its specificity, or the percentage of healthy individuals who have a normal test. By knowing the prior probability of the condition in the population under study, it is possible to use the sensitivity and specificity to calculate the predictive value of a positive or negative test. The predictive value of a positive test refers to the percentage of patients with a positive test who actually have the disease. The predictive value of a negative test refers to the percentage of patients with a negative test who do not have the disease. When screening for an unlikely occurrence, it is important to have a test with very high sensitivity and specificity, or most positive tests will be false positives (Table 54–1). These concepts are very important for understanding the utility of tests. A good general discussion of the topic can be found in a small volume by Galen and Gambino.[5]

History and Physical Examination Versus a Screening Questionnaire

Most authors agree that the most important preoperative evaluation is a thorough history and physical examination. Compiling a complete history and doing a physical examination are a relatively labor-intense undertaking, which costs a significant amount of money and may be unnecessary. One retrospective study[9] demonstrated that an internist's evaluation did yield important information for an unscreened group of patients over the age of 50 years undergoing routine cataract surgery. Fifty-nine conditions that were considered significant were identified in 258 patients. More than half of these conditions (e.g., severe chronic lung disease, atrial fibrillation) would have been identified by a simple questionnaire and a determination of the rate and rhythm. Most of the other conditions would probably have been found, but this is not clear from the paper.

The question that needs to be addressed is: Are a complete history and physical examination always necessary? In ostensibly healthy individuals, there is reason to believe that the first important screening test could be a simple questionnaire. If no abnormalities are found via the questionnaire, the complete history and physical examination are probably unnecessary. The use of a history and physical examination added little to an anesthesiologist's estimation of risk for patients who had all negative responses for the questionnaire in Figure 54–1.[18] During the physical examination, a few patients were hypertensive. Pulse

1. Do you feel unwell?	Yes	No
2. Have you had any serious illness in the past?	Yes	No
3. Do you get more short of breath on exertion than other people of your age?	Yes	No
4. Do you have any cough?	Yes	No
5. Do you have any wheeze?	Yes	No
6. Do you have any chest pain on exertion (angina type)?	Yes	No
7. Do you have any ankle swelling?	Yes	No
8. Have you taken any medicine or pills in the last 3 months? (including excess alcohol)	Yes	No
9. Have you any allergies?	Yes	No
10. Have you had an anesthetic in the last 2 months?	Yes	No
11. Have you or your relatives had any problem with a previous anesthetic?	Yes	No
12. Observation of serious abnormality from "end of bed" (which might affect anesthetic)	Yes	No
13. Date of last menstrual period		

Other Comments:

Figure 54–1. Questionnaire designed to elicit patients' preoperative health status. Adapted from Wilson ME, Williams MB, Baskett PJF, et al. Br Med J 1:509–512, 1980, with permission.

1.	Do you have any major illness other than the one for which surgery is being considered?	Yes	No
2.	Do you take any medications? If yes please list.	Yes	No
3.	Can you climb 10 steps without becoming short of breath?	Yes	No
4.	Can you lie flat without becoming short of breath?	Yes	No
5.	Do you have a cough?	Yes	No
6.	Do you ever wheeze?	Yes	No
7.	Do your ankles ever swell up?	Yes	No
8.	Do you get chest pain with activity?	Yes	No
9.	Have you ever experienced excessive bleeding from prior surgery, injury, or dental work?	Yes	No
10.	Have you or your relatives had any problems with anesthesia?	Yes	No
11.	Do you drink more than an average of 10 drinks per month? (1 drink = 1 beer, 1 glass of wine, 1 oz of hard liquor)	Yes	No
12.	(When appropriate) Date of last menstrual period	_____	

Figure 54–2. *Proposed screening questions used to identify individuals who do not require a complete history and physical examination. It is used only for patients who say that they are healthy.*

and blood pressure determinations should therefore be used with the questionnaire. Anemia was also noted in two patients (see later part of the chapter for a discussion of hemoglobin determinations). In this study, no other evaluation of the patients, including a complete history and physical examination, laboratory tests, and review of the medical record, added significantly to the anesthesiologist's estimation of surgical risk.

The questionnaire in effect was used to place a patient in the class I risk category. The American Society of Anesthesiology does not offer any specific criteria for making this classification and states only that the patient should be healthy. I suggest the use of a questionnaire similar to that shown in Figure 54–2.

Questionnaires have also proved useful in screening patients to see if an electrocardiogram (ECG) should be performed. When all the responses to the questions in Figure 54–3 were negative, obtaining an ECG caused the delay or cancellation of surgery in only 1 in 200 patients. This study was performed with an unscreened population, and it is conceivable

that had the population been screened by such routine measures as palpation of the patient's radial pulse, the abnormal detection rate would have been improved.

One may reasonably conclude that for patients who appear outwardly healthy who are being considered for low risk surgical procedures, the surgeon should consider administering a standardized questionnaire such as that shown in Figure 54–2 and checking the patient's pulse and blood pressure. If the responses on the questionnaire do not suggest any medical illness, the patient can undergo surgery without a complete medical evaluation. If any questions are raised by the patient's responses, he or she should be thoroughly evaluated by the surgeon or referred to another physician for this evaluation.

Before routine acceptance of a questionnaire to take the place of a complete history and physical examination, further validation should be carried out. Inclusion of a history of bleeding disorders with prior surgery or dental extraction seems reasonable. The research protocol for evaluating the accuracy of a questionnaire should be straightforward, but

1.	Have you any chest pain?	Yes	No
2.	Have you experienced breathlessness on exertion?	Yes	No
3.	Have you experienced breathlessness when lying flat?	Yes	No
4.	Has any form of heart disease ever been diagnosed?	Yes	No
5.	Have you had rheumatic fever?	Yes	No
6.	Have you ever been found to have a heart murmur?	Yes	No

Figure 54–3. *Questionnaire to be completed before the ECG is performed. Adapted from Paterson KR, Kaskie JT, et al. Scott Med J 28:116–118, 1983, with permission.*

unfortunately this evaluation has yet to be undertaken. Until a reasonable prospective trial has been published, the busy clinician will be forced to deal with the medical-legal climate that exists and use complete histories and physical examinations. The questionnaire will eliminate the necessity of these measures only if all of the questions are answered negatively. In patients who have obvious medical problems, it will be of no use at all.

Chest X-Ray

The rate of abnormal chest x-rays increases with age, from less than 1% in individuals under the age of 30 years to more than 40% in those over the age of 70 years. In many individuals with abnormal chest x-rays, these abnormalities might have been predicted on clinical grounds. Likewise, the finding of an abnormal chest x-ray does not necessarily increase the patient's risks at surgery.

Recent reviews of the utility of routine preoperative chest x-rays have appeared on both sides of the Atlantic. Pooled data from a number of studies showed that only 2 of 1718 preoperative screening chest x-rays yielded "unexpected radiographic abnormalities with implications for patient care."[16] The authors concluded that screening preoperative films seldom enhance patient care. Similarly, a British reviewer[4] concluded, "there is little doubt that routine preoperative chest x-rays offer little benefit to the patient in terms of increasing life expectancy and preventing morbidity. They also have minimal yield of unsuspected clinical abnormalities and have a negligible effect on patient management." His review of the literature supports the 1984 guidelines offered by the Royal College of Radiologists, which are outlined in Figure 54–4.

It is important to consider whether elderly preoperative patients, over age 65 or 70 years, represent an exception to the above-stated rules. Elderly patients have an increased incidence of pulmonary disease and an increased risk of complications. There is a consensus in the literature on the high likelihood of finding abnormalities on routine chest x-rays in the elderly (40 to 50%), but the utility of this information is open to discussion. To better quantify the benefit of routine preoperative chest x-rays in the elderly population, it is necessary to estimate the incidence of surgical complications. Even with a statistically significant increased complication rate in individuals with abnormal chest x-rays, the predictive value of chest x-ray abnormalities varies greatly with the expected complication rate. If one expects a low complication rate, on the order of 1%, the predictive value of an abnormal result is only 4%; that is, of 100 individuals with abnormal chest x-rays suggesting cardiac disease, only 4 actually develop these complications (based on data of Seymour,[12] with a sensitivity of 33% and a specificity of 83%). If the projected cardiac complication rate from surgery is 10%, an abnormal chest x-ray has a positive predictive value of 20%. Carrying this argument one step further to an estimated complication rate of 25%, the predictive value of an abnormal chest x-ray suggestive of cardiac disease rises to 40%. Surgery in the upper abdomen or thorax may be expected to generate these complication rates.

These mathematical manipulations demonstrate that it is the base-line risk of the surgical procedure in the ostensibly healthy elderly individual that helps to define the need for a routine preoperative chest x-ray. For very low risk procedures, the x-ray is still not indicated even in the elderly patient. As the risk of the procedure increases, it becomes more important to obtain a chest x-ray. One must choose one's own cutoff point. The chest x-ray is very

---

Routine preoperative chest x-ray is no longer justified. However, preoperative chest radiography may be clinically desirable in certain patients in the following categories:

1. *Those with acute respiratory symptoms*
2. *Those with possible metastases*
3. *Those with suspected or established cardiorespiratory disease who have not had a chest radiograph in the previous 12 months*
4. *Recent immigrants from countries where tuberculosis is endemic who have not had a chest radiograph within the previous 12 months*

It should be noted that none of the above categories is routine, and the reasons for examination should, therefore, always be given in the usual way.

Figure 54–4. *Guidelines for preoperative chest x-ray use among patients admitted for elective noncardiopulmonary surgery. Adapted from reference 11, Roberts CJ. J R Coll Physicians London 18:62–65, 1984, with permission.*

useful if one predicts a 25% complication rate. A choice of 5% is very conservative, and most positive results are false positives.

The Electrocardiogram

There is general consensus that an ECG is indicated in any patient who has a history of cardiovascular disease before surgery. The same is true of any individual in whom cardiac abnormalities are detected during the physical examination. A problem arises when considering the patient who is deemed healthy by the history and physical examination before a surgical procedure. The relatively high false-positive rate for ECGs significantly increases the clinical relevance of this question. The not infrequent findings of left ventricular hypertrophy by voltage criteria or nonspecific ST-T wave changes may precipitate costly and time-consuming further evaluations.

The utility of routine ECGs before surgery has recently been reviewed.[6] Data from the Framingham studies suggest that the semiannual incidence of unrecognized myocardial infarction based on ECG criteria reaches a maximum of 0.3% in elderly individuals, that it is impossible to date the time of these infarctions by ECG alone, and that there is a significant false-positive rate for diagnosing recent asymptomatic myocardial infarctions. Thus, the use of a routine ECG as a case-finding technique for delaying surgery is unreasonable. The routine ECG may be useful for screening for rhythm abnormalities, but many of these can be discovered by simple palpation of the radial pulse. Even if arrhythmias are noted, there is no conclusive evidence that treating them preoperatively decreases cardiac risk at the time of surgery.

Discovery of conduction defects before surgery is of little value. A review of the literature suggests that surgery is never an indication for the placement of a temporary transvenous cardiac pacemaker. If a pacemaker is indicated, it is a permanent one, regardless of the proposed surgery. Therefore, a diagnosis of asymptomatic left bundle branch block or bifascicular block is of no utility in the preoperative period.

Once again, the subset of elderly patients raises specific questions vis-à-vis the routine preoperative ECG. As with the chest x-ray, a high incidence of abnormalities can be anticipated in the elderly population. Abnormalities are frequently reported in excess of 50%. The clinical significance of these abnormalities in predicting postoperative complications must be interpreted as a function of the anticipated rate of complications. The predictive value of a positive result associated with a low incidence of complications is miniscule. If one expects a 25% cardiac complication rate, the predictive value of an abnormal ECG in an elderly patient is approximately 31% (data from Seymour[12]). Gallbladder, intrathoracic, and intracranial procedures may generate these high cardiac complication rates in elderly patients.

The choice of doing an ECG before any procedure with greater than a 5% cardiac complication rate is very conservative. Most positive results are false positives, but until good preoperative studies are carried out this is probably a safe choice. Few elective procedures cause such a high expected cardiac complication rate in the healthy patient.

The other question that is frequently raised about ECGs is the importance of having a base-line ECG. Opinion differs on this question. Goldberger and O'Konski[6] argue against obtaining ECGs for this purpose. Seymour, who has written extensively about surgery in the elderly patient, believes that this is an indication for obtaining a preoperative ECG. I believe that it may be important to have a base-line ECG, but only when we can predict a high incidence of postoperative cardiac complications.

If it were clinically and legally possible, it might be useful to obtain a preoperative ECG and not evaluate it unless the patient developed postoperative complications. The danger in obtaining a preoperative ECG for a base line is that many of the "soft" findings that are highly likely to be present are used as justifications for further investigations or for a delay of surgery. Taking an ECG and not evaluating it would make it available if a postoperative ECG were required. (Note: This may make good medical sense but could be legally risky.)

Pregnancy Tests

Any patient who may be pregnant at the time of surgery should have this possibility evaluated. The population at risk has been shown to have approximately a 1.5% incidence of occult pregnancy. The original research was done with urine pregnancy tests, but either urine or serum tests with high sensitivity and specificity ($\geq 99\%$) would be acceptable. This 1.5% risk justifies pregnancy testing in any sexually active premenopausal woman who has not undergone surgical sterilization (surgical sterilization of the patient's partner in monogamous relationships would also suffice).

Hematologic Tests

Partial Thromboplastin Time

A number of years ago we reviewed more than 1000 activated thromboplastin time results and concluded that the test was of no use in screening asymptomatic individuals. All of the unexpected positive results were false positives. In a recent, more elegant study, Suchman and Mushlin[15] looked at the activated partial thromboplastin time in low risk surgical patients in relation to quantifiable surgical outcomes in a definite hemorrhage group and a statistically defined hemorrhage group based on a high transfusion rate or procoagulant administration. Even with this generous definition of bleeding complications, they found that nothing is added to the physician's ability to predict perioperative hemorrhage by the test. (The predictive value of a positive test is less than the prior probability that one assumes.)

Suchman and Griner[14] reviewed the diagnostic use of the activated partial thromboplastin time and the prothrombin time. They enlarged on the poor utility of the partial thromboplastin time to include the prothrombin time by pointing out that the activated partial thromboplastin time can identify all bleeding tendencies that the prothrombin time can identify, with the exception of an isolated deficiency of factor VII. The incidence of this condition is, at most, three per million. They concluded, "we do not recommend preoperative screening with either the APTT or PT test for patients without clinical evidence of a coagulation disorder."

Bleeding Time

Barber and colleagues[1] reviewed the bleeding time in 1800 preoperative patients. They found 6% had a prolonged bleeding time. By a review of patients' charts, they found that only two of the patients with bleeding time of greater than 20 minutes would have been unsuspected. Of the entire population, 1.4% had minor (< 20 minutes) unexpected prolongation. Surgery was performed on 46 patients who had abnormally elevated bleeding times. Blood loss was less than 100 ml in all patients having minor surgery in spite of the prolonged bleeding times. Some patients with bleeding times greater than 20 minutes did have excessive blood loss with major surgery, but there were no deaths or significant complications noted. The odds of identifying a patient at risk of a bleeding complication by using the bleeding time are less than 1 in 1000, and even if these patients do have a statistically significant increased blood loss, it appears to be non–life-threatening.

I conclude that the bleeding time should not be used as a screening test. If there is any suspicion of abnormal bleeding or possible drug ingestion, it is a useful test. It is necessary to perform this test only in situations where surgical control of blood loss may be less than optimal (e.g., a vaginal hysterectomy). Before a surgical procedure with expected high blood loss in a patient taking aspirin or other medications that prolong bleeding, evaluation of the bleeding time should be considered. One must then weigh the risks—psychologic, economic, and medical—of delaying surgery until the medication can be eliminated from the patient's system.

Platelet Count or Estimate

The best data on platelet counts come from the work of Kaplan and colleagues.[7] These authors reviewed the screening of preoperative laboratory tests carried out on 2000 elective surgical patients. They agreed on indications for preoperative testing of platelet counts and removed these patients from the screening population. They then identified the patients with abnormal test results and attempted to determine how these results affected the decisions to operate or the operative outcome. The results of their series are presented in Table 54–2. They noted 2 per 1000 unsuspected low platelet counts that might have been of potential surgical significance (95% confidence interval 0 to 1.4%). Turnbull and Buck[17] found no abnormal platelet counts in 1005 otherwise healthy patients undergoing elective cholecystectomies.

In patients who are undergoing major surgical procedures where surgical hemostasis may be difficult, a screening platelet estimate should be considered. According to data of Kaplan and colleagues,[7] the cost of identifying one patient with unsuspected thrombocytopenia would be approximately $7,000.

Table 54–2. Predictive Value of Tests as Screens for Complications of Surgery

Test	No. of Tests in Sample	Percentage of Tests Without Indication	Percentage of Potentially Surgically Significant Abnormal Results	True Fraction of Unindicated Surgically Significant Abnormal Results: 95% Confidence Limits	Predictive Value of a Positive Result
Prothrombin time	201	77	0	0–1.8	
Partial thromboplastin time	199	77	0	0–1.8	
Platelet count	407	90	0.2	0–1.4	
Platelet count*	1005	100	0		0
Complete blood cell count	610	48	0	0–0.6	
Differential cell count	390	83	0	0–0.9	
Six-factor automated multiple analysis	514	34	0.2	0–1.1	
Glucose level	464	78	0.4	0–1.6	
Hemoglobin*	1005	100	1.4		29%
Urinary white blood cell count	995	99+	4.2		11%

Adapted from Kaplan EB, Sheiner LB, Boeckmann AJ, et al. JAMA 1985, 253:3578–3581, Copyright 1985, American Medical Association and *Turnbull JM, Buck C. Arch Intern Med 147:1101–1105, 1987, with permission.

Complete Blood Counts, Hemoglobin Assays, and Hematocrits

Turnbull and Buck[17] reported the predictive value of a low hemoglobin result as 29% for related complications in patients undergoing elective cholecystectomies. They identified 7 patients of 1005 with abnormally low hemoglobin values. In two of these, they reported complications. Unfortunately, the authors considered postoperative anemia, which is a self-fulfilling prophecy, a complication. Two of the patients with low hemoglobin values did receive preoperative blood transfusions. A much higher percentage of patients with low hemoglobin values had related postoperative complications defined as hypotension and anemia than patients with normal preoperative hemoglobin values.

Based on clinical judgment, with little supporting scientific evidence, it appears that if blood loss is anticipated from surgery, it is appropriate to measure the hemoglobin or hematocrit before surgery. If minimal blood loss is anticipated, a quantification of hematocrit or hemoglobin is no more indicated before surgery than as a routine screening test in an asymptomatic individual.

Turnbull and Buck[17] identified 1 patient of 1005 with a low white blood cell count. No complications developed in this patient. Kaplan and colleagues[7] also found the white blood cell count to be of very little use (see Table 54–2).

Glucose Determination

There have been no good studies of the value of preoperative glucose determinations in the asymptomatic patient that include in-depth evaluations of postoperative complications. Kaplan and coworkers[7] did find 0.4% "potentially surgically significant abnormal results" (95% confidence interval 0 to 1.6%). They did not analyze outcomes in enough depth to assess the effect of moderately high unsuspected glucose level on surgical complications. It is hard to know what they considered to be potentially surgically significant. The question of surgical significance is addressed in an abstract published by Levine and colleagues.[8] They looked at a series of 267 procedures and found no correlation between the markers of diabetic preoperative control and any of the operative complications.

On a theoretical basis, a glucose determination does not fulfill conditions 2 or 3 mentioned in the introduction to this chapter. Asymptomatic hyperglycemia has not been shown to significantly affect morbidity or mortality of surgery. Unless knowledge of the fact that an asymptomatic patient had hyperglycemia would cause cancellation of surgery, there appears to be no indication for this test.

Electrolyte and Renal Function Determinations

Data concerning these tests come from the work of Turnbull and Buck[17] and Kaplan and colleagues[7] as well as from theoretical considerations. Increased creatinine or abnormal electrolyte levels may have a significant effect on surgery, and we would like to make these determinations preoperatively. We[10] suggested on theoretical grounds that an undiagnosed elevated creatinine level would be present in 0.3% of the population. (We based this on the incidence of new onset renal disease and on the prevalence of renal disease.) Kaplan and colleagues used a six-factor automated electrolyte and creatinine analysis and identified 0.2% of their population as having a potentially surgically significant abnormal result (95% confidence interval 0 to 1.1%). Turnbull and Buck *again* identified 0.2% of their population as having elevated creatinine values. Two patients with an elevated creatinine level had surgery without comment and without complication.

Turnbull and Buck also identified 14 cases of hypokalemia (1.4%). In only four of these cases was the hypokalemia corrected preoperatively. No cardiac complications occurred in any of the patients.

With this low incidence of increased creatinine level, the decision to test or not to test should be based on the risk of the surgical procedure. If any risk of intraoperative hypotension is anticipated or if any potentially nephrotoxic drug will be used, preoperative screening for renal failure may be appropriate, even with a relatively high cost for each potentially abnormal laboratory test. In the otherwise healthy patient who is not using diuretics, testing for hypokalemia does not appear to be indicated.

Urinalysis

Data concerning the value of urinalysis comes from the work of Turnbull and Buck.[17] The only part of the urinalysis that they found possibly useful was testing for pyuria. They detected pyuria in 4.3% of their cases. Forty-two patients had no history of prior urinary tract infections, and none of these patients were treated with antibiotics preoperatively. Five developed postoperative urinary tract infections. This compares with 42 patients with a negative urinalysis who developed postoperative urinary tract infections. If one excludes the one patient with a significant history, the predictive value of an abnormal urinalysis for postoperative urinary tract infections was 11%. Most individuals with an abnormal urinalysis do not develop these infections.

The surgeons performing the cholecystectomies in London, Ontario, did not treat asymptomatic pyuria before surgery. If that is the standard of care, there is no indication for a preoperative urinalysis. If the standard of care is to delay surgery and treat asymptomatic pyuria before an elective operation, the urinalysis may be of some value. I would recommend that if a prosthesis or foreign body is going to be inserted during surgery, urinalysis should be carried out and asymptomatic pyuria should be treated preoperatively to prevent possible bacteremia from infecting the prosthesis in the perioperative period. Most surgery of this type is accompanied by antibiotic prophylaxis. If for psychologic, financial, or medical reasons surgery is urgently needed, antibiotic prophylaxis can be started 12 to 24 hours earlier with a drug that is effective against the usual urinary pathogens.

Conclusion

I have suggested that very few routine screening tests are indicated preoperatively in healthy individuals (Table 54–3). The fundamental arguments used to draw these conclusions are based on the premise that these are truly screening tests used in healthy patients. Any suspicion on the part of the surgeon or physician seeing the patient that there may be an abnormality will negate many of the arguments put forward earlier. The very nature of screening tests makes them less than ideal in this population. When the incidence of a condition we are screening for is low, e.g., less than 1%, the specificity and the sensitivity of the test employed need to be extremely high. The low sensitivity and specificity of such tests as ECGs, chest x-rays, and partial thromboplastin time in predicting surgical complications greatly diminish their usefulness. The terrible curse of the routine preoperative screening tests is their high false-positive rates. The added expense and emotional trauma of further testing and delay of surgery are of paramount importance when we consider preoperative tests.

The only tests that should be strongly considered before surgery are the hemoglobin or hematocrit for surgery where blood loss is anticipated (note the specificity and sensitivity of these tests for anemia are, by definition, 100%); pregnancy test, with its extremely high sensitivity and specificity; and possibly a platelet estimate. Under certain conditions where we anticipate a high complication rate in a specific area, a chest x-ray, ECG, and serum creatinine and electrolyte assays may be indicated. These tests have some usefulness as

Table 54–3. *Recommended Preoperative Evaluation in Patients Who Say That They Are Healthy*

Test	When or for Whom Test Should Be Performed
Blood pressure	Everyone
Pulse	Everyone
Screening questionnaire	Everyone
History and physical examination	Only if abnormalities found on any of the above
Pregnancy test	Women who may be pregnant
Hematocrit or hemoglobin	For surgery with expected major blood loss
ECG	Expected cardiac complication rate > 5%* or irregular pulse
Chest x-ray	Expected pulmonary complication rate > 5%
Creatinine level	Expected hypotension or use of nephrotoxic medication
Glucose level	If surgery would be cancelled if elevated glucose value
Electrolyte level	Only if diuretics are used
Prothrombin time/partial thromboplastin time	Never if questionnaire answers are negative
Bleeding time	Never if questionnaire answers are negative
Platelet estimate	If questionnaire answers are positive or if minor bleeding would be life-threatening

*A 5% expected complication rate yields approximately a 10% predictive value of a positive test. This is a conservative choice. At any level less than this the false-positive rate would be much too high. One reasonably could choose a 20 or 25% complication rate.

base lines if the anticipated complication rate is high enough to offset the negative influence of the usually unacceptably high false-positive rate.

References

1. Barber A, Green D, Galluzzo T, et al. The bleeding time as a preoperative screening test. Am J Med 78:761–764, 1985.
   This is the best available reference I could locate on the use of the bleeding time as a preoperative screening test. It is retrospective, not prospective, but looks at a large population of patients and uses the chart review method to look for bleeding complications. Bleeding complications in patients with normal bleeding times are not analyzed. It is therefore not possible to calculate the predictive value of an abnormal bleeding time.
2. Blery C, Chastang C, Gaudy J-H. Critical assessment of routine preoperative investigations. Effective Health Care 1:111–114, 1983.
3. Blery C, Szatan M, Fourgeaux B, et al. Evaluation of a protocol for selective ordering of preoperative tests. Lancet 1:139–141, 1986.
   The authors of references 2 and 3 from the Hospital Rothschild in Paris have undertaken to limit preoperative screening tests in their hospital since 1981. They do not offer any in-depth studies to show a lack of increased complications, but it is useful to see that no great problems have developed from using a restrictive protocol for preoperative assessments.
4. Fowkes FGR. The value of routine preoperative chest x-rays. Br J Hosp Med February:120–123, 1986.
   Fowkes reviews a large body of data on the usefulness of the preoperative chest x-ray. This British perspective is derived from a number of references not frequently quoted in U.S. literature. Fowkes comes to conclusions similar to those of Tape and Mushlin, who emphasize a different body of literature.
5. Galen RS, Gambino SR. Beyond Normality: The Predictive Value and Efficiency of Medical Diagnoses. New York, John Wiley & Sons, 1975.
   Many other discussions of sensitivity, specificity, and predictive value have come out since publication of this small book, but it still provides one of the best, clearest discussions of how to interpret and use tests. It gives concrete examples and clear definitions of terms.
6. Goldberger AL, O'Konski M. Utility of the routine electrocardiogram before surgery and on general hospital admission. Ann Intern Med 105:552–557, 1986.
7. Kaplan EB, Sheiner LB, Boeckmann AJ, et al. The usefulness of preoperative laboratory screening. JAMA 253:3578–3581, 1985.
   This is one of the best in-depth studies of the usefulness of preoperative screening tests. It surveys laboratory data on more than 2000 patients who were operated on at the University of California San Francisco Medical Center.
8. Levine SS, Oboler SK, Bleiden MA, et al. Surgical outcome in diabetic patients and its relation to diabetic control. Clin Res 35:353a, 1987.
   So far this work has only been published in abstract form, but it is the largest study I can find that discusses diabetic control and surgical complications.
9. Levinson W. Preoperative evaluations by an internist: are they worthwhile? West J Med 141:395–398, 1984.
   Levinson tried to assess the usefulness of internists to the evaluation of preoperative patients. This is an intriguing question that has not been looked at by many investigators. Levinson's conclusions are open to challenge based on the methodology she used, but the concept is a reasonable one. The evaluations by internists cannot clearly be classed as screening because no "less invasive technique" had been used first to ensure that the patients were considered healthy.
10. Robbins JA, Mushlin AI. Preoperative evaluation of the healthy patient. Med Clin North Am 63:1145–1156, 1979.
   These data are somewhat dated. This review offers the background and theoretical framework for much of the work that has come after it. Many of the good

studies on preoperative evaluation have appeared since 1979 and are not referenced in this review. It is more useful for the theoretical considerations than for actual data.

11. Roberts CJ. The effective use of diagnostic radiology. J R Coll Physicians London 18:62–65, 1984.

    Roberts reviews arguments about the use of diagnostic x-rays including preoperative chest x-rays advanced by the Royal College of Radiologists' Working Party on the Effective Use of Diagnostic Radiology.

12. Seymour G. Medical Assessment of the Elderly Surgical Patient. Rockville, MD, Aspen Systems Corp., 1986.

    This is the most complete book on surgical assessment of this important population. Seymour references his sources very well. He has also done significant work himself on preoperative ECGs and chest x-rays.

13. Sox HC, ed. Diagnosis and Treatment. Annals of Internal Medicine Series. Philadelphia, American College of Physicians.

    Three pertinent articles have appeared in this series as of this writing. They each have provided an in-depth review of the subject with pertinent references. See references 6, 14, and 16.

14. Suchman AL, Griner PF. Diagnostic uses of the activated partial thromboplastin time and prothrombin time. Ann Intern Med 104:810–816, 1986.

15. Suchman AL, Mushlin AI. How well does the activated partial thromboplastin time predict postoperative hemorrhage? JAMA 256:750–753, 1986.

16. Tape TG, Mushlin AI. The utility of routine chest radiographs. Ann Intern Med 104:663–670, 1986.

    These authors carried out an in-depth retrospective chart review that was assisted by computerized case finding. They surveyed a large population of patients from the University of Rochester Strong Memorial Hospital and were able to demonstrate the lack of usefulness of the activated partial thromboplastin time in preoperative screening.

17. Turnbull JM, Buck C. The value of preoperative screening investigations in otherwise healthy individuals. Arch Intern Med 147:1101–1105, 1987.

    This is a retrospective study of the usefulness of various laboratory screening tests in patients undergoing cholecystectomies. Unfortunately, the authors do not give us enough information to judge for ourselves whether we consider the postoperative complications that they have chosen as significant. What makes the paper very useful is the fact that the charts of patients with normal laboratory tests were also reviewed for complications. This information makes it possible to calculate predictive values for positive and negative screening tests in this population.

18. Wilson ME, Williams MB, Baskett PJF, et al. Assessment of fitness for surgical procedures and the variability of anaesthetists' judgments. Br Med J 1:509–512, 1980.

    This is the best reference on the usefulness of a questionnaire for preoperative assessment. It is not a definitive study in the field, but very few investigations have been done of this intriguing mechanism for decreasing physician labor.

PART FOURTEEN

Ethics

55

Deciding about Life-Sustaining Treatment

BERNARD LO, M.D.

Life-sustaining treatments present ethical dilemmas about what care is humane and appropriate. In a critically ill patient, an acute episode like pneumonia may be reversible, whereas restoring function and improving the underlying disease may not be. General internists can play an important role in making such decisions and in discussing them with patients.

Shared Decision-Making

Ideally, decisions should be made jointly by physicians and informed, competent patients. The doctor should define the benefits and burdens of treatment and the alternatives. Caregivers are not obligated to provide medically futile treatments, even if requested to do so by the patient or family. On the other hand, competent, informed patients may decline treatment, even if family members, friends, or caregivers consider such refusal unwise or even if their lives might be shortened. An active role for the patient is justified by the ethical principle of respecting the autonomy of individuals and by the legal doctrine of informed consent.

Physicians must determine the benefits and burdens of treatment for each particular patient. This determination requires sound information about prognosis and about the indications for treatment. In discussions about life-sustaining treatment, terms like extraordinary or heroic care are often used. Advanced technological, expensive treatments like dialysis or mechanical ventilation are sometimes regarded as extraordinary, as opposed to ordinary care like antibiotics and intravenous fluids. Such distinctions, however, are ambiguous and confusing. All medical treatments have benefits and burdens. The appropriateness of a treatment depends not on the nature of the treatment but on whether the benefits for the individual patient outweigh the burdens.

Sometimes respecting a patient's wishes appears to harm the patient. In such cases, caregivers may educate, counsel, negotiate, and check that patients are informed. However, caregivers should not override refusal of care by informed, competent patients, no matter how strongly they disagree.

Incompetent Patients

Patients may not be mentally competent to make decisions about life-sustaining treatment. In acute care hospitals, about one half of decisions not to resuscitate patients in the case of cardiopulmonary arrest concern incompetent patients. Although a treatment should not be imposed on patients simply because they are incompetent, such patients require additional protection because they are vulnerable.

Strictly speaking, patients should be considered competent unless they are declared incompetent by the courts. In reality, doctors often make determinations that a patient is incapable of giving informed consent or refusal. Competency is usually questioned because a patient declines a treatment that is considered beneficial. Mere refusal of treatment, however, does not imply incompetency. Caregivers often regard as incompetent patients who perform poorly on mental status tests. But a more valid standard is whether the patient understands the nature of the treatment, the risks and benefits, and the alternatives.

Even if patients are not capable of giving

truly informed consent, their assent to treatment may still be needed. Uncooperative patients who thwart treatments, for example, by pulling out intravenous lines, may be restrained or sedated. Insisting on treatment may not be justified if the patient is subjected to indignity and cannot comprehend the reasons for treatment.

In making decisions concerning incompetent patients, physicians must address two questions: what standards should be used and who should make the decisions. A medical, ethical, and legal consensus recommends that decisions follow preferences that the incompetent patient previously expressed while competent. Such prior wishes are called advance directives. Following patient preferences, even when patients are not able to express them directly, is consistent with the ethical principle of respecting patient autonomy.

If advance directives are not available or are unclear, decisions should be based on the best interests of the patient. In deciding what is best for a patient, caregivers must assess the patient's pain and suffering, safety, and loss of independence, privacy, and dignity. Often these considerations are summarized in the ambiguous term quality of life. Problems may arise when judgments about quality of life are made by someone other than the patient. Caregivers may project their own values onto the patient. Life situations that would be intolerable to young, healthy people may be acceptable to older, debilitated patients. Bias and discrimination may occur, especially if quality of life includes economic value to society. Caregivers may not realize that they are making value judgments about quality of life and may mistakenly believe that they are making objective medical judgments or following the patient's wishes. Implicit judgments about the quality of life are more likely to be discussed openly if people with different viewpoints are represented in deliberations, including nurses, social workers, and family members.

The second question regarding an incompetent patient is who should act as surrogate decision maker. Traditionally, the family fills this role and makes joint decisions with physicians because it is presumed that relatives act for the patient's benefit. However, patients may have no family, or family members may decline to make a decision, disagree with each other, or find decisions difficult because of ambivalence, guilt, or grief. Moreover, a conflict of interest may occur because of an inheritance, pension, or the stress of caring for an incapacitated patient. Family members may base decisions on what is best for themselves rather than on what is best for the patient.

These problems with decisions by families have led to alternative approaches. Physicians sometimes make unilateral decisions about what is best for the patient. However, decisions require not only scientific expertise but also value judgments, and the preferences of physicians may differ from those of patients or families. The judicial system may be an impartial forum to determine the patient's best interests. However, it is too cumbersome to be used routinely, and the adversarial system may polarize families and physicians. Institutional ethics committees have been suggested to review cases and make recommendations, especially when there is no one to act as the patient's surrogate. However, more needs to be learned about what kinds of ethics committees improve decision-making and in what situations.

Because of possible problems with determining what is in the best interests of the patient or who should act as a surrogate for the incompetent patient, physicians should encourage patients who are still competent to make advance directives.

Types of Advance Directives

Informal discussions with health care providers, family, or friends may serve as evidence of a patient's preferences. However, people who had talked with the patient may not be available when decisions must be made, and observers may disagree over what the patient said. Physicians should document such informal discussions in the medical record. The note should include an assessment of the patient's medical condition, competency, and understanding of the issues as well as the patient's specific preferences. Direct quotations by the patient are helpful. Subsequent discussions should also be noted. It is not necessary to ask the patient to sign the medical record.

Living will, natural death, death with dignity, or right to die laws have been passed in 37 states in the United States. These laws allow patients to direct their physicians to withhold or withdraw life-sustaining treatment if they should become terminally ill. Caregivers who follow such directives are granted immunity from criminal or civil liability. Because specific provisions and procedural requirements vary, caregivers and patients need to be familiar with the laws in their states.

Despite extensive legislation, there remain fundamental problems with living wills. Many important terms, such as terminal illness, are difficult to define operationally. Because living wills apply only to terminal illness, they do not help with decisions regarding incompetent patients who might survive for months or years, such as patients with severe dementia or irreversible coma.

The *durable power of attorney for health care* is more flexible and comprehensible than the living will. It allows a competent patient to appoint a surrogate, presumably a trusted relative or friend, to make decisions in case he or she becomes incompetent. The proxy takes precedence over family members who traditionally make decisions for incompetent patients. While the patient is still competent, he or she continues to give informed consent or refusal. The surrogate makes medical decisions in all situations in which the patient is incompetent, not just during a terminal illness.

Only a few states have passed laws explicitly authorizing the durable power of attorney for health care. California has the most comprehensive law. The surrogate is required to follow the patient's prior wishes or, if those wishes are unclear or unknown, the patient's best interests. The law also establishes procedural safeguards, requires physicians to follow the proxy's decisions, and guarantees legal immunity for physicians. In a few other states, living will laws also permit the patient to appoint a surrogate decision maker. Although patients in other states may still execute a durable power of attorney, explicit laws may encourage this procedure.

Several important limitations of advance directives should be noted. Physicians are not obligated to follow all directives by patients. Requests for treatment that has virtually no prospect of benefit, that falls below accepted standards of care, or that is unorthodox, and requests for active euthanasia need not be honored. Similarly, refusals of treatment that might jeopardize third parties (such as refusal of therapy for tuberculosis) cannot be accepted. In such cases, the caregiver should discuss the disagreement with the patient as soon as possible. If a compromise acceptable to both parties cannot be negotiated, transfer of care may need to be arranged.

Discussions with Patients

Improved communication between doctors and patients can resolve many problems with decisions about life-sustaining treatment. Most patients with chronic illness want to discuss such treatment with their physicians. Physicians should educate patients about life-sustaining treatments, discuss issues, negotiate, and make recommendations. Such discussions help protect patients from unwise or ill-considered decisions. Because discussions are impossible after patients become incompetent, they are especially important when advance directives are made.

Physicians should invite patients with chronic illness to discuss life-sustaining treatment. Such discussions might be considered part of the routine evaluation. Straightforward questions may broach the topic: "Would you like to talk about how we should make decisions about your medical care in case you become too sick for me to talk with you directly?" Although most patients welcome such discussions, consistent reluctance to discuss such issues should be respected. Specific questions can then be asked about what care they would want if they developed common complications of their diseases. For instance, for patients with chronic obstructive lung disease or with acquired immunodeficiency syndrome, knowledge of preferences about intubation and mechanical ventilation would be important. In addition, if patients became severely, irreversibly demented, would they want intensive care, cardiopulmonary resuscitation, antibiotics for infection, or feeding tubes? Physicians can ask patients to clarify vague or ambiguous statements: "Can you tell me what you mean when you say, 'No heroics'?" They can also ask patients to think about the issues and discuss them again later.

Although specific directives are important, advance directives also need to be flexible because not all future situations can be anticipated or discussed. Physicians can ask how much discretion the surrogate should have in interpreting the patient's wishes and how preferences might change if significant medical discoveries occurred.

Discussions about life-sustaining treatment need to be repeated over the course of the patient's illness. Repeat discussions are generally easier once the topic has been broached. Preferences that differ from previous decisions or statements deserve further discussion. A patient's values may change because of progression of illness or new experiences. Caregivers, however, should check that changes of mind are not caused by reversible medical, psychologic, or social problems.

Patients may have unrealistic expectations about life-sustaining treatment, as when they request mechanical ventilation for respiratory failure caused by metastatic cancer. As with any disagreement, physicians should elicit the patient's concerns with open-ended questions: "What do you think happens to patients whose cancer spreads like that?" In some cases, physicians may need to explain that the patient's goals are impossible. "I wish that were the case. Unfortunately, when cancer spreads that much, even breathing machines don't help patients live much longer."

Emotional reactions need to be discussed explicitly. Patients generally feel relieved and in control when discussing life-sustaining treatment, but negative reactions may also occur. Leading questions may elicit such reactions: "Many patients feel sad thinking about life support. Do you ever feel that way?" These reactions need to be acknowledged as normal; patients who experience them report that they still want to discuss life-sustaining treatment with their physicians.

Discussions about limiting treatment should maintain a positive tone. Otherwise, patients may feel abandoned or believe that nothing more could be done. Although the explicit purpose of discussions about life-sustaining treatment is to elicit the patient's preferences, another purpose is to communicate caring and concern. Supportive care should be discussed, including seeing the patient regularly and controlling pain and other symptoms. Letting the patient cry, holding the patient's hand, or simply being with the patient often is helpful.

If the patient is incompetent, asking family members to report the patient's previously stated wishes rather than their own preferences may reduce guilt. The physician might say, "We'd like to do what your mother would want. Did she ever talk about what care she would want in a situation like this?"

Eliciting the perspective of the patient or family about the illness allows caregivers to correct misunderstandings, explain how care will fulfill their goals, or address their concerns. It can be therapeutic for patients and families to feel that caregivers understand their concerns and expectations.

Specific Clinical Decisions

Medical, legal, and ethical writings agree that a range of treatments may be withheld or withdrawn, including surgery, mechanical ventilation, dialysis, cardiopulmonary resuscitation (CPR), transfusions, medications, and artificial feedings.

Do Not Resuscitate Orders

Although CPR may be effective treatment for unexpected sudden death, it may not be appropriate for patients with terminal or chronic progressive illness whose death is expected. For certain acutely ill patients, CPR may be medically futile. In one prospective study, Bedell showed that no patient with metastatic cancer, pneumonia, acute stroke, or oliguria who suffered cardiac arrest in an acute care hospital was discharged alive after successful CPR. Such information may help physicians and patients assess the usefulness of CPR.

When a do not resuscitate (DNR) order is considered appropriate, the attending physician should write a formal order in the medical record together with a progress note indicating the reasons for the order and plans for further care and summarizing discussions with the patient or family and with other caregivers. Oral DNR orders invite confusion, errors, and legal difficulties.

Strictly speaking, a DNR order means only that CPR will not be performed. Although a DNR order does not necessarily imply limiting other treatments, it is reasonable to review the total plan of care. A patient with a DNR order might still receive antibiotics, other treatments, or even intensive care. Supportive care to relieve symptoms like pain is always indicated, no matter what other treatment is withheld. Discussions with house staff, nurses, and consultants can ensure that there are no misunderstandings about the meaning of the DNR order.

Limited Resuscitation Efforts

The concern that resuscitation may lead to restoration of cardiac function in a patient who has suffered severe brain damage sometimes leads caregivers to consider intermediate steps between full resuscitation and a DNR order. Such efforts are variously called limited, slow, or partial codes. CPR is initiated, but drugs are not administered, intubation is not performed, or resuscitation is stopped after a predetermined period of time. Such limited codes generally cannot be justified because they reduce the possibility of successful resuscitation. Limited codes, however, are appropriate if the patient had agreed to them. For example, a patient with severe chronic obstructive lung disease may not want intubation and mechanical ventilation in case of respiratory failure. Limited codes are sometimes intended to reassure the family that everything was done. Perfunctory CPR, however, cannot be justified because it offers no benefit to the patient and causes cynicism in medical and nursing staff.

Tube Feedings

Tube feedings when severely demented patients cannot take adequate nourishment by hand are a controversial and emotional issue. Some people consider adequate nutrition humane, ordinary care that must always be given. Feeding may symbolize caring and affection. However, recent court decisions have ruled that artificial feedings are like other medical treatments. The burdens of feeding must be weighed against the benefits for each individual patient. The benefits may be small when patients consistently refuse feedings by hand. It is unlikely such patients suffer from hunger or thirst. In addition, demented patients cannot appreciate why the artificial feedings are being given. The burdens may be particularly onerous when patients are sedated or physically restrained because they repeatedly pull out feeding tubes. Such measures, which compromise the dignity and independence of these patients, are difficult to reconcile with the goal of humane care.

Withholding versus Withdrawing Treatment

Many caregivers find it emotionally more difficult to discontinue treatment than not to initiate it in the first place. However, there is no legal or ethical distinction between stopping treatment and not starting it. It is not obligatory to continue treatment just because it has been started. Indeed, there is stronger justification for discontinuing treatment after it has proved unsuccessful.

Discussions with the Health Care Team

Although attending physicians have ultimate responsibility for decisions about life-sustaining treatment, it is advisable for them to discuss decisions with nurses, social workers, house officers, and medical students, who carry out orders. Caregivers who have close contact with patients and families may provide information about the patient and family or raise new considerations and viewpoints.

Disagreements among caregivers may be caused by misunderstandings, different personal values and backgrounds, and previous experience with similar decisions. Stress and personality conflicts may aggravate disagreements. Any caregiver may feel defeated and helpless when life-sustaining treatment is withheld.

Lack of agreement should be recognized and discussed openly. Arguments, public confrontations, and accusations of insubordination usually only inflame the situation. Individual discussions or staff meetings may help the staff understand the medical situation and the reasons for the decision. In addition, emotions, beliefs, and values that underlie decisions can be discussed. Attending physicians may be unwise to insist on decisions in the face of persistent, thoughtful disagreement. Such disagreements should be considered a warning to reconsider the decision.

Economic Considerations

Efforts to curb the rising cost of health care, for example, through Medicare diagnosis-related groups (DRGs), may pressure physicians to limit life-sustaining treatments. Doctors can respond to modest resource constraints on a case by case basis without adversely affecting patient outcomes. If intensive care unit beds are scarce, physicians can provide appropriate care to all patients who need it by adjusting the threshold for admitting patients to the intensive care unit or for transferring them out of the unit. Such decisions use medical resources more efficiently without withholding care from patients who might benefit from it. Because the risk of harming patients is small, it seems reasonable to leave such decisions to physicians.

Although reducing care that is unnecessary or redundant raises no ethical dilemmas, physicians may believe that they are asked to limit care that may benefit patients. Physicians should appreciate that prospective payment under DRGs is based on statistical averages for length of stay and cost of hospitalizations. The relative reimbursement for various DRGs is not based on health care needs or priorities. Some patients exceed the average length of stay, and hospitals cannot reasonably expect to make a profit on every patient or on every DRG. Patients may be harmed if doctors fail to realize that DRG reimbursements are not norms for good care.

In decisions about life-sustaining treatment, the primary responsibility of the physician should remain to the patient, not to the hospital, prepaid group, or society at large. Because illness can render patients vulnerable and dependent, they trust that physicians' knowledge and skills are used for their benefit. Even the suspicion that in clinical decisions physicians give more weight to the economic rewards to an institution or to themselves than to the welfare of patients may have adverse long-term consequences. The public may regard doctors as self-interested business people rather than as professionals devoted to the welfare of their patients. Such loss of trust may in turn harm the quality of medical care.

Conclusion

Decisions about life-sustaining treatment should be made jointly by physicians and informed competent patients. For incompetent patients, decisions should follow the wishes that the patient previously expressed while competent. If these wishes are unclear or unknown, decisions should be based on what is best for the patient. Caregivers should encourage competent patients to give advance directives indicating what care they would want and whom they would want to act as surrogate decision makers if they became incompetent. Attention to communication with patients, families, and other caregivers can improve decision-making.

Bibliography

Brennan T. Ethics committees and decisions to limit care. JAMA 260:803–807, 1988.
The author reviews the 13-year experience of the Massachusetts General Hospital ethics committee and identifies six major types of ethical issues that confronted the committee.

Buchanan A, Brock DW. Deciding for others. Milbank Q 64(Suppl 2):17–94, 1986.
Good discussion of decision-making for incompetent patients.

Drane JF. Competency to give an informed consent. JAMA 252:925–927, 1984.
Discussion of how to assess competency.

Jackson DL, Younger S. Patient autonomy and "death with dignity." N Engl J Med 301:404–408, 1979.
Warning that patient refusals may be caused by reversible medical or psychosocial conditions.

Jonsen AR, Siegler M, Winslade WJ. Clinical Ethics. New York, Macmillan Publishing Co., 1986.
Concise survey of medical ethics for the physician.

Lo B, Jonsen AR. Clinical decisions to limit treatment. Ann Intern Med 93:764–768, 1980.
Acceptable justifications for limiting treatment.

Lo B, McLeod G, Saika G. Patient attitudes towards discussing life-sustaining treatment. Arch Intern Med 146:1613–1615, 1986.
Although most patients want to discuss life-sustaining treatment with physicians, few have done so.

President's Commission for the Study of Ethical Problems in Medicine and Biomedical and Behavioral Research. Deciding to Forego Life-sustaining Treatment. Washington, DC, U.S. Government Printing Office, 1983.
Comprehensive report of an influential Commission.

Shmerling R, Bedell S, Lilienfeld A, et al. Discussing cardiopulmonary resuscitation. J Gen Intern Med 3:317–321, 1988.
This study found that the majority of elderly outpatients had clearly defined opinions about CPR and welcomed the opportunity to discuss issues regarding resuscitation with their physicians.

Veatch RM. An ethical framework for terminal care decisions. J Am Geriatr Soc 32:665–669, 1984.
Guidelines for making decisions for incompetent patients.

56

Informed Consent: An Ideal and a Standard of Practice

STEVEN H. MILES, M.D.

There is moral, legal, and social agreement that patients should participate in decision-making about medical treatment and ultimately direct their medical care. Morally, this view is based on a respect for personal autonomy and a belief that each person's decisions should be determined by his or her unique subjective view of the condition, options, and prognosis. Legally, this view is supported by a right to privacy and to be secure in one's person. Finally, Americans overwhelmingly affirm a wish to be fully informed about their medical condition and options and to be allowed to make treatment decisions for themselves. This support for patients' making choices about their health care is summarized in the concept of informed consent.

Informed consent is both a legal standard for practice and an incompletely realized ethical ideal. The legal concept of informed consent has been articulated in malpractice actions that were brought by patients who were injured in the course of medical treatment. The courtroom process has overemphasized the aspect of consent that pertains to informing patients of the risks and uncertainties of single medical treatments. The substantive aspect of consent—agreement on the philosophy and goals of the treatment plan—has correspondingly been underemphasized. This treatment philosophy includes agreement about how the benefits of treatment are reconciled with the uncertain possibilities of risks or no benefit. Requirements for courtroom evidence of consent have stressed the importance of documented evidence of a patient's consent. The definition of consent that has emerged from malpractice actions has led some clinicians to

mistakenly conclude that informed consent is a legal ritual that is satisfied by obtaining the patient's signature on an unreadable but comprehensive list of risks and authorizations for each element of a treatment plan.

Physicians are acutely aware of how elusive the ideal of informed consent can be in clinical practice. Physicians usually possess a greater understanding of the medical facts of a patient's condition and of the possible treatment choices. A patient's decision about a treatment may be swayed by transient fears or by an unpredictable reaction to being sick and in an unfamiliar situation. Even so, each patient has a unique perspective on how the benefits and burdens of treatment correspond to her or his own preferences and values.

In this situation, consent seems to be an unsolvable riddle. An informed agreement between a patient and a physician is not an entirely rational contract between equally situated parties. The modern rejection of paternalism constrains physicians who see their role as simply convincing a patient that a treatment is medically indicated. The ideal of professional patient advocacy constrains the physician from accepting at face value a patient's initial choice that seems opposed to the patient's long-term interests.

Informed consent requires mutual deference and responsibilities. Patients must at some level trust their physician's judgment and concur with his or her values. Physicians must strive to enhance their patients' autonomy by eliciting the patients' values as treatment approaches are considered and by helping patients to thoughtfully evaluate the treatment options in light of those values.

A newer view of consent in the physician-patient relationship has been proposed by ethicist-physician Siegler and endorsed by the 1982

Dr. Miles is a Henry J. Kaiser Family Foundation Faculty Scholar in General Internal Medicine.

President's Commission on medical ethics. At the center of this model is a view of shared decision-making by the physician and the patient. This physician-patient accommodation encompasses an agreement on treatment goals that the physician believes are achievable and that the patient views as desirable. The shared decision also represents an agreement on the burdens acceptable to the patient in pursuing those goals.

This broad physician-patient accommodation provides a framework by which the desirability of the many treatments that comprise a treatment plan are to be evaluated. Thus, it is broader and more therapeutically focused than the narrow emphasis on the risks of single treatments that emerges from medical-legal concerns. In its focus on a patient-centered view of goals and burdens, this model attempts to bridge the gap between medical indications and how the treatment affects a patient's life. The process of shared decision-making asks the physician to listen, elicit the patient's values, and suggest how the treatment options may be reconciled with them. This view is more clinically relevant than the concepts of moral philosophers. Shared decision-making is mutually voluntary: either the patient or the physician may withdraw from the treatment relationship if the treatment plan is personally unacceptable.

Consent: The Physician's Duties

The physician's responsibility for obtaining proper consent to proceed with therapy generates several duties. First, the physician should determine whether the patient has decision-making capacity. If the patient lacks this capacity, an appropriate proxy decision-making process must be sought. Second, the physician is responsible for counseling the patient with information that is material to the patient's decision. Third, the physician should be sensitive to remediable external constraints on a patient's choices.

1. *Determining decision-making capacity* is a difficult task. In part, it is an assessment of the patient's psychiatric and neurologic function. In part, it requires considering whether complex medical information has been adequately interpreted for the patient. Determining incapacity is rendered more difficult by the recognition that patients may make decisions that seem contrary to the way that health professionals have been trained to view the

patient's interests. The problem of incompetence is further confused by laws defining certain persons, like teenagers or persons unable to manage their finances, as incompetent even though some individuals may have cogent preferences for medical treatment.

Patients are said to lack decision-making capacity when they are unable to coherently relate information about their treatment options to their values and goals for continued care. Patients may be unable to receive information because of disorders of consciousness (coma), attentiveness (delirium), or communication (aphasia or deafness and blindness). Some, like a newborn baby, may not have acquired values or preferences. Some patients may be incapable of relating their values to information about their various treatment options because of disorders of cognition or because of life experiences such as a complete unfamiliarity with medical treatment.

Decision-making capacity (or incapacity) is task specific:

- Persons unable to care for themselves may be able to participate in deciding about other living arrangements.
- Persons unable to participate in decisions about other living arrangements may be able to designate a trusted friend or family to make decisions on their behalf.
- Persons unable to designate a proxy may be able to describe their experience in a way that is helpful to other decision makers.

Physicians should separate the treatment plan decisions to allow patient input for the portions of the treatment plan in which they are capable of participating.

The conclusion that a patient is incapable of decision-making creates secondary responsibilities. Alternative means of making decisions need to be found, as discussed later. Health professionals need to be sensitive to the enhanced vulnerability of persons who are judged unable to speak on their own behalf.

2. The physician is obliged to counsel a patient about information that is *material* to their decision about medical treatment. Malpractice cases, initiated because of injury and tried with perfect hindsight, have disproportionately defined "material" information to include information about the risks and uncertainties of a medical treatment. Material information is not just an enumeration of risks; it is information that a patient needs to fully

evaluate a treatment plan in light of personal goals and values.

The physician's responsibility to provide material information encompasses a duty to explain treatment issues in clear, jargon-free language. This includes information about the patient's medical condition and likely course with and without the preferred treatment. Material information also concerns the availability and effect of alternative therapies (even those that a physician would not recommend or participate in). Material information includes the predictable consequences of a therapy that might have a bearing on a patient's decision. For example, the eventual need for blood transfusions as a consequence of chemotherapy should be explained in advance to a member of Jehovah's Witnesses who is considering consent to chemotherapy. In addition to prognostic information, material information now includes a duty for physicians to help patients anticipate and plan for their incompetence and disability. Patients should be told of the availability of living wills and proxy designations and of the need to discuss such directives with their family and their physician.

Whether or not information is material to a decision is determined in the give and take of shared decision-making. As the physician encourages the patient to articulate the values and concerns that are relevant to medical decisions, the patient's view of material information is revealed. As the patient's values, goals, and fears are identified, the physician should encourage the patient to ask questions to clarify the treatment issues related to these values. The personal nature of material information means that the informing physician must listen with the ear of the counselor rather than merely comprehensively list the effects of treatment.

3. The essence of patient consent is that it is *voluntary*. The patient chooses voluntarily rather than acquiescing in a necessary or inevitable course of action.

Voluntariness may be compromised when patients are manipulated by incomplete information or biased presentation of information. Thus, patients who consent to coronary artery bypass surgery without being informed of the often equally satisfactory option of medical management have not given a fully voluntary consent. Likewise, patients with acquired immunodeficiency syndrome who direct that they should not be connected to a respirator because they are "terminally ill" but who have not been told that a substantial minority of such persons can enjoy a good quality of life after temporary respirator support during treatment of *Pneumocystis* pneumonia have not given voluntary consent. The failure to discuss alternative treatments or to allow patients to balance the benefits and burdens of the treatment are common counseling faults.

Voluntariness is also compromised when patients are compelled by unnecessary institutional policies or health provider practices. Thus, clinics or practitioners who do not allow patients to include nonfamily members in treatment discussions needlessly constrain the patients' approach to decision-making. Likewise, clinics or practitioners who do not treat patients who are known to be taking privately acquired homeopathic substances that are not known to interfere with the prescribed therapy also needlessly limit the patients' autonomy. The physician, as the patient's advocate, should be sensitive to such remediable constraints on patients' autonomy and should strive to address them.

Consent for Persons with Impaired Decision-Making Capacity

The care of patients who are unable to comprehend treatment decisions presents vexing ethical and legal problems. The medical tradition that would provide care according to such patients' best interests, perhaps ratified by families, no longer seems adequate. Lawyers and ethicists have stressed that the patient's subjective view must take precedence over a physician's or family's so-called objective view of the patient's interests. Physicians fear lawsuits from mentally ill persons who actively resist treatments and threaten those who are trying to act in their interests. The perception of physicians' impartiality is compromised by new practice arrangements whereby physicians are financially affected by decisions to provide or withhold care for irreversibly incompetent patients.

The decision-making principles for incompetent patients are similar to those for competent patients:

- Decisions should conform as closely as possible to what is known about the patient's personal views and values.
- Disabled persons should not have treatment withheld in an arbitrary or discriminatory manner.

- The presumption in favor of prolonging life and the difficulty of decision-making for these patients should not lead the clinician to discount discoverable information about how a patient would weigh the burdens and benefits of therapy in choosing a treatment course.

Patients who are unable to express their views may suffer a loss of autonomy as they are subjected to the views of providers and other persons involved in their care. Physicians may feel obliged to provide life-prolonging care as the standard of care despite the fact that such care is contrary to the patient's previous wish or that treatment imposes severe suffering with little chance of success. Providers may subordinate a patient's wishes to their desire to minimize theoretical risks of legal action or public controversy. Strong-willed families may demand treatment that differs from an incompetent patient's previously expressed preferences or interests.

The clinical nature of a patient's impaired decision-making ability affects the clinical approach to these decisions.

- If the patient may be reversibly incompetent and explicit advance directives are not available, the physician would usually strive to restore the patient to decision-making capacity. This most frequently applies to emergency or acute illness of a new patient, when providers know little about a patient's condition and when advance directives are rarely available.
- If decision-making capacity is only recently impaired, the physician or another member of the health care team should search for the patient's previously expressed values and preferences. Such a patient may have authored advance directives (see Chap. 55) in anticipation of the situation. Clinicians should also interview persons with recent, intimate knowledge of the patient to learn of values and preferences that are relevant to the issues at hand. Such directives and recalled information should be conscientiously interpreted in light of the pressing treatment issues (see section on substituted judgment in Chap. 55).
- If the patient is permanently incompetent with family who have been caringly involved in his or her life, such families may ratify treatment decisions that would be customarily provided in light of the patient's situation and previously expressed wishes. Common law and ethical support for personal decision-making usually support the inclusion of the knowledge of patient preferences by intimate friends of the patient. State laws on this matter vary, but most states are less concerned with the degree of relationship of proxies than with a conscientious effort to obtain information about the patient's preferences. The treatment preferences of a guardian or a person with a medical durable power of attorney would ordinarily determine treatment decisions whatever the family's preferences.

Those who have been impaired for their entire lives and are without family present the most difficult problem. Because such persons are often institutionalized, they are rarely seen in ambulatory care. These persons are especially vulnerable; they may require legal guardians, involvement of state agencies, or other protections that are beyond the scope of this chapter.

Informed Consent and the Vulnerable Patient

Informed consent is not only a way to advance patient autonomy in the face of entrenched medical paternalism. An alternative view understands informed consent as a crucial protection for persons who are vulnerable to having their medical interests compromised by social prejudices or interests. This view of informed consent was born in reaction to the abuses of Nazi physicians that were described at the Nuremberg trials. It is echoed in the concerns that led to institutional review boards for research and in more recent efforts for procedural protections for medical decisions for handicapped persons.

Persons without decision-making capacity are vulnerable to treatment decisions that may not serve their interests or represent their values.

- First, health professionals may underestimate a disabled patient's quality of life and then use this mistaken estimate to decide that a person would not want therapy.
- Second, these persons are often isolated, without family or intimate friends to vigorously speak to their interests. If there is

no personal advocate, professionals may not work as well on behalf of these persons' needs and interests.

- Third, these persons may belong to groups that society or some professionals may be less inclined to treat. Such groups might include older persons, prisoners, drug addicts, human immunodeficiency virus–infected persons, disabled persons, racial minorities, poor persons, or hateful patients. An incompetent person belonging to these groups is doubly disadvantaged.
- Finally, persons with impaired decision-making capacity are more likely to be dependent on public or private funds. The health care provider's desire to use costly resources wisely can lead to decisions that inappropriately compromise the interests of these persons.

Decision-making processes for persons without decision-making capacity should take account of the vulnerability of these persons. In addition to incorporating the patient's values and preferences into treatment decisions, physicians should take care that such persons have equal access to health care. To this end, physicians should be sensitized to the needs of these persons and to the potential conflicts of interests that are inherent in these situations. Special procedural safeguards including guardians, second opinions, ethics committees (separate from cost containment committees), and even court hearings might be advisable when patients are especially vulnerable and their fundamental interests are at stake.

Conclusion

Informed consent is both an ideal and a standard of medical practice. The legal definition of informed consent has tended to obscure the nature of informed consent as signifying respect for patient autonomy and a desire for a partnership between patient and physician in determining medical treatments.

In obtaining informed consent, the physician has several duties: to determine whether the patient has decision-making capacity, to counsel the patient about the treatment issues, and to be sensitive to remediable external constraints on a patient's choices.

Decision-making capacity is the ability to coherently relate information about treatment options to the patient's own values and goals for continued care. Decision-making capacity

or incapacity is task specific: persons incapable of one aspect of their treatment planning may well be capable of other types of treatment decisions.

The care of patients without decision-making capacity presents vexing ethical and legal problems. Reversibly impaired patients without previously expressed wishes should be restored to competence. Decisions for irreversibly impaired persons should conform as closely as possible to what is known about their personal views and values as expressed in advance directives or as recalled by those with an intimate knowledge of the patients' views. Physicians should also be sensitive to the vulnerability of persons with impaired decision-making capacity. Social or personal prejudices or an unjustly applied desire to conserve costly resources can distort treatment decision-making for these persons. Procedural safeguards should be appropriate to the vulnerability of these persons and the seriousness of the personal interests at stake.

Bibliography

Goodin RE. Protecting the Vulnerable: A Reanalysis of Our Social Responsibility. Chicago, University of Chicago Press, 1986.
  This book is the most complete balanced discussion of the problem of vulnerable persons in health care and human services that is currently available.
Groves J. Taking care of the hateful patient. N Engl J Med 298:883–887, 1978.
  This article alerts physicians to how their negative reactions to certain patients can affect their care of these persons.
Katz J. The Silent World of Doctor and Patient. New York, The Free Press, 1984.
  This book, by a physician, is a splendid discussion of the history of informed consent and of physicians' uneasy acceptance of this idea.
Lidz C, Appelbaum P, Meisel A. Two models of implementing informed consent. Arch Intern Med 148:1385–1389, 1988.
  The authors propose a "process model" to implement the doctrine of informed consent. This particular model tries to integrate informing the patient into the continuing dialogue between physician and patient that is a routine part of diagnosis and treatment.
President's Commission for the Study of Ethical Problems in Medicine and Biomedical and Behavioral Research. Making Health Care Decisions: The Ethical and Legal Implications of Informed Consent in the Patient-Practitioner Relationship. Washington, DC, U.S. Government Printing Office, 1982.
  This lucidly written, comprehensive, and thoughtful book discusses the legal and ethical theory of informed consent, the problem of impaired decision-making capacity, and the clinical aspects of patient-physician communication in discussions. It is an essential core text written for the general practitioner and medical student.

Schneiderman LJ, Arras JD. Counseling patients to counsel physicians on future care in the event of patient incompetence. Ann Intern Med 102:693–698, 1985.

This is an excellent discussion of the information that a physician should give to patients to allow their treatment preferences to be honored in the event of their future incompetence.

Siegler M. The physician-patient accommodation: a central event in clinical medicine. Ann Intern Med 142:1899–1902, 1982.

The most accessible and completely thought-out version of Siegler's views on the physician-patient relationship. This model was the basis for the President's Commission's discussion of consent.

Starr TJ, Pearlman RA, Uhlmann RF. Quality of life and resuscitation decisions in elderly patients. J Gen Intern Med 1:373–379, 1986.

This intriguing study compared the assessment of quality of life by older patients and physicians and showed how the physicians' lower assessment of the patients' quality of life influenced the physicians' inclination to propose resuscitation for such persons.

Thomasma D. Beyond medical paternalism and patient autonomy: a model of physician conscience for the physician-patient relationship. Ann Intern Med 98:243–248, 1983.

This thoughtful essay examines the tension between medical paternalism and patient autonomy in the application of the ideal of informed consent to clinical practice.

Index

Note: Page numbers in *italics* refer to illustrations; page numbers followed by the letter t refer to tables.